ESSENTIALS OF HAND SURGERY

ESSENTIALS OF HAND SURGERY

Kevin C. Chung MD, MS
Chief of Hand Surgery, University of Michigan Health System
Charles B. G. de Nancrede Professor of Surgery
Professor of Orthopaedic Surgery
Assistant Dean for Faculty Affairs
Associate Director of Global REACH
Section of Plastic Surgery, Department of Surgery
University of Michigan Medical School
Ann Arbor, Michigan
USA

JP medical publishers

London • Philadelphia • New Delhi • Panama City

Published by JP Medical Ltd, 83 Victoria Street, London, SW1H 0HW, UK
Tel: +44 (0)20 3170 8910 Fax: +44 (0)20 3008 6180
Email: info@jpmedpub.com Web: www.jpmedpub.com

ISBN: 978-1-907816-32-1

British Library Cataloguing in Publication Data
A catalogue record for this book is available from the British Library

Library of Congress Cataloging in Publication Data
A catalog record for this book is available from the Library of Congress

Publisher: Geoff Greenwood
Development Editor: Thomas Fletcher
Design: Designers Collective Ltd

Preface

Impaired function as a result of injury to the hand is a major challenge for for patients, especially those in developing countries where this might affect their ability to work. Failing to understand the basic principles of hand surgery can result in suboptimal treatment and impede patients' rehabilitation.

This book provides an understanding of the functional anatomy, physiology and biomechanics that underlie the principles of hand surgery. It is written clearly and concisely to enable complex concepts to be understood easily, with a large number of clinical photos and artworks to illustrate the anatomy and surgical procedures.

The book is split into three sections. The first focusses on the basic principles that underpin hand surgery: the anatomy, imaging studies and fundamentals of treatment. The following two sections include chapters that explore the common conditions of the hand and upper limb. These are organized into those that require emergency surgery and those that are treated on an elective basis.

The ability to restore function to the hand is the most gratifying aspect of being a hand surgeon. I hope that by focussing on the fundamental principles of hand surgery this book will be used by trainees and practicing surgeons to consolidate their knowledge, enabling them to provide treatments that yield optimal outcomes for the patient, even in resource-poor countries.

Kevin C. Chung
November 2014

Acknowledgements

I wish to acknowledge all my contributing authors who have devoted a substantial amount of effort to make this book a reality. I would also like to thank my colleague Sandeep Sebastin, consultant at National University of Singapore, who provided thoughtful guidance throughout the conceptualization, organization and production of this book. I would also like to acknowledge Geoff Greenwood and Thomas Fletcher from JP Medical who had confidence in my ability to undertake this project. Finally, I am grateful to two of my staff, Evan Kowalski and Evan McGlinn, whose dedication made this book a reality.

KCC

Contents

Contributors

Oluseyi Aliu MD MS
Resident, Section of Plastic Surgery, Department of Surgery, University of Michigan Medical School, Ann Arbor, Michigan
USA

Praveen Bhardwaj MS (Ortho) DNB (Ortho) FNB (Hand and Microsurgery) PGDip (Hand Surgery)
Consultant, Hand and Reconstructive Microsurgery, Department of Plastic Surgery, Hand Surgery, Reconstructive Microsurgery and Burns, Ganga Hospital, Coimbatore
India

Matthew D. Chetta MD
Resident, Section of Plastic Surgery, Department of Surgery, University of Michigan Health System, Ann Arbor, Michigan
USA

Alphonsus Chong MBBS MRCS (Ed) MMed (Orth) FAMS (Hand Surgery)
FAMS Senior Consultant and Head, Department of Hand and Reconstructive Microsurgery, National University Hospital; Assistant Professor, Department of Orthopaedic Surgery, Yong Loo Lin School of Medicine, National University of Singapore
Singapore

Aaron WT. Gan MBBS (S'pore) MRCSEd MMed (Surgery)
Associate Consultant, Department of Hand and Reconstructive Microsurgery, National University Hospital
Singapore

Aviram M. Giladi MD
Resident, Department of Surgery, Section of Plastic Surgery, University of Michigan Health System, Ann Arbor, Michigan
USA

Teemu Karjalainen MD PhD
Senior Consultant, Department of Surgery, Central Hospital of Central Finland, Jyvaskyla
Finland

Evan J. Kowalski BS
Research Associate, Section of Plastic Surgery, University of Michigan Health System, Ann Arbor, Michigan
USA

Amitabha Lahiri MBBS MS MCh FRCS FAMS
Consultant, Department of Hand and Reconstructive Microsurgery, National University Hospital
Singapore

Ellen Y. Lee MD
Medical Officer, Department of Hand and Reconstructive Microsurgery, National University Hospital
Singapore

Li Sihui Eileen PGDipMedTech
Neurology Diagnostic Laboratory, National University Hospital
Singapore

Martins Kapickis MD
Consultant Plastic, Hand and Reconstructive Microsurgeon, Latvijas Plastiskās, Rekonstruktīvās un Mikroķirurģijas Centrs, Riga
Latvia

Aymeric Lim FRCS (Glas)
Associate Professor, Department of Orthopaedic Surgery; Senior Consultant, Department of Hand and Reconstructive Microsurgery, University Orthopaedics, Hand and Reconstructive Microsurgery Cluster, Yong Loo Lin School of Medicine, National University of Singapore
Singapore

Kay WP. Ng MBBS MRCP (UK)
Associate Consultant, Division of Neurology, Department of Medicine, National University Hospital
Singapore

Yeong-Pin Peng MBBS FRCS FAMS
Senior Consultant Hand Surgeon, Hand Surgery Associates, Mount Elizabeth Novena Specialist Centre
Singapore

Mark Puhaindran MBBS MMed MRCS (Edin)
Consultant and Head, Division of Musculoskeletal Oncology, Department of Orthopaedic Surgery; Consultant, Department of Hand and Reconstructive Microsurgery, National University Hospital
Singapore

Shady A. Rehim MB BCh MSc MRCS
Specialist Registrar, Department of Plastic and Reconstructive Surgery, Aberdeen Royal Infirmary, Aberdeen
UK

Jeanne M. Riggs OT CHT
Clinical Specialist in Occupational Therapy, Department of Physical Medicine and Rehabilitation, University of Michigan Health System, Ann Arbor, Michigan
USA

Erika D. Sears MD MS
Resident Surgeon, Section of Plastic Surgery, Department of Surgery, University of Michigan Health System, Ann Arbor, Michigan
USA

Sandeep J. Sebastin MCh (Plastic Surgery) FAMS (Hand Surgery)
Consultant, Hand and Reconstructive Microsurgery, National University Hospital
Singapore

Maneesh Singhal MBBS MS MCh FACS
Additional Professor, Department of Surgical Disciplines, All India Institute of Medical Sciences, New Delhi
India

Ter Chyan Tan MBBCh BAO (NUI) MMed (Ortho) MRCS (Edinburgh) FAMS (Hand Surgery)
Specialist Hand Surgeon, Hand Surgery Associates, Mount Elizabeth Novena Specialist Centre and Gleneagles Medical Centre; Visiting Consultant, Department of Hand and Reconstructive Microsurgery, National University Hospital; Visiting Consultant, Department of Orthopaedic Surgery, Tan Tock Seng Hospital
Singapore

Aravinda K. Therimadasamy BSc
Neurophysiology Technologist, Neurology Diagnostic Laboratory, Department of Medicine, National University Hospital
Singapore

Kris Tong DL BOccThy
Senior Occupational Therapist, Department of Rehabilitation, National University Hospital
Singapore

Hari Venkatramani MS MCh DNB EDHS
Senior Consultant, Plastic and Trauma Reconstructive Surgery, Department of Plastic Surgery, Hand and Reconstructive Surgery, Ganga Hospital, Coimbatore
India

Jennifer F. Waljee MD MS MPH
Assistant Professor of Surgery, Section of Plastic Surgery, Department of Surgery, University of Michigan Medical Center, Ann Arbor, Michigan
USA

Keming Wang MD
Attending Physician, 17th Department of Plastic Surgery, Plastic Surgery Hospital, Chinese Academy of Medical Sciences, Peking Union Medical College, Beijing
China

Yirong Wang MD
Plastic Surgery Hospital, Chinese Academy of Medical Science, Peking Union Medical College, Beijing
China

Einar P. Wilder-Smith MD DTMandH (London) FAMS (Neurology)
Senior Consultant, National University Hospital, Yong Loo Lin School of Medicine
Singapore

Section 1

Basic principles

Chapter 1 Anatomy of the upper limb

Shady A. Rehim, Kevin C. Chung

INTRODUCTION

The upper limb, especially the hand, consists of multiple structures that together form a unique and versatile part of the body. To have a better understanding of the pathologic conditions compromising the function of the upper extremity, it is essential to have a detailed and in-depth appreciation of the normal patterns and functions of the anatomic constituents of the hand and the upper limb. In this chapter, we will discuss the relevant surface anatomy, skeletal framework, articular, musculotendinous, vascular, and nervous systems of the upper limb, with a particular emphasis on the anatomy of the hand.

TERMINOLOGY

First, it is important to be familiarized with the general terms and phrases used to describe joints movement, as well as the anatomic and topographic features of the upper limb. The use of a standardized terminology facilitates communication and avoids confusion between hand surgeons and between surgeons and other health-care professionals when describing upper limb pathology (**Figure 1.1a** and **b**).

Palmar/volar surface

This is the anterior surface of the hand, incorporating thick glabrous (hairless) skin with noticeable skin creases over the palm and fingers. More proximal, the anterior surface of the wrist and the forearm is known as the volar surface.

Dorsal surface

This is the posterior surface of the hand and forearm. In the hand, the dorsal surface is covered with thin mobile skin containing hair follicles.

Radial and ulnar borders

The radial border of the hand/upper limb is the side that is furthest away from the midline of the body containing the thumb, whereas the ulnar border of the hand/upper limb is the side closest to the midline and contains the small finger.

Abduction and adduction

Abduction is moving a body part away from the midline, whereas adduction is the opposite and means moving toward the midline. In the hand, the long finger is considered the midline of the hand, and therefore, finger abduction is spreading the fingers away from the long finger, whereas finger adduction is bringing the fingers together toward the long finger.

Flexion and extension

By definition, flexion is a bending movement that decreases the angle between two body parts, whereas extension is a straightening movement that increases the angle between body parts (e.g. wrist joint flexion and extension movements).

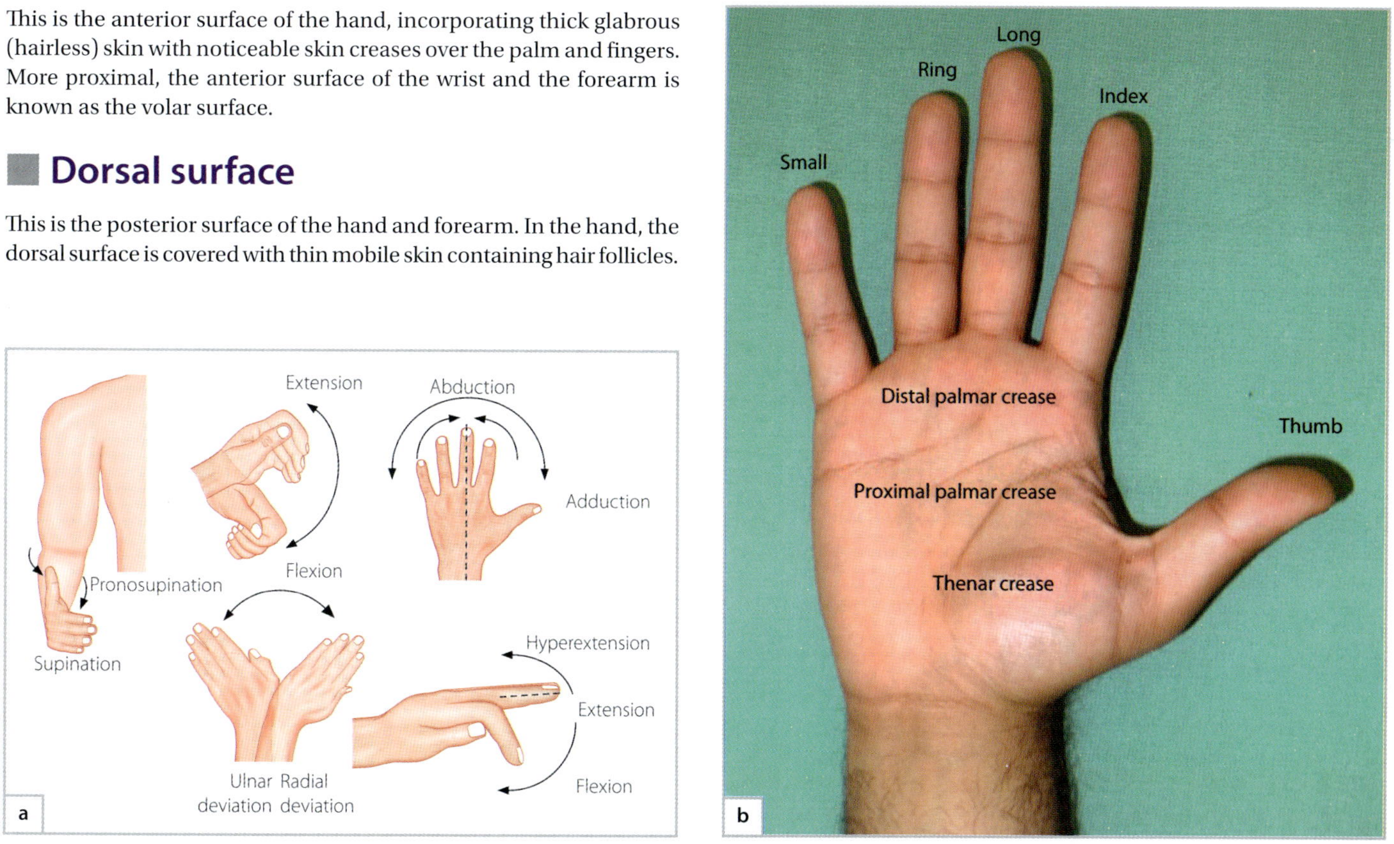

Figure 1.1 (a) Normal range of motion of the hand and forearm. (b) Standard nomenclature and palmar surface of the palm.

Pronosupination

This describes the inward (pronation) and outward (supination) rotation of a joint along its longitudinal axis, and is often used to describe the rotatory movement of the forearm at the proximal and distal radioulnar joints (DRUJs) (**Figure 1.1a**).

EXTERNAL ANATOMY OF THE HAND

Skin and hand creases

Each hand consists of five rays/digits (standard nomenclature: thumb, index, long, ring, and small fingers), a palmar and a dorsal surface, attached proximally to the wrist joint, and is covered by a specialized skin envelope. Besides being a protective layer against infections and other types of injuries, the skin coverage of the hand has a remarkable ability of functional adaptation, and one of its major roles is enhancing the prehensile ability of the hand when executing daily activities.

The palmar and dorsal skin of the hand is functionally and anatomically different, each serving a specific purpose. On the palm, the skin is composed of thick keratinized papillary squamous epithelium that helps it withstand the shearing forces resulting from daily use of the hand. The dorsal skin is supple, thin, and mobile to allow the unrestricted movement of the underlying joints. By looking on the palm, one can see three distinct types of skin lines (**Figure 1.1b**).

- Thick skin creases: Seen over the wrist joint (proximal and distal wrist creases), the palm (three palmar skin creases), and over the metacarpophalangeal (MCP) and interphalangeal (IP) joints of the fingers. These skin creases are tethered to the deep fascia, which stabilize the palmar skin and prevent skin gliding over the hand when handling objects. Additionally, these skin creases are sometimes referred to as the skin joints or folds; this is clinically important, because if a flexion crease is absent, this means that the underlying joint has not been moving, often seen in congenital conditions such as arthrogryposis when the joints are not developed normally.

A fine network of prominent skin folds known as the papillary ridges. The skin papillary ridges serve two important functions: first a tactile function (sense of touch) and second a mechanical function. A moist palm due to secretion of sweat together with these papillary ridges creates a friction coefficient that prevents slipping of objects during prehension. Tension skin lines, also known as Langer lines. It is postulated that along these lines, skin incisions would result in the least amount of scarring when the skin is closed by primary intention.

Underneath the skin is a layer of a fatty tissue, which is divided into fat lobules by fibrous septa extending from the skin to the deep fascia. This creates areas of prominent fat pads that are most noticeable over the hypothenar muscles, thenar muscles, the metacarpal arch, and over the fingers in between joint creases. The fat cushions/pads protect the hands against external forces and allow the hands to conform nicely around objects of various shapes, thus improving the act of prehension.

On the dorsum of the hand, the skin is thin owing to the much thinner dermis and epidermis as well as the lack of fat pads, when compared with the palmar skin. Additionally, the dorsal skin is very mobile due to the loose attachment it has with the deeper tissue. In spite of this great mobility, the skin on dorsum of the hand becomes maximally stretched when making a fist. It is important to realize this limitation when reconstructing soft tissue defects over the dorsum of the hand, as solely relying on skin mobility may not be sufficient to cover or reconstruct wound defects over the dorsum of the hand.

Arches of the hand

When the forearm is supinated and the hand is resting on a flat surface, a concavity is seen on the palmar surface of the hand. Three arches form the shape of this concavity: (1) The proximal transverse arch; (2) longitudinal arch(s); and (3) distal transverse arch, spanning the palmar surface of the hand (**Figure 1.2**).

1. Proximal transverse (carpal arch): A concave curvature formed at the level of distal carpal row. The keystone (apex of the arch that bears maximum force) of this arch is the capitate bone
2. Longitudinal arch(s): a carpometacarpophalangeal arch(s) that extends from the crease of the wrist through the four digital rays. The keystone of this arch is the MCP joint
3. Distal transverse (metacarpal arch): A concave curvature formed at the metacarpal heads of the index, long, ring, and small fingers. The keystone of this arch is the head of the 3rd metacarpal bone

The longitudinal and distal transverse arches of the hand are mobile, whereas the proximal transverse arch is fixed/nonmobile. The mobility of these arches further deepens the concavity of the palm to accommodate for objects of different sizes (e.g. holding a ball using one hand, **Figure 1.2**). Besides the skeletal framework described above, the curvature of the palm is also maintained by the functional tone of intact intrinsic muscles. Thus, conditions that result in intrinsic muscle paralysis such as ulnar nerve palsy would consequently alter the shape of the hand due to the loss of the muscular tone. Another muscle is the palmaris brevis, which is innervated by the ulnar nerve. The palmaris brevis muscle arises from the transverse carpal ligament (TCL) and palmar aponeurosis (PA)

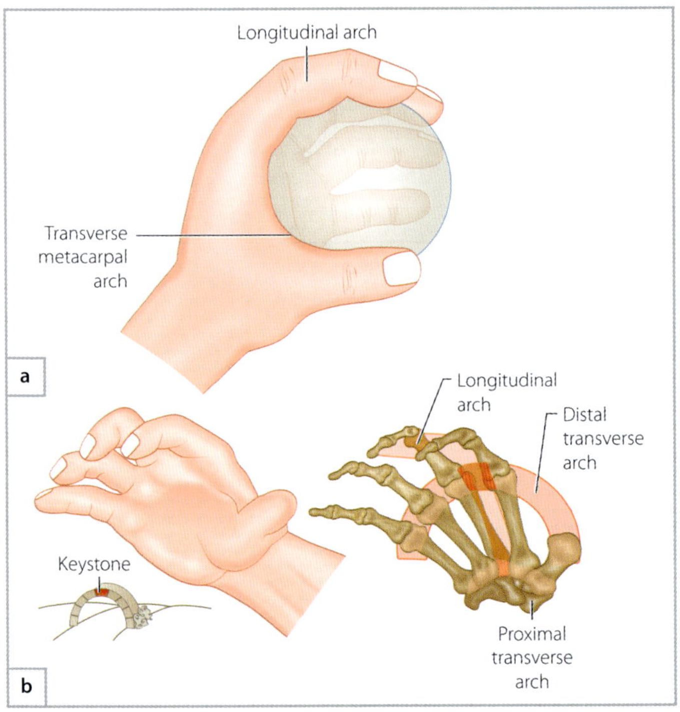

Figure 1.2 (a) Arches of the hand. (b) Mobility of the arches of the hand allows us to handle larger objects.

and inserts superficially into the dermis of the skin. Contraction of this muscle results in cupping of the palm when grasping an object or drinking using the hands.

Surface landmarks

Knowledge of the surface anatomy is essential in the examination of the hand and for planning surgical incisions to avoid iatrogenic injuries of deep vital structures. On the palmar aspect of the hand, one can identify the approximate location of deeper structures using the Kaplan cardinal line. Although several definitions exist, Kaplan described the cardinal line as a line drawn from the junction of the MCP joint line of the thumb at the first interdigital fold to a point 2 cm distal to the pisiform. The proximal intersection of perpendicular lines drawn from the ulnar and radial borders of the long and ring fingers with Kaplan line provide an estimated location of the important structures of the hand (**Figure 1.3**). There is no general consensus on the accurate location of these structures; however, the following are useful measurements to identify pertinent deep structures of the hand based on the above description:

1. Scaphoid tubercle: Palpable at the distal wrist crease just radial to the tendon of the flexor carpi radialis (FCR) muscle
2. Pisiform: Palpable at the distal wrist crease on the ulnar side at the insertion of the flexor carpi ulnaris (FCU) muscle
3. Hook of hamate: Located approximately 1 cm distal and slightly radial to the pisiform bone
4. Motor branch of ulnar nerve: Located midway between the pisiform and hook of hamate lying deep in the Guyon canal
5. Median nerve: The median nerve lies directly under the palmaris longus (PL) muscle (when present), ulnar to the FCR tendon
6. Motor recurrent branch of median nerve: the motor recurrent branch of the median nerve emerges from under the distal edge of the TCL at the thenar skin crease to supply thenar muscle mass. 1 cm distal and slightly ulnar to the scaphoid tubercle is the ridge of trapezium. The distal edge of the TCL runs along a line between the hook of hamate and ridge of trapezium

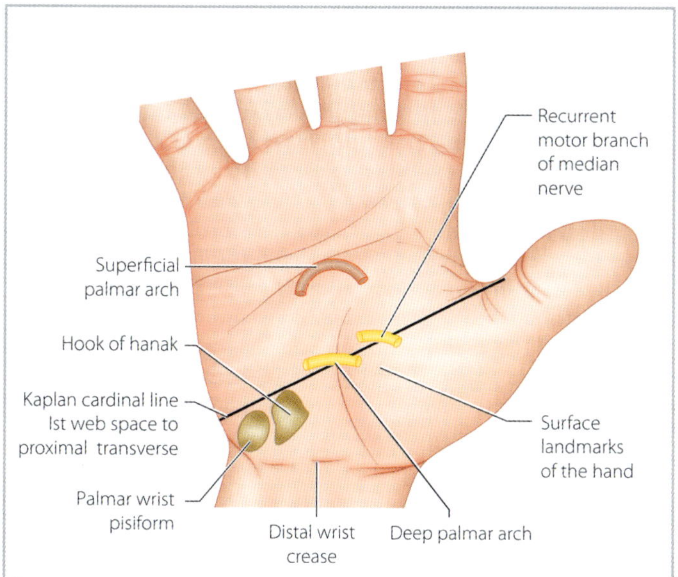

Figure 1.3 Kaplan cardinal line and its anatomical relationship to pertinent deep structures of the hand.

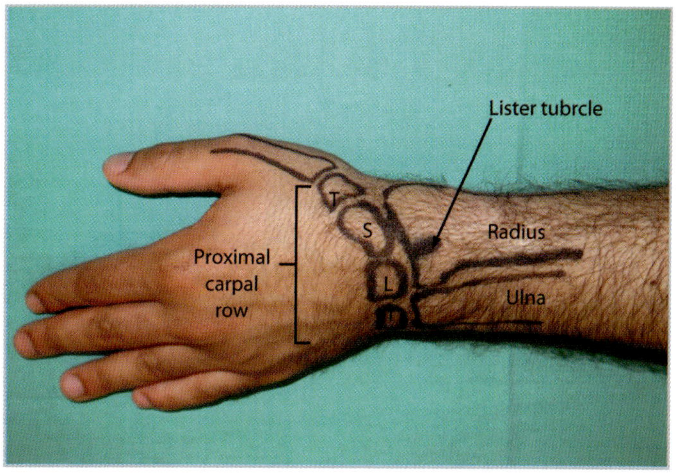

Figure 1.4 Demonstrating the proximal carpal row, radiocarpal, ulnocarpal, and distal radioulnar joints. Additionally, Lister tubercle is marked on the dorsum of the radius.

7. Superficial palmar arch (SPA): located approximately 1 cm distal to the distal edge of the TCL

On the dorsum of the hand, the following locations are useful to identify the following structures (**Figure 1.4**):

1. Lister tubercle: A bony prominence on the dorsum of the distal radius that is palpable midway between the radial styloid and the DRUJ
2. Body of the scaphoid: The scaphoid and trapezium are palpable on the floor of the anatomical snuffbox, which is located between the tendons of the extensor pollicis longus (EPL) and extensor pollicis brevis (EPB) on the radial side of the distal forearm
3. Other important landmarks located on the dorsum of the hand including the radiocarpal joint, the lunate bone, and the scaphoid lunate joint are shown

INTERNAL ANATOMY OF THE HAND

Palmar aponeurosis (PA, Figure 1.5)

Following dissection of the skin and fat tissue, the next layer is the PA, also known as the palmar fascia. The PA is a triangular structure formed of tough connective tissue lying in the center of the palm, and is a continuation of the deep fascia of the forearm. The triangular fascia extends from its apex at the distal wrist crease to its base at a level just distal to the distal palmar crease. On the radial and ulnar sides, the PA joins the fascial covering of the thenar and hypothenar muscles, respectively. Proximally, the fascia gives an insertion to the tendon of the PL muscle (if present).

The PA consists of three layers running in different directions. In the sagittal plane, the layers of the PA are arranged as follows, from superficial to deep:

1. Superficial longitudinal fibers: The superficial fibers of the PA fan out from the PL muscle at the level of the wrist crease and continue in the fingers as the pretendinous band, the superficial transverse ligament (natatory ligament), the spiral fibers, and the lateral digital sheet. The superficial layer also attaches to the overlying skin by multiple vertical septa, thus contributing to the stability of the palmar skin

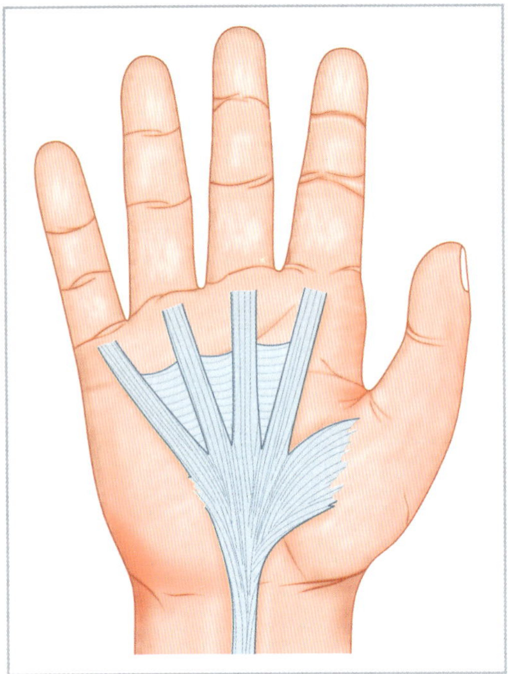

Figure 1.5 Palmar aponeurosis.

2. Transverse fibers: The transverse and deep portions of the PA are anatomically indistinct and can be considered as an extension of the TCL into the palm
3. Deep fibers: The fibers of the deep layer assume a crisscross configuration. Thick fibrous bands (paratendinous bands) extend vertically from the deep surface of the PA to the volar interosseous fascia, forming tunnels that separate flexor tendons from the neurovascular bundle on the ulnar side and lumbrical muscles on the radial side of each finger (**Figure 1.6**)

The PA is a protective layer over the flexor tendons, neurovascular bundles, and other vital structures of the hand, as well as a stabilizer of the palmar skin of the hand. Good knowledge of this complex anatomy, especially of the superficial layer of the PA, is critical to the understanding and treatment of patients with Dupuytren disease.

Carpal tunnel (Figure 1.7)

The carpal tunnel is a fibro-osseous tunnel that forms a passage or an inlet for many of the long flexor tendons as well as the median nerve, when crossing the wrist joint from the forearm to the hand. The tunnel has a dorsal aspect formed by the concavities of the proximal and distal carpal bones, and a palmar aspect covered by the TCL (flexor retinaculum). On the radial side, the TCL attaches to the scaphoid tubercle and trapezium and ulnar to the hook of hamate and the pisiform. The TCL keeps tendons close to the volar side of the wrist and prevents bowstringing of the flexor tendons during wrist and finger flexion.

The carpal tunnel contains 10 structures: 4 tendons of the flexor digitorum superficialis (FDS) muscle, 4 tendons of the flexor digitorum profundus (FDP) muscle, the median nerve, and 1 tendon of the flexor pollicis longus (FPL) muscle. The superficialis tendons to the long and ring fingers are in the top layer, the superficialis tendons of the little and index fingers are in the middle layer, and all of the profundi are lined up in a row in the deep layer. The FPL runs separately. As the flexor tendons emerge from the carpal tunnel on their way to the fingers, the tendons of the FDP pass through a split opening of the FDS known as the Camper chiasm (over the proximal phalanx) to insert into the base of the distal phalanx, whereas the tendons of the FDS reunite and insert onto the base of the middle phalanx of each finger. Therefore, the FDS flexes the proximal interphalangeal (PIP) and MCP joints, whereas the FDP flexes the whole finger, including the distal interphalangeal (DIP) joint and both flexors of the wrist joint. The FPL tendon runs over the palmar aspect of the thumb to insert into the base of the distal phalanx and is responsible for thumb flexion.

Superficial to the TCL passes the palmar cutaneous branch of the median nerve to provide cutaneous innervation to the central area of the palm. During carpal tunnel surgery, the palmar cutaneous branch is rarely seen; however, if encountered it is best to preserve it to avoid the development of a painful neuroma.

Guyon canal

The Guyon canal, sometimes referred to as the ulnar tunnel, is a passage where the ulnar nerve and vessels travel through as they cross

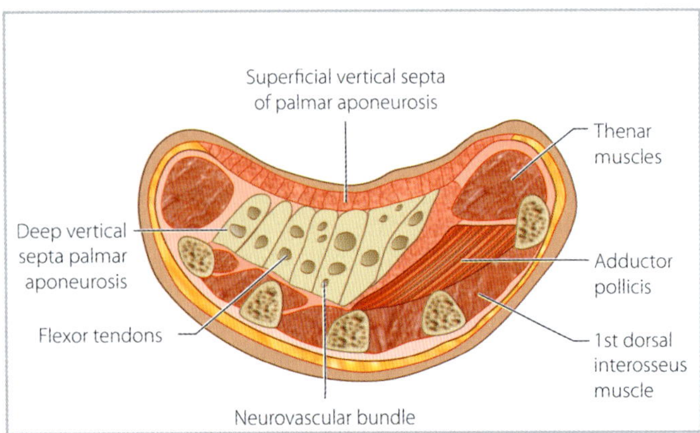

Figure 1.6 A cross section at the level of the mid-palm demonstrating vertical fibrous extensions from the palmar aponeurosis to the interosseous fascia, as well as the arrangement of flexor tendons and their relationship to the neurovascular bundle and intrinsic muscles of the hand.

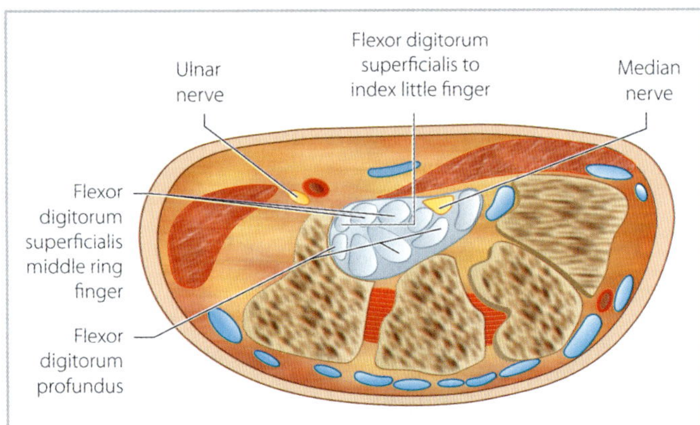

Figure 1.7 A cross-sectional anatomy of the carpal tunnel.

the wrist joint from the forearm to the hand. The canal is approximately 4 cm long and is bounded by the hook of hamate on the radial border and the pisiform bone and the muscle belly of the abductor digiti minimi (ADM) on the ulnar side. The floor of the canal is formed by the TCL (flexor retinaculum); thus, the ulnar nerve and vessels cross superficially and are not part of the contents of the carpal tunnel. The roof of the canal is formed by a fascial expansion known as the volar carpal ligament as well as the pisohamate ligament. The ulnar nerve passes through the Guyon canal and split into two branches: the superficial and deep ulnar nerves. The superficial branch supplies the palmaris brevis muscle and gives off cutaneous to the palm and the digits, whereas the deep branch supplies most of the intrinsic muscles of the hand (see below).

Digital flexor sheath and pulley system

The digital flexor sheath is a closed synovial system consisting of membranous and retinacular portions. The membranous portion is made up of visceral and parietal layers that invest the FDP and FDS tendons in the distal aspect of the hand, and contains synovial fluid that provides tendon nutrition through the process of synovial diffusion. The synovial sheaths of the index, long, and ring fingers extend from the base of the distal phalanx and end at a point near the level of the neck of the metacarpal bones. In the thumb and the small finger, the synovial sheath extends into the carpal tunnel and for approximately 2.5 cm into the distal forearm (**Figure 1.8**). Proximal communication between the tendon sheaths of the little finger and the thumb may occur at a level of proximal wrist crease also known as the space of parona. This is clinically important, as distal infections (originating in the fingers, e.g. septic tenosynovitis) may spread down along the course of the flexor tendon sheath resulting in pain and tenderness and/or collection of pus that can be palpable at the space of parona.

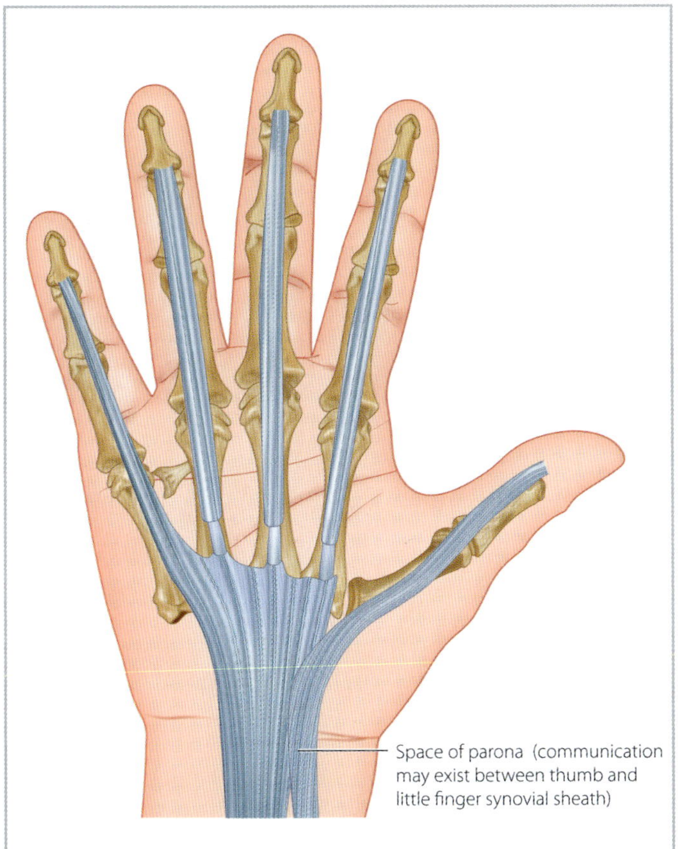

Figure 1.8 Anatomy of the digital flexor sheath.

The retinacular aspect of the flexor sheath consists of a series of transverse annular and cruciate pulleys (fibrous bands) that overlay the flexor tendons and synovial sheaths, and extend from the palmar surface of the MCP joint to the DIP joint. The dorsal aspect of this tunnel is formed by the deep transverse metacarpal ligament, palmar plates of MCP and interphalangeal (IP) joints, and the palmar surfaces of the proximal and middle phalanx. There are five annular pulleys (A1–A5) and three cruciate pulleys (C1–C3) in the index to small fingers. However, in the thumb there are two annular pulleys (A1 and A2) and one oblique pulley. The main function of these retinacular pulleys is to prevent the forward displacement (bowstringing) of flexor tendons during fingers flexion. Keeping tendons close to the volar surface of the fingers concentrates the force of the flexor tendons during finger flexion, thus optimizing flexion movement and enhancing handgrip. Appreciation of the anatomy and biomechanics of the finger pulley system is important during flexor tendons repair and reconstruction procedures. The pulley system of the fingers and vinacular blood supply of the flexor tendons are depicted in **Figure 1.9a** and **b**.

Extensor tendons

On the dorsum of the hand, the extensor retinaculum, also known as the dorsal carpal ligament, keeps the extensor tendons in close proximity with the dorsum of the wrist joint and prevents tendon bowstringing during wrist extension. The extensor retinaculum is a fascial condensation that is analogous and continuous with the TCL, and extends obliquely from the radial side of the distal radius to insert into the sheath of the FCU, the pisiform, the pisometacarpal ligament, and the base of the 5th metacarpal on the ulnar side of the wrist. The space between the retinaculum and the wrist joint is divided by five fibrous septa, creating six dorsal compartments (5 fibro-osseous and 1 fibrous tunnel, fifth compartment, **Figure 1.10**). This is the only area on the dorsum of the hand where the extensor tendons are covered with a synovial sheath, and thus they are prone to inflammatory synovitis due to inflammatory conditions such as rheumatoid arthritis, which may result in dorsal swelling of the wrist and spontaneous tendon rupture. The compartments of the extensor retinaculum (**Figure 1.11**), as well as the associated pathologic conditions of tendons within each compartment, are summarized in **Table 1.1**.

Upon emergence from the extensor retinaculum, the extensor tendons diverge to their respective fingers. Studies have found several variations in the anatomical arrangement of extensor tendons over the dorsum of the hand. Nevertheless, the most common pattern of extensor tendons on the dorsum of the hand is as follows: a single tendon of the extensor digitorum communis (EDC) to the index and long fingers, a double EDC tendon to the ring finger (a slip of ring finger tendon often powers the little finger), and an absent EDC tendon to the little finger. Additionally, a single extensor indicis proprius (EIP) tendon that lies ulnar and deep to the EDC of the index finger and a double extensor digiti minimi/quinti (EDM/EDQ) tendon that has a double insertion on the small finger. Because the index and the small finger are powered by additional (EIP and EDM) tendons, these two fingers can be extended independently from the other fingers. For example, pointing toward an object using the index finger while

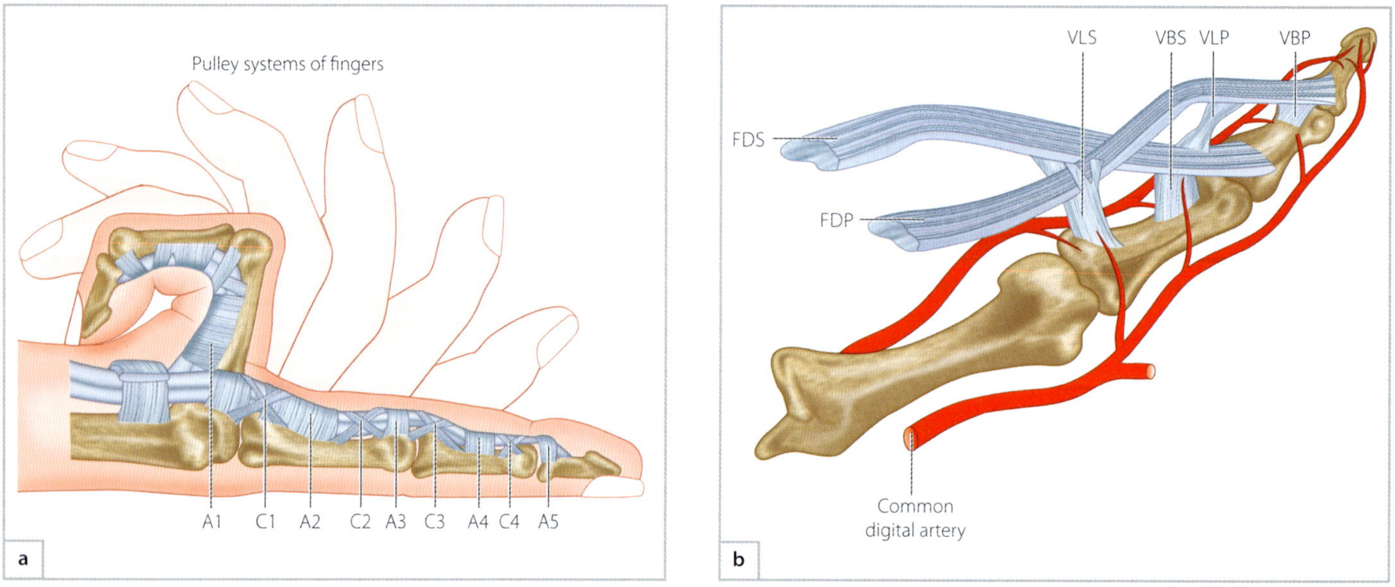

Figure 1.9 (a) Annular and cruciate retinacular pulley system. (b) Vinacular blood supply of flexor tendons. FDS, flexor digitorum superficialis; FDP, flexor digitorum profundus; VBP, vinculum breve profundus; VBS, vinculum breve superficial; VLP, vinculum longus profundus; VLS, vinculum longus superficial.

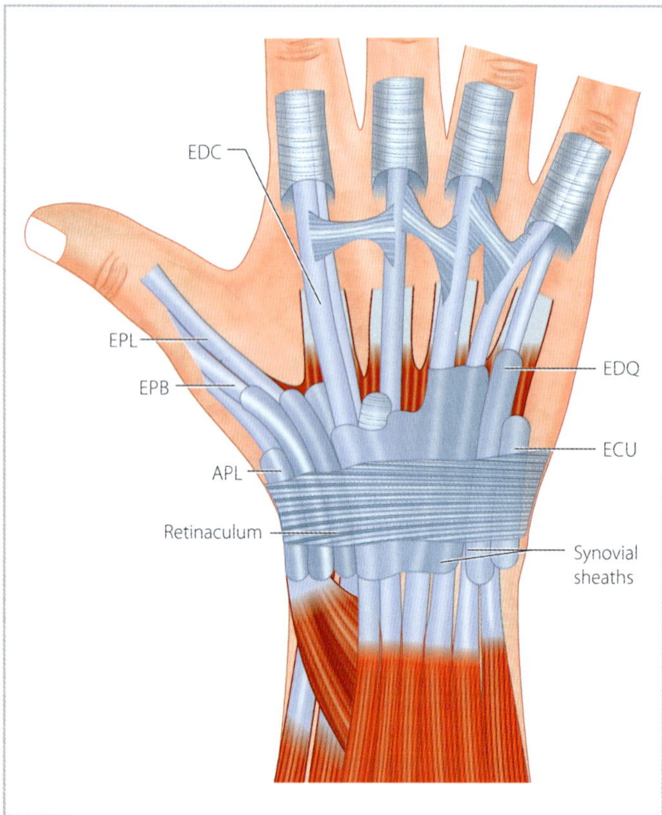

Figure 1.10 Long extensor tendons on the dorsum of the wrist and hand.

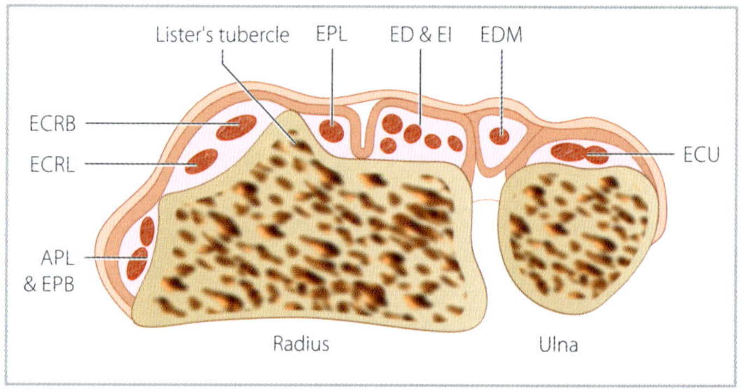

Figure 1.11 Compartments of the extensor retinaculum. APL, abductor pollicis longus; EPB, extensor pollicis brevis; ECRL, extensor carpi radialis longus; EPL, extensor pollicis longus; EDC, extensor digitorum communis; EIP, extensor indicis proprius; EDM, extensor digiti minimi; ECU, extensor carpi ulnaris.

Table 1.1 Extensor retinaculum compartments and associated disease

Compartment	Tendon(s)	Associated disease
1	Extensor pollicis brevis Abductor pollicis longus	De Quervain tenosynovitis
2	Extensor carpi radialis longus Extensor carpi radialis brevis	Intersection syndrome
3	Extensor pollicis longus	–
4	Extensor indicis proprius Extensor digitorum communis	Extensor tenosynovitis
5	Extensor digiti minimi	Vaughn–Jackson syndrome
6	Extensor carpi ulnaris	Extensor carpi ulnaris tendinitis

the rest of the fingers are in flexion. This posture demonstrates an extension of the index finger by the EIP tendon only. Even so, the EDC is the main extensor of the index to small finger. At a level near the MCP joints, the tendons of the extensor communis are joined by fibrous interconnections called tendon juncturae tendinum (**Figure 1.10**). It is because of these fibrous interconnections the long and especially the ring fingers have limited independent extension. However, the role of these connections becomes evident when an extensor tendon is completely divided proximal to the level of the juncturae. Despite a complete division of a tendon, the neighboring extensor tendon can achieve extension of the MCP joint that corresponds to the divided tendon, by powering the distal end of the severed tendon via the juncturae.

Perhaps the most complicated part of the extensor tendon anatomy is the composition of the extensor mechanism of the finger (**Figure 1.12**). On the dorsum of the proximal phalanx, the EDC trifurcates into a central tendon and two lateral slips. The central tendon becomes the central slip and inserts onto the base of the middle phalanx, while the two lateral slips join the lateral bands of the intrinsic muscles (interossei and lumbricals) to become the conjoined lateral bands on the radial and ulnar sides of the fingers, respectively. The conjoined lateral bands then unite to form a terminal tendon that inserts on the dorsum of the distal phalanx of each finger. At the MCP joints, the extensor tendons are encircled by the sagittal bands, which centralize the tendons over the dorsum of MCP joints. The sagittal bands arise from the palmar plate and span both sides of the MCP joint to insert with oblique and transverse fibers into the joint's collateral ligaments and the extensor tendons. When the central extensor tendon contracts, it moves proximally and lifts up the proximal phalanx through the insertion of the sagittal bands onto the palmar plate of the MCP joint (**Figure 1.13**). Along this extensive network of tendons, there are three ligaments on the dorsum of the fingers that interconnect components of the extensor mechanism, and each serves a specific function:

- Triangular ligament: A ligament that holds the lateral bands together on the dorsum of the finger and prevents their volar migration
- Transverse retinacular ligament: Arises from the flexor tendon sheath and spans over the sides of the finger to insert on the edge of the lateral bands. The transverse retinacular ligament prevents dorsal subluxation of the lateral bands during PIP joint extension. Dorsal subluxation of the lateral bands may lead to a finger deformity known as swan-neck deformity (discussed in Chapter 25)

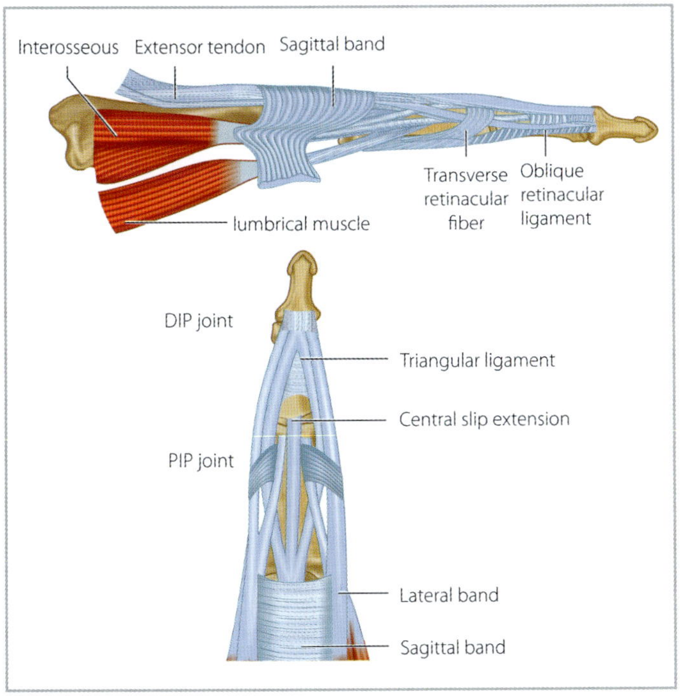

Figure 1.12 Anatomy of the extensor tendon over the dorsum of the fingers and associated ligaments.

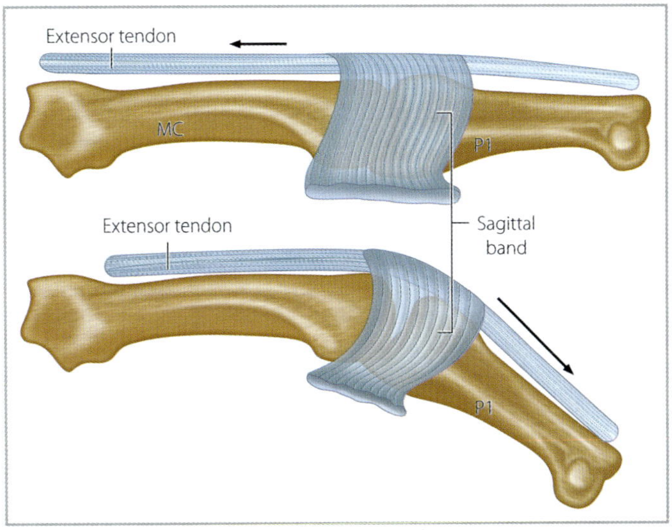

Figure 1.13 Anatomy of the sagittal band.

- Oblique retinacular ligament (ORL): Arises from the flexor tendon sheath at the level of the PIP joint, spirals dorsally, and inserts distally with the terminal tendon on the dorsum of the distal phalanx. Because of its spiral structure as well as its course from the palmar to dorsal side of the finger, the ORL synchronizes the movement between the PIP and DIP joints so that the joints of the fingers flex and extend seamlessly. When the PIP joint extends, the ORL tightens to extend the DIP joint, and when the PIP joint is flexed, the ORL relaxes to allow for the simultaneous flexion of the DIP joint. Detailed illustrations demonstrating the anatomy of the tendons and ligaments over the dorsum of the hand and fingers are depicted in **Figures 1.10** and **1.12**

Intrinsic muscles (Figures 1.14 and 1.15)

These muscles are known as the intrinsic muscles of the hand because they originate and insert within the hand. These include the following groups of muscles:

Muscles supplied by the motor branch of the median nerve

- Thenar muscles (abductor pollicis brevis/APB, flexor pollicis brevis/FPB, and opponens pollicis)
- Radial 2 lumbricals

Muscles supplied by the motor branch (deep branch) of the ulnar nerve

- Interosseous muscles 7 (4 dorsal and 3 palmar)
- Ulnar 2 lumbricals
- Hypothenar muscles (ADM, flexor digiti minimi/FDM, and opponens digiti minimi)
- Adductor pollicis muscle

The interosseous muscles arise from the shafts of adjacent metacarpals and insert by crossing deep to the sagittal bands into the extensor expansion of the extensor tendons and the base of the proximal phalanx of the index to the small finger, and contribute to the formation of the lateral bands with the lumbricals. As the interosseous muscles

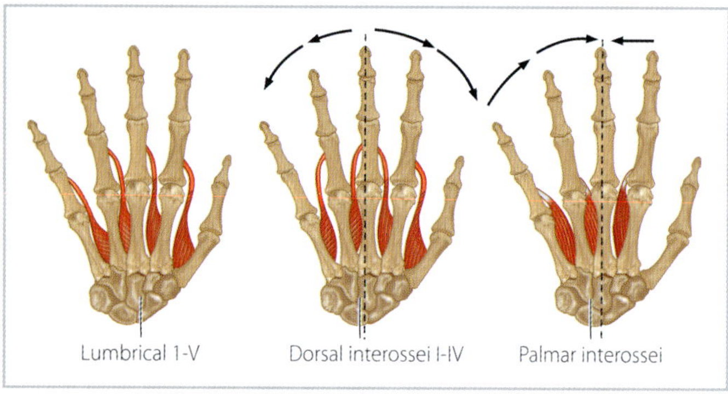

Figure 1.14 Interosseous and lumbrical muscles of the hand.

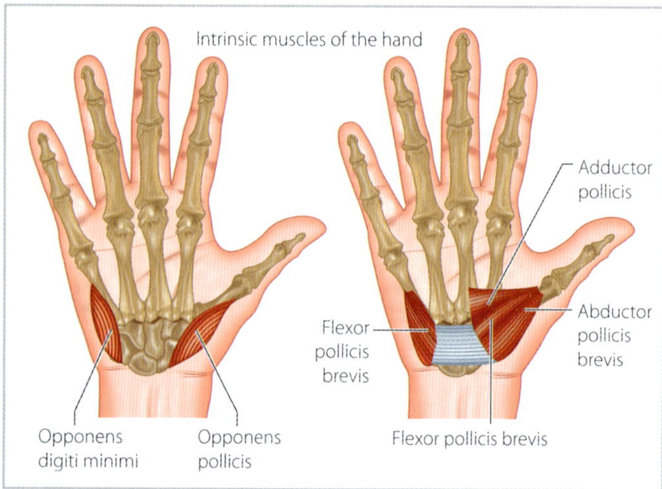

Figure 1.15 Hypothenar and thenar muscle groups.

pass volar to the axis of rotation of the MCP joint, they flex the MCP joint and extend the IP joints. Additionally, the dorsal interossei abducts the fingers (DAB) whereas the palmar interossei adducts the fingers (PAD). The abduction of the little finger is executed by the abductor digiti minimi.

The lumbricals arise from the FDP tendons in the palm and insert into the radial lateral band of the extensor expansion of the index to small fingers by passing deep to the deep transverse metacarpal ligament. The lumbrical muscles are weak flexors of the MCP joints; however, as the lumbricals arise from the flexor tendons and insert into the extensor tendons, they have a unique function of coordinating the fine flexion extension movement of the fingers.

The delicate balance between the intrinsic and extrinsic muscles of the hand may be disrupted by pathologic conditions leading to the development of various deformities. For example, paralysis of the intrinsic muscles as a result of ulnar nerve palsy may lead to varying degrees of finger clawing, depending on the level of nerve injury (i.e. high vs. low ulnar nerve palsy). Finger clawing (aka. intrinsic minus deformity) is characterized by hyperextension of the MCP joint and flexion of the IP joints. This deformity is a result of weakness of intrinsic muscle function, which subsequently results in an unopposed extension of the MCP joints by the long extensors and flexion of the IP joints by the long flexors. In contrast, intrinsic muscle tightness/contracture, which occurs with conditions such as rheumatoid arthritis, is often associated with intrinsic plus deformity, characterized by flexion of the MCP joints and extension of the IP joints (see chapter on Stiff Digit for more details).

Skeletal framework of the hand

The hand and wrist consist of several articular surfaces connecting 27 bones that are stabilized by the normal joint architecture, intact restraining ligaments, and a complete balance of the musculotendinous system of the extrinsic and intrinsic muscles. Alteration to any of these structures can compromise hand function.

The metacarpophalangeal joint (MCP joint, Figure 1.16a and b)

The MCP joint is formed by the articular surfaces of the metacarpal head and the base of the proximal phalanx. The MCP joint is a condyloid joint that allows movement in two planes (flexion/extension, abduction/adduction). A surrounding capsule, collateral ligaments, accessory collateral ligaments, and a palmar plate stabilize the joint. The collateral ligaments arise from the dorsum and sides of the metacarpal heads, and run downward and forward to insert on the palmar aspect of the base of the proximal phalanx and joint's palmar plate. Because the metacarpal head has an asymmetric configuration of 'volar flaring', this creates a Cam effect where collateral ligaments are tightened by joint flexion and loosened by joint extension. The Cam effect is best described as a widening of the interarticular space between the metacarpal head and the base of the proximal phalanx due to the above-described asymmetry that exerts tension on the collateral ligaments during joint flexion.

The proximal interphalangeal joint (PIP joint, Figure 1.16a and b)

The PIP joint is formed by the articular surfaces between the proximal and middle phalanges. The PIP joint is a hinge joint that allows flexion and extension only. The joint can be described as a box shape surrounded by a joint's capsule that is adherent to extensor tendon dorsally, and the palmar plate and the check-rein ligaments on the palmar side. The check-rein ligaments are volar extensions arising proximally from the palmar plate of the PIP joint and insert onto the palmar surface of the proximal phalanx. As their name implies, the check-rein ligaments together with the palmar plate keeps the PIP joint in 'check' and prevents joint hyperextension. Laterally, the joint is supported by collateral and accessory collateral ligaments as well as the fibers of the oblique retinacular ligament of Landsmeer (ORL).

The distal interphalangeal joint (DIP joint, Figure 1.16a and b)

The DIP joint is formed by the articular surfaces between the middle and distal phalanges. The DIP joint is a hinge joint that allows flexion and extension, and the joint is surrounded by a joint's capsule. Laterally, the joint is supported by collateral and accessory collateral ligaments, whereas on the palmar side the joint capsule attaches to the palmar plate.

The wrist joint

The wrist joint connects the forearm to the hand and is a transitional anatomical and functional region that allows the hand a great freedom of mobility, from a relatively limited pronosupination movement

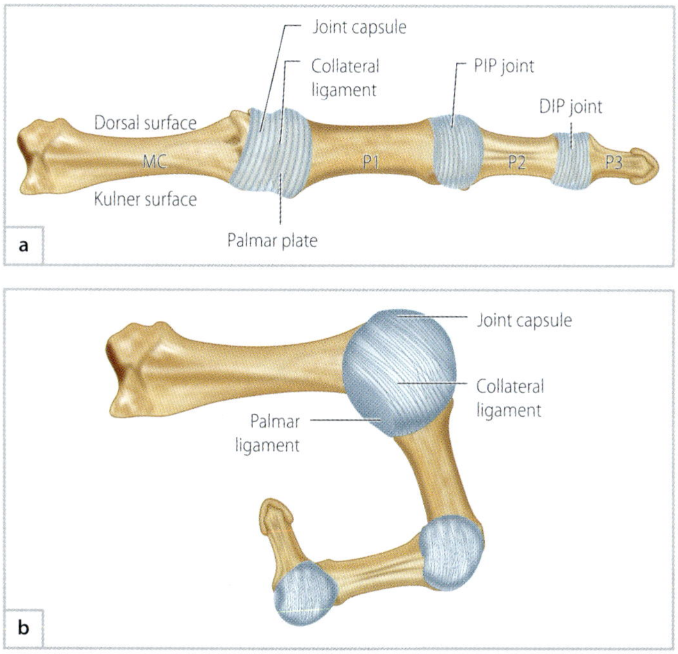

Figure 1.16 (a) metacarpophalangeal (MCP), proximal interphalangeal (PIP), and distal interphalangeal (DIP) joints in extension. (b) MCP, PIP, and DIP joints in flexion.

at the distal forearm to almost any degree of movement, including wrist flexion, extension, radial deviation, ulnar deviation, and circumduction.

The wrist is fairly a complex geometrical structure that is composed of eight carpal bones articulating among each other and also with the distal radius and ulna proximally and distally with the metacarpal bones. The carpal bones are arranged into two rows: the proximal carpal row that consists of the scaphoid, lunate, triquetrum, and pisiform bones and a distal row that is formed by the trapezium, trapezoid, capitate and hamate bones. Between the two carpal rows is the midcarpal joint that permits flexion and extension movement. The articular surface of the distal radius has two bony depressions: the scaphoid fossa and lunate fossa that accommodate the scaphoid and lunate bones, respectively and are known as the radiocarpal joint. On the ulnar aspect of the distal radius, the sigmoid notch articulates with the distal ulna head to form the DRUJ. The DRUJ permits pronosupination of the forearm. There is a discrepancy between the circumference of the sigmoid notch of the radius and that of the ulnar head. This mismatch results in joint incongruity, subsequently resulting in translation and rotation of the ulna during pronation and supination. The ulna translates dorsally in pronation and volarly in supination. However, the DRUJ is stabilized by several structures often referred to as the static and dynamic constraints. The static constraints include the triangular fibrocartilage complex (TFCC), the dorsal radioulnar ligament and volar radioulnar ligament, the ulnar collateral ligament, and the joint capsule. The dynamic muscle stabilizers include the extensor carpi ulnaris (ECU) tendon and the pronator quadratus (PQ) muscle.

At the ulnocarpal joint, the distal ulna is covered by triangular fibrocartilage, which is together with the ulnocarpal ligaments and the sheath of the ECU, forms theTFCC. The TFCC arises from the lunate and distal end of radius and inserts into the base of the ulnar styloid process. The peripheral part of the TFCC is well vascularized, whereas the center of the TFCC is an avascular load bearing part that articulates with the distal ulna and triquetrum. The intricate assembly of the carpal bones is supported by a number of volar and dorsal ligaments. The ligaments of the wrist are divided into extrinsic and intrinsic ligaments as described by Taleisnik. Extrinsic ligaments connect the distal radius and ulna to the carpal bones, and intrinsic ligaments connect carpal bones together, as they have their origins and insertions within the carpal bones.

Blood supply of the hand

An abundant network of arteries arising from the radial and ulnar arteries (branches of the brachial artery) supplies the hand. The radial artery enters the hand passing along the floor of the anatomical snuffbox, then pierces the dorsum of the first webspace (between the two heads of the first dorsal interosseous muscle) to enter the palm of the hand after giving off the princeps pollicis artery to the thumb. The anastomosis between the radial artery and the deep branch of the ulnar artery forms the deep palmar arch (predominately from the radial artery), which lies at the base of the metacarpals. Branches of the deep palmar arch include the radialis indicis artery, palmar metacarpal arteries, perforating arteries to the dorsal system, and recurrent branches to the palmar carpal arch. The SPA (see surface marking in **Figure 1.3**) lies just beneath the PA and is prone to injury due to its relative superficial location in the hand. The SPA (predominantly from the ulnar artery) is formed by the anastomosis between the ulnar artery and the superficial palmar branch of the radial artery. The major branches of the SPA are the common digital arteries (**Figure 1.17**).

On the dorsum of the hand, the posterior interosseous artery and the perforating branches of the anterior interosseous artery (branches of the common interosseous artery that arise from the ulnar artery at the level of the radial tuberosity proximal in the forearm) form the dorsal carpal arch. The 2nd, 3rd, 4th, and 5th dorsal metacarpal arteries branch from the dorsal carpal arch (**Figure 1.18**) and are the source of the blood supply of many of the local flaps performed on the dorsum of the hand (dorsal metacarpal artery system). The dorsal metacarpal arteries bifurcate to give off the dorsal digital arteries, which communicate with the palmar digital arteries in the fingers.

Distal in the palm, the common digital arteries bifurcate into the proper palmar digital arteries. The proper digital arteries run dorsal to their corresponding radial and ulnar digital nerves, respectively (**Figure 1.19**) and anastomose by perforating branches with the dorsal digital arteries. The venous drainage of the hand corresponds to these arteries; however, a superficial network of superficial veins is obvious on the dorsum of the hand that confluences to form the cephalic and basilic veins on the radial and ulnar sides of the dorsum of the hand, respectively. Finally, one must realize that there are large anatomical variations in the blood supply and venous drainage of the hand.

Nerve supply of the hand

The upper limb and the hand are innervated by branches arising from the roots, trunks, and divisions of the brachial plexus. In this section, we will discuss the sensory and motor innervation of three nerves: the radial, median, and ulnar nerves (**Figure 1.20**):

The radial nerve arises from the posterior cord (C5-T1) of the brachial plexus. In the arm, the radial nerve runs in the spiral groove of the humerus and supplies the triceps and anconeus muscles.

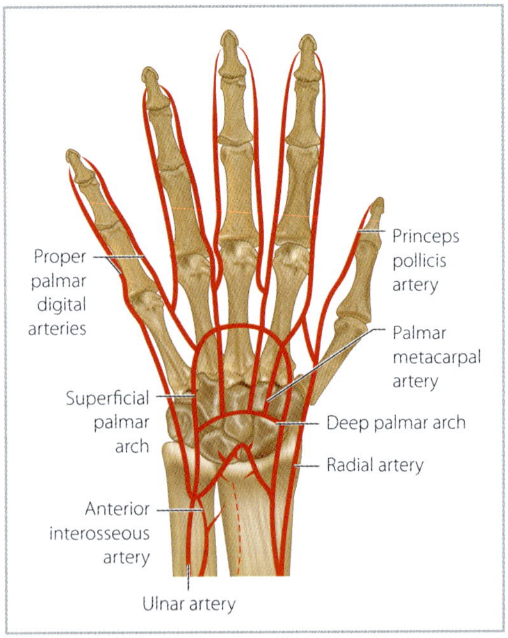

Figure 1.17 Blood supply of the hand (superficial and deep palmar arches).

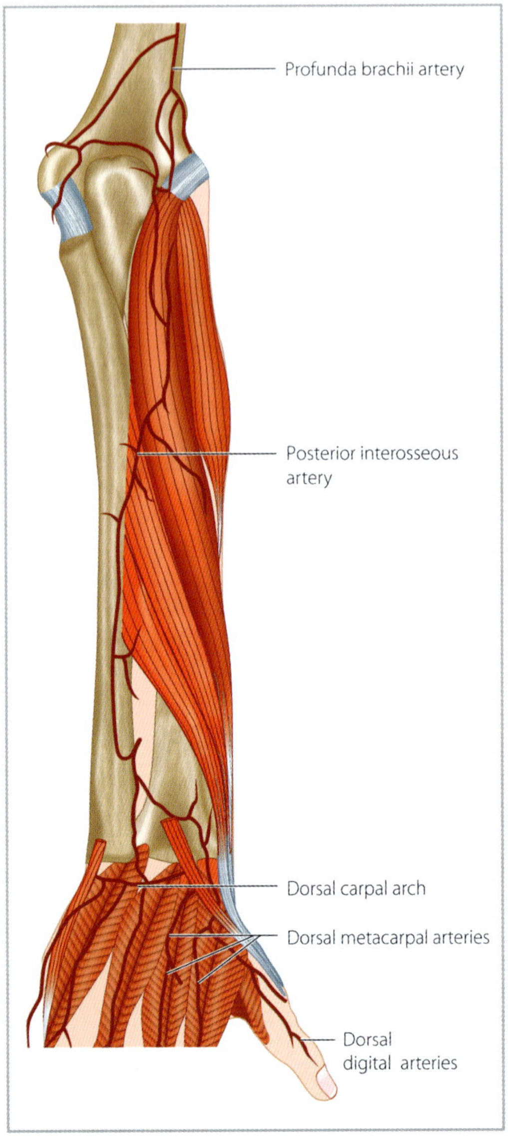

Figure 1.18 Anatomy of the dorsal carpal arch and dorsal metacarpal circulation.

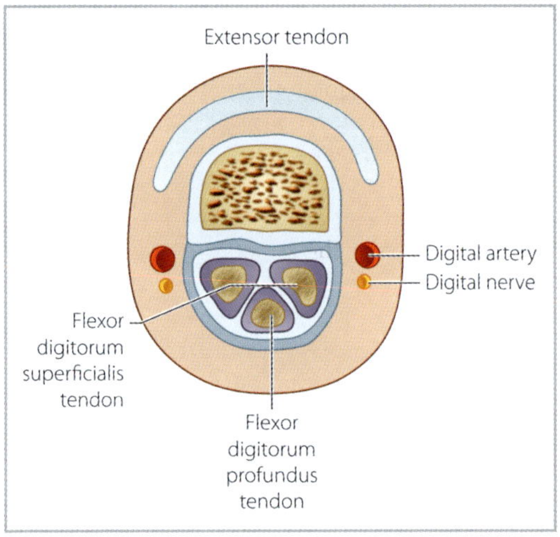

Figure 1.19 Cross section of the finger. Note that the digital arteries lie immediately dorsal to the digital nerves.

The radial nerve then pierces the lateral intermuscular septum of the arm to run in the anterior compartment of the arm. The radial nerve enters the forearm anterior to the lateral epicondyle of the humerus and divides into two branches: a deep branch called the posterior interosseous nerve (PIN) that is a motor branch and supplies most of the extensors of the forearm below the elbow and a superficial sensory branch. The superficial radial nerve is a sensory branch and provides cutaneous innervation over the anatomical snuffbox and the 1st dorsal webspace of the hand (**Figure 1.21a** and **b**).

The median nerve is formed by contributions of the medial and lateral cords of the brachial plexus (C6-T1). The median nerve runs in the anterior compartment of the arm and through the cubital fossa (a triangular space on the volar side of the elbow joint) medial to the brachial artery. The median nerve enters the forearm by passing between the two heads of the pronator teres (PT) muscle (see anatomy of the forearm below). In the forearm, the median nerve gives off two branches: the anterior interosseous nerve (a motor branch) and a sensory palmar cutaneous branch. The median nerve then continues its course and passes through the carpal tunnel to supply the muscles and skin of the hand. The sensory distribution of the median nerve in the hand involves the palmar side of the radial three and a half fingers (thumb, index, long fingers, and radial half of the ring finger) as well as the skin over the dorsum of the distal phalanges, including the nail bed.

The ulnar nerve arises from the medial cord of the brachial plexus (C7-T1). The ulnar nerve initially runs in the anterior compartment before piercing the medial intermuscular septum to enter the posterior compartment of the arm. The ulnar nerve then enters the forearm behind the medial epicondyle by passing through the cubital tunnel (potential site of nerve compression). In the forearm, the ulnar nerve runs underneath the FCU alongside the ulnar artery. The ulnar nerve gives motor innervation to the medial half of the FDP and the FCU muscles. Along its course, the nerve is accompanied by the ulnar artery and both enter the hand by passing through the Guyon canal. Before entering the hand, the ulnar nerve gives off a dorsal and a palmar cutaneous branch that supplies the skin of the ulnar one and a half fingers (small and ulnar half of the ring finger). In the hand, the ulnar nerve supplies the intrinsic muscles of the hand as mentioned previously.

The nerves of the upper limb travel a long distance from the upper arm to the hand, thus they are prone to mechanical compression at several anatomic locations that leads to several clinical sequelae that are discussed in detail in later chapters of this book.

ANATOMY OF THE FOREARM

The forearm extends from the elbow joint proximally to the wrist joint distally. The skeletal framework of the forearm consists of two bones: the radius and the ulna. The two bones are joined together by a fascial condensation called the interosseous membrane, sometimes referred to as the interosseous ligament, and articulate at the proximal and DRUJs along the longitudinal axis. The muscles of the forearm are arranged into two groups on the volar and dorsal sides of the forearm and are surrounded by a tight investing fascia (antebrachial fascia) that gives off deep intermuscular septa that enclose the muscles of the extensor compartment and surround the flexor compartment. Thus, the muscles of the forearm are confined within a tight fascial space, and are therefore prone to the development of compartment syndrome due to a dramatic rise of the intracompartmental pressure following trauma or a reperfusion injury.

On the radial border of the forearm lies a long muscle known as the brachioradialis muscle, which arises from the lateral supracondylar ridge of the humerus and inserts into the lateral side of the distal radius. The brachioradialis is the main flexor of the elbow joint and overlays the radial side of both the dorsal/extensor and volar/flexor compartments of the forearm. The muscle belly of the brachioradialis is noticeable when the elbow is in flexion against resistance while the forearm is in a neutral position.

On the dorsum of the forearm, we can find that the muscle bellies of the extensor compartment are arranged in layers and parallel to each other, this is also true when we will look later at the muscles of the flexor compartment of the forearm. The muscles of the superficial layer of the extensor forearm arise from a common extensor origin, which is the lateral epicondyle of the humerus. From radial to ulnar, the muscles are arranged as follows: extensor carpi radialis longus (ECRL), extensor carpi radialis brevis (ECRB), EDC, EDM/EDQ, and the ECU. With the exception of the supinator muscle, which inserts proximally on the dorsum of the forearm, the extensor muscles of the forearm pass underneath the extensor retinaculum as described previously to insert into the hand. A clinical caveat: most of the muscles of the extensor compartment of the forearm are supplied by the PIN except two muscles, the ECRL and brachioradialis, which are supplied by the radial nerve at a level above the elbow joint. Thus, with radial nerve palsy at the forearm, such as in PIN syndrome, the synergistic action of the extensor muscles is lost and wrist extension is achieved mainly by the ECRL, which results in extension and radial deviation of the wrist joint. A clinical distinction between high or low radial nerve palsy can be made based on the knowledge of this anatomy. In high radial nerve palsy, there is a wrist and finger drop deformity due to the paralysis of all of the muscles of the extensor compartment, whereas in low radial nerve palsy (i.e. below the elbow

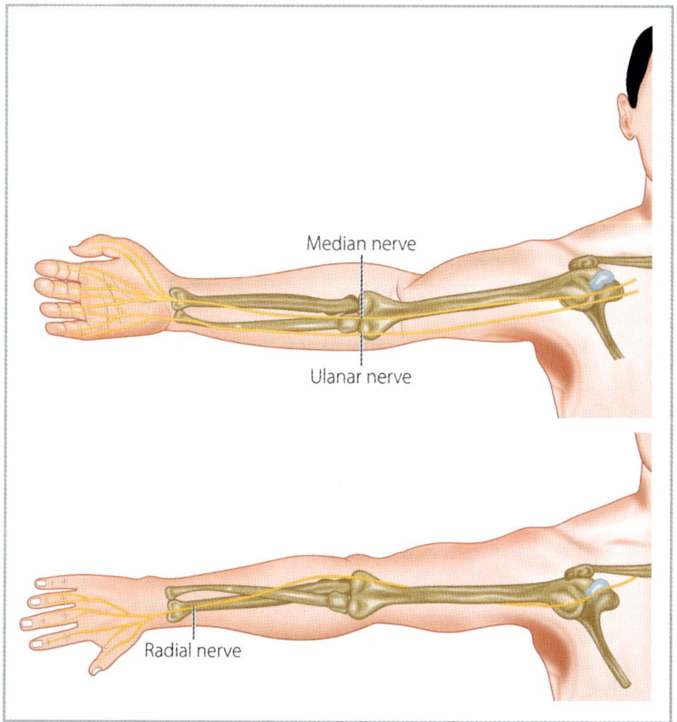

Figure 1.20 Radial, median, and ulnar nerves of the upper limb.

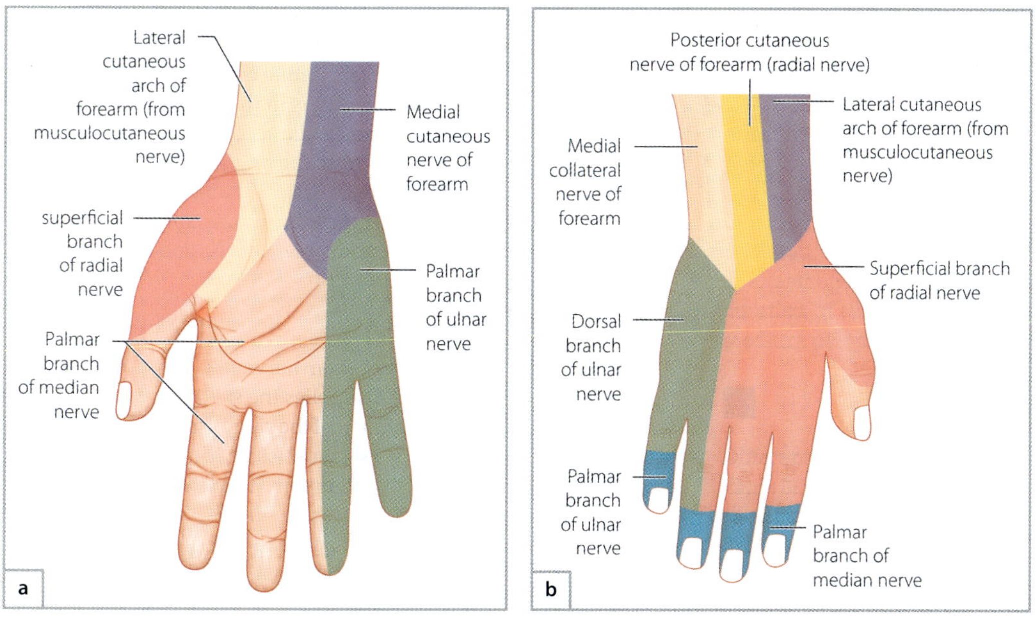

Figure 1.21 (a) Distribution of sensory innervation of the palm. (b) Distribution of sensory innervation on the dorsum of the hand.

joint such as in PIN syndrome) there is only a finger drop deformity as the ECRL muscle is spared.

In the next layer of the extensor compartment of the forearm, the following muscles lie from radial to ulnar; the APL, EPB, EPL, and the EIP. The APL, EPB, and the EPL form the medial and lateral borders of the anatomical snuffbox, respectively, which is located over the radial side of the distal radius and carpal bones. The EPL tendon courses at an acute angle around a bony prominence on the dorsum of distal radius called the Lister tubercle (see surface marking above) to reach the dorsum of the thumb. This sharp angulation around the bony protuberance creates tension on the EPL tendon and may precipitate tendon attrition rupture. The layers of the extensor muscles of the forearm are shown in **Figure 1.22**.

On the flexor side of the forearm, the muscles are arranged from superficial to deep into three layers, with the FCR, the PL, and the FCU being the most superficial layer of the volar forearm. More proximal on the volar side of the forearm is the PT muscle. The PT, FCR, PL, FCU, and FDS all have a common flexor origin arising from the medial epicondyle of the humerus. The next layer is the FDS muscle belly as well as the FPL muscle. Underneath the FDS muscle lies the median nerve after emerging from between the two heads of the PT muscle. The median nerve (and its motor branch, AIN) supplies all of the muscles of the forearm except the FCU and medial part of the FDP (ring and small fingers) that is innervated by the ulnar nerve. In the distal forearm, the median nerve continues as described previously deep to the PL and ulnar to the tendon of the FCR to enter the carpal tunnel after giving off the palmar cutaneous branch of the palm approximately 5 cm proximal to the distal wrist crease. The ulnar nerve and ulnar artery lie deep and ulnar to the FCU tendon and superficial to the muscle belly of the FDP to enter the hand above the TCL by passing through the Guyon canal. In the deepest layer of the forearm, tendons of the FDP and the PQ muscle are found. The PQ muscle, together with the PT, pronates the forearm (**Figure 1.23**).

ANATOMY OF THE ARM

Last but not the least is the anatomy of the upper arm. On studying the anatomy of the upper extremity, one must appreciate that the whole limb work as a functional unit and deformities of proximal joints would affect the distal ones. Similar to the other parts, the upper arm is divided into an anterior and a posterior compartment by an intermuscular septum. The anterior compartment of the arm is the flexor compartment, whereas the posterior compartment is the extensor compartment. In addition to the nerves and vessels described in the previous sections, the anterior compartment of the arm includes the biceps brachii muscle, the brachialis, and the coracobrachialis that are all supplied by the musculocutaneous nerve (MCN). The MCN arises from the lateral cord of the brachial plexus, and as the name implies serves as a motor nerve in the arm and continues as a sensory nerve to supply the lateral aspect of the forearm. The biceps muscle is the main supinator of the forearm and together with the brachialis and brachioradialis it flexes the elbow joint. On the posterior compartment are the three heads of the triceps muscle and a small muscle called the anconeus, both of which are supplied by the radial nerve. The triceps is the main extensor of the elbow joint with a less than modest contribution from the anconeus muscle. The muscles, nerves, and vessels of each compartment are demonstrated by the cross-sectional anatomy shown in **Figure 1.24**.

SUMMARY

A good knowledge of the functional anatomy of the upper limb sets the stage for understanding kinematics of the hand and pathological conditions affecting the function of the upper limb. Having gained such knowledge, a surgeon would feel more comfortable and confident when dissecting through the anatomical planes of the upper limb to deliver an efficient and safe surgery.

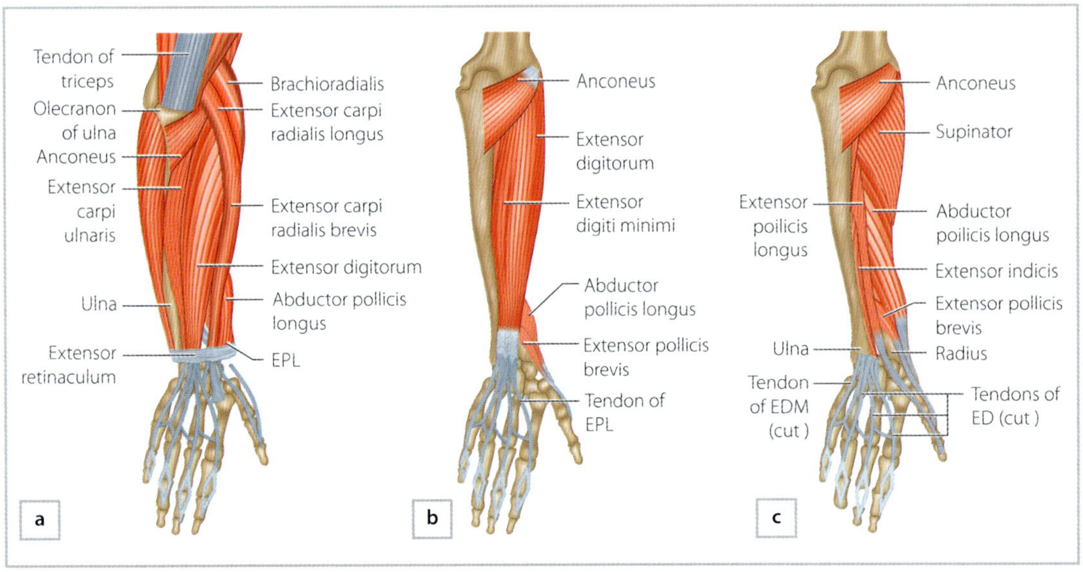

Figure 1.22 Muscles of the extensor compartment of the forearm: (a) superficial, (b) middle, and (c) deep layers. ED, extensor digitorum; EDM, extensor digiti minimi; EPL, extensor pollicis longus.

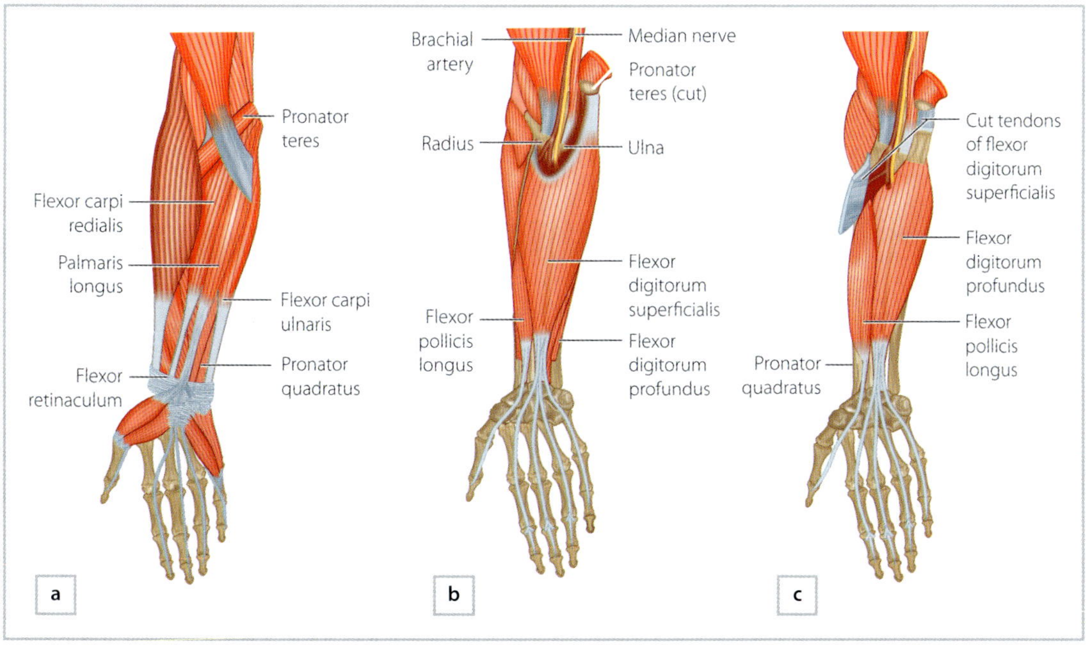

Figure 1.23 Muscles of the flexor compartment of the forearm: (a) superficial, (b) middle, and (c) deep layers.

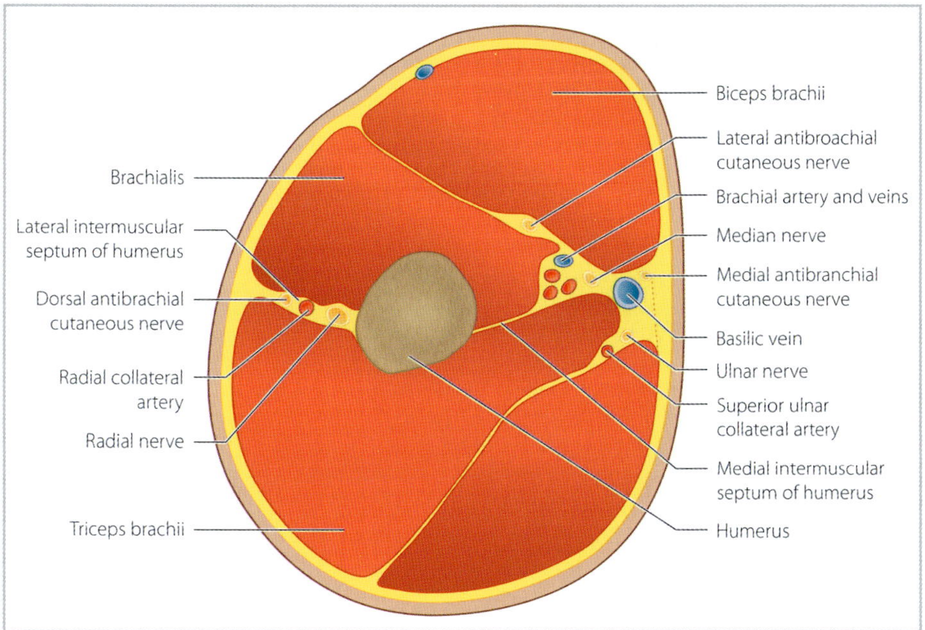

Figure 1.24 Cross section of the muscles and compartments of the arm.

SUGGESTED READING

Doyle JR. Anatomy of the finger flexor tendon sheath and pulley system. J Hand Surg Am 1988; 13:473–484.
A cadaveric study performed on 61 fingers by Dr Doyle who was the first to describe and recognize the anatomical and functional importance of the pulley system of flexor tendons. The outcome of this study has reinforced our understanding of the anatomy of the pulley system as explained in this chapter and addressed other issues such as correct terminology of flexor tendons pulleys and their anatomic variation in the human hand.

Frank H. Netter. Atlas of human anatomy. Chapter 7, Upper Limb p. 293–346.
A comprehensive atlas that includes detailed illustrations and descriptions of the anatomy of the upper limb.

Kareklas K, Nettle D, Smulders TV. Water-induced finger wrinkles improve handling of wet objects. Biol Lett 2013; 9:20120999.
This study sheds light on the role of papillary ridges of the palmar skin. The study compares the transit time of handling wet objects between two groups of healthy volunteers. Results show that wrinkled damp skin has a better ability to grasp wet objects than dry nonwrinkled palmar skin. The outcome of this study provides a new perspective on the understanding of the role of papillary skin ridges during prehension.

Palmer AK, Skahen JR, Werner FW, Glisson RR. The extensor retinaculum of the wrist: an anatomical and biomechanical study. J Hand Surg Br 1985; 10:11–16.
An anatomic and biomechanical study performed on 65 cadaveric specimens to evaluate the anatomic variation and biomechanics of the extensor retinaculum.

Sangole AP, Levin MF. Arches of the hand in reach to grasp. J Biomech 2008; 41:829–837.
A study investigating the biomechanics and kinematics of the arches of the hand during grasping motion. This study provides a clear anatomical description of the arches of the hand and thoroughly investigates the influence of motion on altering arches and the shape of the hand.

Young CM, Rayan GM. The sagittal band: anatomic and biomechanical study. J Hand Surg Am 2000; 25:1107–1113.
A cadaveric study performed on 12 specimens to evaluate extensor tendon instability anatomy associated with the mechanical disruption of the sagittal bands.

Chapter 2 Objective evaluation of hand function

Jeanne M. Riggs, Kevin C. Chung

INTRODUCTION

A basic skill in the clinical evaluation of the hand is critical prior to the development of an appropriate treatment plan for a patient. This chapter reviews the objective measures available for assessment of hand function.

INITIAL EVALUATION

Pain (0–10 ascending scale)

- Pain should be rated by the patient using the visual analog scale (VAS)
- Information on pertinent pain relievers/exacerbating activities is sought, as well as the location, frequency, and description of the pain (burning, aching, stabbing, tingling, constant)
- Is the pain causing the patient to have trouble sleeping?

FUNCTIONAL LIMITATIONS (ACTIVITIES OF DAILY LIVING)

Function can be evaluated using a simple patient-rated questionnaire such as one listed below:

Michigan Hand Outcomes Questionnaire (MHQ)

The MHQ measures several important patient outcomes and includes subscales on overall hand function, activities of daily living, work, pain, aesthetics, and satisfaction with function. This is a tool that is capable of measuring health status domains that are important to patients with hand dysfunction. Raw scores are normalized and presented on a 0–100 scale, where 100 indicates no disability (the exception is the pain domain, where 0 indicates no pain). The MHQ has been translated into Chinese (traditional and simple), Dutch, Japanese, Korean, Spanish, and Turkish.

Refer to the following website for additional information: http://sitemaker.umich.edu/mhq/mhq

OBJECTIVE

Sensory testing

Functional tests are useful in evaluating peripheral nerve function and can be a basis for discussion of sensory precautions that the patient should follow if deficits are found. Sensory precautions include the use of vision when around objects that are sharp, hot, extremely cold, or automated that could cause harm to an insensate area of the hand.

Table 2.1 Static 2-point discrimination scorings

Normal	<6 mm
Fair	6–10 mm
Poor	11–15 mm
Protective	One point perceived
Anesthetic	No points perceived

- Static 2-point discrimination: Assesses a patient's ability to perform tasks requiring precision grip, such as writing. Testing is performed with instrument initially set 6–8 mm between the 2 points. The instrument is placed on the fingertip parallel to the long axis of the digit (proximal to distal). The patient must accurately discriminate between 1 and 2 points in 2 of 3 trials before the distance is reduced
- Moving 2-point discrimination: Assesses a patient's hand function that requires moving touch, such as the fine manipulative task of buttoning. Testing begins with the instrument set 6–8 mm between the 2 points and is moved proximal to distal on the fingertip perpendicular to the long axis of the digit (testing ends side-to-side). The patient must accurately discriminate between 1 and 2 points in 2 of 3 trials before the distance is reduced. Results are documented in **Table 2.1**
- Moberg pickup test: Patient is asked to pick up a number of everyday objects and put them into a small box, first with the involved hand and then with the uninvolved hand, first with eyes open and then with vision occluded. Time required and manner of prehension are noted

Threshold tests

- Sharp/dull test: This is useful in assessing the return of sensibility following a nerve laceration in the early months of initial treatment, and is used to assess pain perception using a dull end pin such as the end of a paper clip. The pin is applied to the skin with enough pressure to indent the skin and cause slight blanching, while the patient responds to the sharp or dull stimulus by reporting what is felt, responding with either 'sharp' or 'dull.' Vision is occluded and the stimulus is applied beginning distally at the fingertips and is progressed proximally
  - Results are documented as follows:
    - Normal: 3/3 correct responses
    - Diminished: 1–2/3 correct responses
    - Absent: 0/3 correct responses
- Hot-cold test: This test is helpful in determining the need for protection from thermal or cold injury due to systemic diseases or peripheral nerve injury. The cold stimulus should be 40°F and the hot stimulus should be 115–120°F. With vision occluded, the temperature stimulus is applied to the fingers from distal to proximal

- Results are documented as follows:
  - Normal: 3/3 correct responses
  - Diminished: 1–2/3 correct responses
  - Absent: 0/3 correct responses
- Vibration (30 and 256 Hz) test: A tuning fork is used for vibratory perception testing and is useful in diagnosing digital nerve injuries, detecting the earliest sensory changes due to nerve compression, and useful in documenting nerve function return following a repair. The tuning fork should be warmed to ensure the patient is not responding to the coldness rather than the vibration. A comparison to the uninvolved side is made and the most distal area where the vibration is felt to be the same on both areas is documented

Objective tests

Wrinkle test for children (O'Riain): Used to evaluate sympathetic nerve function in children and cognitively impaired adults; this test is most useful following a recent nerve laceration. Both hands are immersed in 108° water for approximately 20–30 minutes. Denervated skin will not wrinkle as normal skin will wrinkle.

Range of motion (ROM)

To evaluate ROM, compare the ROM of the injured limb with the uninvolved limb. In addition, note any discrepancies between passive and active range of motion, as well as any fixed joint contractures. There are several other examinations that are useful to evaluate ROM:

- Goniometer use (**Figure 2.1**):
  - Goniometers come in a variety of sizes and materials, from the large international circular bodied goniometer used to measure the shoulder and elbow to the small plastic half circle goniometer used to measure digital joint motion
  - There are five variables that directly affect the reliability of ROM measurements:
    - Size and design of the goniometer
    - Type of ROM (AROM, PROM)
    - The amount of force applied
    - The method of documentation
    - The placement of the goniometer
  - Generally, measurements are taken using a dorsal placement of the goniometer. Most importantly, the axis of the goniometer needs to be at the axis of the joint being measured and the arms of the goniometer aligned with the long bones. With edema and severe joint contractures, lateral placement of the goniometer may provide a more accurate measurement. The alternate placement should be documented for consistency in future ROM testing
- Thumb opposition: Assess patient's ability to oppose their thumb to each fingertip
- Tip to palm distance: The distance from the fingertip to the distal palmar flexion crease may be documented in mm to provide a gross measurement of digital flexion
- Total active motion (TAM): This is the summation of the joint flexion measurements in a composite fist minus the summation of the joint extension deficits in a digit. Total passive motion (TPM) can be calculated as well in a similar fashion. Normal ranges are shown in **Table 2.2**.

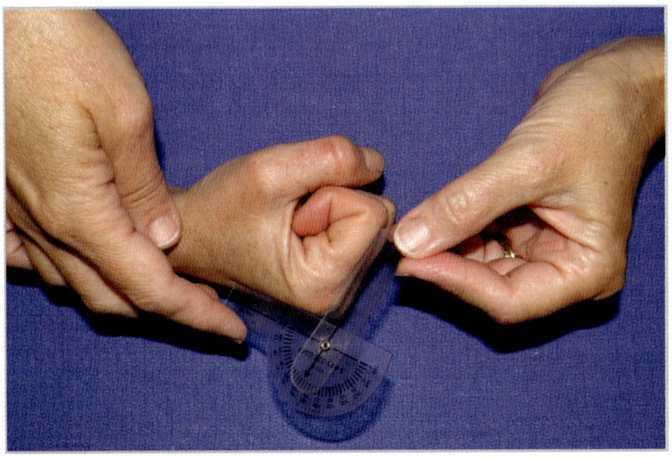

Figure 2.1 Goniometric measurement of metacarpophalangeal joint flexion.

Table 2.2 Normal active range of motion of the upper extremity

Supination	80°
Pronation	80°
Wrist ulnar deviation	30°
Wrist Radial deviation	20°
Wrist extension	70°
Wrist flexion	80°
Digital metacarpophalangeal	0/90
Digital proximal interphalangeal	0/100 TAM=280
Digital distal interphalangeal	0/90
Thumb metacarpophalangeal	0/50
Thumb interphalangeal	0/80
Thumb abduction	70°

Strength

- Manual muscle testing (MMT): This is a method for evaluating gross muscle function that is useful in differential diagnosis, prognosis, and treatment of musculoskeletal and neuromuscular disorders. Proper positioning of the patient and the extremity being tested, as well as stabilization of the extremity proximal to (or adjacent to) the tested extremity is critical. Pressure must be applied gradually, to allow the patient to 'get set and hold.' There is no 'gravity

Table 2.3 Scale for muscle strength (Medical Research Council)

5	The muscle contracts normally against full resistance. 'Normal' differs for each muscle group and in persons of different ages, sex, and occupation
4	Muscle strength is reduced but the muscle contraction can still move the joint against resistance
3	Muscle strength is further reduced; the joint can be moved only against gravity without any additional resistance. The examiner's resistance is completely removed
2	The muscle can move only if the resistance of gravity is removed. As an example, the elbow can be fully flexed only if the arm is maintained in a horizontal plane
1	Only a trace or flicker of movement is seen or felt in the muscle or fasciculations are observed in the muscle
0	No tension is palpated in the muscle or tendon; no movement is observed

factor' in grading (**Table 2.3**) the muscles of the hand, wrist, and forearm rotation because the weight of the extremity is so small in comparison to the strength of the muscle

- Dynamometer: The Jamar dynamometer is considered the most accurate tool to assess grip strength, using a hydraulic system that allows direct measurement of force rather than pressure. Norms are based on using the second handle position, and the mean of three successive trials is used. To control variables that may alter measurement reliability, testing is performed in a seated position, with the shoulder adducted and neutrally rotated, elbow flexed, forearm in a neutral position, and wrist in 0–30° of extension. The right and left hands are tested alternately, and there is usually a 5–10% difference between the normal dominant and normal nondominant hand, according to C. Bechtol
  - If submaximal effort is a concern, grip testing may be performed in all five handle positions, with a bell-shaped curve expected as the results. Grip strength should be highest with handle positions 2 and 3
  - Another technique to detect submaximal efforts is the rapid exchange grip (REG), in which a positive test is found when the REG score equals or is greater than the static score
- Pinch meter:
  - There are three types of pinch strength that may be evaluated using a pinch gauge:
    - Chuck or three-fingered pinch
    - Lateral or key pinch
    - Tip pinch, involving only the index and thumb

Edema

It is important to determine the presence of edema, and there are several easy ways to do this.

- Circumference: Measurements are taken at landmarks such as the elbow flexion crease, wrist flexion crease, and metacarpophalangeal joints and compared with the uninvolved extremity
- Volumeter:
  - Water is poured into the volumeter until overflow occurs and the overflow is discarded
  - The patient then slowly lowers his/her hand until the third web rests on the stop dowel
  - The displaced water is measured in a graduated cylinder and the patient's hand is removed from the water

Wound/Scar

- Assessment of a wound should include documentation of its location, size, color, presence of odor, drainage, and if there is exposure of underlying structures such as tendon and/or bone
  - The color of a closed wound or tissue surrounding an open wound may be described as having redness or erythema, ecchymosis, dusky/whitish, purple/blue, or black (indicating necrotic tissue)
  - Open wounds may be categorized as red, yellow, or black (as described in Chapter 7)
- Assessment of a scar should include location, size, color, pliability, presence of keloid, and presence of hypersensitivity
  - Color may be normal or demonstrate either hypopigmentation or hyperpigmentation
  - Pliability can be scored on a scale of normal, supple, yielding, firm, banding, or contracture

Fine motor coordination

- Nonobjective clinical assessments:
  - Place several coins on the table for the patient to pick up using their affected hand
  - Place several coins in the patient's palm and ask him/her to hand them back to you one-by-one, which requires the patient to manipulate the coins from the palm, radially to the tips of the radial digits
  - Ask the patient to sign their name if the involved limb is their dominant hand
  - Ask the patient to unbutton and then button their shirt button or inquire about difficulty the patient has with such tasks as buttoning, using a key, opening containers, using snaps, fastening their belt, or preparing food
- 9-Hole peg test:
  - This is one of the most commonly used assessment tools for finger dexterity, and consists of a plastic or wooden board with 9 holes and a shallow round dish or a square box to hold 9 pegs
  - A stopwatch is used to time the patient's performance in placing each peg in the board one by one and replacing the pegs back into the container as quickly as possible
  - Bilateral measurements are taken and norms are available

SUGGESTED READING

Dawson C, Mudgal CS. Staged description of the Finkelstein test. J Hand Surg 2010; 35:1513–1515.
A brief, concise description of a staged test, including a pictorial depiction that the authors find reliable and minimally painful for the diagnostic testing of deQuervain syndrome.

Haug A, Bartels A, Kotas J, Kunesch E. Sensory recovery 1 year after bridging digital nerve defects with collagen tubes. J Hand Surg 2013; 38:90–97.
This scientific article provides information on a battery of sensory tests assessing both basic and more complex sensory functions.

Horng Y, Lin M, Feng C, et al. Responsiveness of the Michigan Hand Outcomes Questionnaire and the Disabilities of the Arm, Shoulder, and Hand questionnaire in patients with hand injury. J Hand Surg 2010; 35:430–436.
Self-assessment questionnaires are compared for responsiveness in patients with hand injuries.

Valdes K, LaStayo P. The value of provocative tests for the wrist and elbow: a literature review. J Hand Ther 2013; 26:32–42.
This quantitative narrative review ranks 31 diagnostic studies as far as clinical usefulness and application.

Wang Y, Magasi SR, Bohannon RW, et al. Assessing dexterity function: a comparison of two alternatives for the NIH toolbox. J Hand Ther 2011; 24:313–320.
A single manual dexterity measure is identified for inclusion in the National Institutes of Health (NIH) Toolbox for Assessment of Neurological and Behavioral Function.

Chapter 3 Radiologic studies used in evaluation of the upper extremity

Aviram M. Giladi, Yirong Wang, Kevin C. Chung

INTRODUCTION

Radiographic imaging is an essential component of the evaluation of nearly every hand injury or condition. These studies are not only useful upon initial evaluation but also are equally important for the review of outcomes and results following medical or surgical treatment. There are a variety of viewing orientations that are useful to demonstrate preoperative and postoperative function of the hand and wrist, including those specifically used to evaluate the carpal bones, thumb phalanges, or the metacarpophalangeal (MCP) joints. In addition, computed tomography (CT) scans and magnetic resonance imagings (MRIs) may provide greater detail of structures, deformities, or foreign bodies that cannot be seen with other imaging techniques. In this chapter, we will highlight the different types of radiographic imaging and associated techniques that enable a comprehensive evaluation to be performed.

STANDARD RADIOGRAPHS

In order to ensure that X-rays are consistent and informative, a certain baseline criteria must be met for each radiographic image. The following should be considered to avoid X-rays that are inadequate or provide misleading information:

- All jewelry (rings, watches, etc.) must be removed
- If possible, remove bandages, tape, or other obstructive dressings
- Avoid overexposure (too dark, lose ability to appreciate subtleties) or underexposure (too light/bright, may overaccentuate normal anatomic findings)
- Always obtain image with hand/limb aligned in the proper position and plane – additional details below

In regard to the initial evaluation, at least two views are required, and often three are obtained:

1. Anteroposterior (AP) or posteroanterior (PA) view
2. Lateral view
3. Oblique view with fingers fanned out for minimal overlap

HAND VIEWS

AP/PA and lateral views (Figure 3.1)

These views provide clear visualization of the phalanges, metacarpals, and carpal bones, as well as the MCP, proximal interphalangeal (PIP), and distal interphalangeal (DIP) joints. The AP or PA view should be obtained with the hand held in a neutral position, flat on the X-ray plate. A lateral view, without overlapping of the fingers, is necessary for accurate imaging of each digit.

- Carpal height ratio:
  - This measurement is calculated in the PA view (**Figure 3.2**) and used in the evaluation of wrist disorders such as rheumatoid arthritis or trauma, because it is capable of determining the extent of carpal collapse
  - It is calculated by dividing the carpal height by the length of the middle finger metacarpal; normal ratio is 0.54 ±0.03
  - This ratio can be decreased in scapholunate dissociation, scapholunate advanced collapse (SLAC), and Kienbock disease, occurring because the carpus is collapsed due to a loss of intercarpal stability

Oblique view

The oblique X-ray can be a useful adjunct to the lateral and PA hand views. In particular, this view complements the lateral view for two reasons:

- It provides additional visualization of the metacarpals, MCP joints, and proximal phalanges
- There is decreased overlap of the metacarpals and proximal phalanges when compared with the lateral view.

However, it should be noted that the oblique view cannot replace the lateral view because it does not show small avulsions or the extent of fracture displacement.

WRIST VIEWS

Proper evaluation of many disorders and traumatic injuries requires standard views of the wrist to allow for complete visualization of pertinent wrist structures. In contrast to the standard views of the hand, the PA and AP views are used to demonstrate different anatomic measurements and concepts.

PA view of the wrist (Figure 3.3)

It is critical to avoid ulnar and radial deviation when obtaining PA radiographs of the wrist. The wrist should be oriented so that the ulnar styloid is located ulnarly on the ulnar head and the axis of the radius aligns with the axis of the middle finger metacarpal and phalanges. When obtaining X-rays of the wrist, the PA view is capable of demonstrating true ulnar variance, which the AP view is not able to demonstrate. The true ulnar variance evaluates the relationship between the ulnar head position and the distal radius, comparing relative ulnar and radial length (**Figure 3.4**). The following steps outline the process required to calculate true ulnar variance:

- Draw a line through the ulnar edge of the proximal sclerotic line of the distal radius, perpendicular to the axis of the radius

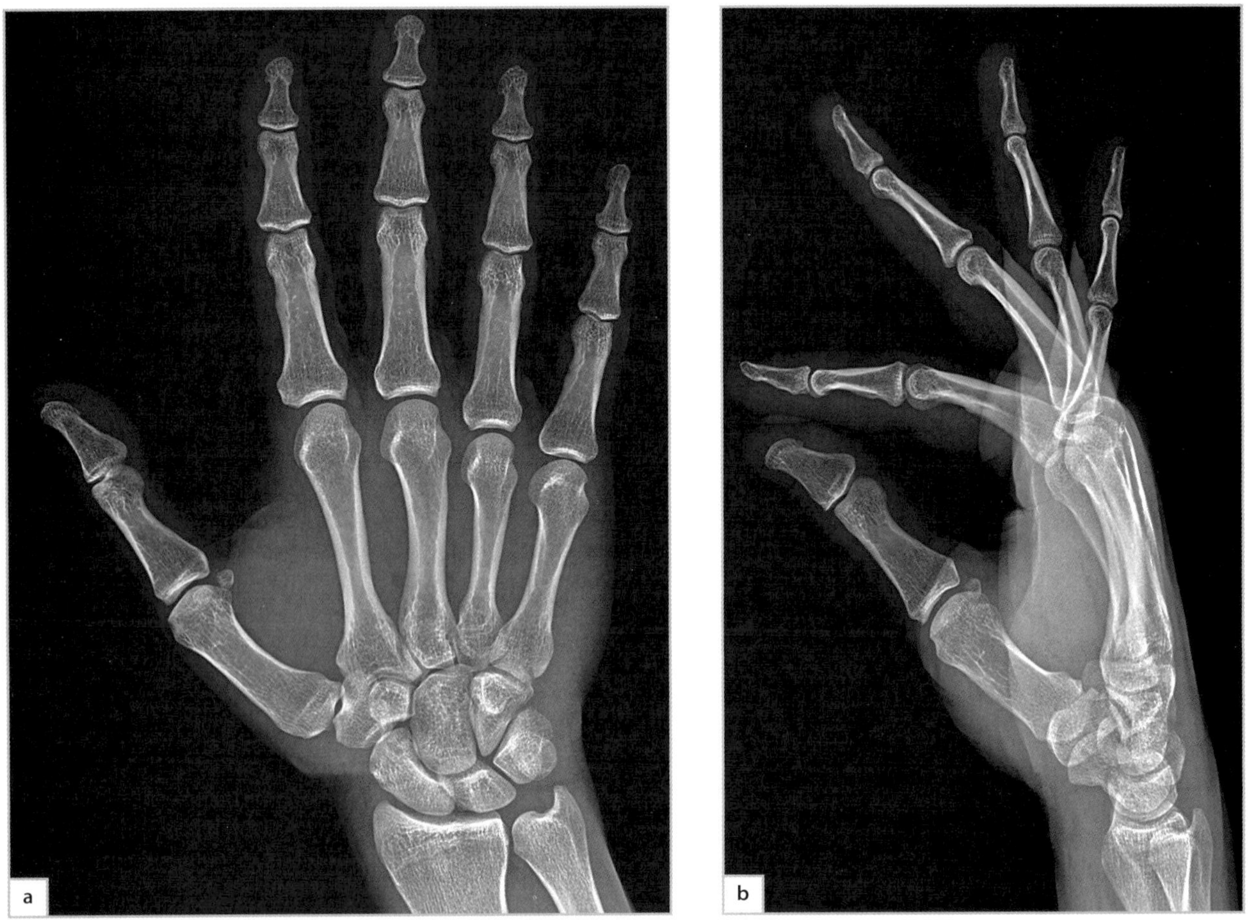

Figure 3.1 Standard posteroanterior and lateral X-rays of the hand. Note fingers fanned in lateral view to minimize overlap and improve visualization (can also be done in oblique view).

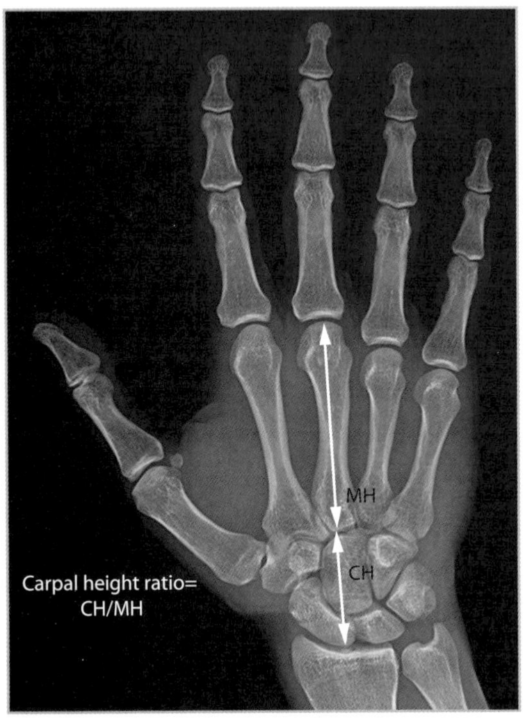

Figure 3.2 Measuring carpal height ratio. Ideal CH/MH = ~0.54.

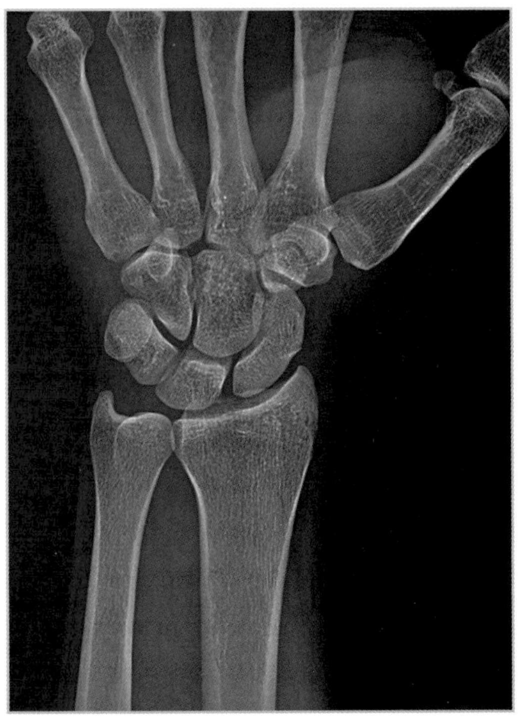

Figure 3.3 Standard postero-anterior X-ray of the wrist (note alignment of radius with middle finger metacarpal).

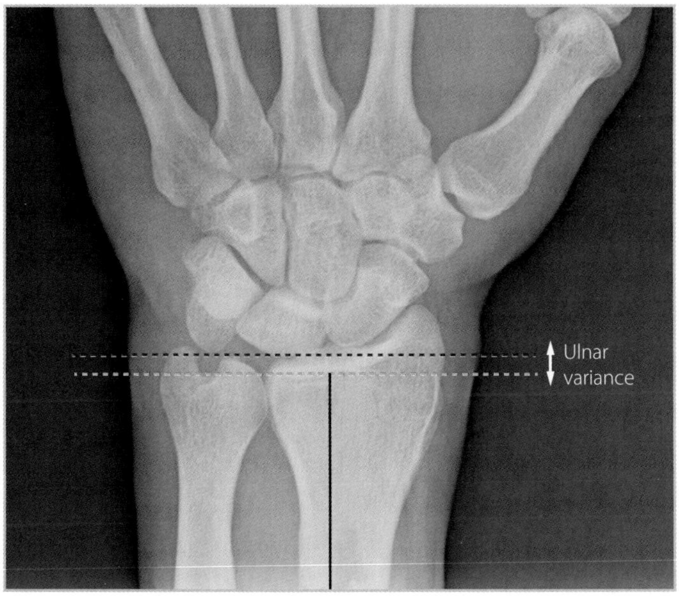

Figure 3.4 Technique for measuring ulnar variance. Black line indicates the longitudinal axis of the distal radius. Dashed green line runs through the proximal sclerotic line of the distal radius. Dashed blue line marks the distal cortical rim of the ulna.

- Variance is the distance between this line and the distal cortical rim of the ulnar dome:
  - Average: –0.9 mm
  - Range: –4.2 mm to +2.3 mm
- Ulnar plus (positive) refers to an ulnar position distal to the sclerotic line of the radius. Ulnar minus (negative) refers to an ulnar position proximal to the sclerotic line of the radius

AP view of the wrist

Proper orientation will position the ulnar styloid centrally over the distal ulna. This view is useful when the intercarpal joints need to be examined, because they are seen more clearly in the AP view than in the PA view.

- Gilula's lines can be seen on the PA and AP views of the wrist: (**Figure 3.5**)
  - The 'lines' represent three parallel arcs outlining the carpal bones. These arcs are easy to identify in the smooth, radiolucent spaces formed between the carpal rows:
    - First arc = proximal border of scaphoid, lunate, and triquetrum
    - Second arc = distal border of scaphoid, lunate, and triquetrum
    - Third arc = proximal border of capitate and hamate
  - Disruption in any of these arcs suggests carpal fracture or ligamentous injury

Lateral view of the wrist (Figure 3.6)

A substantial amount of diagnostic evidence can be gained from a true lateral wrist view. In order to obtain a true lateral, the distal radius must be aligned with the middle finger metacarpal and sit along the same vertical axis. The most valuable measurements provided by the lateral view include the intercarpal angles (scapholunate angle, radiolunate angle, and capitolunate angle) and the scapholunate

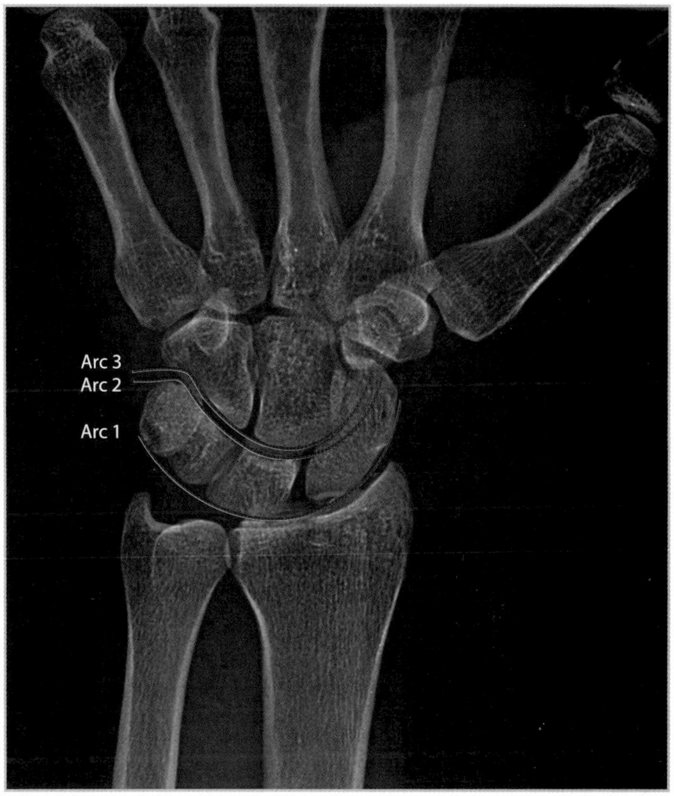

Figure 3.5 Gilula's lines – blue lines marking three carpal arcs, framing the intercarpal lucent spaces.

interval. Intercarpal angles with substantial deviation from the normal values may indicate interosseous ligament disruption. To evaluate these angles, the orientation and position of each carpal bone must be determined by drawing a line through the central axis of the bone.

- Scapholunate angle: measured at the intersection between the long axis of the scaphoid and an axial line bisecting the lunate (**Figure 3.7**). The range for a normal angle = 30–60°
- Radiolunate angle: measured at the intersection between the long axis of the radius and an axial line bisecting the lunate. Normal range = 0±15°
- Capitolunate angle: measured at the intersection between the long axis of the capitate and an axial line bisecting the lunate. Normal range = 0±30°

The scapholunate interval measures the distance between the scaphoid and lunate, and a gap >2 mm is potentially abnormal (see 'Terry Thomas sign' below). It is always helpful to compare this interval with the unaffected side, as the range for a normal scapholunate interval is quite variable.

- Dorsal intercalated segment instability (DISI) (**Figure 3.8**):
  - Often results from scapholunate ligament or volar radiocarpal ligament disruption
  - Lunate extended and scaphoid flexed:
    - Scapholunate angle >60°
    - Radiolunate angle >15° dorsal
- Volar intercalated segment instability (VISI):
  - Often associated with lunotriquetral, dorsal radiocarpal, and/or ulnocapitate ligament disruption
  - Lunate in volar flexion when related to the capitate:
    - Scapholunate angle <30°
    - Radiolunate angle >15° palmar

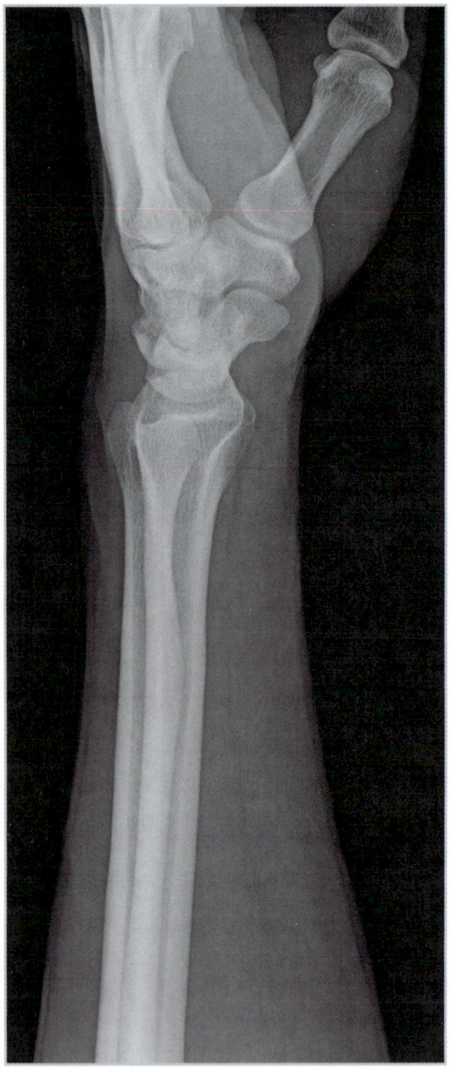

Figure 3.6 Standard lateral X-ray of the wrist.

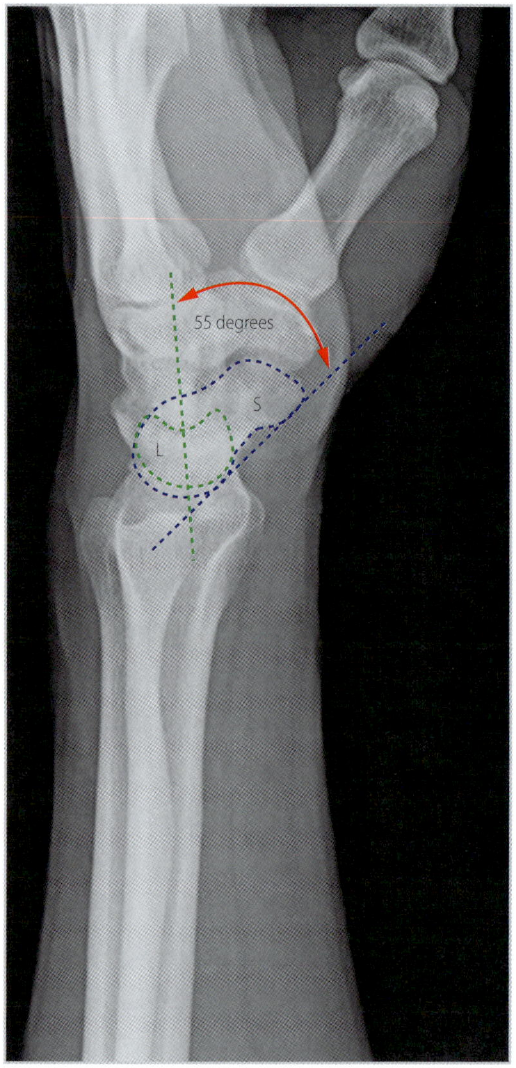

Figure 3.7 Technique for measuring scapholunate angle. Note lunate outlined in green with lunate axis marked by dashed green line. Scaphoid outlined in blue with dashed blue line connecting the most ventral points of the proximal and distal pole, used to represent scaphoid axis (true axis is through midpoint of proximal and distal poles, but this is often difficult to appreciate clearly – the line shown is nearly parallel to the true axis).

THUMB VIEWS

The thumbs views facilitate the evaluation of the bones and associated joints of the thumb.

Roberts view

The Roberts view provides a true AP view of the thumb ray. The beam is centered on the trapeziometacarpal (TM) joint, enabling this view to provide an accurate visualization of the TM joint. To obtain this view, position the hand as follows:

- The forearm in maximal pronation
- Wrist in 15° of extension
- Dorsum of the thumb parallel to the table

Lateral view

Along with the Roberts view, the lateral view can enable visualization of the TM joint, as well as the scaphotrapeziotrapezoidal (STT) joint and trapeziotrapezoidal joint. To obtain this view, position the hand as follows:

- Place the forearm on the table
- Hand pronated 20° with the thumb flat on the table and in line with the forearm
- The X-ray beam centered on the MCP joint

SPECIAL VIEWS

Certain aspects of the hand and wrist are difficult, if not impossible, to evaluate with standard X-ray views. To properly examine these features, the hand must be oriented in a very specific manner that will permit the proper visualization of the aforementioned structures. The following special views can be essential for a comprehensive assessment of the hand and wrist.

Brewerton view

The Brewerton view allows for improved evaluation of the MCP joint and metacarpal head. The positioning for this view minimizes any overlap between the metacarpal head and the base of the proximal phalanx. To obtain this view, angle the X-ray tube 20° and have the patient:

- Flex the MCP joints to 60°

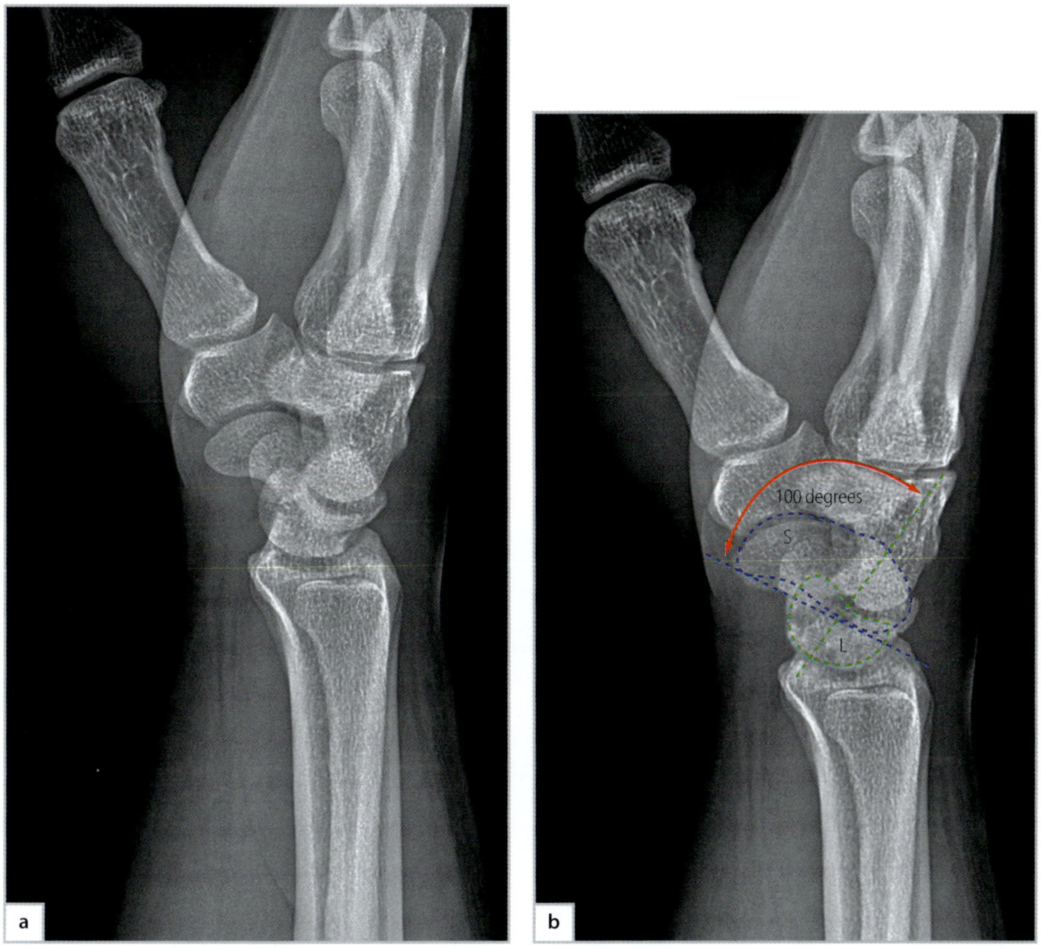

Figure 3.8 Scapholunate angle >60°, supporting the diagnosis of dorsal intercalated segment instability (DISI). Lunate outlined in green with lunate axis represented by dashed green line. Scaphoid outlined in blue with axis represented by dashed blue axis (see Figure 3.7 for explanation of scaphoid axis). Note extended position of the lunate and the flexed scaphoid in DISI deformity.

- Lay the dorsum of the phalanges flat on the film
- Abduct the thumb

Skyline view

This view is generally used to detect fight-bites and other intra-articular lesions of the MCP joint. The skyline view is obtained with the MCP joints and IP joints fully flexed, and X-ray beam parallel to the shafts of the proximal phalanges. By positioning the MCP joints into full flexion, the profile of the metacarpal head can be seen.

Scaphoid view

To accurately X-ray the scaphoid bone, position the wrist in 20° of ulnar deviation in the PA orientation. This view provides a more complete projection of the scaphoid than the standard AP, PA, oblique, or lateral hand and wrist views.

Carpal tunnel view

This view is used for diagnosing fractures affecting the hook of the hamate and pisiform, as well as pisotriquetral arthritis. To obtain the carpal tunnel view, maximally extend the hand while the volar surface of the wrist rests on the table, and direct the beam 15° off the plane of the palm.

DYNAMIC VIEWS

The constant presence of static instabilities in an affected patient allows for them to be recognized upon routine radiographic examination. Dynamic instabilities, on the other hand, are much more difficult to detect because they present transiently and are only produced through stress or motion. The dynamic views of the hand are useful in detecting carpal ligament instability caused by dynamic instabilities. These views are not always comprehensive by themselves, and should be compared with standard neutral PA and lateral views.

Wrist PA radial and ulnar deviation views

Examining the wrist in ulnar and radial deviation improves the evaluation of the motion between the forearm and the carpus and the motion between the proximal and distal carpal rows. These views can be obtained by simply placing the hand and wrist in a standard PA neutral view, and then moving the hand into maximal radial deviation or ulnar deviation. When evaluating the scaphoid in particular, the radial and ulnar views provide several benefits:

- Radial deviation view:
  - Ulnar-sided carpal interspaces are better demonstrated
  - Scaphoid foreshortened
  - Scapholunate interval decreased

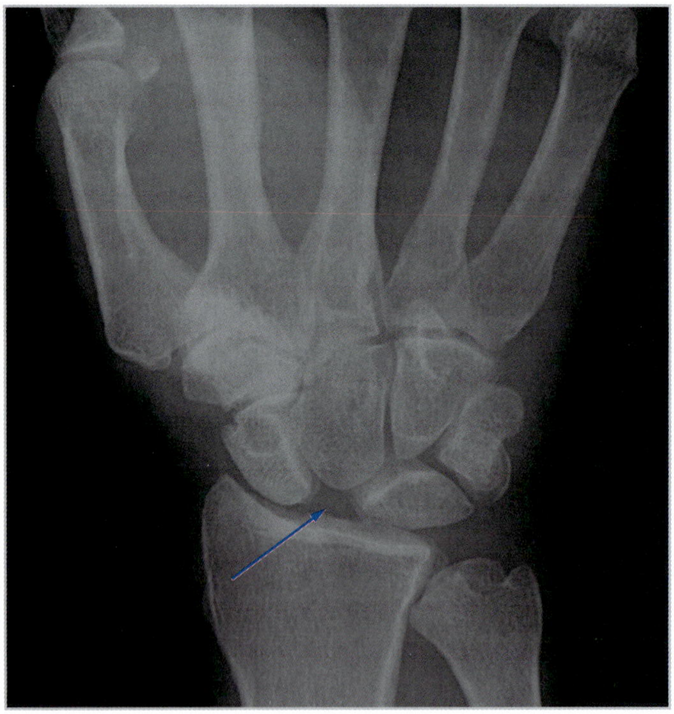

Figure 3.9 Blue arrow identifies a pathologic widening of the scapholunate interval (Terry Thomas sign), indicating probable scapholunate ligament injury.

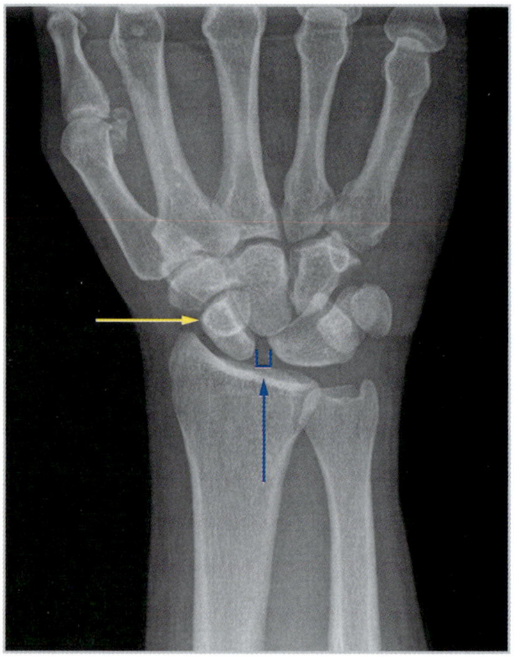

Figure 3.10 Signet ring sign of scaphoid (yellow arrow) with associated scapholunate dissociation (blue arrow and blue bracket).

- Ulnar deviation view:
  - Articular spaces between scaphoid and adjacent carpal bones are better demonstrated
  - Scaphoid elongated
  - Scapholunate interval widened
  - Particularly helpful in detecting scaphoid fractures

These dynamic stress views also may help delineate abnormal features not apparent in other radiographs. For example, a dynamic view may help to better visualize a disruption of Gilula's lines. A gap >2 mm between two carpal bones may be abnormal, such as a Terry Thomas sign of scapholunate dissociation, when a gap between the scaphoid and lunate >4 mm **(Figure 3.9)**. A Signet ring sign, also known as a cortical ring sign, of the scaphoid can be observed with wrist PA radial and ulnar views **(Figure 3.10)**. The cortical ring of the scaphoid is visualized due to a foreshortened appearance as the scaphoid is rotated and flexed volarly on its axis. This is accentuated with a radial deviation view, which adds stress to the scaphoid and augments volar rotation. It is often associated with a scapholunate dissociation that allows for abnormal flexion of the scaphoid.

WRIST PA CLENCHED FIST VIEWS

These views are obtained with the volar aspect of the wrist flat on the table and the hand clenched in a tight fist. Clenching serves to drive the capitate proximally toward the scapholunate joint due to the pull of muscles/tendons across the wrist. For patients experiencing a laxity of the scapholunate ligament, this maneuver can widen the scapholunate joint. This view is commonly used for patients suspected of having a scapholunate ligament disruption. In this view, the distal radioulnar joint (DRUJ) gap distance is a reliable parameter for evaluating distal DRUJ instability **(Figure 3.11)**.

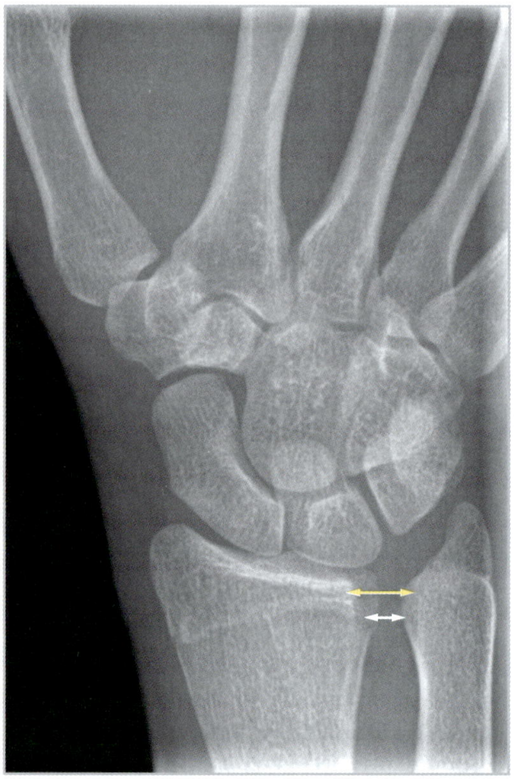

Figure 3.11 Measuring distal radioulnar joint (DRUJ) gap distance. On posteroanterior X-ray, yellow arrow indicates volar gap (measured from radial border of ulnar head to volar rim of sigmoid notch) and white arrow indicates dorsal gap (measured from radial border of ulnar head to dorsal rim of sigmoid notch). The lengths of these two measured gaps are added to give the DRUJ gap distance.

DRUJ gap distance

- Measure the distance between the ulnar head and the volar rim of the sigmoid notch
- Measure the distance between the ulnar head and the dorsal sigmoid notch

- The DRUJ gap is the sum of these two measured distances, and should be compared with the contralateral side to identify an abnormality

A modification, the 'clenched pencil view,' has been described to help diagnose scapholunate dissociation:

- Patient grips a pencil with both fists. The radial border of the right and left index finger is pressed tightly to each other, and the thumb metacarpals are positioned flat on the cassette. Both hands are simultaneously imaged
- The pencil defines a standard reproducible ulnar deviation and pronation angle
- This view more reliably shows a scapholunate gap by eliminating bony overlap
- Clenched pencil view has been shown to be the best stress view to demonstrate dynamic scapholunate instability

THUMB STRESS VIEW

This view is obtained with both thumbs positioned parallel to each other, with the radial aspects of the distal phalanges pressed together. It is used to identify laxity, subluxation, and other joint abnormalities of the thumb carpometacarpal (CMC) joint. Instability of the thumb CMC joint will be demonstrated by the metacarpal displacing from the trapezium in the presence of stress.

VIDEO FLUOROSCOPY

Video recording provides a detailed study for patients who have dynamic wrist instability. Pain and/or audible pathology (e.g. 'clunk') should be reproduced during the study. Includes observation of standard movements:

- Radial and ulnar deviation in the PA view
- Flexion and extension in the lateral view
- Radial and ulnar deviation in the lateral view

ULTRASOUND

Ultrasound is an optimal diagnostic method in many situations. It has the ability to provide detailed information about soft tissues, and is useful for studying structural movement.

Lesions of the hand and wrist

Ultrasound is capable of distinguishing cystic from solid lesions. These lesions can be difficult to differentiate using standard radiographs, making ultrasound a valuable investigative option. In one study, ultrasound correctly diagnosed 87% of cystic lesions and 73% of solid lesions.

Tendon rupture

Ultrasound is able to identify anechoic effusion at the site of a rupture and visualize the blunt torn ends. If the proximal portion retracts, ultrasound can be used to identify it in the retracted/abnormal position. This technique can also identify central slip injuries in the extensor mechanism of the finger. Postoperatively, it can distinguish the rupture of a repaired flexor tendon from a limited range of motion due to adhesions.

Tenosynovitis

In patients with tenosynovitis, anechoic, irregular zones develop around the injured tendon. In advanced cases, synovitis may invade the tendon, and ultrasound can show a thin remaining segment of the partially destroyed tendon.

Foreign bodies

When foreign bodies are suspected but not identified by other imaging methods, ultrasound can often localize them – even those as small as 1 mm. The sensitivity of ultrasound in the diagnosis of foreign bodies in the hand is 94% with a specificity of 99%.

Carpal tunnel syndrome

Ultrasound can be used to confirm the diagnosis of carpal tunnel syndrome. It enables the physician to see the enlargement of the median nerve at the distal wrist crease. A measured diameter >10.5 mm^2 of the median nerve at the level of the distal wrist crease provides a diagnostic sensitivity of 89% and specificity of 94.7%

COMPUTED TOMOGRAPHY

CT scans are often the optimal study for assessing bony anatomy. Most fractures do not need a CT scan, but with certain complex wrist fractures, comminuted fractures of the distal radius or scaphoid, occult fractures, or intra-articular fractures, a CT scan may provide important additional information and imaging details. In addition, a CT scan can be used to evaluate DRUJ instability. It is important to note that a CT scan is inadequate for assessing ligamentous injuries.

CT SCAN PLANES

The different scan planes provide different advantages.

Axial plane

The axial plane is useful for evaluating subluxation or dislocation of the DRUJ, and carpal fractures, especially occult fractures and hook of the hamate fractures. Additionally, it can provide additional details of distal radius fracture patterns. This is especially helpful when the fracture involves the radioulnar and radiocarpal articular surfaces. Scanning in this plane also enables evaluation of the carpal tunnel contents.

Coronal plane

The coronal plane provides a complete view of the radiocarpal, intercarpal, and CMC joints, including the joint space widths. This is especially useful when evaluating Kienbock disease. It is also helpful when it is necessary to measure and quantify the degree of depression or displacement of fracture fragments of the distal radius, especially along the articular surface (**Figures 3.12 and 3.13**).

Sagittal plane

A sagittal plane scan enables the physician to see depression and displacement of distal radius fracture fragments in this plane. It is

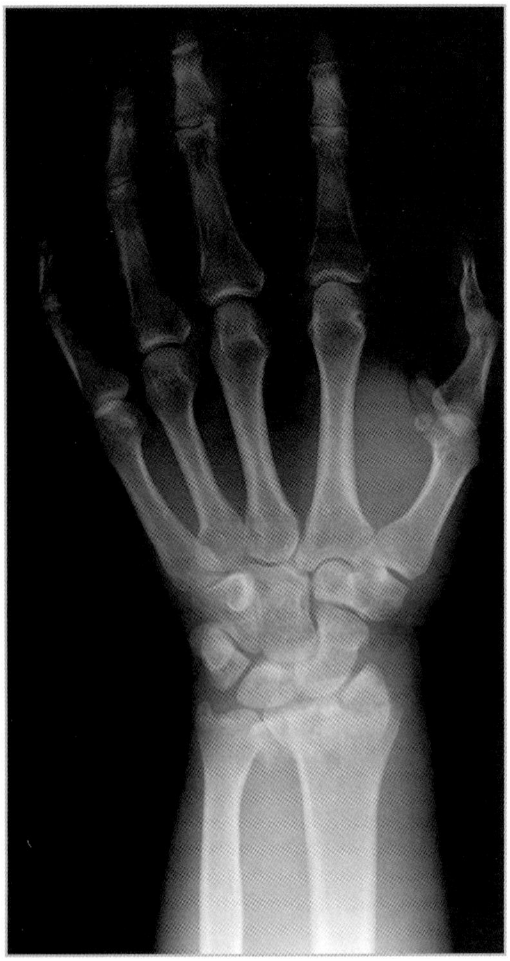

Figure 3.12 Intra-articular distal radius fracture with obvious comminution, difficult to adequately assess in X-ray.

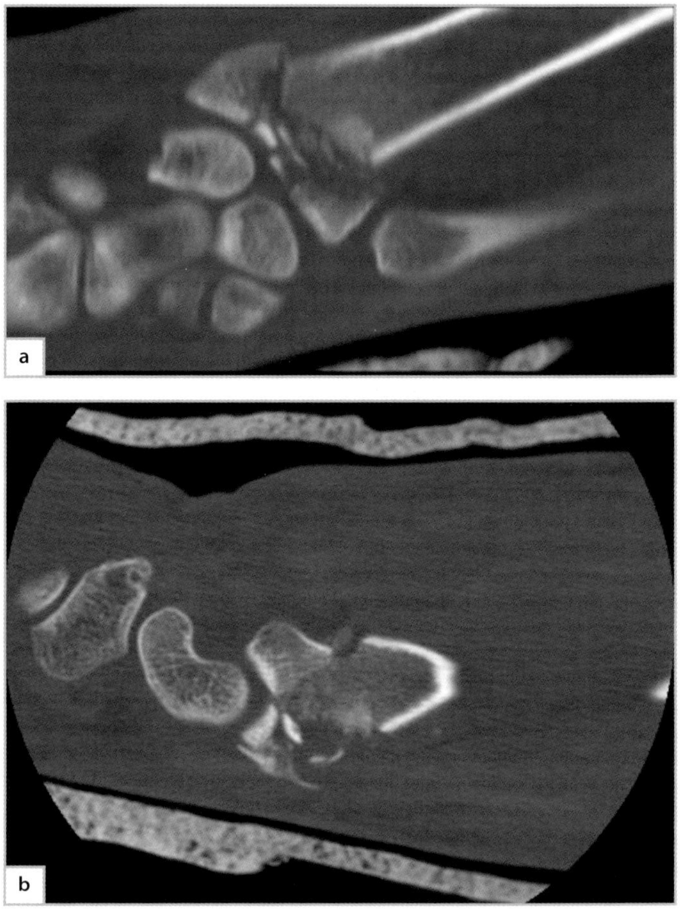

Figure 3.13 Coronal and sagittal computed tomography scan views of the distal radius fracture seen in Figure 3.12, with substantial improvement in clarity and detail of the fracture fragments and displacement.

also useful to identify DISI, VISI, palmar, or dorsal displacement of the carpus. In addition, this scan provides additional structural details for lunate and perilunate fractures and dislocations.

Long sagittal axis of scaphoid plane

Designed to evaluate scaphoid:

- Fracture fragments
- Fracture healing or nonunion
- Status of grafted bone
- Other scaphoid pathology

Three-dimensional CT

A three-dimensional CT scan enables the physician to evaluate the amount of radiocarpal and midcarpal motion in the flexion-extension plane in both stable and unstable rheumatoid wrists. This scan is also useful to identify intra-articular distal radius fracture patterns. Additionally, it provides excellent visualization of carpal bone structure and can aid in the preoperative planning for scaphoid reconstruction.

Scaphoid fracture

CT scans provide information about the architecture or displacement of a scaphoid fracture to guide treatment and provide information about healing. Sagittal images parallel to the long axis of the scaphoid are best for visualizing scaphoid fractures. Increased radiodensity of the proximal pole and absence of any converging trabeculae between fracture fragments in the preoperative CT is predictive of avascular necrosis (AVN) and fracture nonunion. For triage of nondisplaced scaphoid fractures, CT should be used with caution as false-positive results can occur.

Distal radioulnar intra-articular fracture and instability

A CT scan is more reliable for quantifying articular step and gap displacement at the radiocarpal joint, especially for a sigmoid notch fracture. A CT scan is also used (with numerous methods having been described) for quantifying DRUJ subluxation.

MAGNETIC RESONANCE IMAGING

MRI is the best modality to assess ligaments and other soft tissues, joints, lesions, masses, and inflammatory processes, providing images in the axial, coronal, and sagittal planes. Imaging in the axial plane is used to evaluate longitudinal structures such as tendons, nerves, and vessels **(Figure 3.14)**. In addition, the stability of the DRUJ can be evaluated in the axial plane. The volar intrinsic and extrinsic carpal ligaments, as well as triangular fibrocartilage (TFCC) components, can be visualized in the coronal plane. Both the coronal plane and sagittal plane are useful for assessing the integrity and pathoanatomy of the ligaments and TFCC.

MRI pulse sequences

The most frequently employed pulse sequences include T1-weighted, T2-weighted, and short tau inversion recovery (STIR).

- T1-weighted images show bone marrow and subcutaneous fat as bright areas, and can provide some detailed imaging of bony structures (although skeletal imaging is far less detailed than that obtained with CT scans)
- The T2-weighted images show fluid as bright areas against the low-intensity gray images of bone, muscle and other tissues, and dark images of fat. By accentuating the presence of abnormal fluid, the MRI can identify synovitis, edema, or other inflammatory processes
  - Fat-suppressed 'turbo' T2 images identify pus and subacute hematomas
  - Ganglion cysts appear as well-defined high signal intensity areas on a T2 image
- STIR images suppress fat and highlight abnormal lesions or fluid collections

Pathology

Ligamentous perforations or tears appear as a discontinuity in the normal signal intensity of the intact ligaments **(Figure 3.15)**

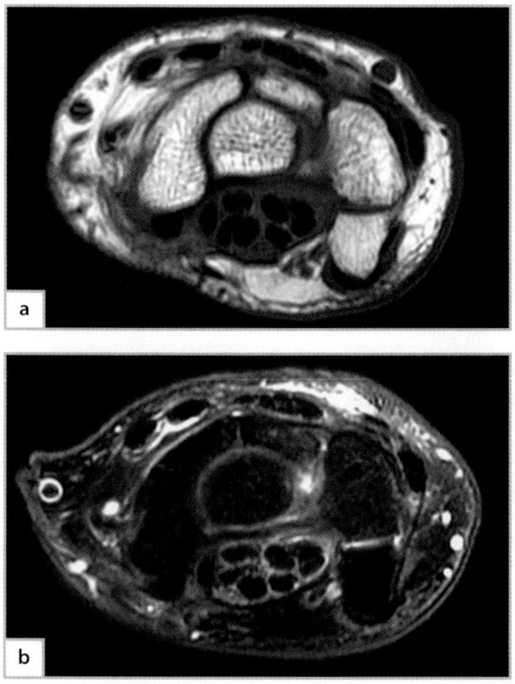

Figure 3.14 Normal magnetic resonance imaging of the wrist, axial plane T1 and T2 weighted, at the level of the carpal tunnel.

TFCC injury

MRI is accurate in identifying certain injuries, including those to the radial attachments and discs of the TFCC. There is also a high incidence of TFCC abnormalities identified in asymptomatic subjects, particularly those over the age of 50.

Scaphoid nonunion (Figure 3.16)

MRI can assess the vascularity of the proximal pole of a fractured scaphoid. Decreased intensity of the proximal fragment of the scaphoid on a T1 image may indicate AVN.

Arthrography

This technique was historically considered to be the standard for assessing carpal ligament injuries, but has now largely been replaced by diagnostic arthroscopy and MRI. Along with high-resolution CT or MRI, arthrography can be used to assess the structural integrity of cartilage and ligaments. For the arthrography technique, the wrist joint is divided in to three major compartments and four minor compartments:

- Normally there is no communication between compartments, with the exception of communication between the midcarpal joint and the common CMC and the second to fifth intermetacarpal joints
- Contrast medium is injected, and dye flow between compartments indicates a tear
  - A negative study helps exclude major ligamentous injury
- Asymptomatic degenerative tears of carpal ligaments are frequent confounders, especially in older adults

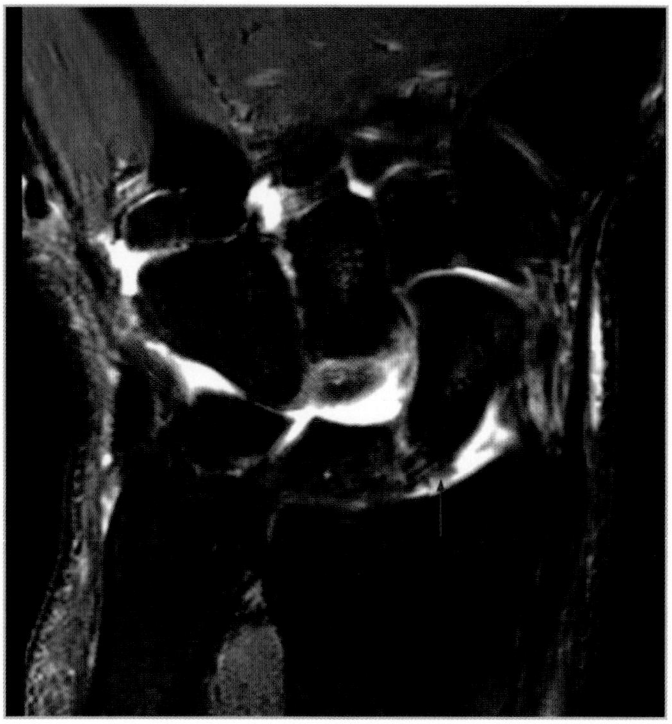

Figure 3.15 T2 magnetic resonance imaging (MRI) view of scapholunate ligament injury (blue arrow) and associated edema in surrounding intercarpal spaces (this MRI is for the same patient with DISI deformity on X-ray in Figure 3.8).

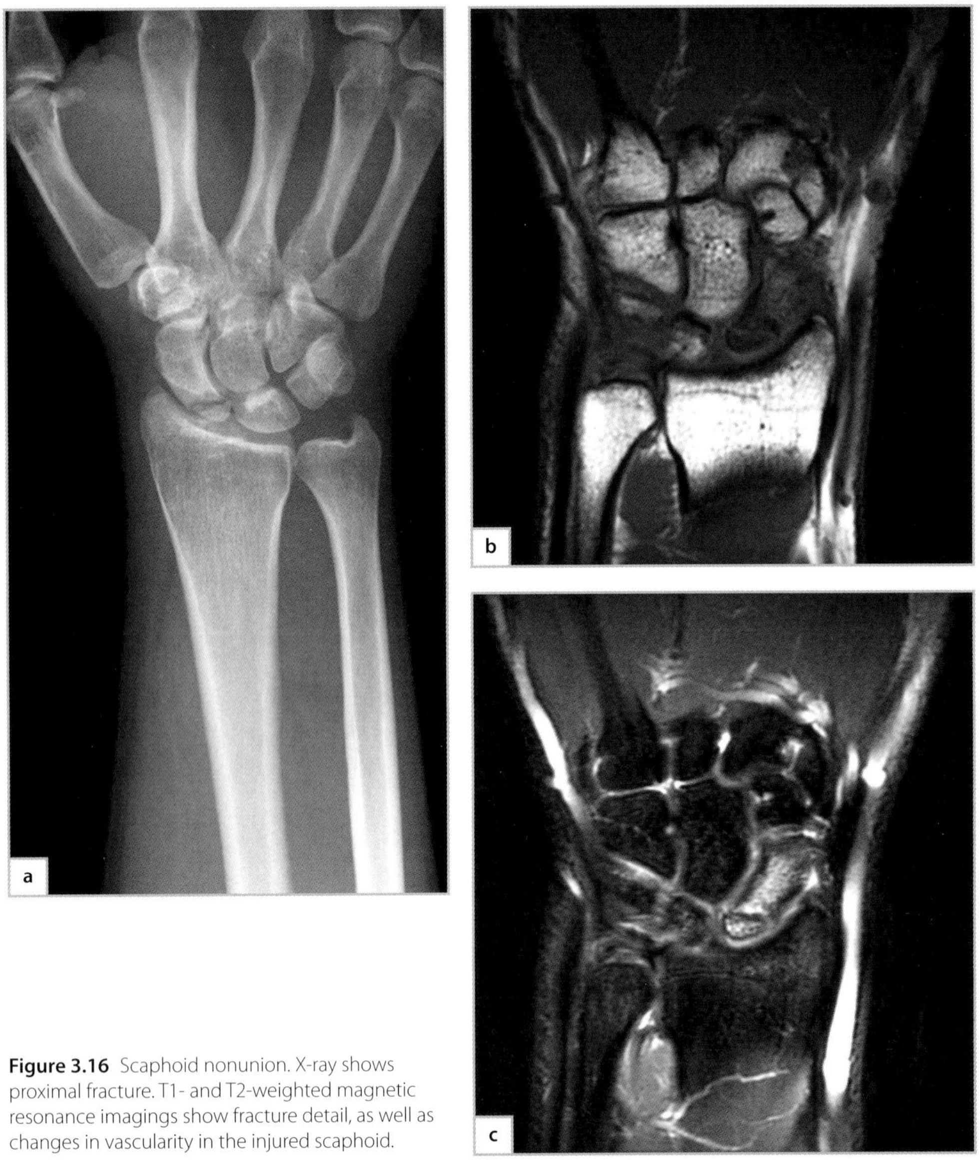

Figure 3.16 Scaphoid nonunion. X-ray shows proximal fracture. T1- and T2-weighted magnetic resonance imagings show fracture detail, as well as changes in vascularity in the injured scaphoid.

Bone scintigraphy

Three-phase technetium 99m bone scanning (TPBS) is a very sensitive technique, but has poor specificity. Despite this drawback, it is helpful to rule out fractures that are difficult to see on standard X-ray images. Three-phases are observed:

- Radionuclide angiogram phase:
  - Radial and ulnar arteries are first visualized on the 5- to 10-second image
  - Then palmar arch blush and early digital perfusion are seen
  - The venous system can be seen on the 15- to 20-second image
- Blood pool or tissue phase:
  - Usually 5–8 minutes later
  - The isotope is mixed into the whole blood pool
  - Distribution of the tracer reflects relative tissue vascularity
- Third phase:
  - A standard bone scan phase
  - Can evaluate radiotracer uptake in bony structures
  - Obtained 3–4 hours after the injection

Fractures have increased uptake within 24 hours after injury, and a negative scan 48 hours or more after injury can exclude a fracture or other significant bony lesions. Focal uptake can also indicate an area of arthritis, whereas diffuse uptake may indicate synovitis. Additionally, bony metastases, osteomyelitis, and inflammatory diseases may be localized by TPBS.

Angiography

Angiography provides a high level of anatomic detail of the vasculature of the hand. Please see Chapter 24 for a thorough review of this technique.

SUGGESTED READING

Horng YS, Chang HC, Lin KE, et al. Accuracy of ultrasonography and magnetic resonance imaging in diagnosing carpal tunnel syndrome using rest and grasp positions of the hands. J Hand Surg 2012; 37:1591–1598.
This paper indicates that by measuring the bowing of the flexor retinaculum in the grasp position, the accuracy of MRI and ultrasound for diagnosing carpal tunnel syndrome can be improved. Techniques for using ultrasonography as a screening method are also described.

Iida A, Omokawa S, Akahane M, et al. Distal radioulnar joint stress radiography for detecting radioulnar ligament injury. J Hand Surg 2012; 37:968–974.
This paper analyzes the use of clenched-fist stress radiographs for evaluation of radioulnar ligament injuries. It concludes that the DRUJ gap distance observed with clenched-fist PA radiography is a reliable parameter, and may be useful for evaluating DRUJ instability.

Lawand A, Foulkes GD. The "clenched pencil" view: a modified clenched fist scapholunate stress view. J Hand Surg 2003; 28:414–418; discussion 9–20.
This paper decribes using the clenched pencil view to investigate scapholunate dissociation. This view combines the dynamic stress of the clenched-fist view with a more optimal standardized and reproducible pronation angle.

Smith ML, Bain GI, Chabrel N, et al. Using computed tomography to assist with diagnosis of avascular necrosis complicating chronic scaphoid nonunion. J Hand Surg 2009; 34:1037–1043.
This paper indicates that the preoperative longitudinal CT of a scaphoid nonunion is of great value in identifying avascular necrosis and predicting subsequent complications. It also describes a new technique of measuring the positon of a scaphoid fracture.

Wolf JM, Oren TW, Ferguson B, et al. The carpometacarpal stress view radiograph in the evaluation of trapeziometacarpal joint laxity. J Hand Surg 2009; 34:1402–1406.
This paper introduces a modified thumb CMC stress view radiograph, useful to evaluate laxity and joint abnormalities at the trapeziometacarpal articulation.

Chapter 4 Electrodiagnostic studies and peripheral nerve ultrasound

Kay WP. Ng, Aravinda K. Therimadasamy, Li Sihui Eileen, Einar P. Wilder-Smith

Nerve conduction studies (NCS) and needle electromyography (EMG) are investigations used to assess patients with neuromuscular conditions. These investigations are valuable in peripheral nervous system (PNS) disorders because they help in

- Localizing the lesion
- Determining underlying pathophysiology
- Following the temporal course
- Assessing severity and prognosis

Ultrasound (US) and magnetic resonance imaging (MRI) are also increasingly used to assess the PNS. These tools are useful to

- Provide supportive evidence of clinical diagnosis
  - E.g. focal nerve enlargement in nerve entrapment
- Help in precise localization of nerve and nerve lesions
- Detect anatomic variations prior to surgical intervention
- Suggest etiology
  - E.g. ganglion, neuroma, and luxation
- Provide information on surrounding structures
  - E.g. muscle, tendon, ligaments, and artery
- Provide information on blood flow to the nerve
  - E.g. to detect inflammation
- Help in guided intervention
  - E.g. nerve blocks

ANATOMY OF THE PNS

The PNS includes the motor, the sensory, and the autonomic systems. The sensory and motor roots combine to form a mixed spinal nerve (**Figure 4.1**). The mixed spinal nerve then divides to form the dorsal and the ventral ramus. The dorsal rami supply the paraspinal muscles, and sensation to the overlying skin. The ventral rami continue as the intercostal nerves in the thoracic region, and in all other regions the ventral rami fuse to form a plexus. The brachial plexus is formed by the ventral rami of the C_5-T_1 roots, whereas the lumbosacral plexus is formed by the ventral rami of the L_4-S_1 roots. Peripheral nerves arise from the plexus to supply different muscles and areas of sensation. These areas can be classified as

- Myotomes (all muscles innervated by individual nerve roots)
- Dermatomes (areas of cutaneous innervation by individual nerve roots)

The autonomic system (sympathetic and parasympathetic) is not under voluntary control. Sympathetic preganglionic cell bodies lie in the lateral horns of the spinal segments T_1-L_2 where these fibers travel a short distance in the mixed spinal nerve. They then exit to enter the sympathetic ganglionic chains that lie paravertebrally from the cervical to sacral region. The parasympathetic preganglionic cell bodies lie in the brain stem in the motor nuclei of cranial nerves III, VII, IX and X, and in the sacral segments of the spinal cord (S_2-S_4), spreading out fibers that synapse near the innervated organ.

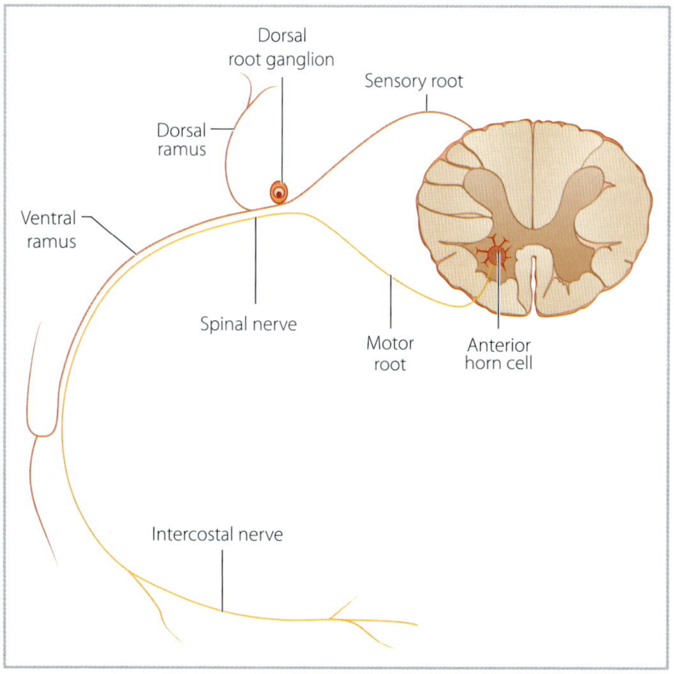

Figure 4.1 The sensory root leaves the cord dorsally, whereas the motor root arises from the anterior horn cells and leaves the cord ventrally. Both combine to form a mixed spinal nerve, which divide to form the dorsal and ventral ramus. The dorsal rami supply the paraspinal muscles, while the ventral rami continue as either intercostal nerves, or fuse to form the brachial or lumbosacral plexus.

PHYSIOLOGY

Each axon has a resting membrane potential (threshold). The membrane is negatively charged internally compared with externally, due to membrane properties and the Na^+/K^+ pump, leading to higher sodium concentrations outside of the membrane. When a current passes through the axon, the axon becomes more positive internally (depolarization) via opening of voltage-gated sodium channels that line the membrane, allowing sodium influx, creating an action potential. Sodium channels are then inactivated, and the threshold re-established.

Propagation of this action potential is very slow without the presence of myelin and the nodes of Ranvier. Conduction velocity is increased substantially by saltatory conduction, which involves action potentials jumping from node to node (**Figure 4.2a**). When the nerve action potential reaches the presynaptic side of the neuromuscular junction, voltage-gated calcium channels open, allowing calcium to enter and triggering the release of acetylcholine across the synapse. Acetylcholine then binds to receptors on the muscle membrane, allowing sodium to enter and depolarizing the muscle fiber. The motor axon, its anterior horn cell, and all of the connecting muscle fibers form a motor unit. A motor unit action potential (MUAP) is created when all of the muscle fibers of one motor unit are depolarized (**Figure 4.2b**). NCS measure mainly the large diameter fibers that have the most myelin, and hence the fastest conduction velocities. Needle EMG studies, on the other hand, analyze the MUAPs.

NERVE CONDUCTION STUDIES

A depolarizing electrical impulse is applied to the skin to stimulate the underlying peripheral nerve, and an electrode records the resultant action potential. NCS may be used for motor, sensory, or mixed nerves.

Motor NCS

The recording electrode is placed over a distal muscle, recording the summation of the individual activated muscle fiber action potentials as a compound muscle action potential (CMAP). The parameters studied in a motor NCS (**Figure 4.3a**) have been summarized in **Table 4.1**.

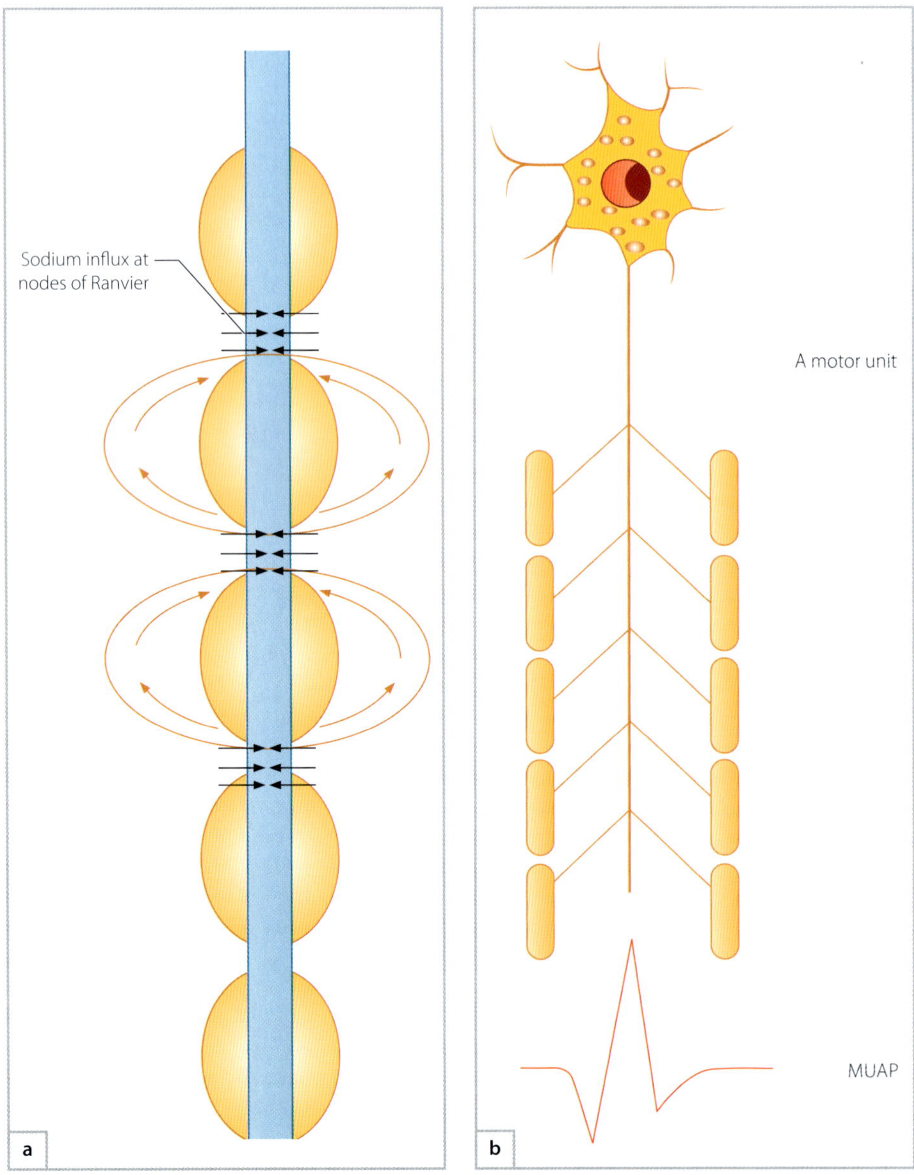

Figure 4.2 (a) Action potentials are created at the unmyelinated areas of the nerve (nodes of Ranvier), and jump over the myelinated portions from node to node, thus increasing conduction velocity. (b) A motor unit action potential is created when all the muscle fibers of one motor unit are depolarized.

Table 4.1 Parameters studied in a motor NCS

Parameter	Description	Significance
dML	Time from the most distal stimulus to initial CMAP deflection from the baseline	Time taken for fastest nerve fibers to conduct. Includes time for neuromuscular transmission and muscle depolarization and activation
Amplitude	From baseline to 'negative' peak (by convention, the upward deflection)	Number of muscle fibers that depolarize, representing the number of conducting axons
Duration	From initial deflection from baseline to first baseline crossing	Extent of synchrony of muscle fiber activation
CV	Calculated by distance between two stimulation sites/difference in latencies between both sites (hence excludes neuromuscular transmission and muscle activation time)	Speed of the fastest conducting motor axons

NCS, nerve conduction studies; dML, distal motor latency; CV, conduction velocity; CMAP, compound muscle action potential.

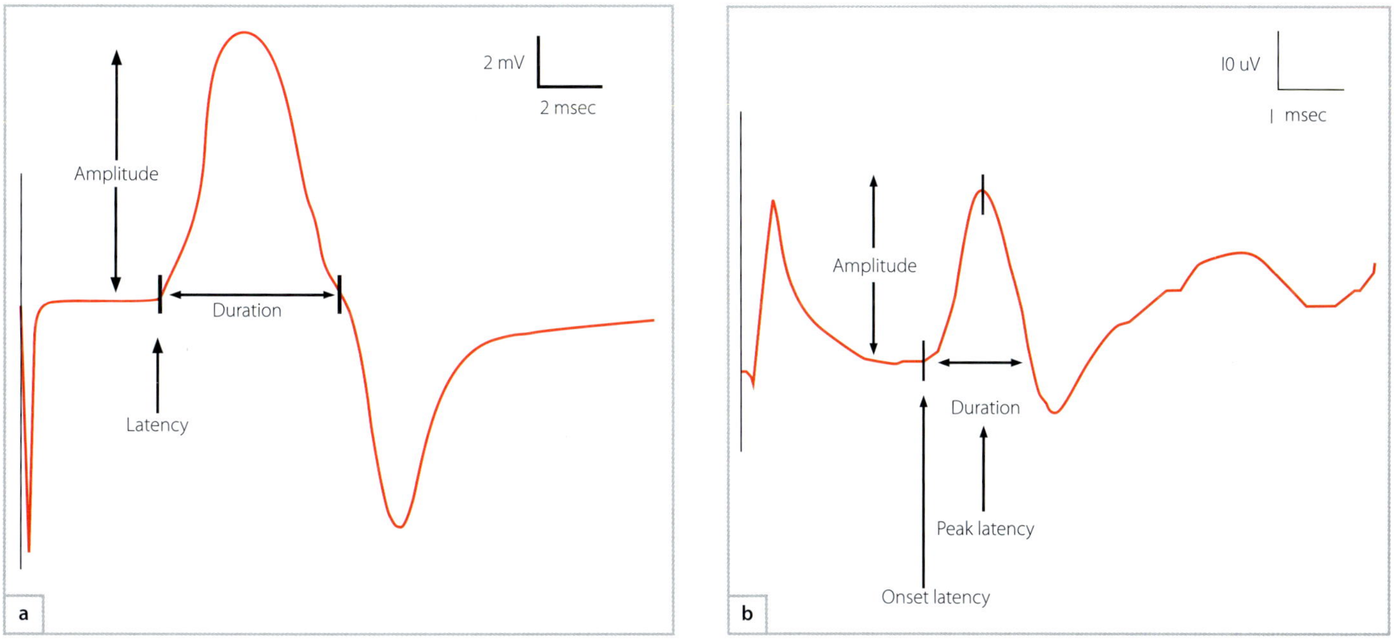

Figure 4.3 (a) Schematic of a compound muscle action potential (CMAP) – Latency (msec): time from stimulus to initial upward deflection of CMAP from baseline. Amplitude (mV): from baseline to peak. Duration (msec): from initial deflection to first baseline crossing. (b) Schematic of a sensory nerve action potential: Peak latency (msec): time from stimulus to first upward peak. Amplitude (µV): from negative peak to positive peak. Duration (msec): from initial baseline deflection to first baseline crossing.

Sensory NCS

Sensory fibers are stimulated and the sensory nerve action potential (SNAP) is recorded with the recording electrode placed either proximally (or orthodromic – direction in which physiologic sensory conduction occurs) or distally (or antidromic – in the reverse direction) to stimulus. The parameters studied in a sensory NCS (**Figure 4.3b**) have been summarized in **Table 4.2**.

Mixed NCS

A mixed nerve action potential (MNAP) reflects the summation of both motor and sensory nerve fiber action potentials. This study assesses the largest and fastest fibers that are the sensory muscle afferents supplying the muscle spindles. For example, MNAP can be used to test the stimulation of the ulnar nerve before the cubital tunnel with a measurement of the nerve potential after the cubital tunnel.

F waves

An action potential is propagated in both directions from the site of stimulus of a motor axon. The proximal impulse conducts to the anterior horn cell, depolarizes the axon hillock, and returns to create a late muscle depolarization (F wave). It is useful in the testing of proximal segments of nerves, is a sensitive indicator of pathology, and tests longer segments of nerves.

Parameters affecting NCS

They include

- Temperature: conduction velocity is slower in lower temperatures
- Age: conduction velocity is slower with increasing age
- Limb length: conduction velocity is slower with increasing length

Table 4.2 Parameters studied in sensory NCS

Parameter	Description	Significance
Peak latency	Time from stimulus to midpoint of first negative peak	Nerve conduction time from stimulus to recording electrodes. Peak latencies preferred over onset latencies as peak more easily identified in sensory studies, due to small amplitudes
Amplitude	From first negative peak to next positive peak	Number of depolarized sensory fibers
Duration	From initial deflection from baseline to first baseline crossing	Extent of synchrony of firing individual fibers (larger fibers conduct faster than smaller ones)
CV	Distance divided by latency	Velocity of 20% largest diameter and fastest conducting fibers that mainly convey fine touch, vibration, proprioception

NCS, nerve conduction studies; CV, conduction velocity.

Interpretation of NCS

Laboratory-specific age-matched 'normal' values are available. The aim of NCS is to determine if the nerve pathology is focal or generalized and if it is axonal or demyelinating. An entrapment neuropathy, e.g. ulnar neuropathy at the elbow from a focal neuropraxia, resulting in demyelination, has a better prognosis than if axonal loss has occurred. The NCS characteristics of axonal and demyelinating lesions have been summarized in **Table 4.3**.

ELECTROMYOGRAPHY

This involves insertion of a needle electrode into muscles selected by an electromyographer based on history and physical examination. This study is used to analyze spontaneous activity (electrical discharge while the muscle is at rest) and MUAPs (when the patient contracts the muscle). The common spontaneous activity and MUAP have been summarized in **Tables 4.4** and **4.5,** respectively.

Table 4.3 NCS characteristics of axonal and demyelinating lesions

Study	Axonal loss	Demyelinating	Apparently normal despite pathology present
Motor studies	Reduced amplitudes Near-normal CV and dML	Reduced CV Prolonged dML Variable amplitude changes Temporal dispersion† Conduction block‡	Hyperacute axonal lesions, e.g. acute nerve transections*
Sensory studies	Reduced amplitudes Near-normal CV and dML	Reduced CV Prolonged dML More prominent temporal dispersion and conduction block	1. Lesion is proximal to the dorsal root ganglion, e.g. radiculopathies 2. Affects only small, unmyelinated, slower conducting fibers

*Stimulating distal to the lesion before Wallerian degeneration has occurred (3–10 days) can yield normal results.

†Temporal dispersion is due to phase cancellation, and is more prominent in sensory nerve action potentials **(Figure 4-4a)**.

‡Where there is conduction failure in some or all of the motor axons, the compound muscle action potential (CMAP) from a proximal stimulation has a reduced amplitude and area compared with the CMAP recorded from a stimulus distal to the lesion. This is called conduction block (more than 50% reduction, without more than 20% increase in duration) **(Figure 4-4b)**.

NCS, nerve conduction studies; dML, distal motor latency; CV, conduction velocity.

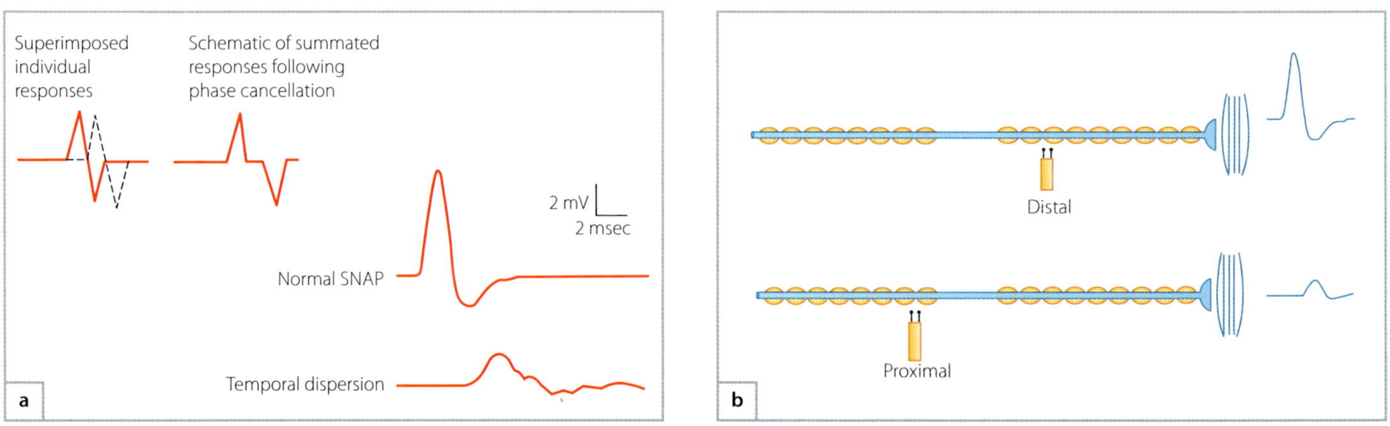

Figure 4.4 (a) In each nerve, fibers conduct at varying speeds, some slower, some faster. With proximal stimulation, as the slower fibers lag further behind the faster fibers, the resulting action potentials created cancel each other out (phase cancellation), resulting in decreased amplitude and increased duration (temporal dispersion). (b) When stimulated across an area of demyelination, the compound muscle action potential (CMAP) of the distal stimulation is normal, whereas the CMAP of the proximal stimulation has reduced amplitude and area due to failure of axonal conduction (conduction block).

Table 4.4 Common abnormal spontaneous activity

Terminology	Description	Significance
Increased insertional activity	Waveforms resulting from needle movement in the muscle that last >300 ms due to depolarization of muscle fibers	Neuropathic disorders Myopathic (mainly inflammatory) disorders
Fibrillation potentials	Spontaneous depolarization of single muscle fibers	Active denervation in neuropathic disorders (3 weeks–3 months post-injury) Inflammatory myopathies/dystrophies
Positive sharp waves	Spontaneous depolarization of single muscle fibers	Active denervation in neuropathic disorders (3 weeks–3 months post-injury) Inflammatory myopathies/dystrophies
Complex repetitive discharges	Depolarization of single muscle fiber with spread to adjacent denervated fibers	Chronic neuropathic and myopathic disorders
Myotonic discharges	Depolarization of muscle fiber but with waxing and waning of amplitude and frequency	Myotonic dystrophy Myotonia congenita Paramyotonia congenita Myopathies (acid maltase deficiency), polymyositis, and myotubular myopathy Hyperkalemic periodic paralysis
Fasciculations	Spontaneous depolarization of individual motor unit	Amyotrophic lateral sclerosis Radiculopathies Polyneuropathies Entrapment neuropathies Benign fasciculations
Myokymia	Grouped spontaneous repetitive discharges of same motor unit	Radiation injury Hypocalcemia Nerve entrapments Radiculopathy

Table 4.5 Common MUAP terminology

Terminology	Description	Significance
Polyphasic	Increased number of baseline crossings of the MUAP	Neuropathic or myopathic disorders
Satellite potentials	Time-locked potential trailing main MUAP	Early reinnervation*
Recruitment	Addition of more motor units with increasing firing rate (normal ratio of 5:1 for firing frequency: number of firing motor units)	Reduced in neuropathic disorders and end-stage myopathies

*By collateral sprouting from adjacent intact motor units.
MUAP, motor unit action potential.

Interpretation of EMG

The EMG provides information that helps in differentiating between neuropathic versus myopathic disorders, localization of a lesion, determining axonal or demyelinating pathology, chronicity, and presence of re-innervation. In a neuropathic disorder (**Figure 4.5**), the recruitment is reduced (due to loss of MUAPs from axonal loss or conduction block). It may be preserved, if demyelination affects only conduction velocity and the number of MUAPs are preserved. Additionally, there is increased fast-firing of MUAPs (reduced number of MUAPs fire at increased rate to exert same force) and altered MUAP morphology in reinnervation (adjacent intact motor units produce collateral sprouts to denervated muscle fibers, leading to fewer, larger motor units). The EMG differentiation between axonal and demyelinating disorders based on chronicity has been summarized in **Table 4.6**.

ELECTROPHYSIOLOGIC FINDINGS (NCS AND EMG)

The electrophysiologic findings in some common upper limb conditions have been summarized below. In all of these conditions, neurophysiology allows localization of the lesion and helps exclude other PNS disorders mimicking the clinical syndrome. It is important to consider the timing from onset of symptoms when interpreting the NCS and EMG findings (**Table 4.7**).

Carpal tunnel syndrome

Carpal tunnel syndrome (CTS) is diagnosed when a patient has the typical clinical symptoms and signs, associated with median nerve entrapment at the wrist. The compression at the carpal tunnel leads to local ischemia and myelin dysfunction, with resultant slowed conduction velocity (CV) and prolonged latencies on NCS, especially on sensory studies, where sensory fibers have a higher proportion of large myelinated fibers. This may be followed by axonal loss. The PNS differential diagnoses to be considered include proximal median neuropathy (e.g. at elbow), brachial plexopathy (upper trunk), cervical radiculopathy ($C_6/_7$), and polyneuropathy. The NCS findings (**Figure 4.6a** and **4.6b**) in CTS include

- Prolonged sensory and motor latencies
- Slow CVs
- Amplitudes decreased if axonal loss or conduction block present
- Prolonged median F wave latencies

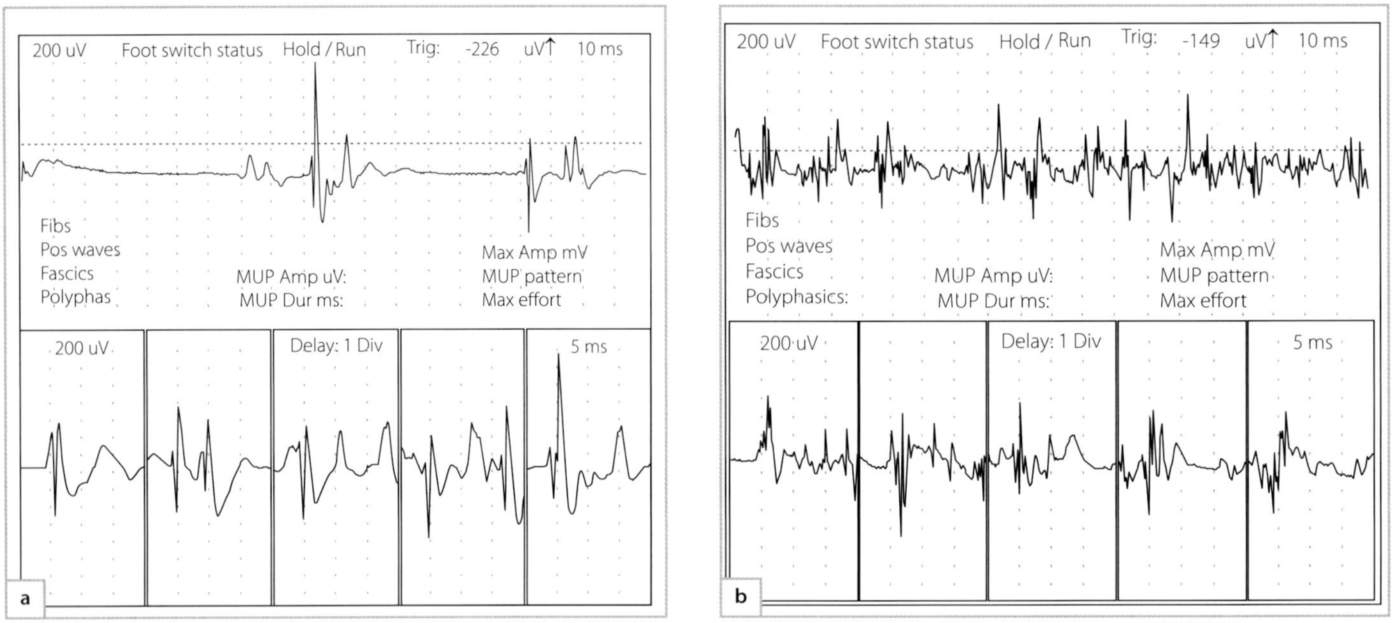

Figure 4.5 (a) Decreased recruitment of motor unit action potentials (MUAPs) due to a neurogenic condition, such as acute nerve damage or neuropraxia. (b) Increased recruitment of MUAPs due to a muscle disease such as myopathy.

Table 4.6 EMG differentiation between axonal and demyelinating disorders

Temporal relationship	Axonal	Demyelinating
Acute	Normal morphology Reduced recruitment Fibrillations, positive sharp waves	Normal morphology (±reduced recruitment)
Chronic with reinnervation	Increased MUAP duration Increased MUAP amplitude Polyphasic Reduced recruitment Satellite potentials Nil spontaneous activity, or complex repetitive discharges	Normal morphology (±reduced recruitment)

MUAP, motor unit action potential; EMG, electromyography.

Table 4.7 The effect of timing on interpretation of electrophysiologic studies

Post-injury/symptoms onset days	Pathological impact on electrophysiologic studies	Interpretation/action
1–10	Wallerian degeneration is still not yet established: be aware that NCS and EMG may be normal	Consider repeat studies, or delaying study till a more suitable time
11–14	Wallerian degeneration established – NCS may be abnormal, or still normal depending on fascicular susceptibility EMG may not show evidence of acute denervation activity, i.e. spontaneous activity of positive sharp waves and fibrillations	May have to repeat studies for conclusive localization
>14	Sufficient time evolved for NCS and EMG abnormalities to manifest	Most accurate information for diagnosis and prognosis

NCS, nerve conduction studies; EMG, electromyography.

- Normal ulnar studies, lateral, and medial antebrachial cutaneous nerve SNAPs, otherwise consider differentials

Additional NCS studies that may be considered in CTS include

- Comparison of median nerve with another nerve – usually median-versus-ulnar comparison
  - Compares the difference in latencies with the recording electrodes equidistant from the stimulating electrodes for both median and ulnar nerves
  - E.g. 2L-INT study (records at the 2nd lumbrical (2L) on stimulating the median nerve, compared with the recording at the interossei (INT) on stimulating the ulnar nerve) (**Figure 4.6c**)
- Inching studies (**Figure 4.6d**)
  - Motor or sensory inching across the wrist at 1-cm intervals to look for an abrupt change in latency or amplitude

The EMG findings in CTS include

- Denervation changes in the abductor pollicis brevis (APB) in more severe cases

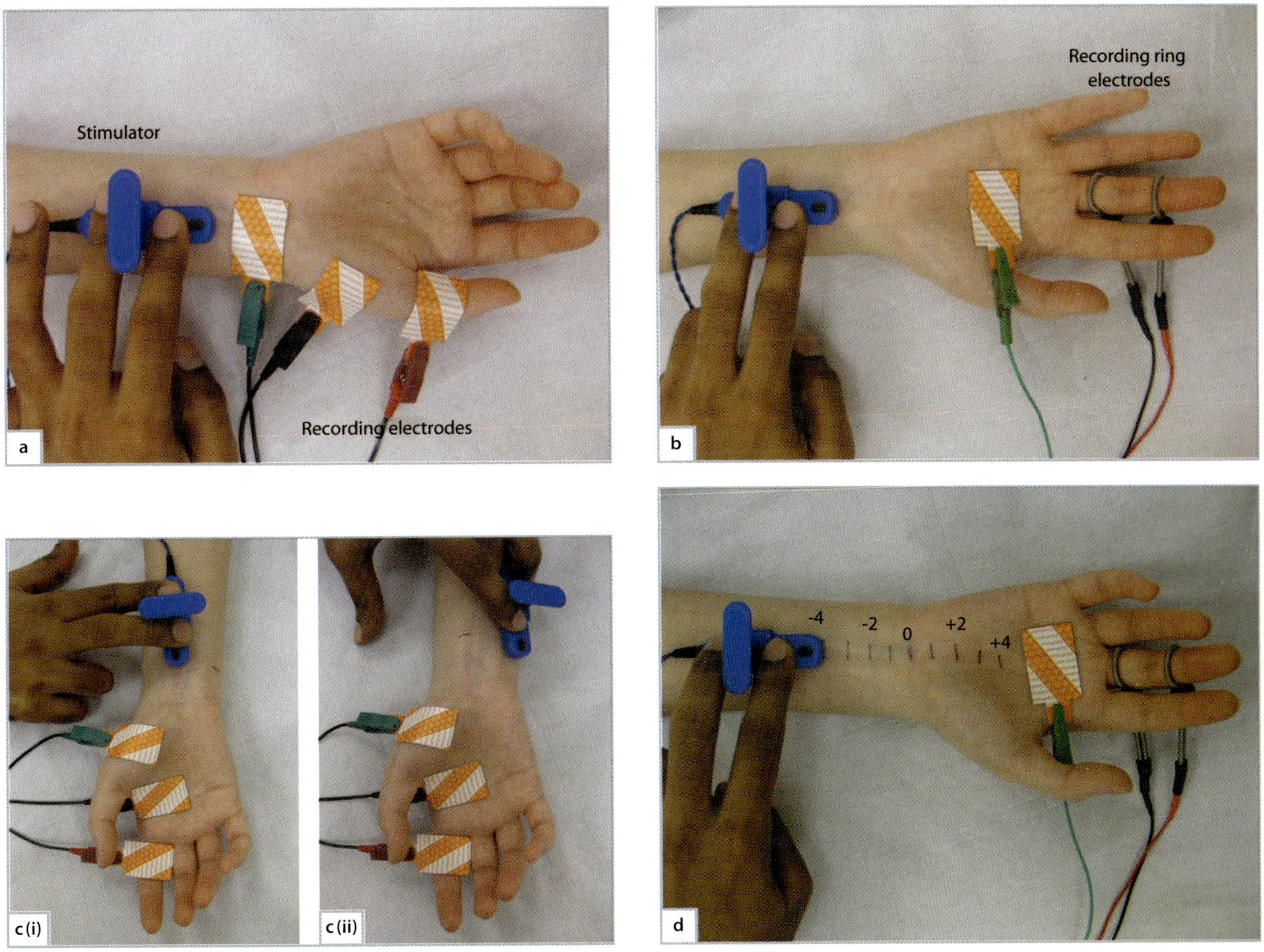

Figure 4.6 (a) Median motor study for carpal tunnel syndrome, stimulating median nerve at wrist, recording electrode over abductor pollicis brevis. (b) Median sensory antidromic study, stimulating over median nerve, recording over middle finger. (c) 2L-INT study, comparing the latencies of (i) (stimulating the median nerve, recording over the 2nd lumbrical, '2L') versus (ii) (stimulating the ulnar nerve, recording over the interossei, 'INT'). (d) Inching studies, stimulating the median nerve at 1 cm intervals looking for an abrupt change in latency or amplitude from the sensory nerve action potential recorded at the middle finger.

- Normal studies in muscles supplied by the median nerve more proximally [flexor carpi radialis (FCR) and pronator teres (PT)]
- Normal studies in C_6/C_7-innervated muscles (PT, triceps, extensor digitorum communis, paraspinal muscles)
- Normal studies in C_8/T_1-innervated muscles [first dorsal interosseous (FDI), extensor indicis pollicis (EIP), paraspinal muscles]

A 7-point scale based on NCS and EMG findings by Bland has been proposed for grading CTS severity. A simplified version is in **Table 4.8**. This scale has been found to correlate with surgical outcomes.

Ulnar neuropathy at the elbow

It is a result of compression or mechanical forces on the ulnar nerve as it passes from the arm to the forearm through the cubital tunnel. Once axonal loss has occurred, it is difficult to localize with NCS alone, and EMG studies are required. The PNS disorder differentials to be considered include ulnar neuropathy at other sites (wrist, rarely forearm), brachial plexopathy (lower trunk or medial cord), cervical radiculopathy (C_8/T_1), and polyneuropathy. The NCS is conducted with the arm in a flexed position (approximately 100°), to stretch out the nerve to its maximal length with stimulation above and below the elbow. The NCS findings in ulnar nerve neuropathy at the elbow (**Figure 4.7a** and **4.7b**) include

- Focal demyelinating lesion:
  - Conduction block: drop in amplitude of the CMAP below the elbow compared with above
  - Reduction of CV: Slowing across the elbow compared with the forearm segment
- Axonal loss: unable to localize – small CMAP amplitudes throughout

Additional NCS studies that may be considered in ulnar nerve neuropathy at the elbow include

- Recording from the FDI, which can increase diagnostic yield due to different fascicle bundles within the same nerve being affected to different degrees (differential fascicular susceptibility)
- Record dorsal cutaneous ulnar nerve SNAP: This sensory branch arises proximal to the wrist, so its absence denotes a lesion above the wrist

Table 4.8 Grading of the severity of CTS based on electrophysiologic studies

Grade	NCS findings	EMG findings
Mild	Isolated prolonged sensory latencies Normal motor studies	Normal
Moderate	Isolated prolonged sensory latencies Isolated prolonged distal motor latency	Normal
Severe (evidence of axonal loss)	Absent/low amplitude SNAP Absent/low amplitude CMAP	Fibrillations Altered MUAP morphology

CTS, carpal tunnel syndrome; NCS, nerve conduction studies; SNAP, sensory nerve action potential; MUAP, motor unit action potential; CMAP, compound muscle action potential; EMG, electromyography.

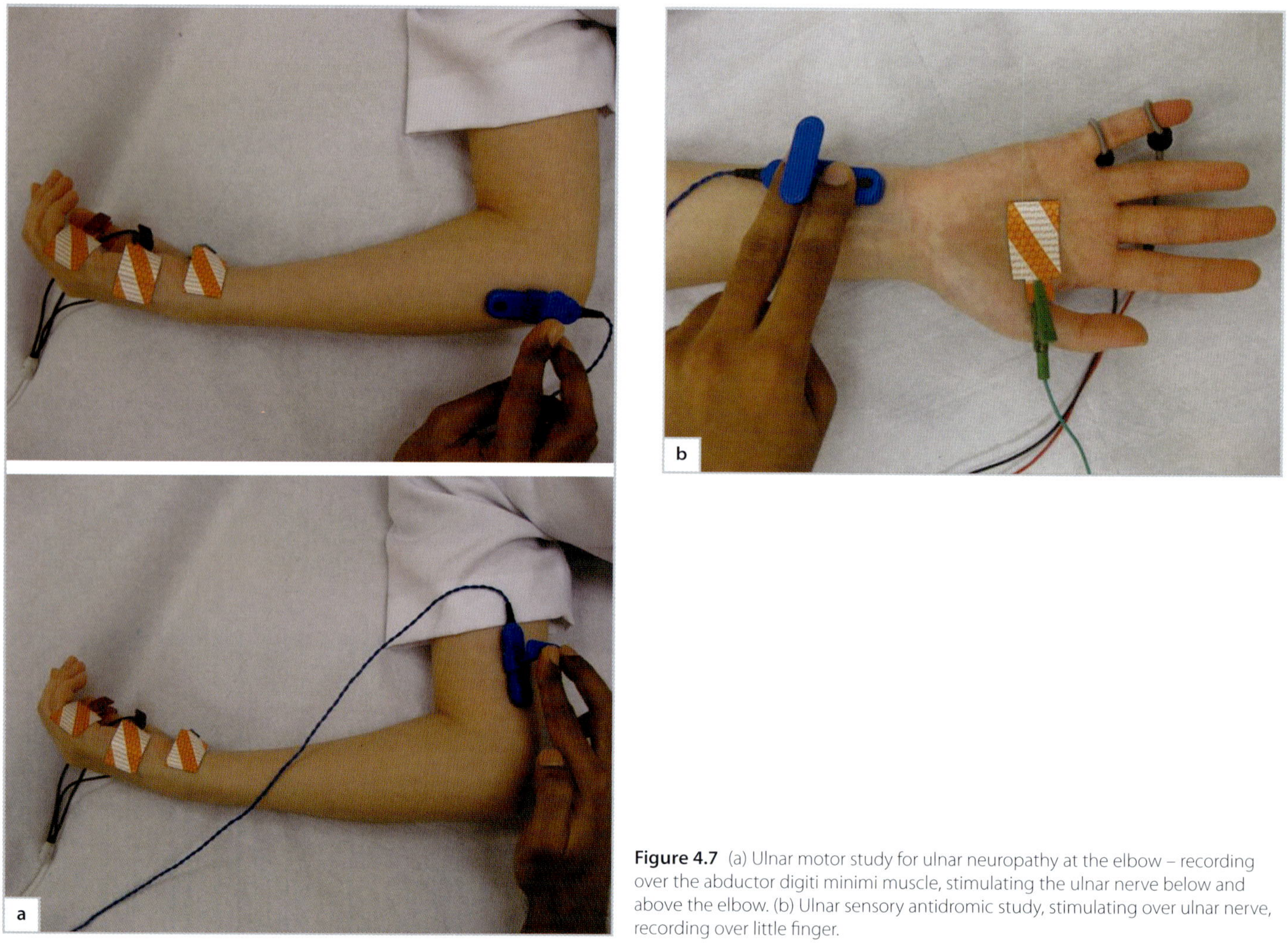

Figure 4.7 (a) Ulnar motor study for ulnar neuropathy at the elbow – recording over the abductor digiti minimi muscle, stimulating the ulnar nerve below and above the elbow. (b) Ulnar sensory antidromic study, stimulating over ulnar nerve, recording over little finger.

The EMG findings in ulnar neuropathy at the elbow include

- Abnormal study in ulnar-innervated muscles: FDI, flexor digitorum profundus to digit 4 and 5, abductor digiti minimi
  - Flexor carpi ulnaris may be normal due to differential fascicular susceptibility
- Normal C8/T1-innervated muscles: APB, flexor pollicis longus, EIP, paraspinal muscles

Radial nerve palsy at the spiral groove

It is the most common site of radial neuropathy and usually results from compression against the humerus from immobilization, e.g. arm hanging over the chair while asleep or drunk! ('Saturday night palsy'). This can also be caused by a fracture of the humerus. The PNS disorder differentials include radial neuropathy at other sites (i.e. axilla), posterior interosseous neuropathy (distal to the lateral epicondyle), brachial plexopathy (posterior cord), cervical radiculopathy ($C_7/_8$), and polyneuropathy. The radial nerve is stimulated above and below the spiral groove and recording is taken from the extensor indicis proprius. NCS findings (**Figure 4.8a** and **4.8b**) include

- Demyelinating lesion: temporal dispersion, conduction block across the spiral groove
- Axonal loss: diminished CMAP amplitudes throughout – will need EMG studies for further localization

Additional NCS studies that may be considered

- Superficial radial sensory nerve study: stimulating nerve over the radius, recording over the extensor tendons to the thumb
  - If absent: axonal loss has occurred
  - If present:
    - Wallerian degeneration has not yet occurred OR
    - Demyelinating pathology OR
    - Posterior interosseous neuropathy

The EMG findings in radial nerve palsy at the spiral groove include

- Abnormal study of muscles supplied by the posterior interosseous nerve: extensor indicis proprius, extensor carpi ulnaris, extensor digitorum communis
- Abnormal study of muscles supplied by nerve distal to the spiral groove: brachioradialis, long head of extensor carpi radialis, supinator muscle
- Normal study of muscles proximal to the spiral groove: triceps
- Normal study of posterior-cord innervated muscles: deltoid, latissimus dorsi
- Normal study of C_7-innervated muscles: FCR, PT, flexor digitorum sublimis, paraspinal muscles

PERIPHERAL NERVE US

US waves are sound waves of a high frequency (>20,000 Hz). The frequency ranges used in medical US range from 2 to 20 MHz. The increasing frequency of US transducers provides better image resolution, but with reduced penetrative ability. For imaging the PNS, US requires frequencies anywhere from 10 to 18 MHz. A generous amount of acoustic coupling gel is required to minimize artifacts from air–skin interface during this study. The advantages of US include easy accessibility, low cost, real time images, and better resolution (than MRI) of peripheral nerves. The main disadvantage is that there is poorer image resolution with deeper imaging, e.g. sciatic nerve.

US imaging technique

In US, B-mode imaging and color Doppler flow imaging are commonly used. In B-mode imaging, transverse and longitudinal images are obtained, allowing assessment of the cross-sectional area (CSA) or diameter, fascicular structure (presence of disruption),

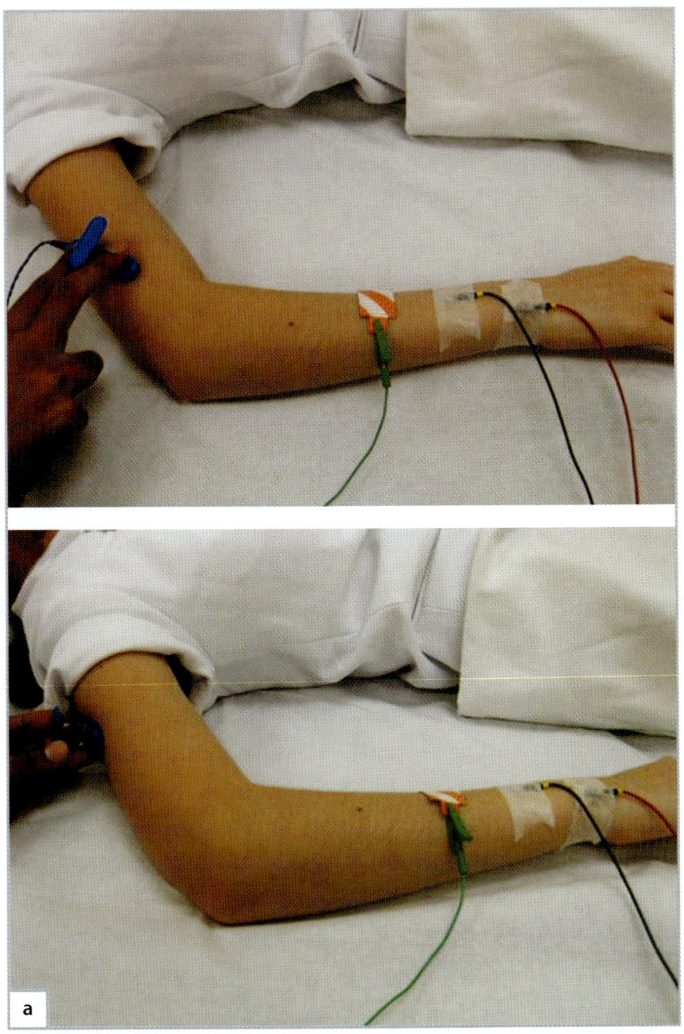

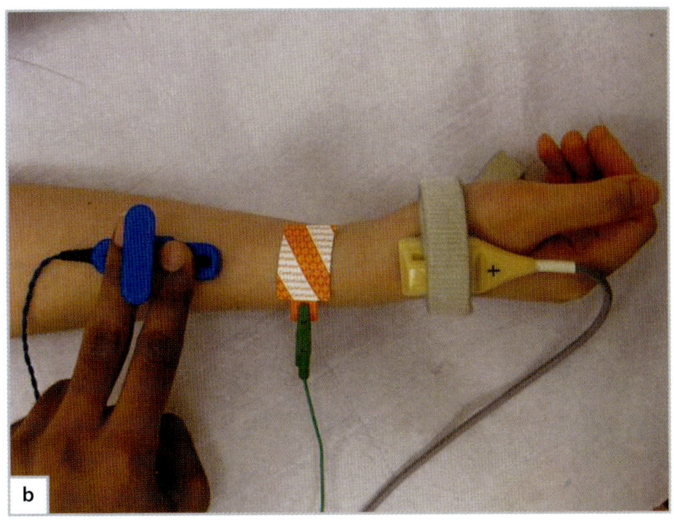

Figure 4.8 (a) Radial motor study across sulcus spiralis, stimulating below and above (b) the spiral groove, recording over extensor indicis proprius. Radial sensory study, stimulating radial nerve over the radius, recording over the radial sensory nerve that is over the thumb extensor tendons.

and echotexture (hypo/hyperintensity). In color Doppler flow imaging, blood flow to the nerve and the surrounding tissues is assessed. In general, transverse imaging is better in identifying focal swelling of nerve fascicles, whereas longitudinal imaging looks for sudden change in diameter of nerve. Doppler flow can be useful in diagnosis of entrapments, inflammatory lesions, postoperative states, and tumors. The findings are compared against the unaffected contralateral side and laboratory-specific normal values (population norms). The features of normal peripheral nerves include (**Figure 4.9a** and **4.9b**)

- More echogenicity than muscles but less so than tendons
- Honeycomb appearance (fascicular structures seen on transverse view)
- Less mobility than tendons

US findings

The US features that suggest nerve anomalies/entrapment include

- Change in CSA:
  - Just proximal to entrapment: increased CSA
  - At entrapment: nerve is flattened
- Change in echotexture:
  - Loss of fascicular discrimination due to nerve edema
- Color Doppler flow
  - Increased nerve blood flow, usually just proximal to entrapment

Carpal tunnel syndrome

US position: transverse and longitudinal scans over the wrist, with arm supinated (**Figure 4.10**).

Sonographic features:

- Enlarged nerve proximal to entrapment (cut-off of 10 mm^2 CSA)
- Loss of median nerve fascicular discrimination (**Figure 4.11**)
- Abrupt change of median nerve caliber (notch sign) (**Figure 4.12**)
- Increased intra- and perineural vascularization (**Figure 4.13**)

Additional US features:

- Detects secondary causes of CTS, e.g. tumors and ganglia
- Detects persistent median artery, which may accompany anatomical variants of median nerve, e.g. bifid nerve

Overall, sensitivity of US for CTS is 77.6%, specificity 86.8%.

Cubital tunnel syndrome

US position: arm extended, to limit traction on ulnar nerve during flexion resulting in nerve flattening in normal subjects (**Figure 4.14**). The nerve is adjacent to the medial epicondyle at level of ulnar groove.

Sonographic features (**Figure 4.15**):

- Increased CSA anywhere along ulnar nerve segment from 4 cm proximal to 4 cm distal to the medial epicondyle (cut-off of 10 mm^2 CSA)
- Thickened cubital tunnel retinaculum
- Loss of fascicular discrimination

Additional useful US features:

- Edema in surrounding soft tissue
- Luxation or subluxation of nerve: during elbow flexion, the ulnar nerve either moves to the tip of the medial epicondyle (subluxation); or over the epicondyle (luxation). This recurrent movement results in wear and tear to the nerve causing ulnar neuropathy at the elbow. Presence of luxation/subluxation affects surgical approach. Note that subluxation or luxation also occurs in healthy controls, so this finding needs clinical interpretation

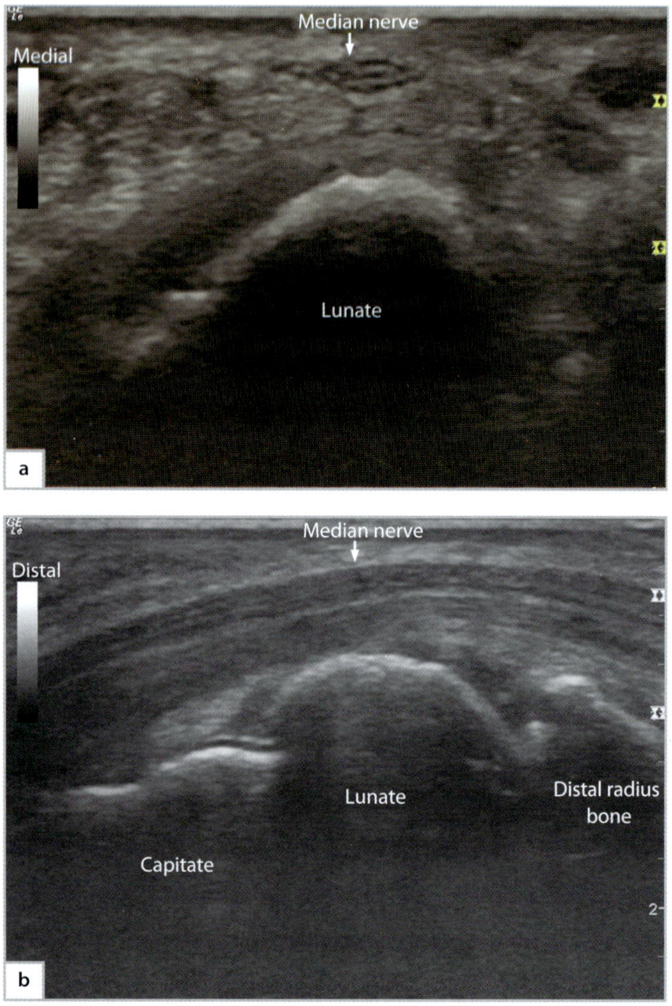

Figure 4.9 (a) Transverse image of a normal median nerve. Note the honeycomb appearance of the fascicles within the nerve. (b) Longitudinal image of a normal median nerve.

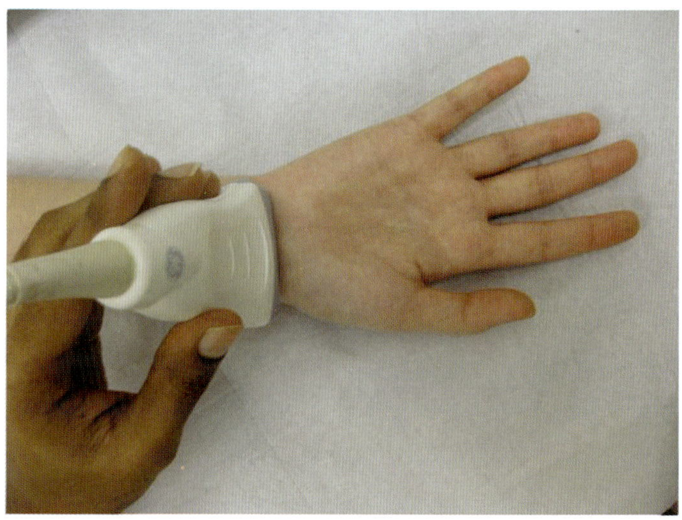

Figure 4.10 Imaging for carpal tunnel syndrome – transverse imaging over patient's wrist, arm supinated.

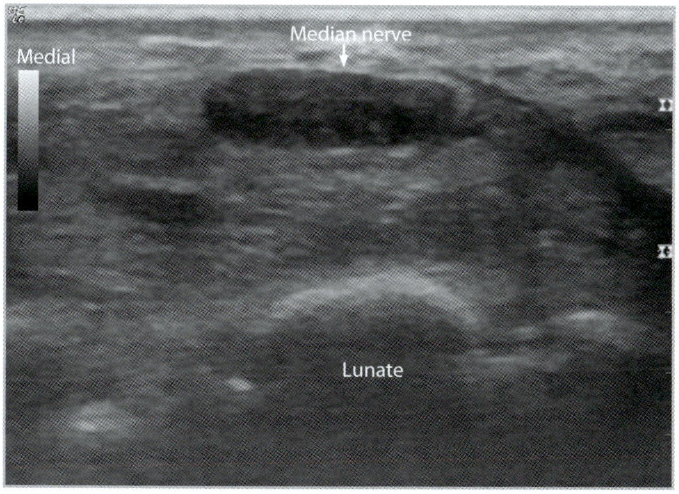

Figure 4.11 Sonographic appearance of median nerve at the wrist in a patient with carpal tunnel syndrome. Note the enlarged nerve, with loss of fascicular discrimination.

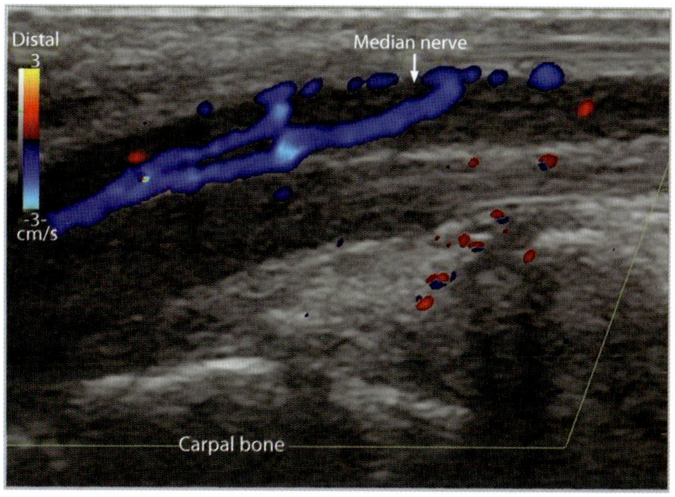

Figure 4.13 Longitudinal image of the median nerve with color Doppler flow imaging showing increase in intra- and perineural vascularization.

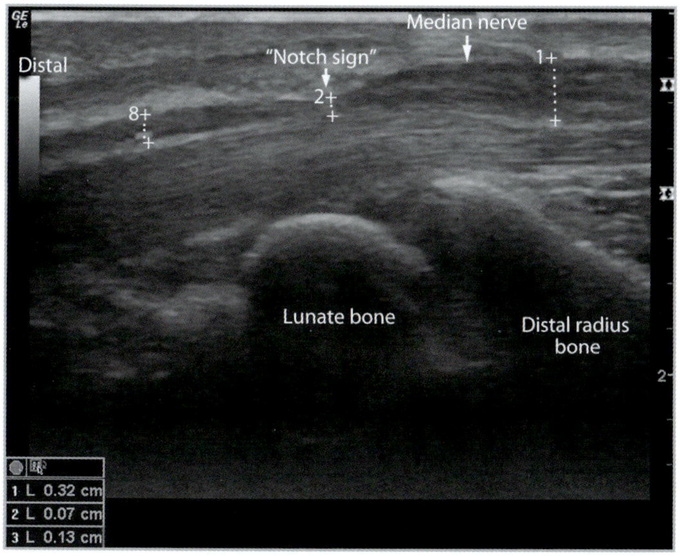

Figure 4.12 Longitudinal image of the median nerve showing the 'notch sign' where there is an abrupt change in caliber.

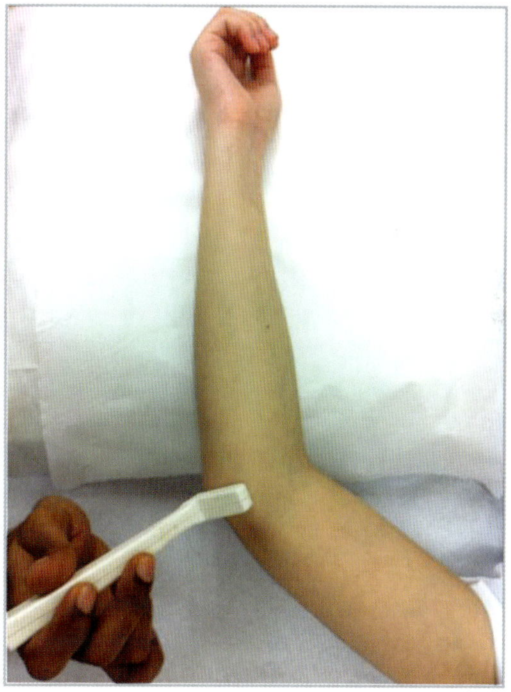

Figure 4.14 Sonography of ulnar nerve at cubital tunnel, with arm in extended position.

- Masses like ganglia, osteophytes, tumors, and rare reports of lymphoma, intraneural perineurioma, etc.

The sensitivity of US for the diagnosis of ulnar nerve compression at the elbow is generally >80%.

Radial neuropathy at the spiral groove

US position: The nerve is detected at mid-humerus level and color Doppler is used to identify the deep brachial artery as a guide.

Sonographic features of radial neuropathy are relatively less well-studied, with laboratory-specific CSA cut-offs. The features include:

- Swelling proximal to compression site
- Hypoechogenicity with loss of fascicular discrimination
- Increased epineural vascularity

Additional US features:

- Etiology – neuroma, etc.
- Assesses continuity of nerve, e.g. for nerve trauma

Nerve trauma

The sonographic features suggesting nerve trauma include

- Axonal swelling
- Nerve discontinuity
- Neuroma formation (**Figure 4.16**)

US is used as a complementary investigation with electrodiagnostic studies:

- Aids in differentiating complete nerve transection versus partial discontinuity

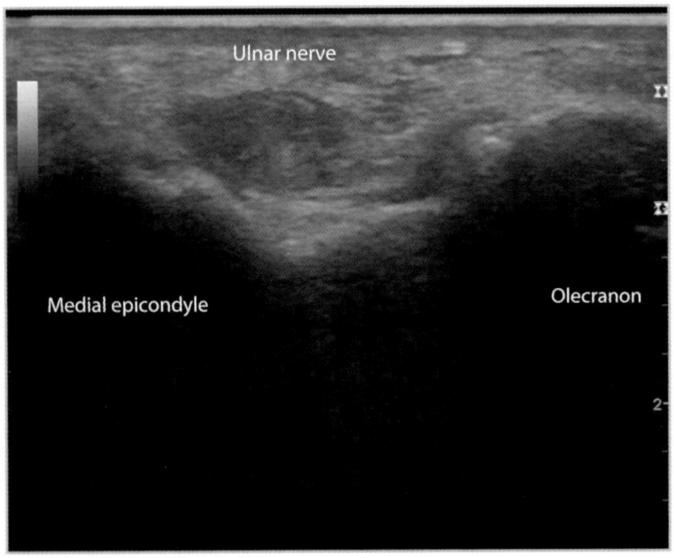

Figure 4.15 Sonography of the ulnar nerve at the cubital tunnel in a patient with cubital tunnel syndrome. Note the enlarged nerve with loss of fascicular discrimination.

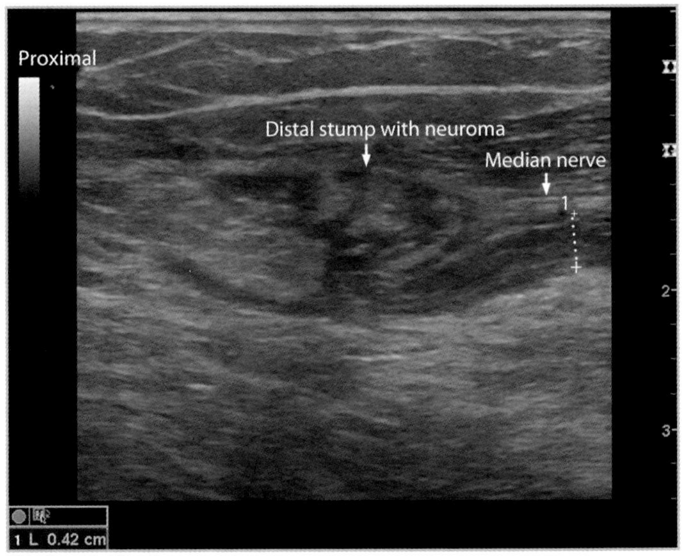

Figure 4.16 Nerve discontinuity and neuroma formation of the median nerve in the forearm following nerve trauma.

- Obtains information immediately and considerably earlier than electrodiagnostic studies (EDx), due to time lag required for visible changes in the NCS and EMG
- Aids in early decision for surgical versus conservative treatment
- Aids in localizing lesion

Nerve tumors

Some of the common nerve tumors that have been described using US include schwannomas and neurofibromas. US determines the location of the tumor (intra versus extra-neural), extent of vascularity, and consistency (cystic or solid).

Nerve inflammation

Well described in chronic demyelinating neuropathies, e.g. Charcot–Marie–Tooth 1A, chronic inflammatory demyelinating polyneuropathy (CIDP), and multifocal motor neuropathy. US shows a marked increase in nerve size from inflammatory cells and edema outside typical sites of nerve entrapment. In Hansens disease (leprosy), a multifocal inflammatory disease, the nerves appear focally enlarged, with increased vascularity.

Role of US in comparison with electrodiagnostic studies for assessing nerve diseases

US has a complementary role and can impact diagnostic and therapeutic decisions in approximately 40% of cases, with confirmatory role in 40%. It enhances diagnostic information and follow-up provided by EDx by providing information on nerve morphology and surrounding structures.

SUGGESTED READING

Beekman R, van der Plas JP, Uitdehaag BM, et al. Clinical, electrodiagnostic, and sonographic studies in ulnar neuropathy at the elbow. Muscle Nerve 2004; 30:202–208.
Good review of what is known (and not known) in the evaluation of ulnar neuropathy.

Daube JR, Rubin DI. Needle electromyography. Muscle Nerve 2009; 39:244–270.
Excellent and detailed review on the principles and uses of EMG in peripheral nerve and muscle disorders.

Fowler JR, Gaughan JP, Ilyas AM. The sensitivity and specificity of ultrasound for the diagnosis of carpal tunnel syndrome: a meta-analysis. *Clin Orthop Relat Res* 2011; 469:1089–1094.
Timely meta-analysis of the value of ultrasound in the evaluation of CTS. The paper emphasizes the need for a structured approach to ultrasound investigation of entrapments.

Padua L, Liotta G, Di Pasquale A, et al. Contribution of ultrasound in the assessment of nerve diseases. Eur J Neurol 2012; 19:47–54.
In this article, the authors assess the practical value of adding ultrasound to the routine neurophysiological examination of peripheral nerve disorders.

Werber RA, Andaray M. Electrodiagnostic evaluation of carpal tunnel syndrome. Muscle Nerve 2011; 44:597–607.
All you need to know in the evaluation of CTS using nerve conductions.

Chapter 5 Use of locoregional anesthesia and tourniquet in the upper limb

Shady A. Rehim, Kevin C. Chung

INTRODUCTION

The majority of upper limb procedures have traditionally been performed under general anesthesia. The development of modern techniques of local and regional anesthesia as well as advances in ultrasound imaging to visualize the nerves during regional anesthesia have led to an increased number of surgical procedures performed without subjecting patients to the systemic complications, prolonged hospitalization, and higher costs associated with general anesthesia.

INDICATIONS OF LOCOREGIONAL ANESTHESIA

Several factors and clinical indications may influence the decision of using local and/or regional anesthesia over general anesthesia when performing surgery of the upper limb. These factors may include

- An isolated upper limb/hand injury
- Patients deemed high risk for general anesthesia (e.g. ASA grade ≥3)
- Procedures of a relatively short duration that may be suitable for local or regional anesthesia
- Patients may wish to undergo surgical procedure(s) under local or regional anesthesia instead of general anesthesia

ANESTHETIC AGENTS

The agents used for locoregional anesthesia consist of two groups: an aromatic group and an amine group separated by an intermediate chain. The chemical bond that links the aromatic group to the intermediate chain (usually an ester or amide) determines the class of the drug. Examples of anesthetic esters and amides are as follows:

- Amino esters: procaine, chloroprocaine, and tetracaine
- Amino amides: lidocaine, mepivacaine, bupivacaine, and prilocaine

MECHANISM OF ACTION

The mechanism of action of anesthetic agents is illustrated in **Figure 5.1**. In clinical practice, it is difficult to produce an adequate sensory block without affecting a patient's motor function. Nevertheless, an experienced anesthetist or surgeon can titrate the dose of anesthesia according to the type and length of the surgical procedure required. For example, a carpal tunnel decompression procedure would require less time and anesthesia compared with a longer procedure such as a tendon or joint reconstruction that may require more time and anesthesia.

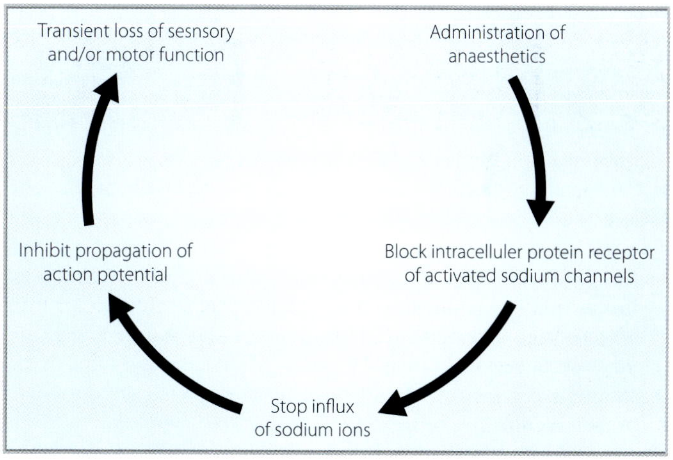

Figure 5.1 Mode of action of local anesthesia.

Nerves are categorized according to their diameters. The largest diameter nerve fibers are responsible for conducting pressure and motor function (type A). The smallest diameter nerve fibers are myelinated and are responsible for transmission of pain and temperature (type C), and these nerves are the most sensitive to anesthetics. Thus, the order of sensory loss following the administration of local anesthesia is loss of

1. Pain
2. Temperature
3. Touch
4. Motor function

Anesthetic agents are alkaline in nature; the presence of an infection produces an acidic medium that ionizes (charge) alkaline anesthetics and when anesthetic drugs become ionized they cannot penetrate the membrane efficiently and become less effective. Apart from tissue penetration, there are other factors that affect the pharmacokinetics of anesthetic medications that may alter drug potency, onset, and duration of action. Those factors include drug-lipid solubility, drug-medium pH (p*K*a), and vascularity of the injected site.

DRUGS AND DOSAGE

Different procedures may be performed using different anesthetics. **Table 5.1** summarizes the recommended dosage, onset, and duration of action of commonly used anesthetic agents. Additionally, the following precautions should be thought and applied when necessary to avoid undesired situations:

- Allergic reactions: the metabolism of amino esters produces PABA derivatives that may stimulate an allergic systemic response.

Table 5.1 Commonly used anesthetics

Drug	Dose (with adrenaline)	Onset	Duration	Comments
Amino amides				
Lidocaine	3–4 mg/kg (7 mg/kg)	Fast	Short	Most commonly used anesthetic
Mepivacaine	4 mg/kg (7 mg/kg)	Fast	Moderate	
Prilocaine	3 mg/kg (6 mg/kg)	Fast	Moderate	Least toxic therefore more frequently used with IV administration (e.g. Bier block).
Bupivacaine	1.5 mg/kg (3 mg/kg)	Slow	Long	Cardiotoxic. Sensory >motor block
Amino esters				
Procaine	8 mg/kg (10 mg/kg)	Slow	Short	Rarely used nowadays, as they were largely replaced by amino amides due to safer drug profile and less risk of allergic reactions.
Chloroprocaine	10 mg/kg (14 mg/kg)	Fast	Short	
Tetracaine	1.5 mg/kg(2.5 mg/kg)	Slow	Long	

*Doses above are suitable for adults' ≥18 years, must be reduced for children and elderly. Drug dosage obtained from the British National Formulary March 2012 edition.

Therefore, it is better to use amino amides such as lidocaine to avoid precipitating allergic reactions

- Significant comorbidities: bupivacaine is a markedly cardiotoxic anesthetic; hence, it is advisable not to administer in patients with a significant history of cardiac disease
- Combining anesthetic medications: administrating mixtures of fast-acting (e.g. lidocaine) and long-acting (e.g. bupivacaine) anesthetics provide rapid onset anesthesia and adequate postoperative pain control. However, when using mixtures of the same class of anesthesia, care must be taken not to exceed the safe maximum dose, as the mixed agents will have a cumulative effect.

Role of adrenaline

Using anesthetic preparations containing adrenaline induces a potent vasoconstriction effect within the operative field. This has the following advantages:

- Decreases the rate of anesthetic absorption into systemic circulation, thereby decreasing the risk of systemic toxicity
- Retains anesthetic molecules within the operative field, thus prolonging the action and duration of the anesthesia
- Provides temporary hemostasis

Adrenaline must be used in low concentrations when administered with local anesthetics, and the total dose should not exceed 500 µg. A commonly used adrenaline concentration is 1:200,000 (1 mg/200 mL); however, other concentrations are also available. The absolute contraindications of using anesthetics containing adrenaline include

- Peripheral vascular disease
- Pheochromocytoma
- Thyrotoxicosis
- Cardiac dysrhythmias

Contrary to traditional teaching, the use of adrenaline containing preparations is not considered as an absolute contraindication in digital anesthesia. However, it is well acknowledged that adrenaline containing anesthesia may cause digital gangrene/necrosis. Hand experts may argue the safety of this mixture when used in digital nerve blocks, but it is not advisable to perform these types of procedures without adequate experience and training, especially with the use of an adrenaline antagonist (phentolamine) to reverse the effect of epinephrine.

Toxicity and adverse effects

The adverse effects of anesthetic drugs can be classified as local or systemic effects.

Local adverse effects include

- Skin and soft tissue necrosis
- Puncture site infection and hematoma formation
- Intraneural injection and nerve injury

Systemic adverse effects include

- Hypersensitivity reactions, mostly related to PABA derivatives of amino esters
- Central nervous system: initial excitation (lightheadedness, restlessness, perioral numbness, blurry vision) followed by depression (respiratory depression, convulsions, and coma)
- Cardiovascular system: hypotension, myocardial depression, arrhythmias, and cardiac arrest

The mainstay of treatment for anesthetic toxicity is supportive management. This includes the following:

- Stop administration of anesthesia and call for help
- Support and manage patients' airway
- Control seizures (e.g. by administering benzodiazepines)
- Manage cardiac arrhythmias
- Administer inotropes for anaphylaxis or circulatory collapse
- Consider intravenous lipid emulsion (interlipid 20%), which binds to circulating anesthetics, thus preventing their redistribution in the body

LOCAL ANESTHESIA

The term 'local anesthesia' commonly refers to a type of anesthesia that is applied directly to a relatively small anatomical area of the body to induce a transient loss of sensation. The types of local anesthesia include

- Direct infiltration
- Peripheral nerve block
- Topical anesthesia

Direct infiltration

This is the simplest type of local anesthesia, and mastering this technique is essential prior to performing more complex types of anesthesia. The key steps for direct infiltration include

- Use a small-sized needle to infiltrate the anesthetic solution
- First inject a small amount intradermally to create a skin wheal
- Gently advance the needle toward the subcutaneous tissue
- Aspirate to ensure that you are not injecting into a blood vessel then infiltrate the rest of the anesthetic solution
- Infiltration is performed in a circular fashion around the area to be anesthetized to achieve the desired effect

A hematoma block is a special type of direct infiltration technique in which the local anesthetic agent is infiltrated around a fracture site (usually into the hematoma surrounding the fracture). This allows painless manipulation of closed fractures, e.g. distal radius, metacarpal, and phalangeal fractures. The key steps for hematoma block include

- Position the needle over the fracture site
- Advance the needle until it is in contact with the bone
- Aspirate a few milliliters of the formed hematoma surrounding the fracture to ensure correct positioning of the needle and gradually inject the anesthetic
- Allow a few minutes for the anesthetic to work, then manipulate and reduce the fracture and immobilize in a satisfactory position

Peripheral nerve block

This method uses a similar technique as direct infiltration described above to achieve an adequate sensory block of the peripheral nerves. This is performed by directly infiltrating the anesthetic solution around the nerves you wish to block. The most common drawback while performing peripheral nerve blocks is the injection of anesthetics intraneuraly, which can be harmful to the nerves. To avoid inflicting this type of injury ask the patient as you are advancing the needle if he/she is experiencing an electrical type of 'sharp shooting pain' (paresthesia) and reposition the needle if necessary. The following types of peripheral nerve blocks are commonly performed in the upper limb.

- Digital block (**Figure 5.2a–c**): Each digit has four digital nerve branches: two palmar and two dorsal branches. The palmar branches arise from a common digital nerve (median and ulnar nerves) and the dorsal branches arise from the superficial radial nerve and dorsal branch of the ulnar nerve. One should avoid circumferential blocks around the base of the digit because this can lead to compression of the vascular supply. The different approaches for digital nerve blocks include
  - Dorsal and/or palmar approach
  - Flexor sheath approach
  - Web space approach
  - Intermetacarpal approach
- Wrist block (**Figure 5.3a–c**): The aim of the wrist block is to anesthetize all the three nerves (median, ulnar, and radial) and their branches at the level of the wrist joint. The surface marking and blocking techniques of these nerves are as follows:
  - The median nerve is blocked by infiltrating between the tendons of the palmaris longus and flexor carpi radialis at the level of the proximal wrist crease
  - The ulnar nerve is blocked by infiltrating ulnar and deep to the flexor carpi ulnaris tendon at the level of the proximal wrist crease
  - The radial nerve and its branches are blocked by infiltrating in a wide arc at the level of the radial styloid
  - The dorsal branch of the ulnar nerve is blocked by infiltrating in an arc at the level of the ulnar styloid
- Elbow block: similar to a wrist block, the aim of this type of block is to anasthetize the three nerves (median, ulnar, and radial) at the level of elbow joint. Although this type of block is rarely performed as a primary anesthesia in upper limb surgery, it is usually used to supplement other types of plexus/nerve blocks. The surface marking and technique of elbow block are as follows:
  - The median nerve is blocked medial to the brachial artery just proximal to the antecubital crease, between the medial and lateral epicondyles
  - The ulnar nerve is blocked in the groove behind the medial epicondyle and olecranon

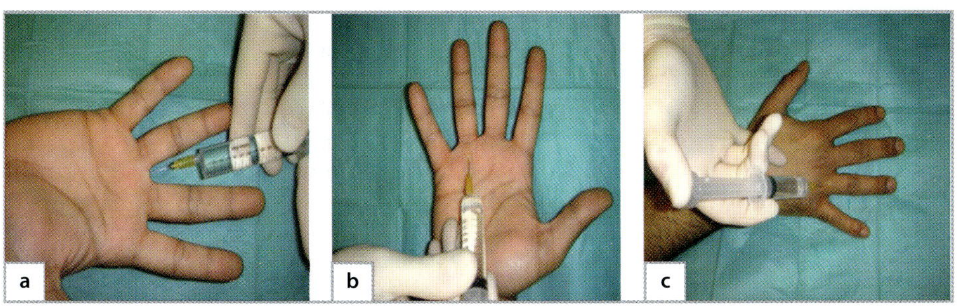

Figure 5.2 (a) Common digital nerve block through web space approach, (b) flexor sheath block, and (c) dorsal digital nerves block.

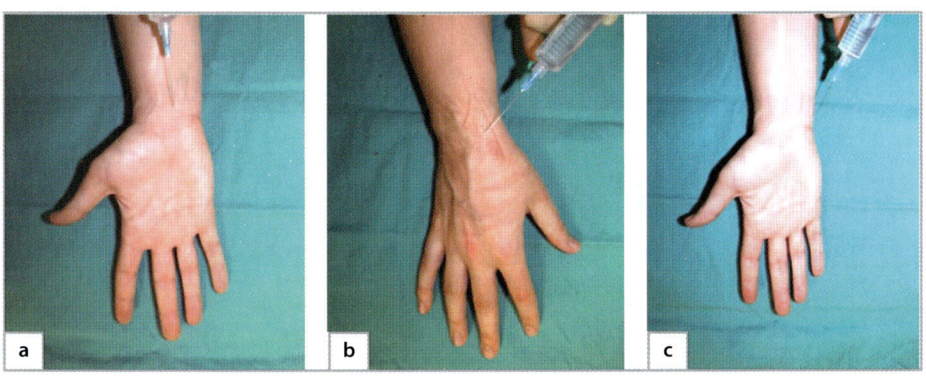

Figure 5.3 Wrist block. (a) Median nerve block, (b) radial nerve block, and (c) ulnar nerve block.

- The radial nerve is blocked 3–4 cm above the lateral epicondyle, between the tendons of the biceps and brachioradialis

Topical anesthesia (Table 5.2)

Topical anesthesia refers to the application of an anesthetic agent over a small surface area of the skin. This is typically applied before minor procedures, and the anesthetic, which is commonly in the form of an ointment, is covered with an occlusive dressing. Topical anesthesia induces superficial analgesia of the epidermis and superficial dermis, and is commonly used in the pediatric age group or with patients suffering from needle phobia.

REGIONAL ANESTHESIA

Regional anesthesia produces temporary loss of sensory and motor function over larger areas of the body. The types of regional anesthesia include

- Intravenous (Bier block)
- Plexus block

Bier block

A commonly used anesthetic technique that is useful for minor procedures performed on the wrist and hand such as manipulation of distal radius fractures (e.g. Colles fracture). The anesthetics are administered intravenously and prevented from reaching systemic circulation by the action of a pneumatic arm tourniquet. The extravasation of anesthetics into the interstitial tissue blocks the surrounding nerves and provides adequate anesthesia. Patients generally are able to tolerate the tourniquet for approximately 30–45 minutes without additional anesthesia or sedation. Using a double tourniquet technique allows the surgery to be extended up to 90 minutes by alternate inflation of the tourniquets. The key steps of Bier block are as follows:

- Two intravenous accesses are established: one on the dorsum of the hand of the affected limb and the other on the opposite noninjured limb
- Elevate and exsanguinate the injured limb. The tourniquet should be inflated to 100 mmHg above the systolic blood pressure. Then inject the anesthetic agent (40 mL of 0.5% lidocaine) intravenously on the same side of tourniquet using the intravenous access established previously
- If the duration of surgery is <20 minutes, the tourniquet should not be released immediately. You should wait for at least 20 minutes before deflating the tourniquet for the drug to become fixed to the local tissues. Otherwise there will be a sudden surge of the anesthetic drug into the systemic circulation resulting in systemic toxicity
- A double tourniquet technique achieves prolonged anesthesia below the elbow. Using a double tourniquet, the proximal tourniquet is inflated first and the local anesthetic is injected. Once the patient starts to complain of pain due to arm compression, the distal tourniquet is inflated and then the proximal tourniquet is released to relief pressure and ease pain
- At all times during the procedure, the physician must ensure that the tourniquet is working well and is maintaining adequate pressures

Plexus block

The brachial plexus is enclosed within a fascial sheath, which extends from the root of the neck to the axilla. Depending on the anatomical location and type of the procedure, different types of blocks can be performed by infiltrating anesthetics around divisions, trunks, and cords of the brachial plexus. A brachial plexus block provides intraoperative as well as postoperative analgesia. It can be given as a 'one-off' (single administration) or by continuous infusion through a catheter such as in chronic pain syndromes. In recent years, ultrasound-assisted techniques have improved the safety profile and efficacy of brachial plexus blocks and are currently considered to be the standard technique when administrating regional anesthesia.

The brachial plexus block can be divided into several blocks given above the clavicle (interscalene and supraclavicular blocks) and below the clavicle (infraclavicular and axillary blocks). Occasionally, an additional block such as the intercostobrachial nerve may be required to anesthetize the arm for the use of arm tourniquet.

- Interscalene block (**Figure 5.4a**): This aims to block the roots and trunks of the brachial plexus (C_5-C_7) located in the interscalene groove between the anterior and middle scalene muscles. This block is suitable for shoulder and arm surgery, but it does not adequately block the ulnar nerve (C_8-T_1) and is therefore not appropriate for surgery of the hand and forearm. The risks associated with this block include
  - Injury of the sympathetic chain (Horner syndrome), recurrent laryngeal, and phrenic nerve
  - Intravascular injection (vertebral artery)
  - Pneumothorax
  - Spinal and epidural block
- Supraclavicular block (**Figure 5.4b**): This blocks the divisions and trunks (C_5-T_1) of the brachial plexus, located above the midpoint

Table 5.2 Commonly used topical anesthetics

Drug	Properties	Indication
LMX 4	Lidocaine 4% cream Onset: 30 minutes	Anesthesia before venepuncture or venous cannulation
EMLA	Lidocaine 2.5% and prilocaine 2.5% cream Onset: 1 hour	Anesthesia before venepuncture and over skin graft donor sites prior to skin harvest
Ametop	Amethocaine 4% (tetracaine) Onset 30–45minutes	As above. Rapidly absorbed, avoid using over traumatized or large surface areas. Lidocaine preparations are considered as safer option
Cryogesic	Ethyl chloride spray. Onset: 10 seconds lasts 2 minutes.	Minor procedures, suitable alternative if allergy to other forms of topical anesthesia exists

[+]Drug dosage obtained from the British National Formulary March 2012 edition.

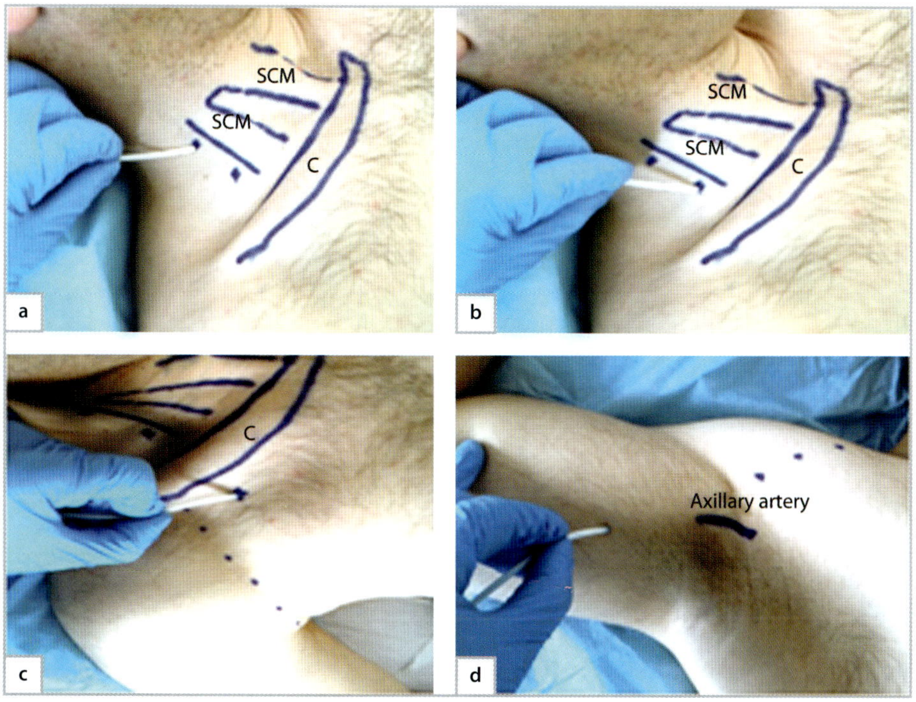

Figure 5.4 Anatomical landmarks of a plexus block: (a) Interscalene block, (b) supraclavicular block, (c) infraclavicular block, and (d) axillary block (surface marking indicating the two heads of sternocleidomastoid, clavicle, and axillary artery).

of the clavicle and lateral to the subclavian artery. It is suitable for procedures performed on the arm, forearm, and hand. The risks associated with this block include
  - Pneumothorax
  - Vascular injury
  - Diaphragmatic hemiparesis
- Infraclavicular block (**Figure 5.4c**): This blocks the medial, lateral, and posterior cords of the brachial plexus, located in the infraclavicular fossa. It is suitable for forearm and hand procedures and does not usually require additional blocks. The risks associated with this block include
  - Vascular injury (axillary artery)
  - Hematoma formation
- Axillary block (**Figure 5.4d**): It blocks the median, ulnar, and radial nerves; the surrounding axillary artery is encased by an axillary sheath. It is the most commonly performed block for surgery of the distal forearm and hand. There is less risk of pneumothorax or neurovascular injury due to a distal relation to the lung and other major structures. An additional block of the musculocutaneous nerve and/or intercostobrachial nerve may be required

SEDATION

Sedation is defined as depression of a patient's level of consciousness without impairment of spontaneous respiratory or cardiac functions. The main purpose of sedation is to alleviate a patients' anxiety and enhance comfort during the procedure. The drugs used for sedation are summarized in **Table 5.3**. Sedatives are not analgesics and are often combined with opioids and nonopioids to produce analgesia, amnesia, and relief of anxiety. The following levels of sedation have been defined:

- Minimal sedation: Normal response to verbal stimuli, patient maintains his/her spontaneous ventilation, and cardiovascular function
- Moderate sedation (conscious sedation): Patient is less responsive, however, able to maintain his/her spontaneous ventilation and cardiovascular function. This type of sedation is the most commonly performed for day-case and outpatient procedures
- Deep sedation: Heavily sedated patient that may not be responsive and may require assistance with his/her ventilation
- General anesthesia: Unarousable patient whom requires ventilation +/– circulatory support

The following safety measures must be undertaken prior to the administration of sedation:

- A comprehensive review of a patient's medical status is required prior to the administration of sedation
- Patient allergies should be checked carefully and documented
- As with regional anesthesia, patients should be instructed to fast prior to the procedure in case conversion to general anesthesia is required
- A qualified personnel or an anesthesiologist who received adequate training on the safe administration of monitored sedation should administer sedatives
- Sedation should be performed in a controlled environment where adequate monitoring (oxygen saturation probe, blood pressure, ECG) and resuscitation equipment is available

TOURNIQUET

A tourniquet is a device for stopping the blood flow through a vein and/or artery by compressing the limb/digit with a cuff or tight bandage. A tourniquet

- Provides a bloodless field for upper limb surgery
- Prevents the spread of local anesthetics into systemic circulation when used with a Bier block
- Allows for temporary control of hemorrhage in the upper limb

The following should be considered with using the tourniquet:

- The tourniquet should be avoided or a special care should be taken in patients with peripheral vascular disease (e.g. diabetes mellitus,

Table 5.3 Drugs used for sedation

Drug	Properties	Dose	Treatment of overdose
Sedative-hypnotics			
Midazolam	Benzodiazepines: Short acting. Induce sedation, amnesia, and relief of anxiety	Initially 1–2 mg IV then by slow infusion approximately 2 mg/minute	May cause profound respiratory depression especially in elderly Treatment: Flumazenil IV 200 μg then 100 μg if required (maximum 1 mg) and supportive management
Propofol	Barbiturate: Most commonly used anesthetic for induction and maintenance of anesthesia. Rapid onset and recovery	Induction: 1.5–2.5 mg/kg at rate of 20–40 mg every 10 seconds Maintenance: 1.5–4.5 mg/kg/hour	Potentially fatal but rare side effect is propofol infusion syndrome (metabolic acidosis, cardiac failure, rhabdomyolysis, hyperlipidemia, and hepatomegaly) Treatment: Supportive management
Thiopental	Barbiturate: Short acting rapid onset and recovery	50–100 mg IV over 10 seconds Max 500 mg	Hypotension, respiratory and myocardial depression, laryngeal spasm Treatment: Supportive
Methohexital	Barbiturate: Ultra-short acting with rapid onset and recovery	20–50 mg IV	As thiopental
Opioid analgesia			
Fentanyl	Rapid onset 1–2 minutes and short duration of action	IV injection 50–100 μg IV infusion 3–4 μg/kg/hour	Respiratory depression is the main side effect of opioid analgesia. Other side effects may include cardiovascular system depression, nausea, vomiting, and laryngospasm Treatment: Naloxone 100–200 μg (100 μg every 2 minutes if required)
Remifentanil	Given at induction and by IV infusion, titrated to response. Reduces dose requirement of other anesthetics. Remifentanil is metabolized by tissue esterases hence little risk of accumulation and residual post-operative respiratory depression	Induction 0.5–1 μg/kg/minute. Maintenance 25–100 nanogram/kg/minute	
Alfentanil		IV injection 500 μg over 30 seconds. IV infusion 30–50 μg/kg	
Nonopioid analgesia			
Ketamine	N-methyl-D-aspartate receptor antagonist. Mainly used in pediatric anesthesia	IV injection 1–4 mg/kg IV infusion 10–45 μg /kg/minute	Hallucination, nightmares, nausea, vomiting, hypertension Treatment: Supportive treatment
Acetaminophen	Effective analgesic and antipyretic. 1st choice for management of acute and chronic pain	0.5–1 g (maximum4 g/day) IV/PO/PR	Hepatotoxicity Treatment: *N*-acetylcysteine
Diclofenac	Nonsteroidal anti-inflammatory drug. Analgesic and anti-inflammatory. Provide effective pain relief that may reduce requirement of opioid analgesia	75–100 mg daily in 2–3 divided doses	Gastrointestinal irritation +/–bleeding

+Doses above are suitable for adults' ≥18 years, must be reduced for children and elderly. Drug dosage obtained from the British National Formulary March 2012 edition.

severe atherosclerosis, severe hypertension, and Raynaud disease), severe crushing injuries with devitalized tissue, lymphoedema, and sickle cell disease.

- In patients suffering an infection or malignancy, do not exsanguinate the upper limb to avoid systemic spread
- To protect the skin from direct contact and pressure generated by the overlying cuff, wrap a soft cast around the arm. A waterproof tape can also be wrapped around the distal end of the cuff to avoid soakage of the tourniquet with antiseptic solutions
- Administration of preoperative antibiotic prophylaxis and marking of skin incisions should be performed prior to inflation of the tourniquet
- Inflate the tourniquet to pressures ranging between 250 and 300 mmHg (100 mmHg above systolic) for adults, and 150–250 mmHg for children
- The use of the tourniquet should be restricted to 120 minutes at most. If a longer duration of tourniquet use is required, one must release the tourniquet at 90–120 minutes and allow tissue perfusion for 20–30 minutes before reinflating the tourniquet
- It is good practice to assess neurovascular status of the limb following the use of a tourniquet and prior to hospital discharge to check for complications (e.g. paresthesia or paresis) that might have been caused by the tourniquet

Types of tourniquet

Finger tourniquet (Figure 5.5a–d)

A constrictive band is applied to the base of the finger that is suitable for procedures performed distal to the proximal interphalangeal joint. Various techniques are available, including application of commercially available tourniquets or by performing the Salem method. In the Salem method, one of the fingers is cut off from a glove and the tip of the finger snipped off. This is then placed over the digit and rolled toward the base. This simultaneously exsanguinates the digit and forms a tourniquet. Regardless of which type of finger tourniquet is used, it is important to ensure that the tourniquet is not left underneath the finger dressing at the end of the procedure. We always place a clamp over the finger tourniquet to remind us to

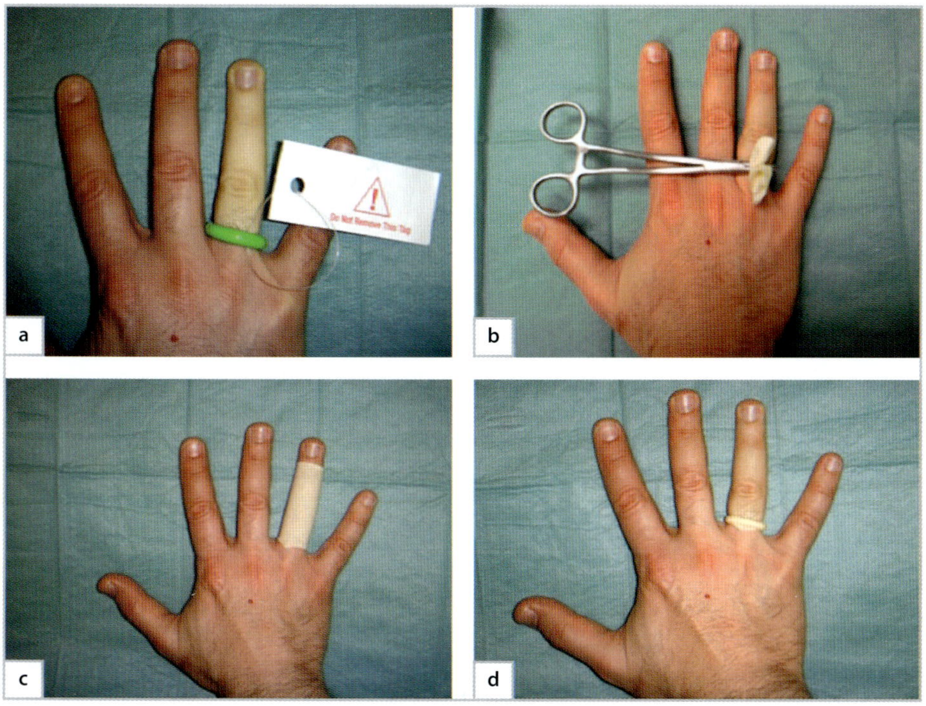

Figure 5.5 (a) Commercially available finger tourniquet, (b) Glove and clamp method, (c and d) Salem method.

remove the finger tourniquet after the end of surgery. Because of the finger is anesthetized, patients often will not complain of tourniquet pain, until it is too late.

Forearm tourniquet

Suitable for procedures performed in the distal forearm and the hand. If applied distally in the forearm where there is less muscle bulk, the patient will be able to tolerate the tourniquet for longer. However, there may be some difficulty in compressing blood vessels between the radius and ulna within forearm compartments. This tourniquet may provide an alternative to the arm tourniquet in a select group of patients (e.g. arteriovenous fistula in upper arm or proximal forearm).

Arm tourniquet

This tourniquet is applied at mid-arm level and provides hemostasis from the level of the elbow to the hand. A sterile tourniquet may be considered if the surgical incision is very close to the tourniquet (e.g. decompression of the ulnar nerve proximal to the elbow) or there is a need to extend the incision proximal to the site of the tourniquet (e.g. elevation of a lateral arm flap).

The complications associated with the use of a tourniquet include

- Skin pressure necrosis
- Chemical and friction burns that may result from poorly fitted tourniquets
- Neurapraxia
- Skeletal muscle ischemia and reperfusion injuries
- Compartment syndrome, rhabdomyolysis, and vascular injuries

SUGGESTED READING

British National Formulary. http://www.bnf.org/bnf/index.htm.
A medical and pharmaceutical reference book that contains a wide spectrum of information and advice on prescribing and pharmacology. This free online resource includes indications, contraindications, and drug interactions of all commercially available pharmaceuticals.

Covino BG. Pharmacology of local anaesthetic agents. Br J Anesth 1986; 58:701–716.
Types and classification of commonly used local anesthetics. Properties, pharmacokinetics, and adverse effects associated with drugs used for local anesthesia.

Lalonde D, Bell M, Benoit P, et al. A multicenter prospective study of 3,110 consecutive cases of elective epinephrine use in the fingers and hand: the Dalhousie Project clinical phase. J Hand Surg Am 2005; 30:1061–1067.
A landmark study to examine prospectively the incidence of digital infarction and phentolamine rescue in a large series of patients in whom local anesthesia with adrenaline was injected electively into the hand and fingers.

O'Donnell BD, Ryan H, O'Sullivan O, Iohom G. Ultrasound-guided axillary brachial plexus block with 20 milliliters local anesthetic mixture versus general anesthesia for upper limb trauma surgery: an observer-blinded, prospective, randomized, controlled trial. Anesth Analg 2009; 109:279–283.
A comparative RCT of outcomes of ultrasound-guided brachial plexus block versus general anesthesia in upper limb surgery. Results suggested analgesic superiority of ultrasound guided anesthesia over general anesthesia technique.

Chapter 6 Surgical instrumentation and magnification

Keming Wang, Evan J. Kowalski, Kevin C. Chung

INTRODUCTION

A collection of precision surgical instruments is essential for a hand surgeon to perform procedures safely, efficiently, and effectively. Although many instruments are considered standard for every hand surgeon, the choice of certain instruments is dependent on individual preference.

Standard requirements for the majority of hand surgical procedures include

- Basic surgical instruments
- Power instruments
- Microsurgical instruments
- Magnification
- Fluoroscopy
- Tourniquet

BASIC SURGICAL INSTRUMENTS

Cutting and dissecting instruments

- Scalpels: A no. 7 handle with a no. 15 blade is the most commonly used scalpel in hand surgery for making incisions and dissecting tissue. The no. 11 blade has a sharp point, making it ideal for stab incisions. The no. 10 blade is twice the size of the no.15, and is used mainly for debridement of wounds
- Small Metzenbaum scissors: These scissors are typically used for delicate soft tissue dissection, and to access small structures just under the skin (**Figure 6.1**). The name is derived from its designer, Myron Firth Metzenbaum, an American oral surgeon. The blade is curved and narrow, with a blunt tip, and the handles are elongated
- Short tenotomy scissors: Tenotomy scissors are used to incise or cut through tendons and are commonly used when precise dissection is required (**Figure 6.1**). The scissors feature an extremely slender blade and a strong handle that provides a steady grip, allowing access to areas with small openings. They may also be known as Stevens scissors, named after a professor of physiology and ophthalmology in New York in 1889, who recommended the use of these scissors for correcting strabismus
- Suture scissors (short straight scissors): Used to cut the ends of sutures without damaging the surrounding tissue (**Figure 6.1**)
- Rongeurs: Used to gnaw and extract tissue and bone (**Figure 6.2**)

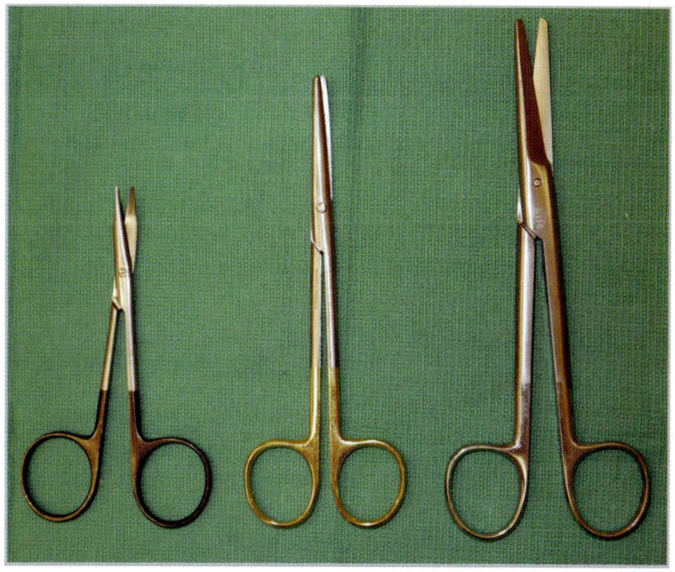

Figure 6.1 From left to right, small Metzenbaum scissors, short tenotomy scissors, and suture scissors.

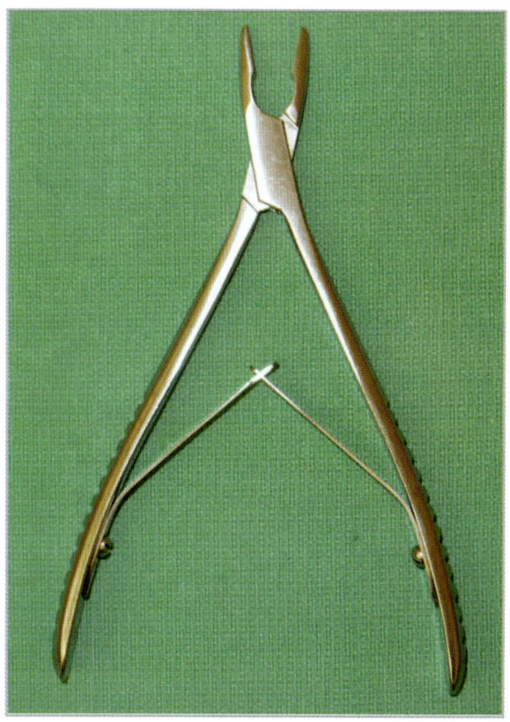

Figure 6.2 Rongeurs.

Retracting and exposing instruments

- Weitlaner retractors: Used to retract shallow incisions (**Figure 6.3**)
- Ragnell retractors: These retractors come in different sizes to enable either shallow or deep retracting. The blunt tip makes this instrument a good choice when retracting close to a nerve (**Figure 6.3**)

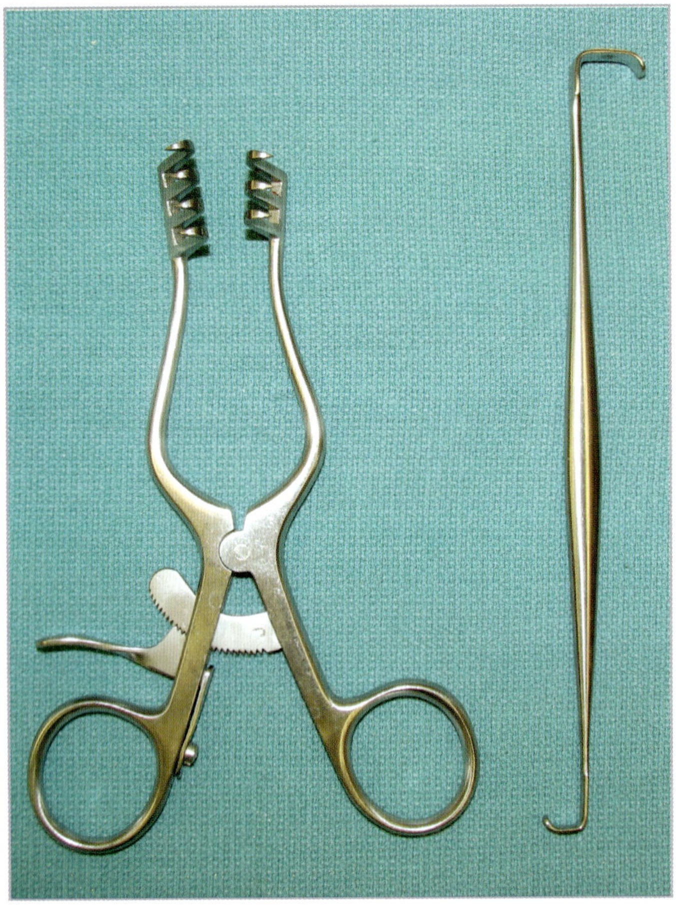

Figure 6.3 On the left a set of Weitlaner retractors, and on the right Ragnell retractors.

- Gelpi retractors: Useful for deeper exposure and retraction of tissue
- Skin hooks: Skin hooks are used for holding skin edges and cause only small points of trauma to underlying tissue. Because tissue trauma induces inflammation that may restrict finger motion, hand surgeons must be particularly conscientious to use instruments that are less traumatic, such as using a knife to expose tissue planes. They are typically used at the beginning of an incision, and come in several different sizes: single skin hooks, small double skin hooks, and Senn retractors (**Figure 6.4**)

Clamping and occluding instruments

- Hemostat clamp: The hemostat clamp is a very important tool for occluding the flow of blood in vessels. They vary in size and shape depending on the surgeon's preference and the type of surgery being performed. The mosquito clamp has a smaller and finer tip. The fine right angle is a type of Mixter clamp that features an aggressive 90° angle with a fine tip that can be used for dissection, occlusion, or grasping in deep layers of tissue

Grasping and holding instruments

- Toothed forceps (e.g. Adson): Used for handling the skin, dermis, or subcutaneous tissue

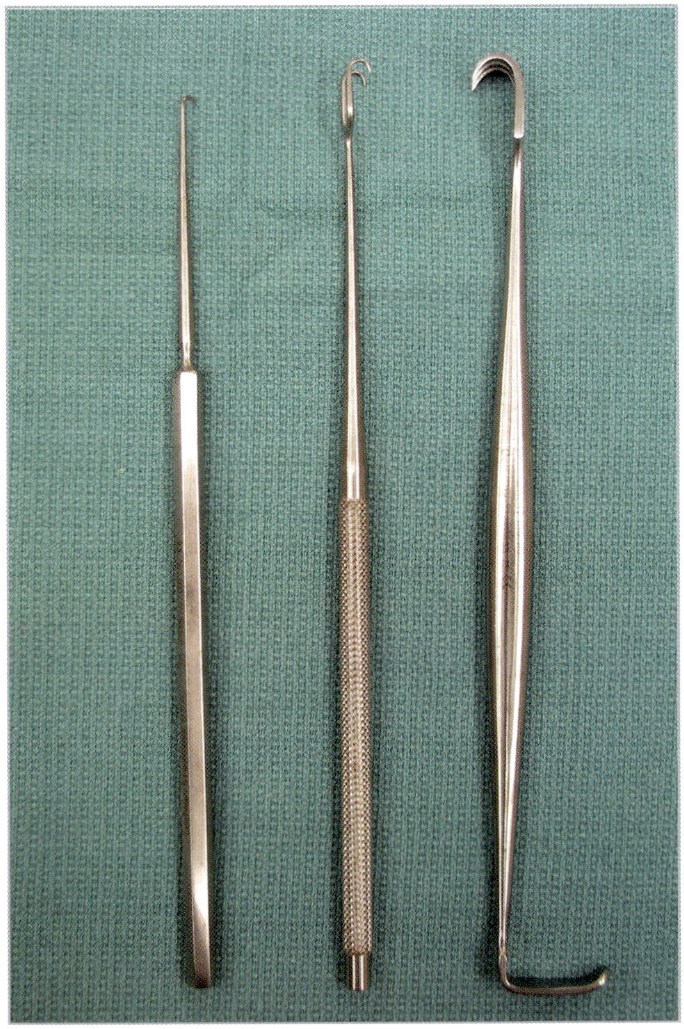

Figure 6.4 From left to right, single skin hook, small double skin hook, and Senn retractor.

- Micro-Adson forceps: These forceps have a more delicate tip than the Adson forceps and cause less tissue damage
- Fine needle holders: Come in sizes of small needle holders, medium needle holders, and large needle holders

Power instruments

- Surgical power drill: A small and easy to handle surgical power drill is essential for drilling holes, but requires water cooling during drilling. 4- or 6-inch double-pointed Kirschner wires are standard lengths for hand surgery applications, and 0.028 inch, 0.035 inch, 0.045 inch, and 0.0625 inch are all appropriate wire sizes. A Kirschner wire cutter should be used to cut the Kirschner wires
- Electrical saw: This tool is essential in hand surgery to provide the ability to perform precise and rapid osteotomy

MICROSURGICAL INSTRUMENTS

A set of microsurgical instruments is essential to perform microsurgery. They should be precise, easily maneuverable, and feature a fine tip. The shorter instruments measuring 11–15 cm are appropriate for superficial surgery, whereas instruments longer than 15 cm are recommended for deeper hand surgery procedures.

Micro-forceps (e.g. Jewelers and Pierce) vary in design and size. Adventitia forceps, also referred to as Pierce forceps, are useful for initial dissection. Smooth-tipped forceps, often called Jeweler forceps, are most commonly used in microsurgery. Tying forceps have a platform near the tip of the forceps, which is helpful to make a knot.

- Microneedle holders (e.g. Castroviejo): These are used for holding tiny needles
- Straight microscissors: Can be used for cutting and freshening the ends of vessels and nerves, or for cutting sutures
- Curved design microscissors: These scissors are mainly used for dissecting nerves and vessels

MAGNIFICATION

Magnification can be a necessity during certain hand surgery procedures, and is available in various combinations of magnification and size of field, ranging from 2.5× to 4.5×. A loupe should be chosen based on utility and comfort level, with comfort level largely dependent on individual preference. A 2.5× magnifying loupe with a wide field of vision is commonly used to perform hand surgery. A 4.5× loupe can be used for microneurovascular dissection and repair when a microscope is not available. The ideal microscope should feature a double-headed binocular unit, so that the assistant is able to participate in the procedure.

FLUOROSCOPY UNIT

A fluoroscopy unit is essential during many hand surgery procedures for accurate assessment during surgical treatment.

Mini C-arm

This form of fluoroscopy has the advantages of a decreased size, reduced radiation emissions, and a more simplistic function than the full-scale unit, and is therefore generally recommended for intraoperative hand treatment over the full-size unit. It is recommended that the surgeon wear a lead apron of 0.5 mm lead thickness to reduce radiation exposure when using fluoroscopy. Athwal et al. reported that when using the mini C-arm, the nursing staff and anesthesiology staff standing 1 m from the center of the hand table received significantly less scatter radiation when compared with surgeons ($P < 0.01$). The authors also determined that standing directly behind the image intensifier aspect of the machine had lower radiation exposure to vital areas (groin, chest, thyroid) compared with the source side of the mini C-arm. The National Council on Radiation Protection and Management (NCRP) recommends that whole-body radiation dose limits should be no greater than 5000 mR per year. The mean in-beam radiation exposure of a mini C-arm is known to be approximately 3720 mR/h.

TOURNIQUET

A pneumatic tourniquet should be placed proximal above the elbow to reduce blood loss during a procedure. A narrow cuff is the recommended size for hand surgery. Estebe compared a wide (14 cm) and a narrow (7 cm) tourniquet cuff size and found that the narrow cuff was less painful than the wide cuff when inflated to a pressure over 100 mmHg. Several layers of soft cast padding should be placed under the tourniquet, with care taken to avoid creases or ridges and a stockinette wrapped around the extremity from the fingertips to the tourniquet for maximum exsanguination of the entire extremity. It is recommended that the inflation time for tourniquet use not exceed 2 hours.

- Pressure:
  - Upper extremity ≤250 mmHg
  - Lower extremity ≤300 mmHg
  - Less pressure is desired for children (180–200 mmHg)

Excessive tourniquet time increases the risk of muscle and nerve-related complications, because nerves are susceptible to pressure injury and muscles are particularly vulnerable to ischemia. For procedures with an anticipated duration of >2.5 hours, the tourniquet should be deflated for 15–20 minutes after 2 hours. For procedures using tourniquet time >180 minutes, a deflation interval of 30 minutes was found to have fewer neurologic complications (22%) than that of an interval time of <30 minutes (39%). Odinsson reported that in 63,484 operations, 26 complications occurred due to tourniquet use, of which 15 were neurological. He also found that 13 of the nerve complications resolved within 6 months.

SUTURE MATERIAL

Various suture materials are available for hand surgery procedures. Different suture properties are appropriate for different clinical applications, but the ideal suture must have a high tensile strength, be easy to handle and use, have high flexibility for security loop formation, cause minimal tissue reaction, and be able to maintain tensile strength during the necessary period of tissue healing.

Suture material can be divided into absorbable and nonabsorbable sutures (**Table 6.1**). In regard to the material structure, sutures can also be divided into two other groups (**Table 6.2**): Multifilament (braided) and monofilament (nonbraided). Studies documenting mechanical analysis have shown that braided sutures were more flexible than nonbraided suture, and had a greater degree of resistance to stretch. Because suture materials are foreign bodies, they can be responsible for inflammatory reactions resulting in redness, edema, and an increased risk of hypertrophic scar formation. The reaction at the wound site is more extensive in absorbable compared with nonabsorbable sutures, and in multifilamentous more than monofilamentous sutures.

Table 6.1 Advantages and disadvantages of absorbable and nonabsorbable sutures

	Absorbable sutures	Nonabsorbable sutures
Advantages	Do not require removal	Less tissue reaction and inflammatory response Cannot be dissolved and keep tensile strength
Disadvantages	More wound reaction Lower time of wound support and loss of tensile strength	Suture sinus and suture extrusion Foreign body left Require removal when used for skin closure

Table 6.2 Advantages and disadvantages of multifilament and monofilament sutures

	Multifilament (braided)	Monofilament (nonbraided)
Advantages	High flexibility and easy handling Better tensile strength and ability to tie secure knots	Reduced tissue reaction and scar formation Lower risk of infection
Disadvantages	More tissue reaction Increased infection risk Scar formation	Stiffness and tendency to untie Decrease the loop tension and knot security

Table 6.3 Sutures classification

Sutures	Multifilament (braided)	Monofilament (nonbraided)
Absorbable suture	Vicryl, polygycolic acid (Dexon), chromic gut	Monocryl, polydioxanone (PDS), polyglyconate (Maxon)
Nonabsorbable suture	Polyester (Ethibond)	Nylon (Ethilon), polypropylene (Prolene),

Absorbable sutures

Absorbable sutures, such as plain gut, chromic gut, and synthetic polymers of polyglycolic acid (Dexon), Vicryl, polydioxanone (PDS), polyglyconate (Maxon), and Monocryl (**Table 6.3**), have the advantage of not requiring removal and may accelerate wound healing due to their biocompatibility. Chromic gut maintains full tensile strength up to 18–21 days, and has an absorption time of approximately 90 days, but incites a greater inflammatory response than other sutures. Polyglycolic acid sutures decrease to 23% of their initial strength at 4 weeks, and are completely absorbed by 60–90 days. One study reported that polyglycolic acid sutures have a higher affinity for bacterial adherence than other absorbable sutures such as PDS, Vicryl, Ethibond, Echilon, and chromic gut; PDS sutures have the lowest affinity bacterial adherence. Vicryl maintains 75% of its initial tensile strength at 2 weeks and 25% at 4 weeks, and is completely absorbed by 57–70 days. PDS retains approximately 75–80% of initial tensile strength at 2 weeks, with 60% remaining at 6 weeks. Monocryl loses 20–30% of its initial tensile strength after 2 weeks, with complete absorption occurring between the 91st and 119th days. Absorbable sutures can be helpful for children and replantation cases for skin closure when it is not desirable to remove sutures following the procedure. Vicryl is mainly used in the deep subcutaneous layer or for dermis closure, whereas Monocryl and chromic catgut can be used as a skin suture when suture removal is impossible.

Nonabsorbable sutures

Nonabsorbable sutures, such as polypropylene (Prolene), stainless steel, Teflon, polyester, Ethibond, Ethilon, and Dacron, are not dissolved by the body and are less likely to elicit an inflammatory response. Nonabsorbable monofilament sutures have a high bending stiffness and tendency to untie, which decreases loop tension. Therefore, they are not appropriate for tendon repair due to the secure knotting required. However, nonabsorbable multifilament sutures, such as Ethibond, with secure knot formation and the ability to maintain a high tensile strength up to 6 weeks, are the ideal sutures for tendon repair. Polypropylene, which causes minimal tissue reaction, is mainly used for vascular anastomoses both in small vessels and large vessels, as well as in neurosurgery. It should be noted that the deeper the suture is buried, the less the extent of tissue reaction and inflammation.

Multifilament and monofilament sutures

- Multifilament (braided):
  - Vicryl, Ethibond, and Dexon
  - Have the advantage of easy handling and the ability to tie secure knots
  - They are more prone to induce tissue reaction and infection
- Monofilament (nonbraided):
  - Maxon, PDS, and Monocryl
  - Reduce the tendency for infection and tissue response as well as decrease scar formation
  - Difficult to handle because of stiffness and an inability to tie secure knots

For skin closure, multiple studies have reported varying results regarding the use of different suture materials.

- Kharwadkar reported on the outcomes of scar formation, including scar tenderness and extent of wound inflammation following open carpal tunnel release. The study determined that polyglactin 910 (Vicryl) and Polypropylene (Prolene) had no significant difference regarding scar formation
- Erel compared nonabsorbable sutures versus absorbable sutures in carpal tunnel release wound closure, and found that Prolene resulted in less wound inflammation than Vicryl. Prolene has the disadvantage of stitch marks and pain on suture removal
- Multiple studies have demonstrated that Monocryl has a lower incidence of hypertrophic scarring compared with Polyglactin 910 (Vicryl). The characteristics of Monocryl include
  - Tensile strength loss of 20–30% after 2 weeks
  - Complete absorption between 91st and 119th day of implantation
  - Minimal tissue reaction

Tendon repair

3-0 or 4-0 braided and nonabsorbable suture (Ethibond) is recommended for tendon repair. Greenwald compared 10 suture materials before and after in vivo incubation, and found that braided polyester (Ethibond) was the only stable suture, maintaining all basic mechanical properties after 6 weeks in vivo.

Nerve repair

A small caliber (8-0 or 9-0) nonabsorbable and monofilament suture is preferred, such as polyamide (Nylon) and polypropylene (Prolene).

Vascular repair

A small caliber (8-0 or 9-0) nonabsorbable and monofilament suture such as Prolene is recommended for vascular repair or anastomosis. **Table 6.4** demonstrates the sutures we recommend for various tissue structures.

Table 6.4 Recommended Sutures for tissues

Tissue layers	Sutures
Skin/subcuticular	Nylon, Prolene, Monocryl (6-0)
Dermal suture	Vicryl, PDS (4-0 or 5-0)
Deep/superficial fascia	Vicryl, PDS (2-0 or 3-0)
Tendon repair	Ethibond (3-0 or 4-0)
Vascular suture	Prolene (8-0 or 9-0)
Nerve repair	Prolene (8-0 or 9-0)

SUGGESTED READING

Athwal GS, Bueno RA Jr, Wolfe SW. Radiation exposure in hand surgery: mini versus standard C-arm. J Hand Surg Am 2005; 30:1310–1316.

Bezwada RS, Jamiolkowski DD, Lee IY. Monocryl suture, a new ultra-pliable absorbable monofilament suture. Biomaterials 1995; 16:1141–1148.
This study compared a new absorbable monofilament suture of Monocryl to PDS, Chromic gut, and Vicryl. They found that Monocryl displayed excellent handling properties, excellent tensile properties, and minimal tissue reaction, with complete absorption at 91st and 119th days of implantation.

Caulfield RH, Maleki-Tabrizi A, Patel H, Coldham F. Comparison of zone1 to 4 flexor tendon repairs using absorbable and unabsorbable four-strand core sutures. J Hand Surg Eur Vol 2008; 33:412–417.
In this study, the authors conducted a retrospective review of 576 Zone 1 to 4 flexor tendon repairs comparing absorbable sutures and nonabsorbable sutures. They found that absorbable and nonabsorbable four strand core sutures had no significant differences in regard to wound infection, tendon ruptures, and tenolysis.

Erel E, Pleasance PI, Ahmed O et al. Absorbable versus non-absorbable suture in carpal tunnel decompression. J Hand Surg Br 2001; 26:157–158.

Estebe JP, Le Naoures A, Chemaly L, et al. Tourniquet pain in a volunteer study: effect of changes in cuff width and pressure. Anaesthesia 2000; 55:21–26.
This study described the relationship between tourniquet cuff size, occlusion pressure, and pain in 20 volunteers. They found that a wide tourniquet cuff (14 cm) was less painful than a narrow (7 cm) cuff when the pressure was less than 100 mmHg. However, if the occlusion pressure inflated to more than 100 mmHg, a small tourniquet was found to induce less pain.

Kharwadka N, Naique S, Molitor PJ. Prospective randomized trial comparing absorbable and non-absorbable suture in open carpal tunnel release. J Hand Surg Br 2005; 30:92–95.
This prospective randomized study showed that at 3-month final follow-up, absorbable sutures resulted in better outcome than nonabsorbable suture in regard to pillar pain. There were no significant differences in scar tenderness and extent of wound inflammation between the absorbable sutures and nonabsorbable sutures in 33 patients who underwent open carpal tunnel release.

Odinsson A, Finsen V. Tourniquet use and its complication in Norway. J Bone Joint Surg Br 2006; 88:1090–1092.
This retrospective study reviewed complications in 63484 operations using tourniquets, and found that the overall incidence of tourniquet complications was 0.04%. Neurological complications were found to account for 58% of all complications.

Chapter 7 Rehabilitation

Jeanne M. Riggs, Kevin C. Chung

The hand therapist may spend considerably more time with a patient than the physician and have the opportunity to observe and monitor their progress, learn about the patient's concerns, and be able to communicate with the physician when deemed necessary. The principles of rehabilitation that will result in better outcomes in patients with hand injuries include

- Effective communication: The physician should communicate any concerns or changes in the patient's status that would affect the therapist's treatment approach. This effective communication between the surgeon/physician and therapist is vital to maximize the best outcome for the patient
- Early intervention in general is the goal of the hand therapist. It can improve the patient's quality of life in the short term (e.g. wearing a splint rather than a cast), manage early edema, and promote wound healing. It also provides vital patient education about their injury and subsequent precautions, promote gliding of adjacent structures with early range of motion (ROM) so as to prevent scar adhesions, and develop a rapport with the involved patient in order to allow them to express their concerns and fears in a therapeutic relationship
- Patient education is provided both verbally, demonstrated, and in writing regarding contraindications and precautions regarding his/her injury or condition. The patient should feel confident in their own ability to protect themselves from further injury, able to manage their symptoms, and welcome to ask questions. The patient is provided with a thorough home exercise program that may include edema, wound, and/or scar management, ROM, splinting, and strengthening among other treatment programs
- Frequent evaluation provides the therapist with information on the patient's progress, necessary data to rationalize ongoing therapy to insurance companies, encourages the patient by demonstrating that his/her efforts are paying off, and provides guidance in adjusting the therapy regime to address status changes
- Sound clinical judgment is based on having all of the facts, having the knowledge base regarding anatomy, therapy protocols, knowledge based on clinical experience, collaborating with colleagues when necessary, and including the patient's input in decision making

THERAPEUTIC INTERVENTIONS

Wound management

A sutured surgical incision will epithelialize within 6–48 hours, and the healing of a noninfected wound by secondary intention is also predictable. Complications may arise due to factors such as malnutrition, irradiation, medication, immunosuppression, or poor local blood supply. A simplified explanation of appropriate wound cleansing is based on the color of the open wound as described by J Cuzzell:

- Black: The presence of eschar or thick necrotic tissue characterizes the black wound. Whirlpool, irrigation, and soap and water scrubs may be used to cleanse the wound. Surgical, mechanical, or enzymatic removal of the eschar is important to allow for cellular migration and proliferation and also reduce a medium in which bacteria can grow. Wet-to-dry dressings or the use of enzymatic ointment or synthetic dressings to promote autolysis are used
- Yellow: The yellow wound is characterized by drainage present that may be purulent with slough that ranges from liquid to semiliquid and has a distinctive odor. Colonization with pseudomonas gives the tissue a yellow-greenish appearance. Soap and water are best with avoidance of antiseptics. Regular cleaning, debridement of nonviable tissue, and use of absorbent dressings are important
- Red: This is a wound that is healing uneventfully, with no signs of infection, and characterized by granulation tissue and definite borders. Sterile saline or water is used and again, antiseptics are avoided. Dressings that may adhere and disturb healthy forming granulation tissue when removed are avoided

Edema control

The following measures are useful in edema control:

- Elevation: A simple yet effective way to enhance venous and lymphatic flow out of an edematous upper extremity is to elevate the hand slightly higher than the wrist, the wrist slightly higher than the elbow, and the elbow positioned and supported slightly higher than the shoulder. This level of elevation is altered to address arterial occlusion to below the heart. Special precautions must be taken with revascularization, replantation, and transplantation patients to avoid stressing the arterial system by elevating the limb at the level of the heart and modifying this according to the patient's vascular status
- Compression: Many commercial dressings are available to provide digital level, hand, and forearm/elbow compression to assist with venous and lymphatic drainage. Dressings are applied distal to proximal. For digital level compression, options include self-adhesive wrap, x-span tubular dressing, and finger socks sewn from Ace wrap. For compression of the hand and forearm, edema gloves, elasticated tubular stockinette (**Figure 7.1a** and **b**), and Ace wrap are available. For more proximal compression, larger elasticated tubular stockinette, and Ace wrap can be used. Custom compression garments are sometimes indicated as well as the use of short stretch bandages for lymphedema
- Cold: Cold packs, ice, a frozen bag of peas, or vapocoolant sprays may be used to facilitate edema reduction as well as pain reduction. When a limb has sensory or vascular compromise, this should be used with caution
- Massage: A variety of techniques can be used to massage excessive tissue fluid and protein from an edematous upper extremity. Retrograde massage, effleurage, and stroking as well as a special manual edema mobilization technique used for lymphedema are some common techniques
- Elevated fist pumping: The patient is instructed to hold their hand above their elbow and their elbow slightly above their shoulder as they repeatedly make a fist and open their hand fully. This may be performed quite often during the day
- Contrast bath: A contrast bath begins and ends in warm water. The patient soaks their hand/wrist in warm water (bathtub

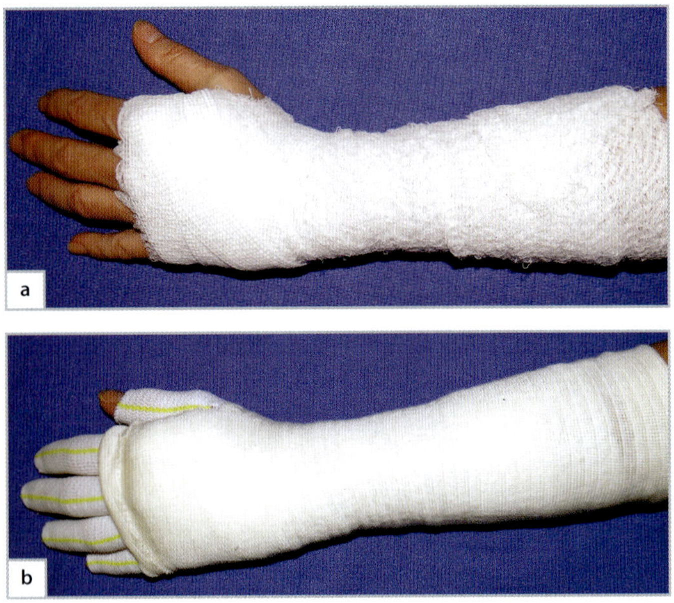

Figure 7.1 Compressive dressing for the hand and forearm.

temperature) for 2–3 minutes followed by a cold water soak (mildly uncomfortable) for 1–2 minutes. The patient alternates between the two soaks for 15 minutes, ending in the warm water

Scar remodeling

The following measures are useful in the management of scars:

- Massage: Following suture removal, massage is initiated several times a day to facilitate the reduction in adhesions between the skin and underlying tissue
- Deep friction massage and retraction: Efforts to separate the skin layer from underlying adhesions are enhanced by using Dycem to offer friction with massage (**Figure 7.2**). Dycem is a soft, flexible nonslip material for use with massage over an adherent scar, performed when the skin is clean and dry
- Gel sheeting/otoform: Silicone Elastomer Sheeting (Silon-SES) is used in the prevention of keloid or hypertrophic scarring and is versatile in use as it may be cut to any size or shape desired. Silicone has the added benefits of hydrating the tissue and softens/smoothes the scar. It is used in combination with compression or splinting and should not be used over a wound. Gel caps (Silopad brand gel caps) are lined with a polymer gel that slowly releases a medical grade mineral oil to soften and moisturize the skin and reduce scarring. A custom insert can be made using Rolyan elastomer putty that takes approximately 5 minutes to cure and offers additional pressure over a scar when used in combination with a compression garment or splint
- Custom compression garments: These are used to provide 200 mmHg of pressure to decrease the inflammatory response and the amount of blood flow to a forming scar. They also reduce itching and swelling. Gloves, gauntlets, or sleeves can be measured and ordered and it is recommended that compression garments are worn for 12–18 months until scars are mature, in the case of a burn scar. The three signs of an immature hypertrophic scar are raised, red, and rigid. Garments are replaced every 8 weeks

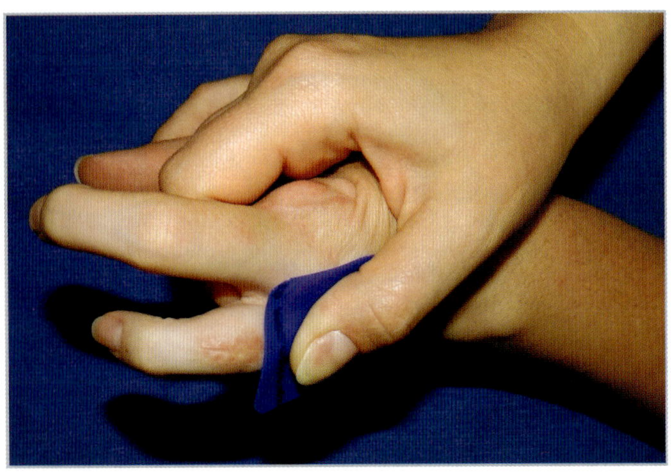

Figure 7.2 Scar retraction with Dycem.

Desensitization

- Textures: Graded from soft to rough, materials are used against the skin until accommodation to the particular texture is accomplished
- Pressure: Light pressure to firmer pressure is used during massage efforts, using the uninvolved hand
- Contact particles: A variety of dry materials such as rice, beans, popcorn kernels, or peas can be used as a medium (**Figure 7.3**). Small objects may be placed in these contact particles and the patient attempts to retrieve them
- Vibration: A battery operated minivibrator may be used to provide vibration, using one of three rubber head attachments

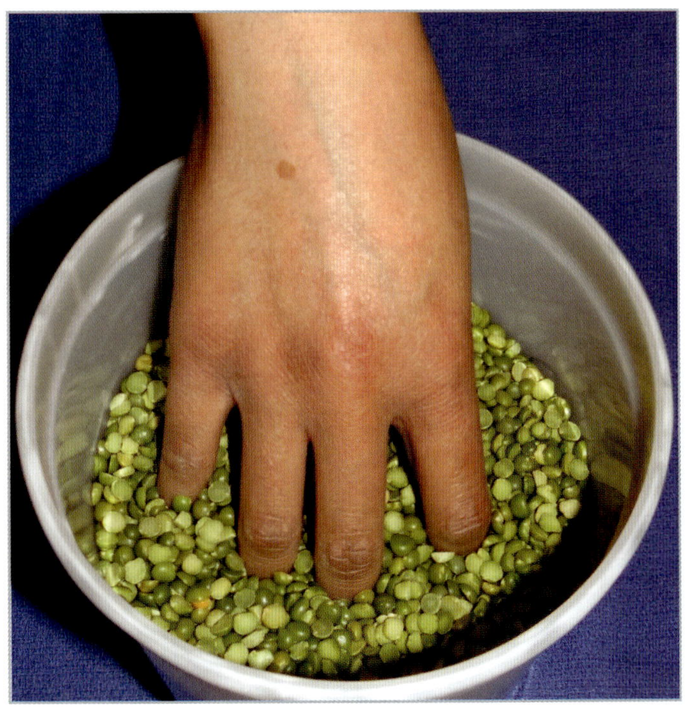

Figure 7.3 Desensitization exercise with contact particles (split peas).

Pain management

- Use of heat: Patients may benefit from the use of heat to relieve pain as well as prior to exercise sessions to increase tissue extensibility and improve performance. Heat comes in many forms such as electric heating pads, microwavable gel or rice packs, a warm damp towel heated either in the clothes dryer or simply using hot water from the sink, paraffin wax, hot water bottle, foot massage bath, or warm water soaks in a sink or bucket. If edema is a concern, heat should be used in an elevated position. If sensory loss is present, close monitoring of skin should take place to prevent a possible burn
- Use of cold: Patients may respond to cold for pain relief as well as to reduce edema, especially following an exercise session that may have increased their pain level. This can be accomplished using an ice pack from the freezer, a homemade slush pack (double bagged solution of one part rubbing alcohol to two parts water) from the freezer, or simply a frozen bag of peas that will conform to the area nicely. A paper cup can be filled with water and frozen and then peeled back to ice directly over the skin

Sensory re-education

The following exercises are recommended to be performed three times a day for 10 minute sessions:

- Localization of touch: Patient closes their eyes as someone touches their hand with the eraser end of a pencil. Patient opens their eyes and points to the spot they felt the eraser. If incorrect, the touch is applied in the same spot but this time with the patient's eyes open. Seeing and feeling where they are touched helps to train the sensory nerves. Again the patient closes their eyes, and someone touches them in the exact same spot again and the patient then points to where they felt the touch. This exercise is performed in different areas of the hand, starting with larger objects and then switching to small objects such as a paper clip as sensation improves
- Discrimination: Patient closes their eyes and feels two different grades of sandpaper with their hand. Patient states if they feel the same or different. If they cannot feel a difference between the two grades, this is done again with their eyes open. Patient closes their eyes and feels the same two grades of sandpaper again and is asked if they can feel a difference
- Fabric swatch matching: Patient closes their eyes and feels a sample swatch of fabric and then feels three choices (1 choice should be the same as the sample) and tries to identify which of the three choices match the sample. As the patient improves, more choices are provided. Patient may attempt to match pairs of matching swatches, initially with only 3 pairs and moving up to 10 pairs
- Other ideas: Patient has someone trace letters, numbers, or shapes on their hand as they try to identify it with vision occluded. Patient is provided with a variety of coins to identify with vision occluded. Patient tries to remove small objects from a bowl of dried contact particles such as rice or beans

Range of motion (ROM) exercises

- Active range of motion (AROM): AROM exercises are performed using the patient's own muscle power through the available arc of motion, without the assistance of any external forces. AROM exercises facilitate tendon gliding and assist in the reduction in edema and pain. Tendon gliding exercises are one type of AROM exercise that move the flexor tendons through their maximum excursion potential (**Figure 7.4a–c**). Intrinsic hand muscle exercises include digital abduction/adduction and metacarpophalangeal (MCP) flexion/extension with interphalangeal (IP) joint extension. Extrinsic hand muscle exercises include tendon glides, taking the digits from full extension, into a 'hook' fist, then a full composite fist, and finally into a flat fist. Thumb active exercises include circumduction of the thumb carpometacarpal joint and radial and palmar abduction/adduction; MCP and IP joint exercises include flexion and extension and opposition, as the patient attempts to oppose each fingertip. Wrist AROM includes wrist flexion and extension exercises that can be performed both with and without a fist, and wrist radial and ulnar deviation. Forearm rotation is performed with the elbow at 90° at the patient's side, to isolate the forearm rotation from any compensatory shoulder rotation. Pronation and supination are then performed

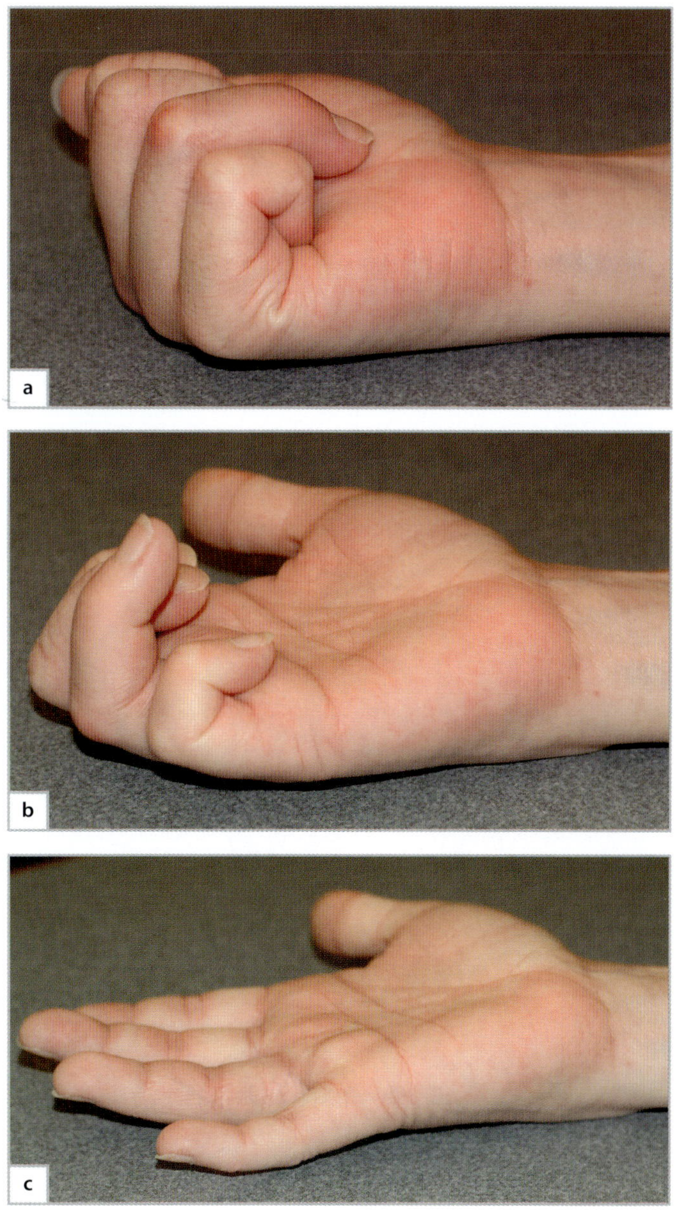

Figure 7.4 Flexor tendon gliding exercises for differential gliding of flexor digitorum superficialis and flexor digitorum tendons.

- Active-assisted range of motion (AAROM) and passive range of motion (PROM): AAROM exercises involve the stabilization of proximal joints to improve the mechanical advantage of the muscles that move the distal joints. PROM exercises are performed when the muscles are relaxed and the joint(s) are moved manually by the patient using the uninvolved hand or when another individual or external force is moving the joint(s). An individual cannot have active motion greater than the allowable passive suppleness of the joints
- Nerve glides: The peripheral nervous system involves excursion or gliding of the nerves during normal joint movement; however, this may be altered due to surgical scarring, edema, compression, or pain that limits normal movement and thus normal excursion. Nerve glides are performed in a pain-free manner to restore mobility and/or improve a patient's tolerance for tension at a remote joint that may assist the nerve in attenuating tension throughout its length and thus improve a patient's pain symptoms
- Sustained stretching: To address limited passive motion of the wrist, a sustained stretch can be provided using 1–3 pounds. The forearm is supported and the wrist and hand hang over the edge of a table or arm of a chair in either pronation (for a wrist flexion stretch) or in supination (for a wrist extension stretch) for at least 5–7 minutes. This can be done in combination with heat to facilitate ROM. A small hammer (12–16 ounces) is helpful in facilitating forearm rotation. The elbow is positioned at 90° at the patient's side and the forearm is supported, while the hammer is held in the hand for 5–7 minutes to allow the head of the hammer to elicit a stretch in either pronation or supination. The grip may progress toward the bottom of the handle to increase torque. A sustained stretch can be provided to the digits compositely using either paper tape or self-adhesive tape as well as a fabricated flexion glove to address extrinsic extensor tightness or joint stiffness (**Figure 7.5a** and **b**). The tape may be used in combination with a heat application and done prior to AROM exercises for 15 minutes. During the taping, layers of tape may be added as the digits accommodate to the stretch and a greater stretch is desired

Strengthening

- Isometric (static) strengthening: When a patient demonstrates a limited arc of motion of a joint due to pain, strengthening may be appropriate, beginning with isometric strengthening in the neutral position. For example, a patient who has healed from a distal radius fracture can benefit from isometric wrist flexion and extension exercises with the wrist in neutral. These are done several times a day, long enough to recruit as many muscle fibers as possible (10 seconds) using maximum contraction or effort
- Eccentric strengthening: Applying resistance during the lengthening phase of a muscle contraction is often tolerated in a patient with pain when concentric strengthening is too painful. Lateral epicondylitis patients often begin with eccentric strengthening of the wrist extensors by holding a 1–3 pound weight in their hand, passively placing the wrist in extension, and then actively bringing the wrist into flexion while the forearm is supported and resting in the pronated position over the edge of a table
- Concentric strengthening: Applying resistance during the shortening phase of a muscle contraction can be done with low-repetition exercises using high tension to gain muscle strength. Progression involves increasing the duration, the intensity (combination of resistance and speed), frequency, or any combination of these
- Grip/pinch strengthening: Strengthening grip and pinch muscles of the forearm and hand can be done simply by gradually resuming normal activities of daily living in an elderly patient, to providing resistive putty, a rubber ball, a spring-loaded gripper, or a rubber band gripper to a patient who progresses with repetitions and resistance levels

Psychological support

An empathic conversation alone has healing power. Be sure to have the patient share with you what their goals are for attending OT and try to understand their perception of their problems. Early on, try to judge their underlying ability to cope with their condition/injury.

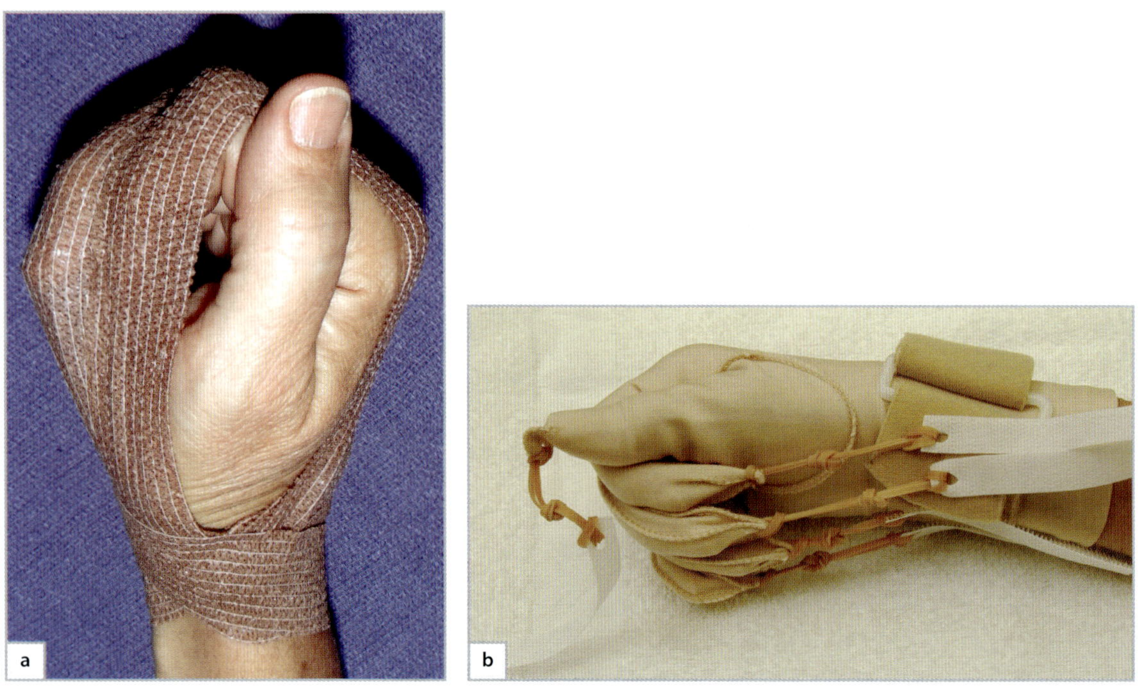

Figure 7.5 Sustained passive digital flexion stretch using self-adhesive wrap or custom flexion glove.

A psychological screening tool can acknowledge the importance of the emotional function of an individual and allow them to feel more comfortable in sharing their true feelings and thoughts. Do not be afraid to discuss depression, loss of interest in family, friends, or leisure activities or if the patient is experiencing thoughts of suicide, because discussing this would not put the idea in a patient's head. Understand that the smallest of scars or perceived injury can easily be magnified in a patient's mind and underappreciated by the therapist and physician.

Orthoses

Orthoses are fabricated to meet the patient's individual needs, designed with an appreciation of the various factors of anatomy, physiology, kinesiology, pathology, rehabilitation goals, occupation, and the emotional status of the individual.

- Static: A static orthosis supports a joint or joints in one position (**Figure 7.6**). The goals of wearing a static orthosis are to immobilize joint(s) to allow them to rest, prevent deformity progression by providing a preferred position when the orthosis is worn, and to prevent soft tissue contracture by positioning the hand in a protected posture. A static orthosis may be serially adjusted to improve joint motion by reheating the orthosis and fitting it to the joint or joints in an improved position following treatment. Some static orthoses are worn for a brief period of time, e.g. for fracture healing, whereas others are worn for months or possibly years, such as a rheumatoid arthritis patient wearing a night resting orthosis for joint protection

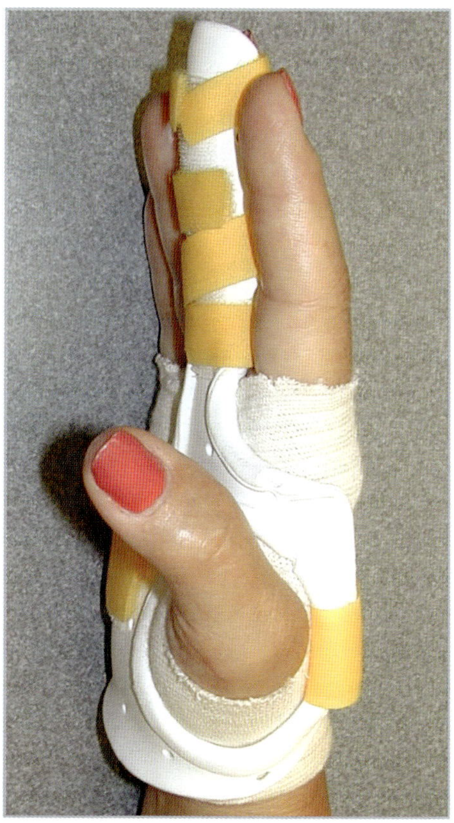

Figure 7.6 Example of a static custom orthosis: hand-based extension gutter orthosis

- Dynamic: A dynamic orthosis provides movement and controlled force to improve the available joint ROM (**Figure 7.7**). Too little force will accomplish nothing and too much force will possibly result in a soft tissue response of pain and edema, further worsening stiffness. There are many principles and methods of fabricating dynamic orthoses to accomplish the goals of orthosis wear. Frequent assessment of changes in ROM, evidence of sheering forces on the skin, pressure points from the orthosis, angle of pull, tension used, and proper donning and doffing of the orthosis by the patient are some of the important guidelines in the use of a dynamic orthoses
- Static progressive: The theory of static progressive orthoses is that by providing the correct mechanical stress to contracted soft tissue structures over a prolonged period of time, you allow for elongation and 'creep' of the contracted structures that provide a permanent length change (**Figure 7.8**)
- Prefabricated orthoses: When a custom orthosis is not needed or not an option, an off the shelf orthosis may suffice to provide support and gentle immobilization to a joint. Orthoses come in neoprene or fabric with elastic and self-adhesive hook and loop strapping, and are typically washable by hand or in a washing machine. Some prefabricated orthoses, such as a wrist orthosis, may have metal stays to provide further support

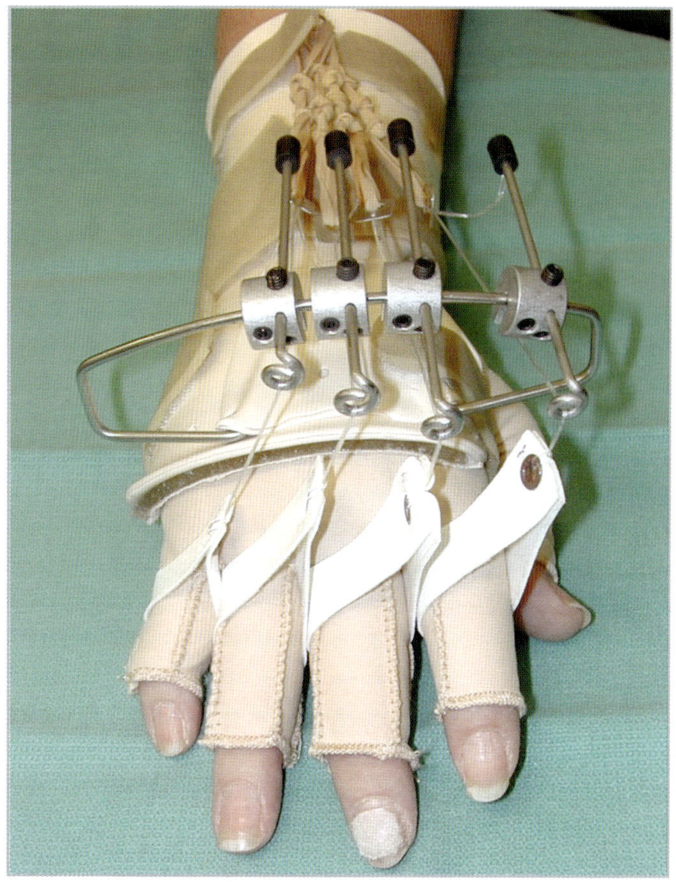

Figure 7.7 Dynamic metacarpophalangeal (MCP) extension orthosis worn following MCP joint arthroplasty.

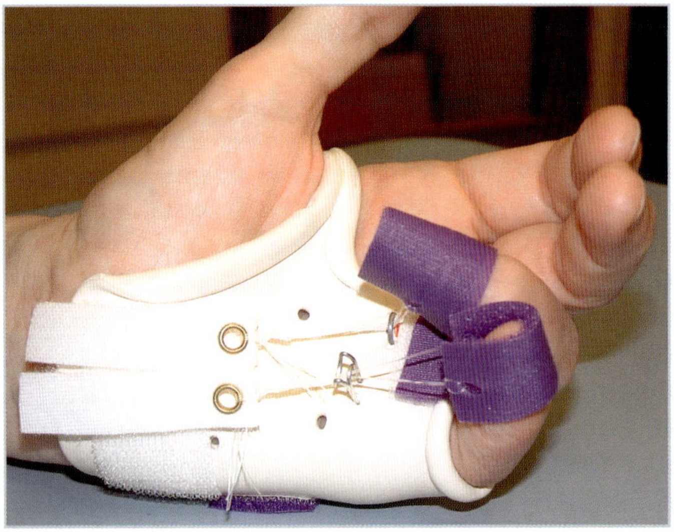

Figure 7.8 Static progressive orthoses for sustained passive IP joint flexion stretching.

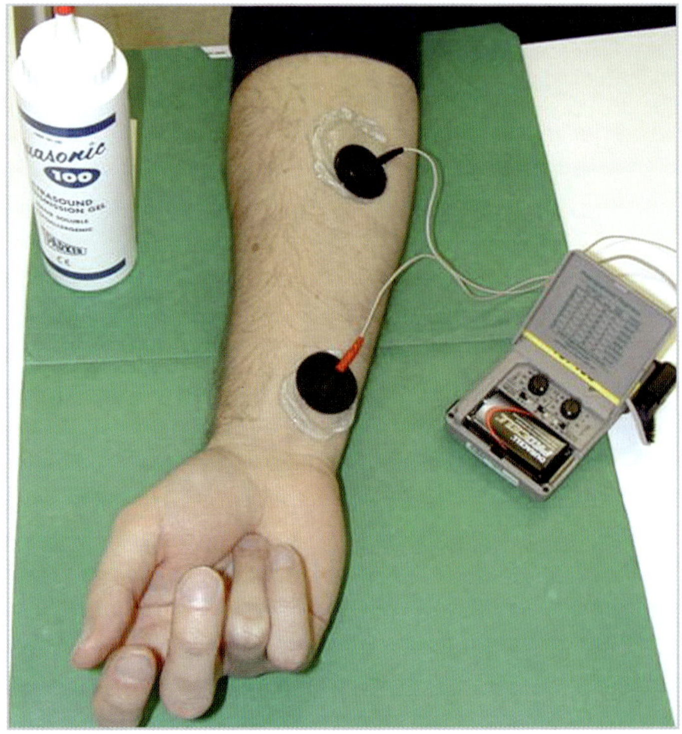

Figure 7.9 Neuromuscular electrical stimulation to flexor digitorum superficialis muscle to facilitate digital flexion.

Thermal modalities

- Heat: The benefits from using heat prior to exercise are well documented. Vasodilation and increased blood flow caused by heat can improve nutrition to healing structures, decrease pain, and increase extensibility of connective tissue. Superficial heat includes the use of moist heat packs, paraffin, electrical heating packs, and Fluidotherapy, whereas deep heat is provided by ultrasound. Patients with sensitivity to heat may benefit from wearing a warm, loose, cotton or plastic glove for 20 minutes prior to exercises and receive the benefit of relaxation when heat application is not possible. In the hand, there is little adipose tissue, therefore superficial heat sources may sufficiently heat the deeper structures such as the joint
- Ice: The use of ice will reduce muscle spasms, inflammatory edema, and pain. Use of cold is contraindicated in patients with Raynaud phenomena, and must be closely monitored in patients suffering from sensory deficits. In addition, the use of cold with scleroderma patients is generally contraindicated as they typically have Raynaud phenomena
- Contrast bath: As previously described, by alternating between warm and cold soaks, vasodilation and vasoconstriction are accomplished, which can be helpful in pain reduction as well as edema control. The patient is to spend approximately 15 minutes alternating between warm water and cold water soaks ending and beginning with the warm water. A ratio of 3:1 in warm and cold allows for 4 warm soaks and 3 and cold soaks. The warm water should be bathtub temperature, whereas the cold water should be mildly uncomfortable with the use of ice cubes permitted

Electrical modalities

- Neuromuscular electrical stimulation (NMES): The use of pulsated current for stimulation of innervated muscles can maintain or gain ROM and facilitate muscle contraction (**Figure 7.9**). NMES selectively stimulates the large muscle fibers and can be a useful adjunct to active exercises for atrophy reduction and increased strength. The units are battery operated and have two to four electrodes to allow for one or two muscle placements during a 15-minute session. One electrode is active and is placed over the muscle belly, while the second electrode is dispersive and is placed in an adjacent area. The on/off cycle is recommended to be a 1:2 or 1:3 ratio to prevent muscle fatigue
- Transcutaneous electrical nerve stimulation (TENS): Electrical stimulation for the use of pain control is known as TENS and works by a 'spinal gating' mechanism of action to block pain signals. The TENS provides a modulated current of bursts with an intensity not strong enough to elicit a contraction of the muscles. Electrode placement generally brackets the painful area or may be used in a clamshell manner such as dorsally and volarly over a painful wrist

SUGGESTED READING

Cuzzell JZ. The new RYB color code. Am J of Nurs 1988; 88:1342–1346.

Evans RB. Managing the injured tendon: current concepts. J Hand Ther 2012; 25:173–189.

A pioneer in tendon repair rehabilitation, Evans provides a thorough look at flexor and extensor tendons from the anatomy and mechanics to current concepts in rehabilitation.

Glasgow C, Tooth LR, Fleming J. Mobilizing the stiff hand: combining theory and evidence to improve clinical outcomes. J Hand Ther 2010; 23:392–400.

The authors provide a narrative review of the evidence behind a variety of therapy interventions for joint stiffness of the hand.

Hannah SD. Psychosocial issues after a traumatic hand injury: facilitating adjustment. J Hand Ther 2011; 24:95–102.

A hand therapist has a unique role in facilitating a patient's psychosocial adaptation and adjustment. Assessment tools, coping strategies, and role change are some of the topics discussed.

Schultz-Johnson K. Static progressive splinting. J Hand Ther 2002; 15:163–178.

The author describes static progressive splinting indications, guidelines for creating a splint wearing regimen, and offers many examples of static progressive splints.

Villeco JP. Edema: a silent but important factor. J Hand Ther 2012; 25:153–161.

Edema and its relationship to the stages of healing are simply explained and the research supporting edema management techniques is reviewed.

Section 2

Emergency hand surgery

Chapter 8 Examination of the traumatized hand

Shady A. Rehim, Kevin C. Chung

INTRODUCTION

Hand injuries account for almost 10% of the total injuries that present annually to emergency room (ER) in the United States. Naturally, the hand is a complex anatomical structure consisting of multiple bones, tendons, nerves, muscles, and blood vessels. As a result of this complex anatomical configuration, the management of hand trauma is often challenging and requires a great level of knowledge and expertise. Physicians involved in the management of hand trauma should therefore develop good history-taking skills and clinical examination techniques as well as a sound knowledge of the basic concepts of management of hand trauma in order to evaluate and manage hand injuries more effectively. The purpose of this chapter is to describe the different patterns of hand injuries and to explain the examination techniques of common hand trauma that is frequently encountered in the ER. It should also be emphasized that despite management of a large number of hand injuries in the ER, emergency physicians, junior residents, and nurse practitioners should always keep a low threshold for making appropriate and prompt referrals to a specialized hand surgeon if necessary.

TYPES OF HAND INJURIES (FIGURE 8.1A–F)

- Laceration injuries
- Crush injuries
- Degloving injuries
- Amputation injuries
- Bite injuries (animal and human bites)
- Electrical and burn injuries
- The mangled hand (a combination of several types of injury patterns present in a single hand)
- Hand injuries can also be classified as open or closed injuries according to the integrity of the overlying skin and soft tissue coverage of the hand. Additionally, hand injuries may be associated with underlying bone injuries, which again can be classified as open or closed fractures

EVALUATION OF HAND INJURIES

The clinical presentation of hand trauma varies widely, from a simple skin laceration that may or may not require further treatment, to more extensive types of injuries that can be life or limb threatening. Because of the large variation in clinical presentation, it is prudent that physicians develop a systematic approach that incorporates pertinent examination techniques when evaluating and treating hand injuries. There are several methods of evaluating hand injuries, but in this chapter we will follow an algorithmic approach (in line with Acute Trauma Life Support-ATLS protocol) to initially evaluate and manage common hand injuries (**Figure 8.2**), in a way that is consistent and universally accepted. In the following sections, we will focus on two areas, namely history taking and physical examination of traumatized hands.

History taking

Good history-taking skills are an integral part of the initial evaluation process of patients with hand trauma. One should start by asking open-ended questions to gather as much information as possible relating to the trauma event. Then, closed ended questions are used to address specific issues related to the unique features of each type of injury. However, with any form of hand trauma, the following aspects should be considered:

- Mechanism of injury: The mechanism of injury helps a physician determine the extent of injury. For example, minor injuries may not require further investigation or treatment if the rest of the clinical examination is unremarkable. However, severe trauma such as amputation or crush injuries should alert physicians to the possibility of coexisting conditions such as compartment syndrome or injuries of the underlying structures such as bones, tendons, nerves, or blood vessels that would require additional investigations (e.g. X-rays, CT, or angiography) to guide further management
- Time of injury: The time of injury helps to distinguish between primary or delayed clinical presentations by estimating the time interval between the initial injury and the time of first medical assessment of that injury. Wounds presenting several days or weeks after the initial trauma are often neglected and contaminated, or even infected. These types of injuries are usually not amenable to primary closure or repair (e.g. definitive soft tissue coverage or primary tendon repair) until the wounds are adequately cleaned and debrided
- Place of injury: It is important to know the environment in which the injury took place. Injuries occurring in farmyards may be grossly contaminated with soil, thus subjecting patients to several types of infections including *Clostridium tetani* infection, which is associated with high mortality. Similarly, injuries occurring in industrial areas should draw physicians' attention to the possibility of exposure to hazardous material such as chemicals. In both scenarios, the treatment should be initiated immediately. It should be noted that chemical burns, in particular, often result in an ongoing process of tissue damage that lasts for several hours following the initial injury. Therefore, with these types of injuries it is essential to fully explore a patient's history and initiate the appropriate management without delay
- To obtain a full patient history, inquire about the following additional information:
  - Patients' age, gender, occupation, handedness, and hobbies

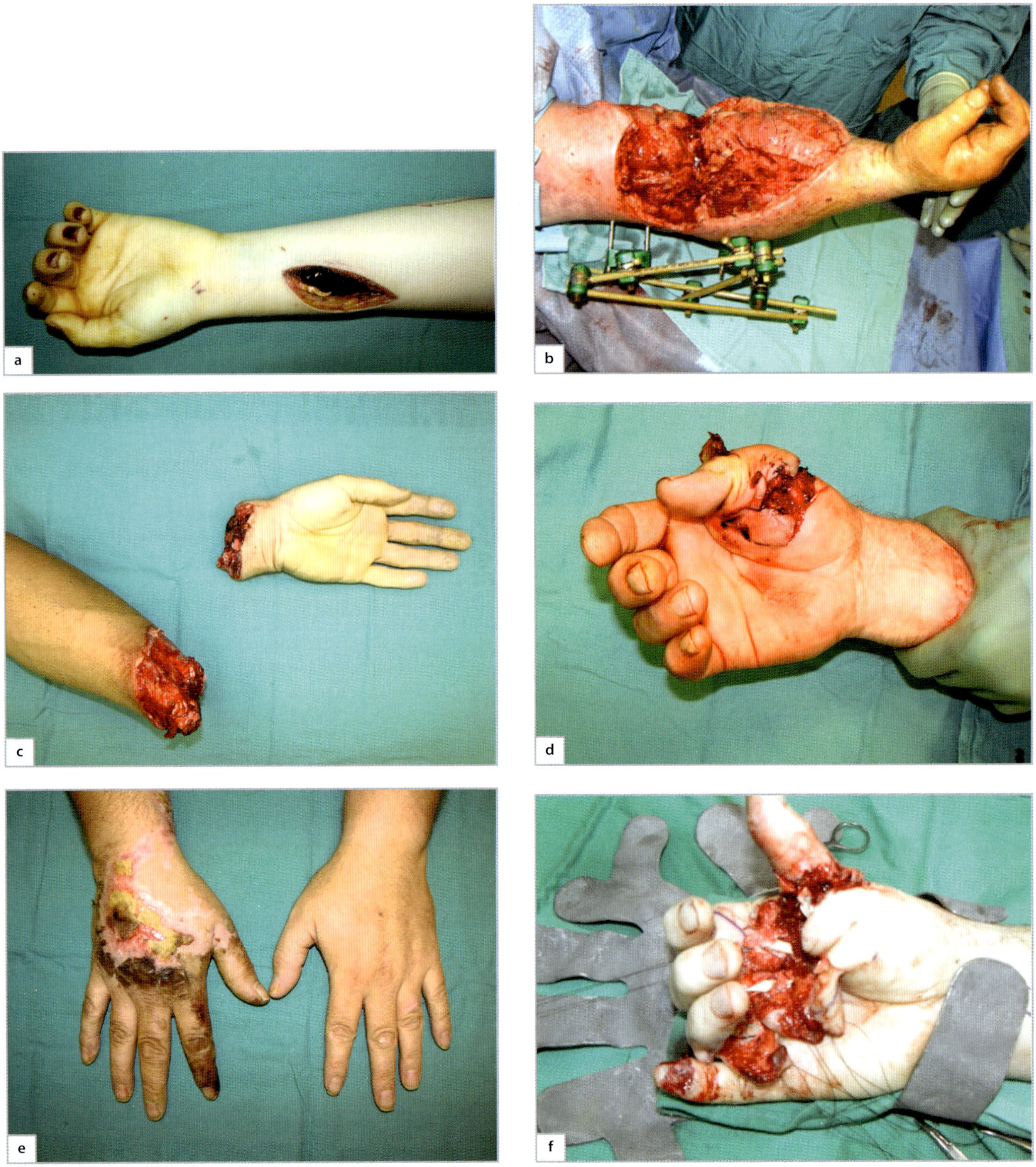

Figure 8.1 Demonstration of different types of injuries: (a) Laceration injuries, (b) degloving injuries, (c) amputation injuries, (d) bite injuries (extensive dog bite), (e) burn injuries, and (f) the mangled hand.

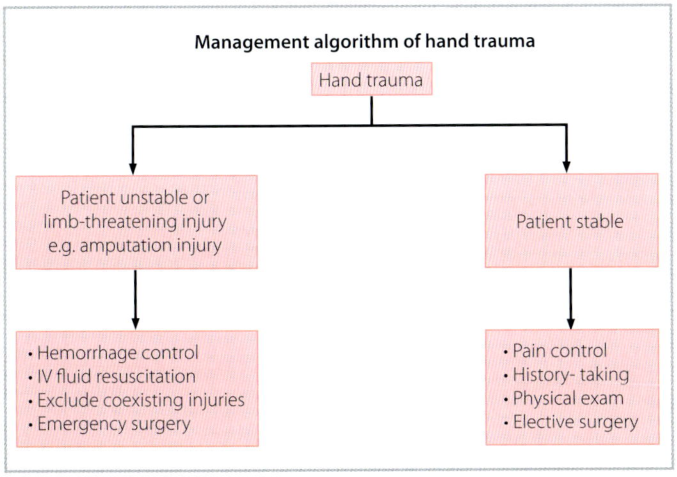

Figure 8.2 A simplified algorithm to prioritize initial management of hand trauma according to the patient's general health condition and presence of coexisting morbidities.

- Patients' allergy status
- Immunization history. This is particularly important, as a tetanus booster/immunization in a nonimmunized patient may prove to be lifesaving
- Past medical and surgical history, including careful documentation of previous injuries, disabilities, or surgeries performed, especially to the affected hand. A patient's eligibility or fitness for surgery should be assessed by establishing the ASA (American Society of Anesthesiologists) grade for each patient. Patients who are considered among the high-risk group (ASA ≥3) from the anesthetic point of view may be candidates for locoregional anesthesia instead of general anesthesia

Physical examination

The physical examination begins by a general 'screening' of a patient's hands to look for obvious injuries or deformities, followed by a specific and detailed examination of the hand to identify injured structures. It is important to compare the injured hand with the contralateral noninjured hand to recognize the 'normal' appearance and function of an individual patient's hands. Before embarking on the physical examination, ensure a patient's comfort by adequately controlling pain using sufficient analgesia. However, local anesthetic given to an injured finger or hand is not advisable, until a full hand examination has been performed by an experienced physician to document potential nerve injuries.

The sequential steps of 'look,' 'feel,' and 'move' that constitute a physical examination help to establish the clinical diagnosis. Even following those simple instructions, aspects of the physical examination may be overlooked or performed that are not clearly documented in a patient's record. For these reasons, it is helpful to have a schematic illustration (hand examination pro forma, **Figure 8.3**) that highlights the essential components of the physical examination used to evaluate hand trauma. The benefit of using hand examination pro forma is twofold:

1. It serves as a reminder of the important steps required to complete the physical examination
2. It is a reproducible (record-keeping) method to help in demonstrating patients' injuries without the need of repeatedly exposing a patient's injury, especially if coupled with clear medical photographs of the wounds

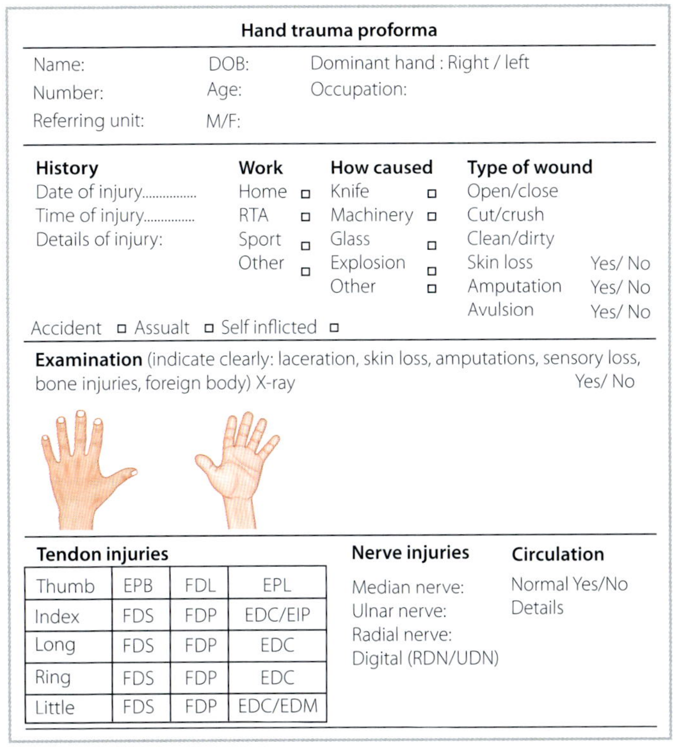
Hand trauma proforma

Name: DOB: Dominant hand : Right / left
Number: Age: Occupation:
Referring unit: M/F:

History
Date of injury...............
Time of injury..............
Details of injury:

Work
Home ☐
RTA ☐
Sport ☐
Other ☐

How caused
Knife ☐
Machinery ☐
Glass ☐
Explosion ☐
Other ☐

Type of wound
Open/close
Cut/crush
Clean/dirty
Skin loss Yes/ No
Amputation Yes/ No
Avulsion Yes/ No

Accident ☐ Assualt ☐ Self inflicted ☐

Examination (indicate clearly: laceration, skin loss, amputations, sensory loss, bone injuries, foreign body) X-ray Yes/ No

Tendon injuries

Thumb	EPB	FDL	EPL
Index	FDS	FDP	EDC/EIP
Long	FDS	FDP	EDC
Ring	FDS	FDP	EDC
Little	FDS	FDP	EDC/EDM

Nerve injuries
Median nerve:
Ulnar nerve:
Radial nerve:
Digital (RDN/UDN)

Circulation
Normal Yes/No
Details

Figure 8.3 Hand trauma pro forma.

Wound inspection

Wound inspection is an invaluable aspect of the evaluation of a traumatized hand. By simply observing the wounds and the shape of the hands at rest, one can identify the following:

- Gross examination: On first glance, look for obvious injuries and gross deformities. Rings and jewelry should be removed at this stage to prevent the development of constriction rings/bands with subsequent edema formation. By carefully looking into the wound, one can also check for the presence of obvious foreign bodies
- Presence of an infection: Look for signs of infection, which include swelling, erythema (redness), cellulitis, abscesses, or discharging sinuses
- Tissue viability: Both the palmar and dorsal sides of the hand and fingers should be fully inspected. By doing so, physicians can assess the viability of soft tissues and rule out the presence of digital ischemia. Healthy tissues appear pink whereas necrotic and devitalized tissues or ischemic digits may look pale white, dusky, or even black in color
- Boundaries of the defect: Inspecting wound site and size can provide important clues regarding any associated injuries of the deeper structures within the vicinity of the original injury. For instance, in wrist lacerations one should always suspect injury to the underlying nerves (e.g. median or ulnar nerves) or blood vessels (e.g. radial or ulnar arteries)
- Tendon injuries: The posture of the hand and/or fingers may indicate the presence of tendon injuries. For example, a finger extension lag can be suggestive of a partial or complete extensor tendon injury if no concomitant injuries (e.g. fractures/ dislocations) are present. Similarly, the inability to flex the fingers

may indicate a flexor tendon injury. In an obtunded patient, the integrity of flexor and extensor tendons can be assessed by the tenodesis effect. This is performed by passively extending and flexing the wrist while observing finger movement. When the wrist is passively extended, the fingers and thumb should fall into flexion, whereas when the wrist is passively flexed the fingers and thumb should move into full extension (**Figure 8.4**)

- Bone fractures/dislocations: Malalignment of the hands or fingertip cascade may also suggest fractures or dislocations of the underlying bone. Rotational deformities of the fingers are frequently observed with metacarpal and phalangeal fractures. In a healthy hand, the fingertips of the index to little fingers should point toward the scaphoid bone (**Figure 8.5**) when patients gently flex their fingers. However, with metacarpal or phalangeal fractures, the affected finger may overlap onto the neighboring fingers (scissoring) and/or angulate along the sagittal plane (rotation).

Palpation

Before palpating the hand, ensure that the patient is comfortable and pain free. The following items can then be examined by palpation:

- Circulation: The hand is well vascularized and contains an abundant network of collateral circulation arising from the radial and ulnar arteries. A vascular compromise to the hands or digits should be treated as a surgical emergency and necessitates urgent revascularization, especially in the event of a complete amputation. When faced with a completely amputated digit, the physician should preserve the amputated digit by taking the following sequential steps:
  - Gently cleanse the amputated digit by using an isotonic solution, such as a Ringer lactate solution
  - Wrap the amputated digit in sterile moist gauze
  - Place the digit in a plastic bag, and then place this bag in another plastic bag, and finally place this bag into a thermally insulated container that contains ice water. Try and avoid filling the container only with ice to prevent freezing of the digit
  - By palpating the hand, tissue perfusion can be assessed using the following methods:
  - Capillary refill time (CRT): Capillary refill is the rate at which blood refills empty capillaries, and is the most sensitive method of assessing tissue perfusion. It can be measured by holding the hand higher than heart level (prevents venous reflux), pressing the finger pulp until it turns white, and taking note of the time needed for the color to return once pressure is released. Normally, the CRT is approximately 2–3 seconds; however, in ischemic hands/digits this duration is prolonged
  - Temperature: A hypoperfused hand or digit will generally feel cold when compared with the noninjured side. However, this should be interpreted with caution, as the hands or digits may be cold if they were exposed to cold weather conditions during the initial injury
  - Pulse: As previously mentioned, the hand is adequately perfused via branches arising from the radial and ulnar arteries, thus the presence of a radial or ulnar pulse usually indicates a good blood supply to the hand. To test for patency of the radial and ulnar arteries, one can perform the modified Allen test (**Figure 8.6**). First ask the patient to make a tight fist so that blood is expressed out of the hand and back into the forearmThen, apply pressure at the wrist to occlude both the radial and ulnar arteries. Ask the patient to reopen his/her fist, and observe blanching (turning white/pale) of the palm. Release finger compression off the radial artery while keeping the ulnar artery occluded and observe for the return of blood flow (color change) into the palm. A color change of the palm from pale white to pink within 5–6 seconds indicates an adequate blood flow to the hand via the radial artery. To test patency of the ulnar artery, repeat the same steps, but release the pressure off the ulnar artery this time while maintaining compression of the radial artery

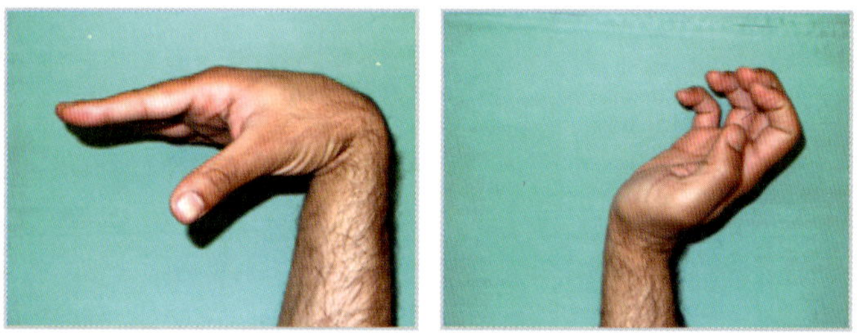

Figure 8.4 Tenodesis test/effect. Note the fingers and thumb extended on passive flexion of the wrist and flex on passive wrist extension.

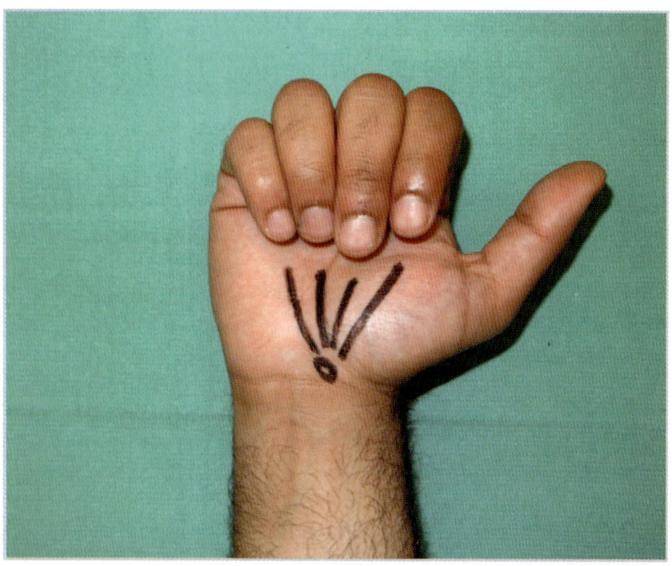

Figure 8.5 Normal fingers cascade; in a healthy hand all fingertips should point toward the scaphoid bone.

Sensory and motor function

- Sensory: The hand is innervated by sensory branches of the median, ulnar, and radial nerves, which are branches of the brachial plexus. The dermatomal distribution of the sensory supply of the hand is shown in **Figure 8.7**. Hand sensation can be assessed using the following methods:
  - Light touch and pinprick: In the hand trauma setting, light touch is the most utilized method of testing sensory function of the hand, whereas the pinprick technique is seldom used in examining hand sensation. By using the edge of a blunt object or a cotton bud, the sensation of the hands and fingers can be evaluated. However, this is a rather subjective and largely inaccurate method of assessing the sensory function of the hand. One way of improving the efficacy of this test is by asking patients to quantify their response to light touch on a scale of 0–10, where 0 is absent sensation and 10 is a full sensory response to light touch. The examiner can touch the patient's face first to establish

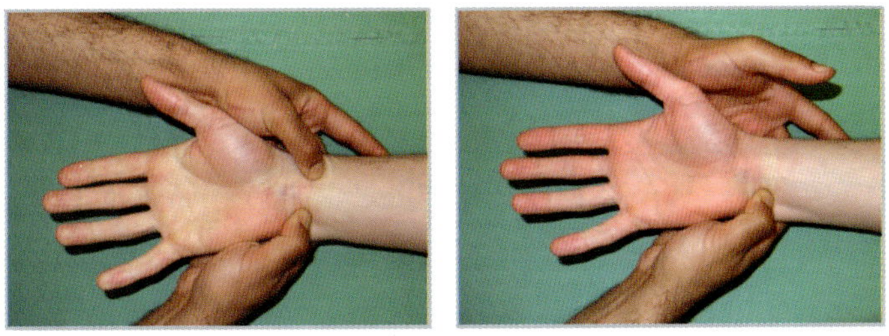

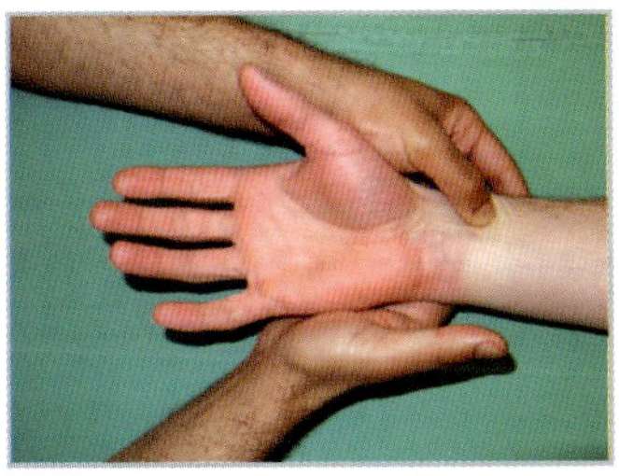

Figure 8.6 Modified Allen test. Note blanching of the palm when the radial and ulnar arteries are occluded and return of blood flow with alternate release of artery compression.

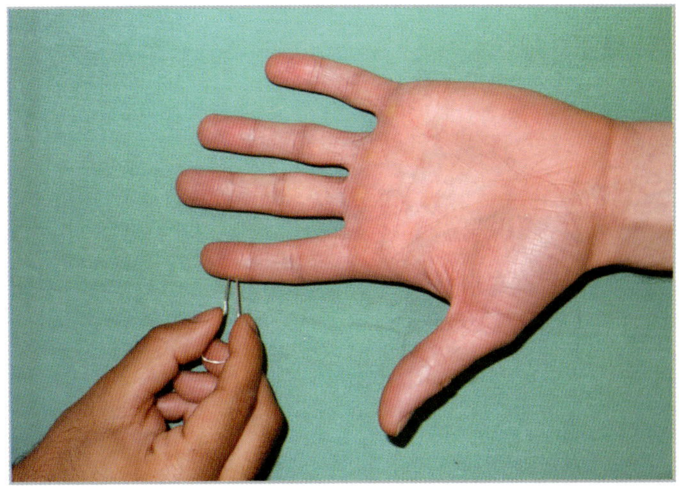

Figure 8.8 Demonstrating two-point discrimination using two blunt ends of a paper clip. It is helpful to explain to the patient how the test works, first by demonstrating the test on a patient's healthy hand with the patient's eyes open, then by repeating the test on the affected hand as described in the text with the patient's eyes closed.

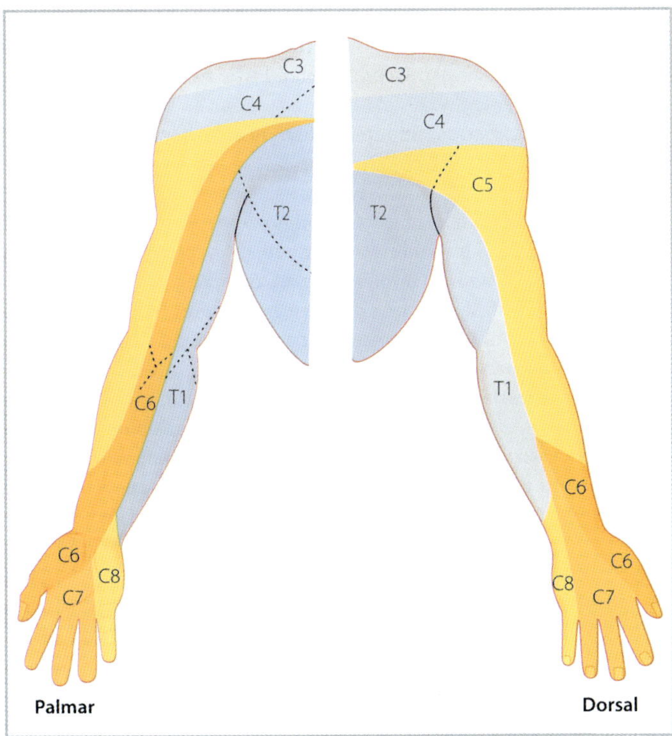

Figure 8.7 Dermatome distribution of sensory nerves of the upper limb.

normal sensation of the face as a 10 to as a reference to help the patient determine the sensation in the digit. In traumatized digits, the radial and ulnar digital nerves are often examined using this method by assessing the sensation on the radial and ulnar borders of individual fingers

- Two-point discrimination (**Figure 8.8**): This technique tests the ability of a patient to differentiate between two nearby objects touching the skin by assessing the patient's ability to determine if they are truly two distinct points and not one. Two-point discrimination is a reliable and objective method of testing hand sensation. It is best to show the patient how the test works beforehand by demonstrating the technique on the noninjured hand to make sure that the patient understands and is compliant with test instructions. To test a desired area, touch the skin using the two blunt ends of a paper clip (approximately 1 cm apart) and move them progressively closer. The distance at which the patient is no longer able to differentiate one from two points is the two-point discrimination result
- Autonomic function: The normal skin sweating ability is lost after sympathetic denervation of the fingers following digital nerve injuries. This can be examined by rolling the sides of a pen over the sides of the fingers. Normally, a resistance is met when the pen rolls over a 'sticky' surface due to the presence of sweat. However, in denervated fingers, the pen will role smoothly over dry skin surfaces

- Motor: In trauma situations, it is not always feasible to test the individual nerves for full motor function. However, performing some key tests would help the examiner to identify injured nerves:
  - Median nerve (**Figure 8.9**): Intact function of the abductor pollicis brevis muscle reliably indicates an intact motor function of the median nerve. To examine the action of the abductor pollicis brevis, lay the dorsum of the patient's hand on a flat surface, then ask the patient to palmarly abduct the thumb against resistance while palpating the muscle belly using your other hand. Another test that evaluates median nerve function is performed by asking the patient to perform the 'OK' sign that tests the opposition of the thumb against the index finger
  - Ulnar nerve: The ulnar nerve supplies most of the intrinsic muscles (palmar and dorsal interossei and the two ulnar lumbricals) of the hand. Asking a patient to demonstrate the action of these muscles will accurately reflect the motor function of the ulnar nerve. The dorsal and palmar interosseous muscles are responsible for finger abduction and adduction movements. To test the function of the interosseous muscles, place the patient's palm on a flat surface and ask them to abduct and adduct their fingers against resistance and to cross their fingers (**Figure 8.10a** and **b**). A weakness of fingers abduction and adduction movement or an inability to cross the fingers is sugges-

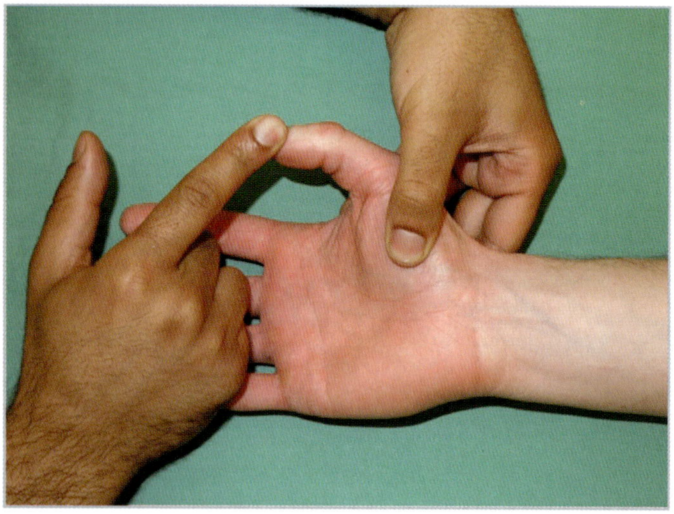

Figure 8.9 Demonstration of how to test action of the abductor pollicis brevis (APB) muscle. First lay the dorsum of a patient's hand on a tabletop then ask the patient to abduct the thumb against resistance. Note that an intact APB reliably indicates an intact motor function of the median nerve in the hand.

tive of an ulnar nerve injury. Another indication of ulnar nerve injury is the presence of Froment sign (**Figure 8.11**). This sign is observed due to weakness of the adductor pollicis muscle that is supplied by the ulnar nerve. To demonstrate this, ask the patient to hold a piece of paper between the thumb and index fingers, then pull the paper out of the patient's hand. A positive test is considered when the patient flexes the interphalangeal joint (distal phalanx) of the thumb using the flexor pollicis longus (FPL) muscle (supplied by the median nerve) instead of adducting the thumb using the adductor pollicis muscle (supplied by ulnar nerve) to hold the paper

- Radial nerve: The distal radial nerve supply of the hand is mainly sensory (dorsum of the 1st web space). However, injury of the radial nerve motor branches higher up in the forearm result in fingers drop deformity, as the radial nerve is the main nerve supply of the extensor muscles of the forearm extensor compartment

Tendon function

Examining function of individual tendons can conducted with asking the patient to flex the distal and proximal interphalangeal (PIP) joints sequentially. One should never probe the wound because it causes pain and all the information on tendon integrity can be obtained by a good hand exam. Within the context of hand trauma, the following examination techniques help to identify commonly injured tendons:

- Flexor tendons:
  - FPL: Hold the thumb metacarpal in extension and ask the patient to flex his/her thumb interphalangeal joint (distal phalanx) against resistance. An inability to flex the distal phalanx of the thumb indicates injury of the FPL
  - Flexor digitorum profundus (FDP of index to little fingers, **Figure 8.12**): Hold the finger metacarpophalangeal joint and interphalangeal joints in full extension and ask the patient to flex the distal phalanx against resistance. The inability to flex the distal phalanx of the finger indicates an injury of the FDP
  - Flexor digitorum superficialis (FDS of index to little fingers, **Figure 8.13**): The FDS is examined by holding the neighboring fingers in full extension and asking the patient to flex the metacarpophalangeal and PIP joints of the affected finger. By extending the neighboring fingers, this blocks the action of the FDP (which may compensate for the action of an injured FDS) as it arises from a common muscle belly. However, in the index finger the FDP arises from a separate muscle belly, and therefore this test is not reliable in testing the FDS function of the index finger
- Extensor tendons:
  - Extensor pollicis longus (EPL, **Figure 8.14**): The EPL tendon can be tested by asking the patient to place his/her palm on top of a flat surface and extend the thumb (tabletop test). The inability to fully extend the thumb indicates and EPL tendon injury. Additionally, an intact EPL tendon can be visualized on the dorsum of the thumb
  - Extensor indicis proprius (EIP, **Figure 8.15**): This tendon is tested by asking the patient to make a fist, and then point toward an object using the index finger. By asking the patient to make a fist, the action of the extensor digitorum communis (EDC) is excluded as it may compensate for an injured EIP tendon

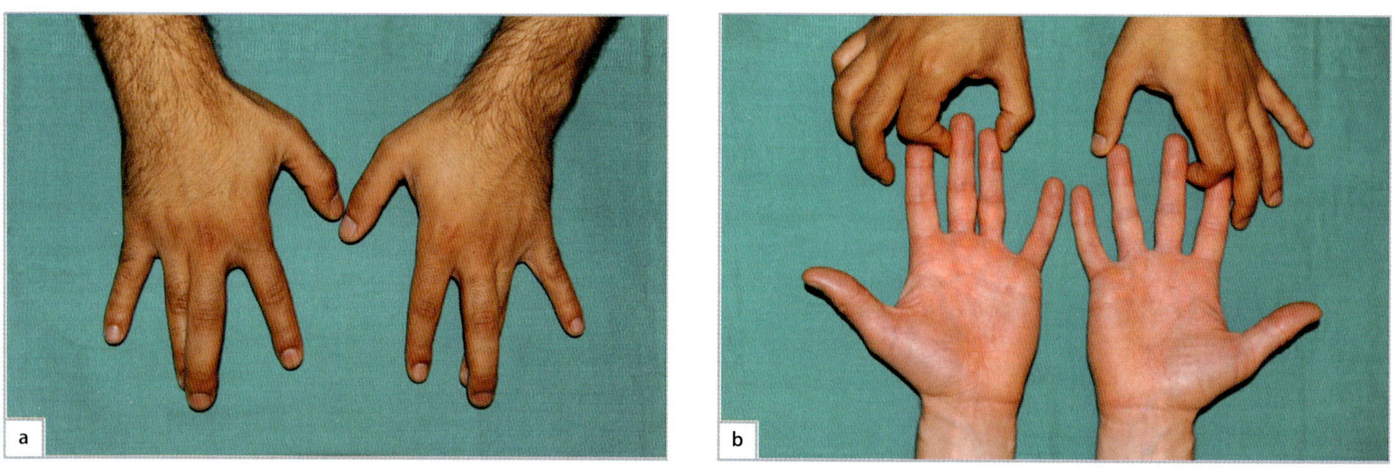

Figure 8.10 Demonstration of crossing of the long finger over the ring finger as well as abduction and adduction of the fingers against resistance; both tests indicate an intact ulnar nerve and interosseous muscle function.

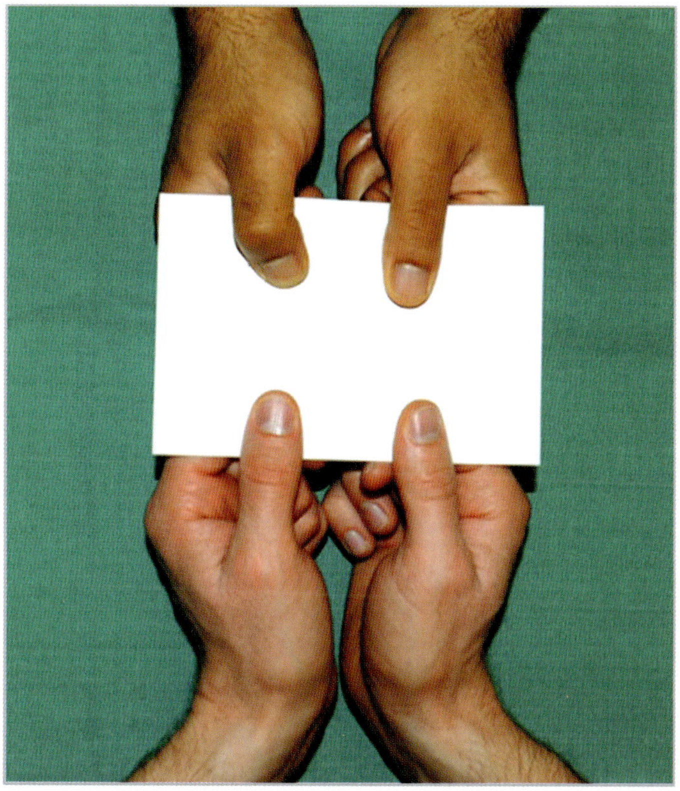

Figure 8.11 Froment sign.

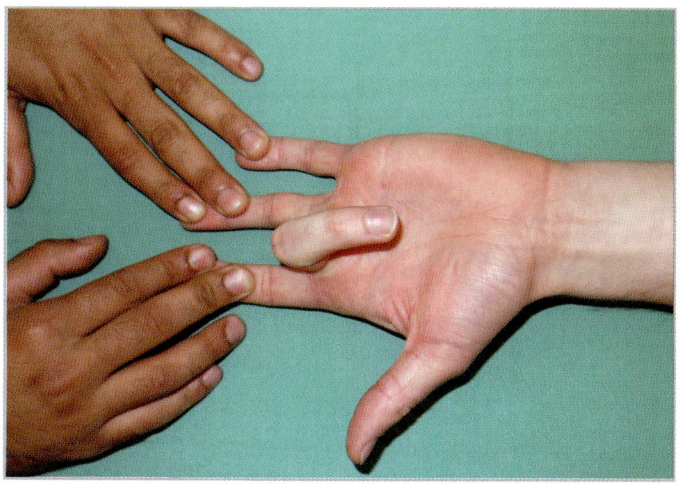

Figure 8.13 Evaluation of tendons of the flexor digitorum superficialis muscle.

- Extensor digiti minimi (EDM): This tendon is tested by asking the patient to make a fist and point toward an object using the little finger. By asking the patient to make a fist the action of the EDC is excluded, as it may compensate for an injured EDM tendon
- EDC (**Figure 8.16**): To test the EDC tendons, ask the patient to fully extend individual fingers against resistance. The inability to extend finger(s) or the presence of an extension lag indicates an extensor tendon injury. To test for central slip integrity, place the patient's fingers (at the level of the PIP joint) on the edge of a tabletop (**Figure 8.17**) and ask the patient to extend the PIP joint.

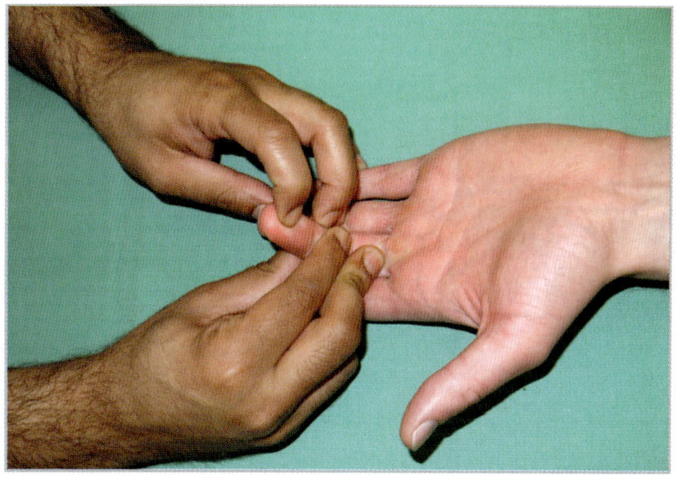

Figure 8.12 Evaluation of tendons of flexor digitorum profundus muscle.

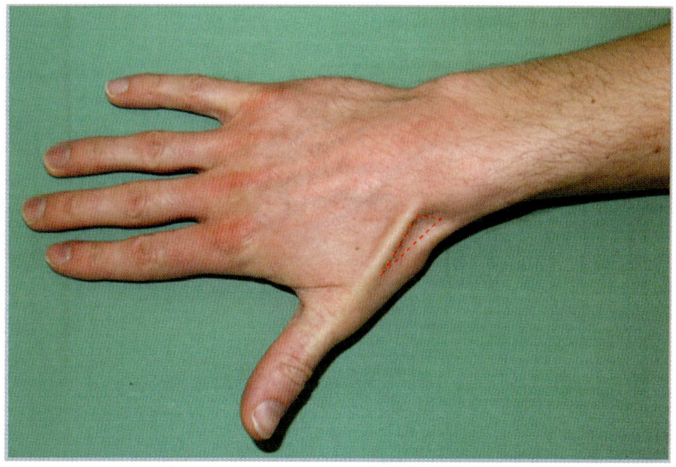

Figure 8.14 Tabletop test to evaluate the integrity of the extensor pollicis longus (EPL) tendon. An intact EPL tendon can be seen on the dorsum of the thumb.

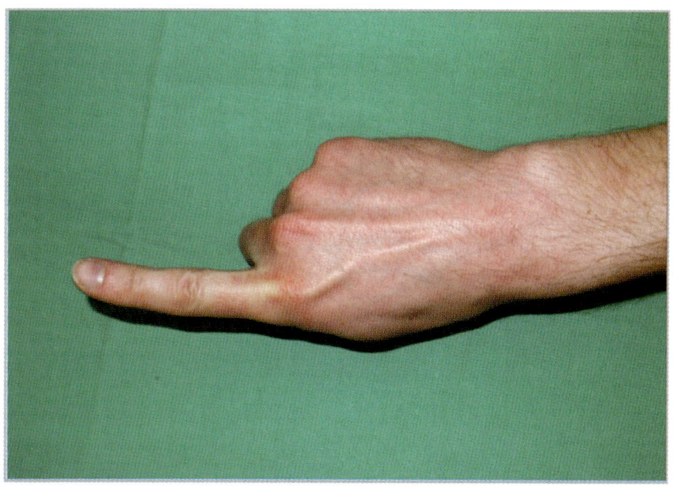

Figure 8.15 The extensor indicis proprius tendon executes independent extension of the index finger when pointing toward an object while the rest of the fingers are flexed.

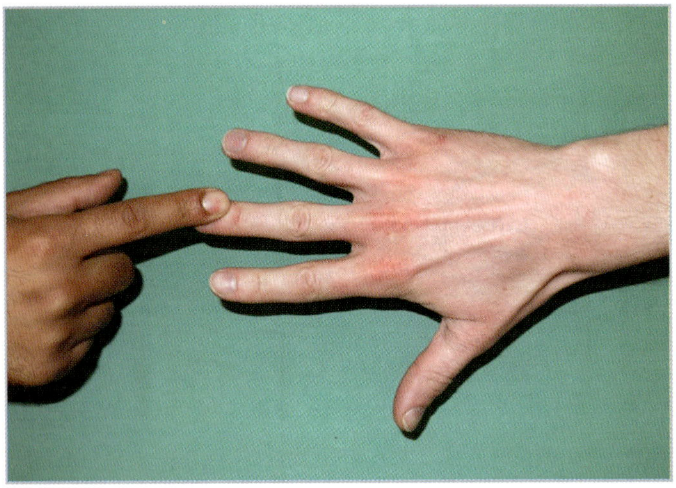

Figure 8.16 Extension of fingers (long finger) against resistance by the extensor digitorum communis tendons. Intact extensor tendons are visible on the dorsum of the hand.

An inability to extend the PIP joint indicates a central slip injury

- Extensor carpi radialis longus (ECRL) and extensor carpi ulnaris (ECU): The tendons of these two muscles can be assessed by asking a patient to extend their wrist and move the wrist joint radially (ECRL) and then ulnary (ECU) against resistance. Weakness or failure to move the wrist in either direction indicates a tendon injury of the corresponding muscle

Radiographic assessment

Radiographic examination completes the assessment of hand trauma. The standard radiographic examination of the hand should

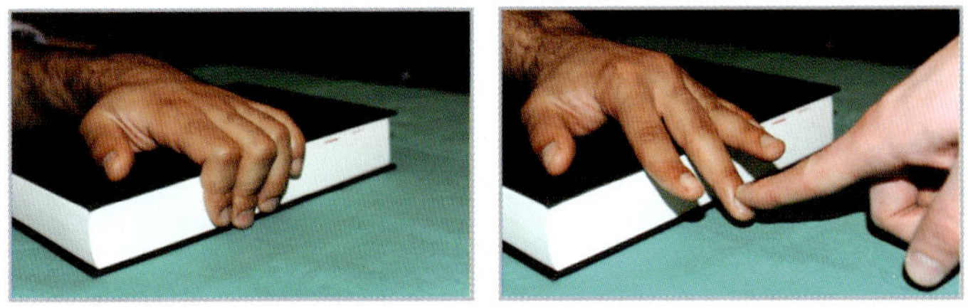

Figure 8.17 Elson test to evaluate central slip integrity.

include posteroanterior, true lateral, and oblique views. X-rays help the examiner to identify the following:

- Fractures: Carpal, metacarpal, and phalangeal fractures
- Fracture pattern: Displaced versus nondisplaced, extra-articular versus intra-articular fractures, simple versus comminuted fractures
- Joint dislocations: Useful to assess joints' congruity, the majority of displaced joints can be successfully reduced and splinted in the ER until formal skeletal fixation
- Complex fractures or dislocations detected by X-rays may require further investigations, e.g. CT or MRI.
- Foreign body: Metal, glass, or retained teeth are identifiable and obvious on X-rays

SUMMARY

Hand trauma may present as an isolated injury or part of multiple trauma. Therefore, physicians are often required to perform several steps simultaneously to evaluate and manage hand injuries. By following consistent hand examination techniques, physicians will be able to refine their examination skills in order to evaluate and manage hand trauma safely and effectively.

SUGGESTED READING

Ootes D, Lambers KT, Ring DC. The epidemiology of upper extremity injuries presenting to the emergency department in the United States. Hand (N Y) 2012; 7(1):18–22.

A one-year (2009) retrospective study analyzing the incidence of traumatic injuries of the upper-limb in the United States. The National Electronic Injury Surveillance System (NEISS) – a database of emergency department visits based on a sample of hospitals selected and weighted to represent the entire US population was examined and a comprehensive list of upper-limb injuries, incidence, and anatomic distribution of injuries was drawn. Results showed that the majority of upper-limb injuries are domestic type injuries and most of the injuries occur in the fingers.

Finnell JT, Knopp R, Johnson P, et al. A calibrated paper clip is a reliable measure of two-point discrimination. Acad Emerg Med 2004; 11:710–714.

A randomized, prospective, blinded, observational study that included 75 subjects to compare two instruments: (1) a paper clip and (2) Disk-Criminator to assess two-point discrimination of the index and long fingers. Paper clips were found to be as effective as Disk-Criminator in measuring the two-point discrimination in fingers of healthy volunteers.

Nassab R, Kok K, Constantinides J, Rajaratnam V. The diagnostic accuracy of clinical examination in hand lacerations. Int J Surg 2007; 5:105–108. Epub 2006 Jul.

A retrospective analysis of 101 patients who presented with hand injuries to the emergency department. In this study, hand surgeons were found to be better than emergency doctors in diagnosing extensor tendon and digital nerve injuries utilizing clinical examination only. The study also highlights the role of hand clinical examination as an indispensable tool in the diagnosis of traumatic hand injuries.

Robins RH. Hand assessment charts. J Hand Surg Br 1986; 11:287–298.

This article summarizes the recommendations of a subcommittee of the British Orthopaedic Association on the design of assessment charts for routine use in accident and emergency departments and in hand clinics. This article also discusses benefits of using hand charts by junior doctors and for training purposes.

Tuncali D, Yavuz N, Terzioglu A, Aslan G. The rate of upper-extremity deep-structure injuries through small penetrating lacerations. Ann Plast Surg 2005; 55:146–148.

A retrospective study including 226 patients with small lacerations who were analyzed for the presence of an associated deep structure injury. Extensor tendons were found to be the most commonly injured structure and 20% of patients presenting with superficial lacerations suffered a combination of injuries to deep structures including tendons, nerves, and vessels.

Chapter 9 Compartment syndrome

Matthew D. Chetta, Kevin C. Chung

DEFINITION

Compartment syndrome occurs when the tissue pressure in a confined osseofascial space rises above the perfusion pressure, compromising the blood flow to vital structures within that compartment. If left untreated, permanent tissue damage may occur, leading to tissue necrosis, fibrosis, functional impairment, and in severe cases renal failure and death.

ETIOLOGY

There are a number of risk factors that may precipitate the development of compartment syndrome. In general, any condition that causes increase in the intracompartmental pressure over the perfusion pressure will result in tissue ischemia and may lead to compartment syndrome in that space or body compartment. The common causes of compartment syndrome are summarized in **Table 9.1**.

PATHOPHYSIOLOGY

Increase in compartment pressure initially obstructs the venous outflow (lower pressure system), while the arterial inflow remains unaffected. This causes development of progressive interstitial edema, which causes a further increase in the compartment pressure. Once the tissue pressure rises above the capillary perfusion pressure, blood flow stops through the capillaries, leaving oxygen and nutrient exchange unable to proceed. At this stage, cellular metabolism changes from aerobic to anaerobic and produces less adenosine triphosphate (ATP) molecules, making it impossible to meet the energy requirements of vital structures. Additionally, the cellular osmolar gradient maintained by the ATP-dependent Na^+/K^+ pump is compromised leading to myocyte damage that worsens the edema. Cellular damage causes release of oxygen-free radicals and degradative enzymes that cause further myocyte damage. This results in a feedback cycle of increasing edema and intracompartmental pressure compounding the original injury. Finally, the damaged myocytes release lactic acid and myoglobin, which then enters circulation and causes metabolic acidosis and myoglobinemia, leading to acute renal failure.

The tissue damage caused by compartment syndrome can be reversible if identified and treated early. However, irreversible damage may occur after 4–12 hours depending on the type of tissue involved and the compartmental pressure. Therefore, prompt treatment should be instituted, which includes urgent release/decompression of the fascial layers of the affected compartment, aggressive hydration with crystalloids, followed by diuresis using mannitol, aiming for a urine output >2–3 cc/kg/h. Alkalinization of urine with sodium bicarbonate has been postulated to protect the kidneys, as urine pH >6.5 may minimize myoglobin breakdown to nephrotoxic metabolites and may reduce uric acid crystallization, though this effect has not been proven. Crippling contractures can develop due to prolonged ischemia called Volkmann contractures (see Chapter 27). If the condition is not reversed, death may occur owing to an infectious etiology or acute metabolic disturbance (e.g. hyperkalemia) causing cardiac arrhythmias.

CLINICAL ASSESSMENT

A careful history and thorough clinical examination are essential to identify compartment syndrome as early as possible. Physicians should be suspicious of any symptoms indicative of compartment syndrome and have a low threshold to initiate the appropriate management, which is primarily surgical. It is always helpful to compare the affected limb with the unaffected limb, fully exposing the limb and making sure to remove all rings and jewelry. The rule of '6 P's' (pain, pressure, paresthesia, pallor, pokilothermia, and pulselessness) may aid in the diagnosis of compartment syndrome:

- Pain: Pain out of proportion to the clinical examination is the hallmark feature of compartment syndrome and should alert clinicians to consider compartment syndrome. Pain is particularly evident and severe on passive flexion and extension of a limb or muscle
- Pressure: A limb that is affected by compartment syndrome usually feels tense, or hard, on palpation due to excess pressure in the compartment. In addition, pressure blisters are frequently present in the area of the compartment
- Paresthesia (altered sensation): Paresthesia is another feature of compartment syndrome that is caused by compression and ischemia of the sensory nerves of the affected compartment,

Table 9.1 Factors leading to compartment syndrome

Internal increase in compartment volume	External restriction of compartment size
• Hemorrhage (hemophilia)	• Military antishock trousers
• Fractures	• Casts/splints
• Medications (aspirin, heparin, thrombolytics)	• Tight dressings
• Muscle edema (crush injury, intense exercise, seizure)	• Burn eschar
• Injection injury	• Closure of fascial defects
• Burns or electrical injuries	• Malfunctioning pneumatic boot
• Envenomation	• Posture (laying on extremity)
• Space occupying lesion (tumor, hemangioma)	
• Hypoalbuminemia (nephrotic syndrome)	

typically affecting the sensory nerves before the motor nerves. It is important to evaluate the nerves that travel through the compartments (i.e. median nerve passing through volar forearm compartment) to complete a thorough examination. However, paresthesia is usually a late sign of compartment syndrome and occurs a few hours after the beginning of pain. Paresthesia is therefore indicative of compartment syndrome but not a reliable sign to make an early diagnosis without the presence of other symptoms

- Pallor: Elevated compartment pressure compromises tissue vascularity causing the skin to appear pale and shiny. Prolonged ischemia eventually leads to a mottled appearance
- Pokilothermia: With further progression of compartment syndrome, pokilothermia will ensue as the extremity experiences a loss of thermoregulation. This can be determined by comparing the temperature to that of the unaffected extremity. If cool to the touch, thermoregulation is no longer functional in the affected extremity. It is worth noting that this feature is also not reliable in the early diagnosis of compartment syndrome, but indicates a more advanced stage of the condition
- Pulselessness: This is the least reliable of the exams. Compartment syndrome is a disorder of the microvasculature, and the major vessels are not usually affected until late in the disease. Tissue damage occurs with an intracompartment pressure >25 mmHg, and if pulselessness is present (i.e. intracompartment pressure higher than the systolic blood pressure) on the clinical examination, a substantial amount of tissue damage may have already occurred

INVESTIGATIONS

Objective measurements

In a conscious patient, the clinical examination is the standard for making the correct diagnosis of compartment syndrome. However, in an obtunded patient, direct compartment measurements must be obtained for definitive diagnosis. Several products are available such as the Stryker (Kalamazoo, MI) needle to directly measure compartment pressures. Alternatively, an arterial line from an anesthesia machine (not licensed) connected to a monitor may be used for this purpose if a specialized needle is not available. Intracompartmental pressure >30 mmHg requires urgent surgical decompression.
Laboratory studies:

- Blood tests:
  - Complete blood count with differential, potassium, creatinine, creatine phosphokinase, myoglobin, prothrombin time, activated partial thromboplastin time.
- Urine tests:
  - Urinalysis, myoglobin, urine toxicology screen
- Imaging studies:
  - X-ray; to evaluate for any underlying fracture
  - Ultrasound; evaluates arterial flow and may locate deep venous thrombosis; however, should not delay the management of compartment syndrome

TREATMENT

Compartment syndrome often happens in the setting of trauma and the principle of 'life over limb' presides. The initial assessment and treatment should be in line with the advanced trauma life support protocol to stabilize the patient first. Early intervention is critical and irreversible tissue damage begins approximately 6 hours after the onset of compartment syndrome. Supportive treatment includes IV hydration aiming for a urine output goal of 2–3 cc/kg/h to prevent myoglobin precipitation in the renal tubules and renal failure. Surgical decompression (fasciotomy) is the definitive treatment of compartment syndrome. The decision for surgical intervention is chiefly based on findings gleaned from the clinical examination.
Indications of fasciotomy:

- Clinical suspicion is the most important indicator
- Elevated compartment pressure (30 or 20 mmHg below diastolic blood pressure)
- Revascularization of a limb (interrupted perfusion >4 hours)
- Consider in full-thickness circumferential burns, which is best treated with escharotomy by releasing the tight eschar, rather than formal fasciotomy

GENERAL PRINCIPLES OF SURGICAL DECOMPRESSION

Position the patient safely on the operating table after he/she is fully anaesthetized. Apply a high tourniquet to the arm or lower limb, and then prepare and drape the extremity in a sterile fashion. Design the skin incisions (as described below) to avoid damage to the neurovascular bundles and tendons. Debridement of necrotic muscle should be performed while the tourniquet is inflated or prior to revascularization to reduce myoglobinemia. The tourniquet should be released intermittently to assess muscle viability. Following fasciotomy, recheck the intracompartment pressure to confirm adequate decompression. Consider a 'second look' within 24–48 hours following initial compartment release to check if additional debridement is required.

The upper extremity

The upper extremity is divided into three parts: the upper arm, the forearm, and the hand. In this section, we will describe the important anatomical landmarks and incisions required for surgical decompression.

The forearm (Figure 9.1)

Consists of three compartments, separated by fascia and interosseous septum:

- Dorsal compartment (extensors of fingers, thumb, ulnar wrist)
  - Test with passive finger, thumb, and wrist flexion
- Mobile wad (brachioradialis, radial wrist extensors)
  - Test with passive wrist flexion
- Volar compartment (flexors of fingers, thumb, wrist)
  - Test with passive finger, thumb, and wrist extension

Surgical incisions of the forearm

- Volar forearm incision:
  - The standard volar incision resembles a lazy S incision (**Figure 9.2**) connecting carpal tunnel release to a curvilinear volar incision. This can leave the median nerve and flexor tendons exposed at the wrist after decompression. The authors' preferred method involves a longitudinal volar radial forearm incision to allow dissection down to the forearm fascia (**Figure 9.3**). This allows access to the mobile extensor wad and the dorsal extensor compartment. Dissection down to the deep volar compartment requires dissecting between the flexor carpi radialis and the palmaris longus

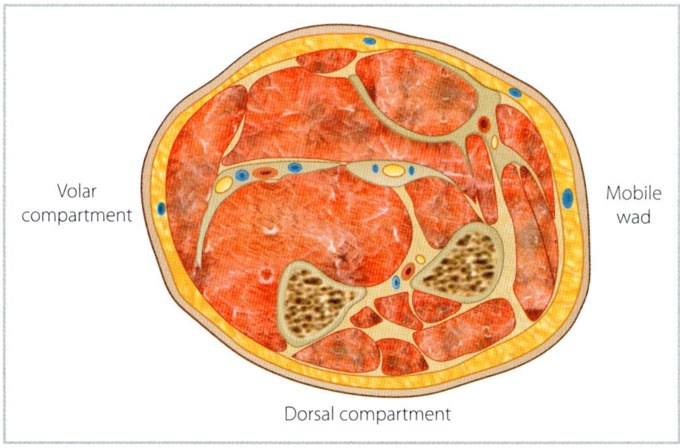

Figure 9.1 Cross section of the three compartments of the forearm.

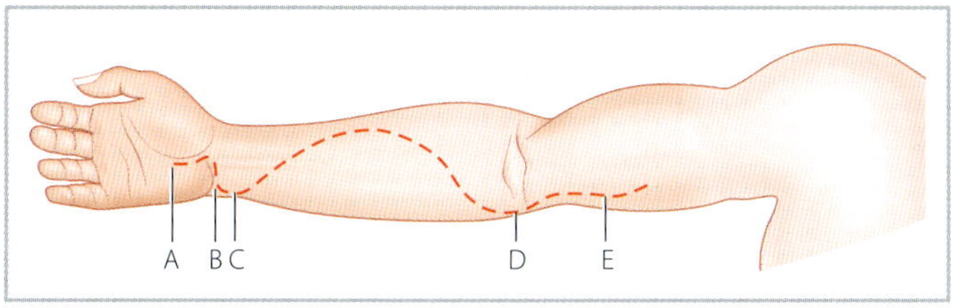

Figure 9.2 The lazy-S incision of a volar forearm compartment release. Beginning at the elbow, the incision extends ulnarly (d), gently curves across to the radial volar forearm, returns to the ulnar side (c), and then extends into the mid palm just ulnar to the thenar crease to allow release of the carpal tunnel (b–a). The incision may extend proximally for upper arm release (e).

- Dorsal forearm incision (**Figure 9.4**):
  - A 10–15 cm longitudinal volar ulnar forearm incision beginning 3–4 cm distal to the medial epicondyle
- Carpal tunnel incision (**Figure 9.5**):
  - Historically, the incision connects to a curvilinear volar forearm incision, but this leaves the median nerve exposed following decompression. Thus, a standard surgical carpal tunnel incision is made between the thenar and hypothenar muscles to expose the palmar aponeurosis and the transverse carpal ligament. The transverse carpal ligament is then divided from distal to proximal making sure to protect the median nerve

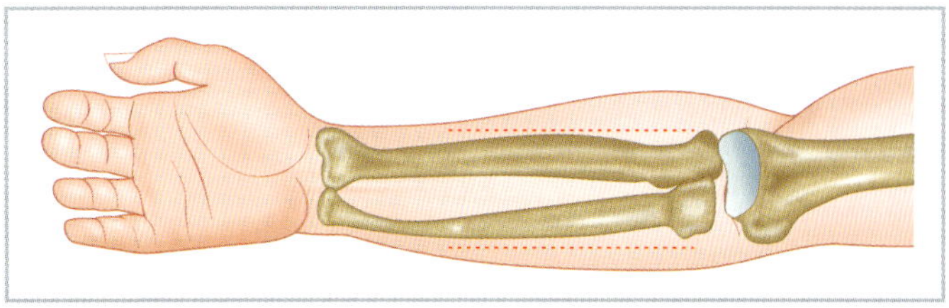

Figure 9.3 Alternate volar incision.

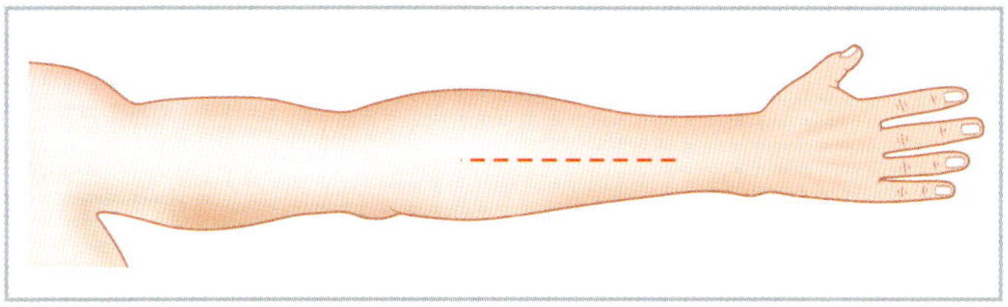

Figure 9.4 Dorsal forearm incision.

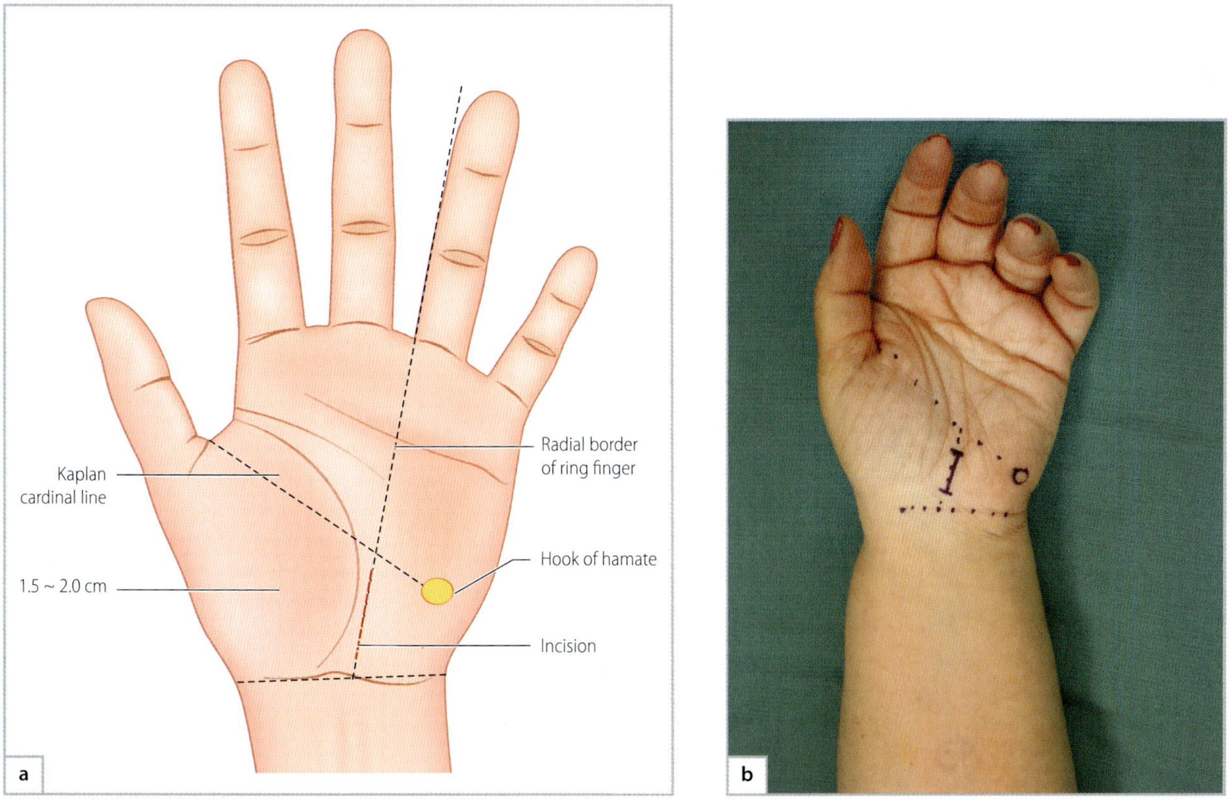

Figure 9.5 (a–b) Incision of carpal tunnel release.

The hand

The hand consists of 10 compartments:

- Dorsal interossei (4)
- Palmar interossei (3)
- Adductor
- Thenar
- Hypothenar

Surgical incisions of the hand

The standard incisions are shown in **Figures 9.6–9.7**. The first dorsal incision is centered over the index finger metacarpal, allowing access to the deep investing fascia of the first dorsal interosseous, the adductor pollicis, the second dorsal interosseous, and the second palmar interosseous muscles. These structures may be approached by dissecting on either side of the metacarpal using tenotomy scissors perpendicular to the horizontal plane of the hand and spreading into each compartment. The deep fascia of the adductor pollicis can be identified radial and deep to the first dorsal interosseous muscle.

The second dorsal incision is centered over the ring finger metacarpal allowing access to the third and fourth interossei compartments and once again by dissecting on either side of the metacarpal bone. The thenar incision should be made in the interval between the dorsal skin and the glabrous skin. The deep investing fascia should be released and the need for individual muscle decompression should be evaluated. The hypothenar incision should be made slightly ulnar to the little finger metacarpal to avoid the motor nerve branch. Once again, evaluate the need for individual muscle decompression.

The upper arm

Consists of two compartments (anterior and posterior, **Figure 9.8**): The anterior compartment is released through a medial incision and the posterior compartment is released through a lateral incision. The ulnar and radial nerves travel through these compartments and at increased pressure will produce symptoms of nerve compression along the areas supplied by their nerve distribution.

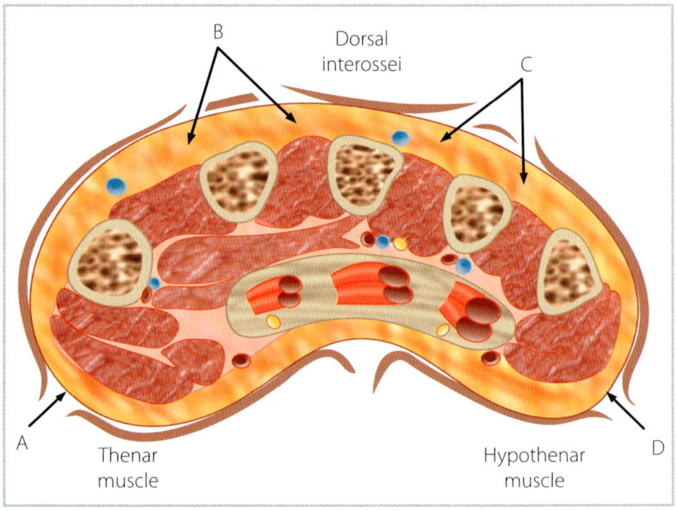

Figure 9.7 A schematic for placement of incisions allowing access to all myofascial spaces of the hand. The arrows b–c represent the plane of dissection through the dorsal incisions, which allows access to the adductor and interosseous compartments. A thenar incision (a) and hypothenar incision (d) to allow access to the thenar and hypothenar muscle bundles, respectively.

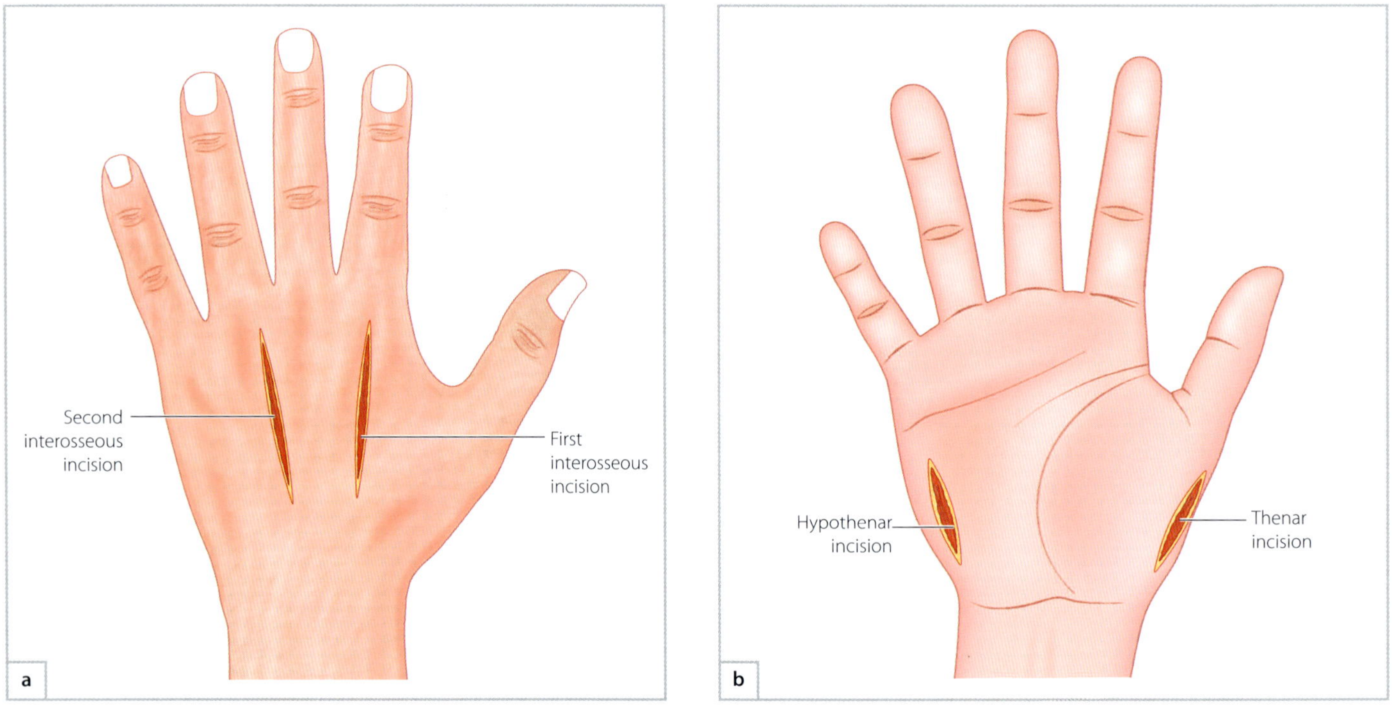

Figure 9.6 (a–b) Hand fasciotomy, demonstrating volar and dorsal incisions of hand compartment release.

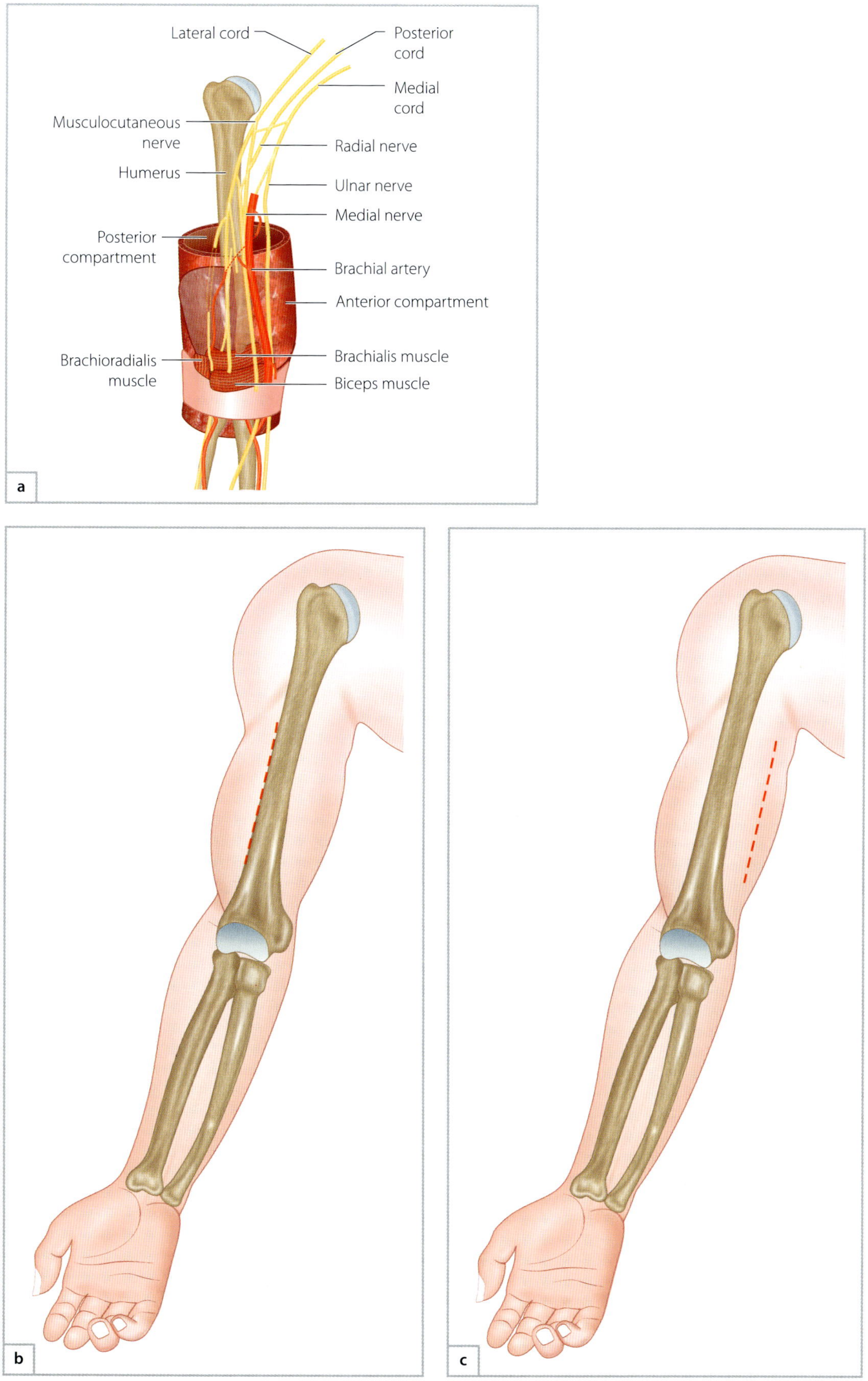

Figure 9.8 (a–c) Upper arm compartments and incisions of compartment release.

POSTOPERATIVE MANAGEMENT

- Wound closure:
  - Fasciotomy wounds should not be closed initially
  - May partially close, or close one side, preferably the flexor surface
  - Thin split-thickness skin grafts to open areas are typically indicated (secondarily contract facilitating later excision/closure).
- Postoperative rehabilitation:
  - Mobilize the limb for 6–12 weeks to prevent adhesions and stiffness after closure/skin graft has stabilized
- Splinting:
  - Full-length splint maintaining a functional position should be worn at night for 4–6 weeks to prevent flexion contractures
- Follow-up:
  - Serial skin graft excision/scar revision can be performed as needed. May need extensive reconstruction (tendon/functional muscle transfer) if a significant loss of flexor or extensor compartments has occurred in the upper extremities

OUTCOMES

- Early intervention is extremely important. A nearly universal recovery of limb function has been reported if fasciotomy is performed within 6 hours of the onset of compartment syndrome
- Complications include permanent nerve damage, infection, cosmetic deformity, loss of limb, and death
- The long-term morbidity includes pain, altered sensation, dry scaly skin, pruritus, wound discoloration, swollen limbs, scar and tendon tethering, and muscle herniation

KEY POINTS

- Pain on passive stretch is one of the earliest and most predictable symptoms of compartment syndrome
- Clinical suspicion is an important indicator for fasciotomy
- Objective direct compartment measurements are critical in establishing the correct diagnosis, especially in obtunded patients. Intracompartmental pressure >30 mmHg requires an intervention
- Best prognosis if fasciotomy is performed within 6 hours

SUGGESTED READING

Bae DS, Kadiyala RK, Waters PM. Acute compartment syndrome in children: contemporary diagnosis, treatment, and outcome. J Pediatr Orthop 2001; 21:680–688.

A retrospective study in pediatric patients (n=33) with compartment syndrome treated from 1992 to 1997. The majority of the compartment syndromes diagnosed (75%) resulted from fracture. The 5 P's (pain, pallor, paresthesia, paralysis, and pulselessness) proved to be unreliable signs and symptoms of compartment syndrome. With early diagnosis and intervention, more than 90% regained full restoration of function (level IV evidence).

DiFelice A Jr, Seiler JG III, Whitesides TE Jr. The compartments of the hand: an anatomic study. J Hand Surg Am 1998; 23:682–686.

An anatomic study of 21 cadaver hands that showed variability in the discrete compartments of the interosseous muscles. Subcompartmentalization of the myofascial spaces must be anticipated and thorough inspection or generous release of the dorsal and palmar compartments along the metacarpal must be performed at time of fasciotomy. (Level V evidence)

Ouellette EA, Kelly R. Compartment syndromes of the hand. J Bone Joint Surg Am 1996; 78:1515–1522.

A retrospective review of patients with compartment syndrome of the hand managed with fasciotomies. Tense, swollen hand and elevated pressure in at least one interosseous compartment were found in each patient. Decompression of the involved compartments as well as carpal tunnel release resulted in satisfactory function in 13 of the 17 patients. The other 4 patients had a poor result. (Level IV evidence)

Ragland R III, Moukoko D, Ezaki M, et al. Forearm compartment syndrome in the newborn: report of 24 cases. J Hand Surg Am 2005; 30:997–1003.

A retrospective review of forearm compartment syndrome at time of birth in 24 children. Only 1 child was treated early with emergent fasciotomy and had a good result. The remaining 23 cases showed tissue loss, compressive neuropathy, muscle loss, and late skeletal changes that led to impaired function and distal bone growth abnormalities. (Level IV evidence)

Chapter 10 Acute hand infections

Jennifer F. Waljee, Kevin C. Chung

OVERVIEW

Acute and chronic hand infections are a frequent cause of morbidity commonly encountered by emergency, primary care, and specialist physicians. Patient risk factors for hand infections include diabetes mellitus, poor nutrition, substance abuse, immunocompromised states or use of immunomodulating medications, and autoimmune disorders (**Table 10.1**). Although antibiotic therapy may be appropriate in early, mild infections, progressive infection may warrant surgical intervention, and associated edema may result in tissue ischemia and necrosis. Treatment is crucial as inadequate treatment may lead to chronic stiffness, joint contractures, and in severe cases, amputation.

CLASSIFICATION

Hand infections may be classified into four categories (**Table 10.2**):

1. Bacterial infections are the most common, and typically caused by *Staphylococcus aureus* (80%), or *Streptococcus* species. Polymicrobial infections are more common in diabetic and immunocompromised patients, as well as traumatic injuries. In recent years, the emergence of antibiotic-resistant organisms (e.g. methicillin-resistant S. *aureus* and vancomycin-resistant enterococci) have resulted in greater morbidity related to hand infections and the need for more aggressive antibiotic regimens
2. Viral infections are relatively uncommon, and the most notable of these is herpetic whitlow, caused by the herpes simplex viruses (HSVs)
3. Fungal organisms are most commonly due to *Candida* species, and may be seen in chronic paronychia infections that are difficult to eradicate. However, they may be a notable cause of fungal hand infections in immunocompromised patients (e.g. patients on immunosuppressive chemotherapy regimens)
4. Atypical (mycobacterial) infections often present in an indolent manner. These infections may be more difficult to eradicate due to the emergence of resistant organisms and the need for prolonged antimicrobial therapy that demands strict patient compliance (e.g. *Mycobacterium marinum*)

Table 10.1 Patient-related risk factors for specific types of hand infections

Patient factor	Unique features
Diabetes	Polymicrobial infections are common More likely to fail conservative measures and require surgical intervention
Immunocompromised individuals (chemotherapy, steroid use, HIV)	Opportunistic infections, atypical pathogens (e.g. Candidal flexor tenosynovitis, disseminated *Neisseria gonorrhoeae*)
Intravenous drug use	Polymicrobial infections resulting in abscesses and flexor tenosynovitis
Marine exposure	*Mycobacterium marinum* infections that cause chronic and indolent hand infections
Sexually transmitted diseases	Flexor tenosynovitis and abscesses due to disseminated *N. gonorrhoeae*)

Table 10.2 Microbiology of common hand infections

Type of infection	Common organisms	Treatment	Caveat
Acute, purulent, soft tissue infections	Gram-positive aerobic organisms	Penicillin, 1st-generation cephalosporins	Monitor closely for failure to improve, which may signal the need for additional surgical drainage or the presence of resistant organisms (e.g. MRSA)
Chronic infections	Mycobacterial infections, fungal infections	Antifungal agents (topical or oral) if fungal infection is present. Antibiotic therapy specific to the organism for mycobacterial infections	Organisms may require advanced culture techniques or prolonged culture
Human bite wounds	α-hemolytic and β-hemolytic *Streptococcus*, *Eikinella*, anaerobes	Prophylactic antibiotics are indicated for all human bite wounds, and should be tailored to the cultured organism	All wounds should be evaluated for the presence of septic arthritis and foreign bodies (teeth)
Fish spine inoculation	*Vibrio* infection	Fluoroquinolones and surgical debridement	Can progress to necrotizing fasciitis
Marine water exposure	*Mycobacterium marinum*	May require treatment with multiple agents for 9–12 months	Can cause superficial verrucous lesions, subcutaneous granulomas, or deep space infections
Rose thorn inoculation	*Sporothrix schenckii*	Antifungal agents	Patients often present with proximal lymphadenopathy

ANATOMY

Bursa of the hand: (Figure 10.1)

The radial bursa is a continuation of the flexor pollicis longus (FPL) tendon sheath beginning at the metacarpophalangeal (MCP) joint through the carpal canal. The ulnar bursa is a continuation of the small finger flexor tendon sheath in 50% of individuals. The ulnar bursa widens proximally over the long and ring finger metacarpals and surrounds (but does not include) the ring and long finger flexor tendons. The radial and ulnar bursas communicate proximal to the transverse carpal ligament, deep to the flexor digitorum profundus, and above the pronator quadratus, an area known as the Parona space.

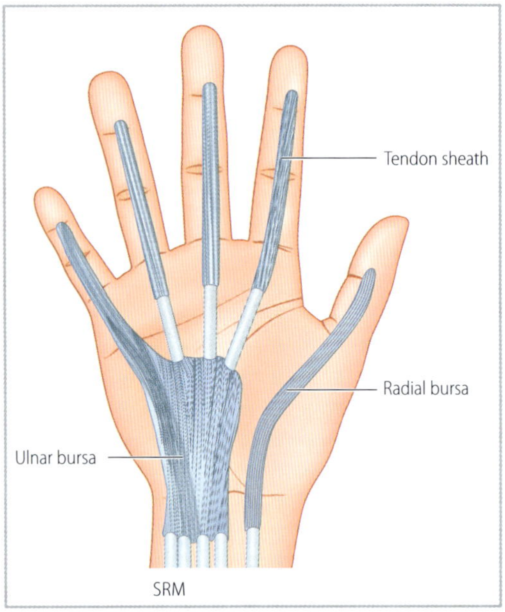

Figure 10.1 Spaces of the hand and wrist.

Potential spaces of the hand (Figure 10.2)

Deep

- Thenar
- Midpalmar
- Hypothenar

Superficial

- Dorsal subcutaneous space
- Dorsal subaponeurotic space
- Interdigital web space

SPECIFIC TYPES OF INFECTIONS

Acute paronychia

Acute paronychia is a bacterial infection of the soft tissue/paronychial fold and is usually preceded by traumatic injury (nail biting, foreign body, instrumentation) causing disruption between the nail fold and nail plate. The most common pathogen is *S. aureus.*

Presentation

Patients present with erythema and tenderness along the paronychial fold and nail plate in early infections. Abscesses may form in those infections that are untreated or failed to respond to therapy, and may track in the nail bed, fingertip pulp, or contralateral nail fold.

Diagnosis

Diagnosis is based on clinical presentation. Radiographs and laboratory markers may be useful options to consider. Consider radiographs to look for the presence of a foreign body in those infections that have failed to respond, and consider laboratory markers (leukocyte count) in those patients with systemic symptoms or those who are immunocompromised.

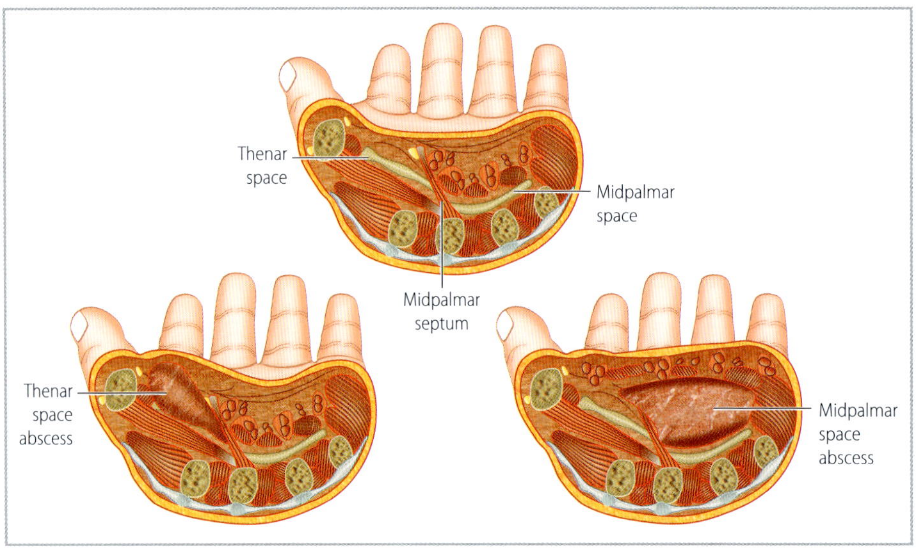

Figure 10.2 Spaces of the hand and wrist.

Treatment

For early infections, treatment may involve warm soaks with dilute betadine or hydrogen peroxide in addition to oral antibiotic therapy directed toward *S. aureus*. For abscess treatment, drainage of the abscess under digital block with partial or complete removal of the nail plate and release of the paronychial fold is required. Avoid incisions directly within or toward the nail matrix to avoid later nail plate deformity.

Prognosis

Failure to respond may be due to the presence of resistant organisms, undrained abscess, osteomyelitis, fungal infection, or presence of a foreign body.

Chronic paronychia

Chronic paronychia typically results from polymicrobial infections including *Candida* and mycobacterial species.

Presentation

Chronic paronychia presents as a chronic induration and nail plate deformity, accompanied by recurrent episodes of inflammation and drainage due to colonization of the eponychium or paronychium (usually *Candida* species). (**Figure 10.3**) Chronic paronychia is more common in women, patients with diabetes, and individuals chronically exposed to water immersion in detergents.

Diagnosis

When diagnosing chronic paronychia, evaluate for underlying systemic conditions. Additionally, radiographs may be useful to evaluate for osteomyelitis or other lesions.

Treatment

Chronic paronychia may be managed both nonoperatively and operatively. Nonoperative management includes oral and topical antibiotics and antifungals, as well as avoidance of the inciting environment. Operative intervention includes marsupialization of the eponychial fold (and nail plate if there is extension under the nail plate or deformity) under digital block with excision of the indurated tissue, avoiding injury to the germinal matrix. The tissue is sent for culture and sensitivity. Dilute betadine or hydrogen peroxide soaks with dressing changes are performed following surgery.

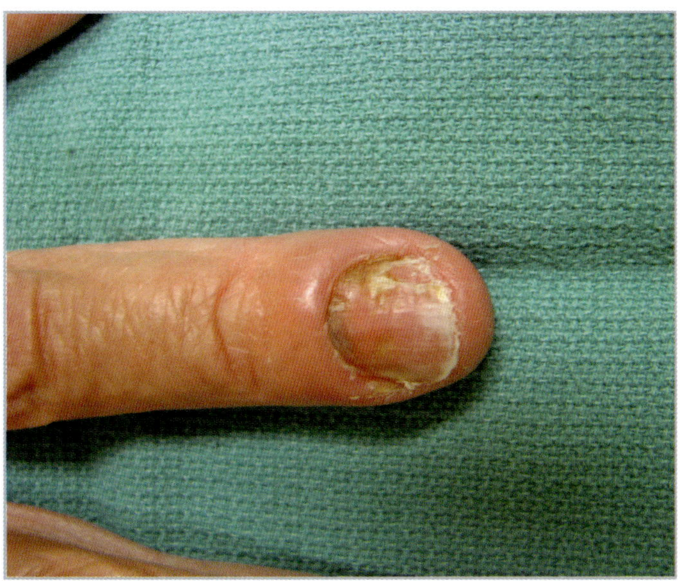

Figure 10.3 Chronic paronychia.

Prognosis

Wounds heal by secondary intention within several weeks, although nail deformities and sensitivity are common complications.

Felon

A felon is a subcutaneous abscess of the fingertip pulp that involves multiple septated areas resulting in a compartment syndrome-like presentation of the distal fingertip. Felons are most commonly due to *S. aureus* and usually seen in diabetic or otherwise immunocompromised patients.

Presentation

Patients present with severe throbbing pain and swelling of the pulp of the distal fingertip that does not cross the DIP joint crease. Felons may be associated with an inciting trauma event, such as a splinter or laceration. In advanced cases, the abscess may involve the distal phalanx and result in osteomyelitis.

Treatment

Early presentation may be treated with close observation, antibiotics, and frequent soaks in warm water. Fluctuance and progressive pain should be treated with drainage under a digital block through a longitudinal incision at the point of maximal tenderness, or along the radial or ulnar aspects of the distal pulp if the point of maximal tenderness is at the center of the pulp. The flexor tendon sheath should not be entered, but all involved septae should be divided for complete drainage. The wound is completely irrigated and debrided, and left to heal by secondary intention. Antibiotics should be directed toward *S. aureus*, and intravenous administration should be considered for patients with severe infections.

Prognosis

Wounds heal within several weeks by secondary intention. Complications include pulp instability, osteomyelitis, nail deformity, and recurrent infection due to incomplete debridement.

Abscess (stiles)

Abscesses are most commonly localized to the subcutaneous space, and usually present in patients who have suffered a recent puncture wound (trauma, insulin injection, laceration, bite) or can be associated with intravenous drug use. The most common pathogen responsible for this infection is *S. aureus*.

Presentation

Simple, subcutaneous abscesses often develop from a simple puncture wound and present with cellulitis and a localized, fluctuant area (**Figure 10.4a**). Patients will present with extreme pain and tenderness over the area, which is relieved with drainage.

Treatment

Surgical exploration and drainage is the foundation of therapy (**Figure 10.4b**). Cultures should be taken at the time of drainage in order to direct antibiotic therapy. The wound should be left to heal by secondary intention and treated with warm water soaks and dressing

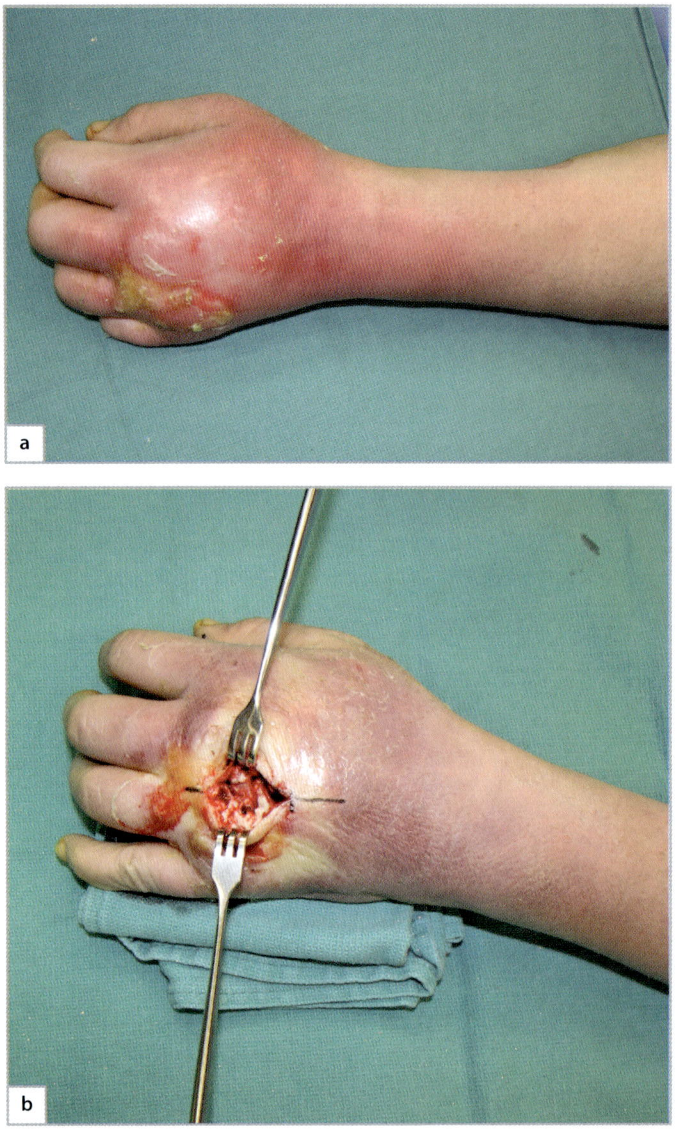

Figure 10.4 (a) Soft tissue abscess. (b) Drainage of soft tissue abscess.

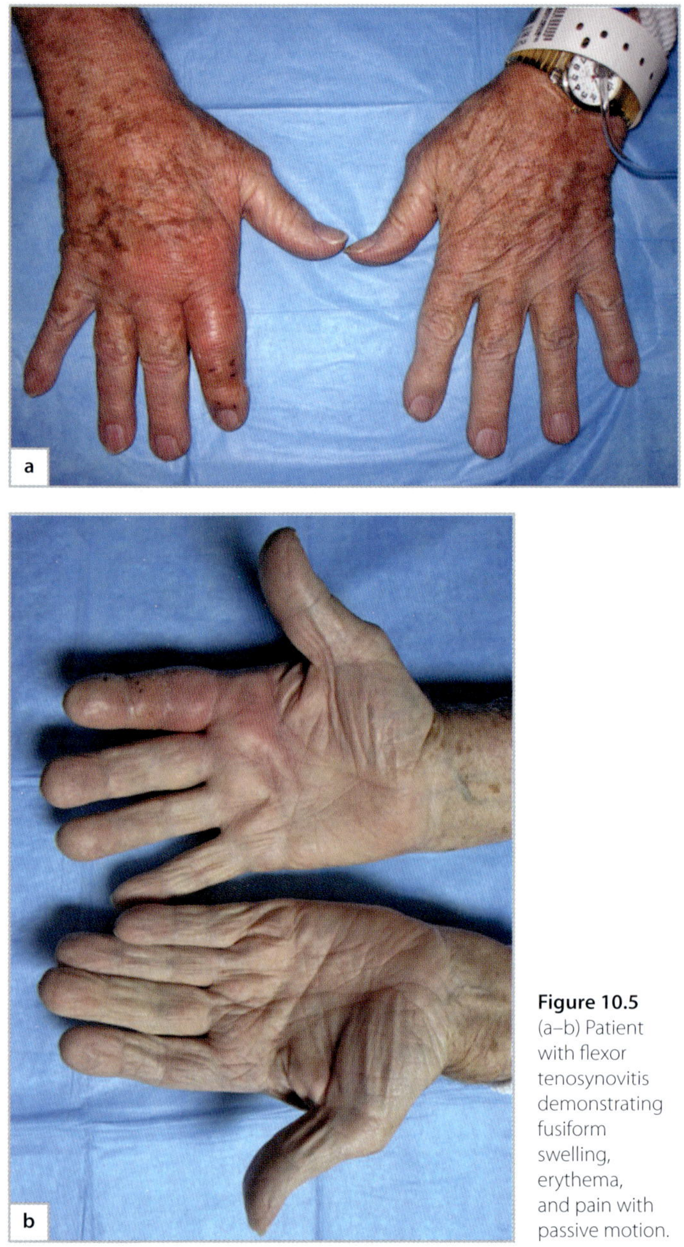

Figure 10.5 (a–b) Patient with flexor tenosynovitis demonstrating fusiform swelling, erythema, and pain with passive motion.

changes. Early range of motion is important to prevent long-term stiffness.

Flexor tenosynovitis

Flexor tenosynovitis results from a bacterial infection of the flexor tendon sheath usually caused through direct inoculation from local trauma. The most common pathogen includes *S. aureus*.

Presentation

Knavel cardinal signs include tenderness over the tendon sheath, flexed finger posture, pain with finger extension, and fusiform swelling of the finger (**Figure 10.5a–b**).

Diagnosis

Diagnosis is based on clinical presentation and should not rely on radiographic imaging or laboratory markers.

Treatment

In early infections, nonoperative management with immobilization, broad-spectrum intravenous antibiotics, and elevation may be attempted with close observation. Patients with an acute presentation or who fail conservative management should undergo immediate exploration and drainage. The digit is explored through an incision at the distal palmar crease at the level of the A1 pulley, a midlateral incision at the distal phalanx, and opening of the A5 pulley. A small, pediatric feeding tube is placed within the sheath and secured. The sheath is then irrigated with 10–20 cc of saline several times per day for 2–3 days. The hand is kept splinted and elevated, and the catheter position should be checked to ensure that it resides in the sheath and not the surrounding tissues to avoid the development of a compartment syndrome. The wounds are left to close by secondary intention.

Prognosis

The majority of patients improve with surgical washout and debridement, but patients should be followed closely and returned for repeat exploration if there is no improvement over 24–48 hours. Long-term complications include stiffness and joint contracture. In rare cases, tendon necrosis can occur, requiring delayed reconstruction.

Radial and ulnar bursa infections

Radial and ulnar bursa infections usually occur in conjunction with flexor tenosynovitis of the thumb and/or small finger.

Presentation

Patients present with signs associated with flexor tenosynovitis of the thumb and/or small finger, as well as swelling and pain over the thenar or hypothenar eminences. The wrist and adjacent fingers are held in a flexed position due to the proximity of the infection. Swelling may be subtle if the bursa ruptures into the surrounding space. A 'horseshoe abscess' occurs when the infection of one bursa extends through the Parona space to the other bursa. Patients may also present with acute median nerve compression due to inflammation and swelling within the carpal tunnel.

Treatment

Patients with radial and ulnar bursa infections require surgical exploration, drainage, and debridement of the involved flexor tendons and bursa. The flexor tendon is explored as described above, and the incision is extended to drain the distal bursa. The proximal bursa is explored through a wrist and forearm incision beginning at the wrist crease, and the flexor tendons and neurovascular structures are mobilized and retracted. Cultures are obtained and all spaces are copiously irrigated. The incisions are left open, or closed loosely over the drains.

Prognosis

Complications for radial and ulnar bursa infections are similar to those associated with flexor tenosynovitis, but the likelihood of chronic stiffness, flexion contractures, and tendon adhesions is higher.

Osteomyelitis

Osteomyelitis is a bony infection resulting from open fractures, hematogenous spread, or extension of a local process. The usual pathogens include *S. aureus* and *Streptococcus* species, but may also include gram-negative, anaerobic, mycobacterial, or polymicrobial infections among patients who are immunocompromised or diabetic.

Presentation

Patients present with pain, swelling, and erythematous joints. Chronic ulceration with underlying exposed structures will often progress to osteomyelitis (**Figure 10.6**). Constitutional symptoms such as fever or malaise are uncommon.

Diagnosis

Radiographic imaging is used to possibly reveal lytic lesions, osteopenia, osteosclerosis, periosteal reactions, or sequestered bone. Laboratory values may reveal an elevated erythrocyte sedimentation rate (ESR), c-reactive protein (CRP), or elevated leukocyte count, but these may also be within normal limits despite the presence of osteomyelitis.

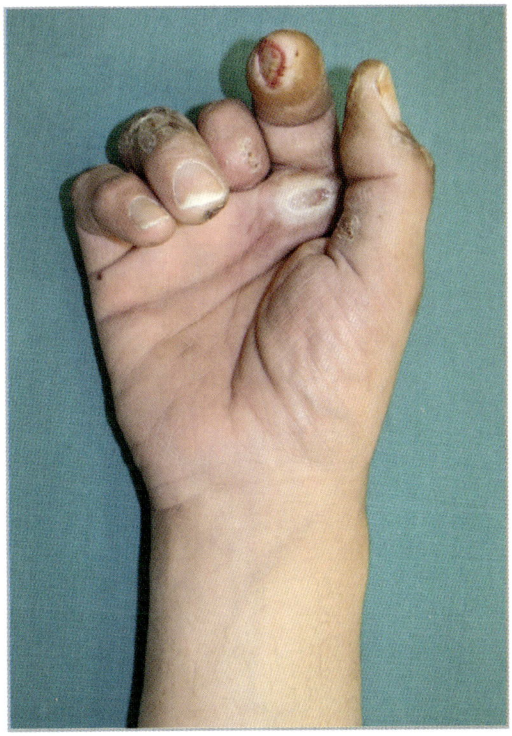

Figure 10.6 Osteomyelitis of the right index finger.

Treatment

Surgical debridement and bony cultures are the mainstay of treatment, followed by an extended course of intravenous antibiotics for 4–6 weeks.

Septic arthritis

Septic arthritis occurs when joint space infections result from direct penetration or trauma, hematogenous spread, or extension of a surrounding process. The inflammation results in cartilage destruction and can progress to osteomyelitis. Typical pathogens include *S. aureus*, *Streptococcus* species, and *Gonococcus*.

Presentation

Patients present with edematous, painful joints, which are classically held in flexion (**Figure 10.7a**). The flexed joint position allows for maximal joint space to accommodate the increased swelling and inflammation. In addition, pain is present with any joint motion.

Diagnosis

Joint aspiration may distinguish septic arthritis from noninfectious inflammation (e.g. gout) if the fluid leukocyte count is elevated beyond 50,000 cells with >75% neutrophils and glucose 40 mg less than fasting serum glucose. Gram stains may or may not reveal the presence of the inciting organisms.

Treatment

Patients with septic arthritis should undergo incision, drainage, and debridement of purulent and necrotic debris. (**Figure 10.7b–c**) Wounds are left open to heal by secondary intention, or closed loosely over a small irrigation catheter. The wrist is drained through an incision between the 3rd and 4th compartments, and the MCP joint is drained through a dorsolateral incision through the proximal sagittal band. The

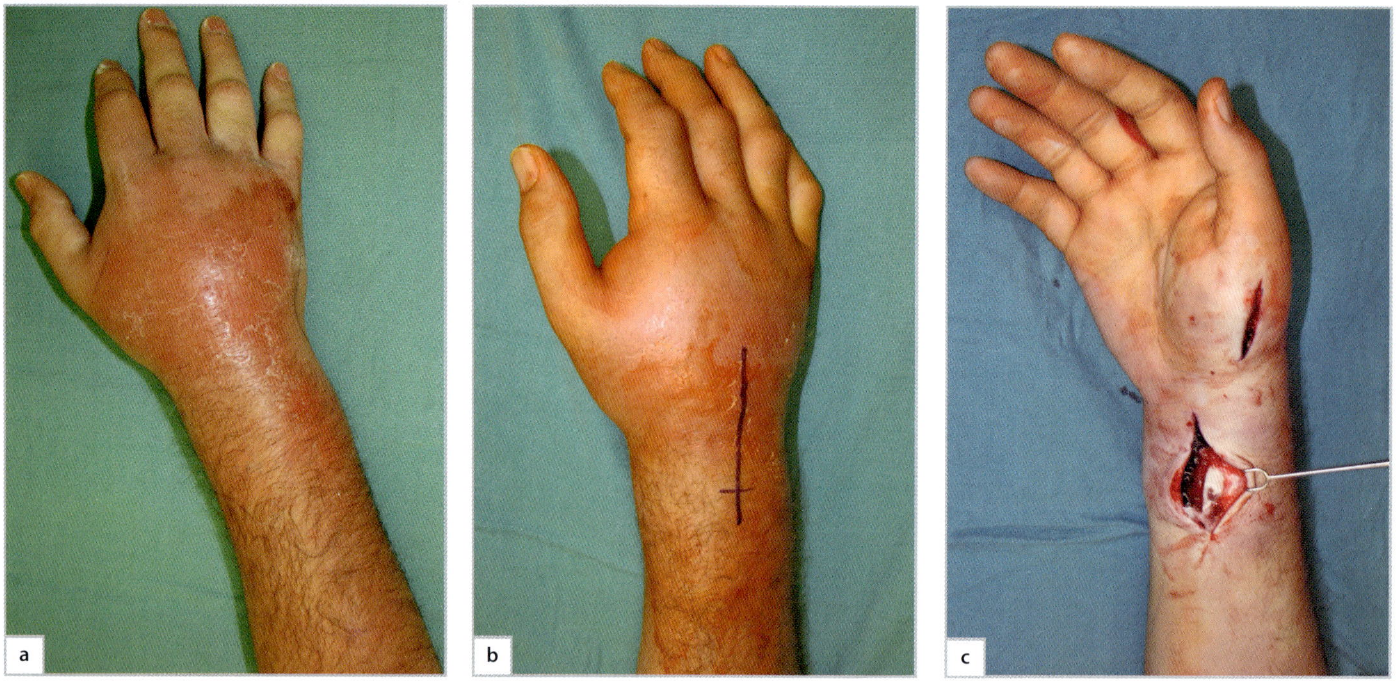

Figure 10.7 (a) Septic arthritis of the right wrist. (b–c) Approach for drainage of septic arthritis of the right wrist.

interphalangeal (IP) joints are drained through a midaxial incision between the volar plate and accessory collateral ligaments. Following drainage, the hand should be splinted and elevated for several days, and active and passive motion should be initiated to prevent stiffness. Patients should be started on broad-spectrum intravenous antibiotics, and the regimen can be tailored appropriately when cultures reveal the responsible organism.

Cellulitis

Cellulitis occurs when inflammation spreads without clear abscess formation, and is usually associated with local trauma. The most frequent pathogens include *S. aureus* and *S. pyogenes.*

Presentation

Patients typically present with pain, swelling, and diffuse erythema. Erythematous streaking may indicate lymphangiolytic spread, and petechiae may indicate a streptococcal infection. The leukocyte count may be elevated in pronounced cases, and patients may present with fever and systemic symptoms. Radiographs may reveal a foreign body if there is a history of local trauma. An ultrasound may be obtained to evaluate for the presence of an abscess, but if an ultrasound is not available, needle aspiration using an 18-gauge needle at the most tender spot may reveal a loculated fluid collection. The involved area should be examined closely to ensure that there is no evidence of abscess or necrotizing infection, which would mandate surgical intervention.

Treatment

Empiric antibiotics are the mainstay of therapy, and the decision between oral and intravenous administration is based on the patient's clinical presentation. Strict hand elevation and placement of a resting hand splint will alleviate the patient's symptoms of discomfort and may help with edema resolution. Following medical treatment, patients should be monitored closely for improvement. Lack of improvement should prompt further investigation for an underlying abscess or other process, or the presence of an antibiotic-resistant infection that would require different therapy.

Necrotizing infections

Necrotizing infections are fast spreading soft tissue infections that occur following trauma (can be minor in nature) and require immediate surgical intervention. Risk factors include substance abuse, malnutrition, and immunocompromised states (e.g. diabetes). Necrotizing infections usually involve polymicrobial infections, but are most commonly associated with *S. pyogenes* (group A *Streptococcus*), anaerobes, *Aeromonas, Clostridium spp., Streptococcus spp.*, and S*taphylococcus spp.* (including methicillin-resistant S. *aureus*).

Presentation

Patients with necrotizing infections typically present with pain out of proportion to examination, ecchymosis, hemorrhagic bullae, epidermolysis, or crepitance, but these symptoms may be more subtle or absent in many patients (**Figure 10.8**). Patients may also present with hemodynamic instability and an altered mental status.

Treatment

Emergent treatment is indicated, and patients should receive aggressive resuscitation and broad-spectrum intravenous antibiotics with planned admission to an intensive care unit. Surgical debridement is mandatory, and all necrotic tissue should be debrided including skin, subcutaneous fat, fascia, and muscle. It is common for patients to require re-exploration and redebridement within 24–48 hours in order to ensure that the infection is controlled and all necrotic, infected tissue is eradicated.

Prognosis

Outcomes depend on the timing and adequacy of debridement, the patient's age, and other comorbidities. Overall mortality rates are

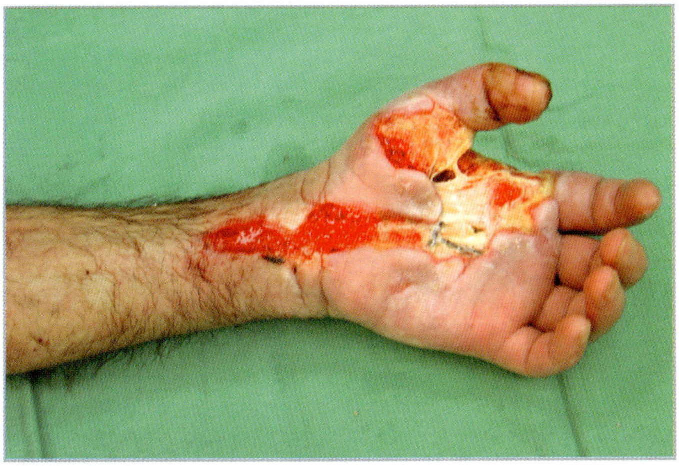

Figure 10.8 Necrotizing soft tissue infection.

approximately 10–50%, and amputation rates remain high for patients with this type of infection.

Herpetic whitlow

Herpetic whitlow is a HSV infection of the fingertip that can mimic a paronychia or felon. This infection is caused by contact with mucosa that is actively shedding HSV, and can be caused by either HSV 1 or 2. Herpetic whitlow commonly occurs in children (thumb-sucking) or adults due to nosocomial contact (e.g. dentists).

Presentation

Herpetic whitlow usually presents in either the index finger or thumb, and has an incubation period of approximately 2 weeks. Erythema, edema, and small vesicles develop over a 1-week period. Patients complain of throbbing pain and tingling in the fingertip, and complaints may be out of proportion to clinical findings in the early stages of the infection.

Diagnosis

Diagnosis is based on clinic presentation, and can be difficult to distinguish from a bacterial infection. When vesicles are present, viral cultures or a Tzanck smear may be performed, but these tests are less sensitive than clinical presentation. If available, serum testing for HSV antibodies may aid in diagnosis.

Treatment

The treatment method for herpetic whitlow is to prevent further inoculation or transmission by covering wounds with a dry dressing. Oral or topical antiviral medications may be administered, but surgical debridement that can cause an open wound and contamination should be avoided. Partial excisions of the nail plate may be performed if lesions are present in the nail bed and cause the patient pain.

Prognosis

The course of herpetic whitlow is self-limiting, but HSV remains latent and approximately 20% of patients will experience a recurrence.

Human bites

Human bites are less common than animal bites, and the true incidence is unknown.

Presentation

Human bites present by four mechanisms:

1. Self-inflicted injury (nail biting, sucking)
2. Traumatic bite amputation
3. Full-thickness bite
4. Clenched fist injury ('fight bite')

Fight bites are the most common bite injury, and any wound over the dorsum of the hand adjacent to the MCP joints should be suspected of a clenched fist injury regardless of the history (**Figure 10.9a**). Patients commonly present with pain, localized swelling, and erythema, but systemic symptoms are rare.

Diagnosis

Patient history may not mirror presentation on clinical evaluation, and patients may present with an extensor tendon injury, infection, or fracture. Septic arthritis of the MCP joint is the most dreaded complication of these injuries due to misdiagnosis or inadequate treatment, and patients should be monitored closely if these injuries are suspected. Physical examination should include a full examination of the area for violation of the joint capsule, sagittal bands, and extensor tendon. Laboratory values should be obtained (complete blood count, CBC, ESR, CRP) but may be normal, and therefore are not considered definitive evidence to rule out human bite infections. Radiographs should be obtained to investigate for fractures or foreign bodies, such as teeth. In rare, delayed circumstances, changes associated with osteomyelitis may be present.

Treatment

Surgical exploration in the operating room is indicated for these injuries in order to prevent ongoing infection (**Figure 10.9b**). During examination, the wound should be widely explored with the digit flexed, in order to assess injury to the joint space. The sagittal band should be released, the joint capsule should be opened, and the articular surfaces visualized. The wound should be copiously irrigated, which can be performed using a 16-gauge angiocatheter, and debrided of all necrotic or grossly infected debris. Extensor tendon injuries should undergo delayed repair, and the wound should be closed loosely or left open. Following surgery, the patient should be initiated on broad-spectrum antibiotic coverage. The most common pathogens isolated include *Staphylococcus* and *Streptococcus* species; however, *Eikinella corrodens* is classically associated with human bite injuries. Antibiotic therapy should cover both gram-positive and gram-negative organisms, and amoxicillin-clavulanic acid, ampicillin/sulbactam sodium, cefoxitin, or moxifloxacin are appropriate choices for antibiotic coverage.

Prognosis

Patients should expect chronic pain and stiffness of the MCP joint even if treated early. Severe complications include injury septic arthritis, flexor tenosynovitis, and osteomyelitis.

Animal bites

Animal bites are most commonly caused by dogs (90%), cats (5%), and other animals such as rodents (5%). Dog bites rarely become infected (<5%), but cat bites develop infection in approximately 50% of injuries, and the bite mechanism influences the propensity for infection. Crushing and tearing (e.g. dog bites) create blunt injuries and open wounds, and bacteria can drain more easily. Sharp, penetrating injuries (e.g. cat bites) create less local trauma and smaller skin wounds, preventing drainage of bacteria, thereby increasing the chance for infection.

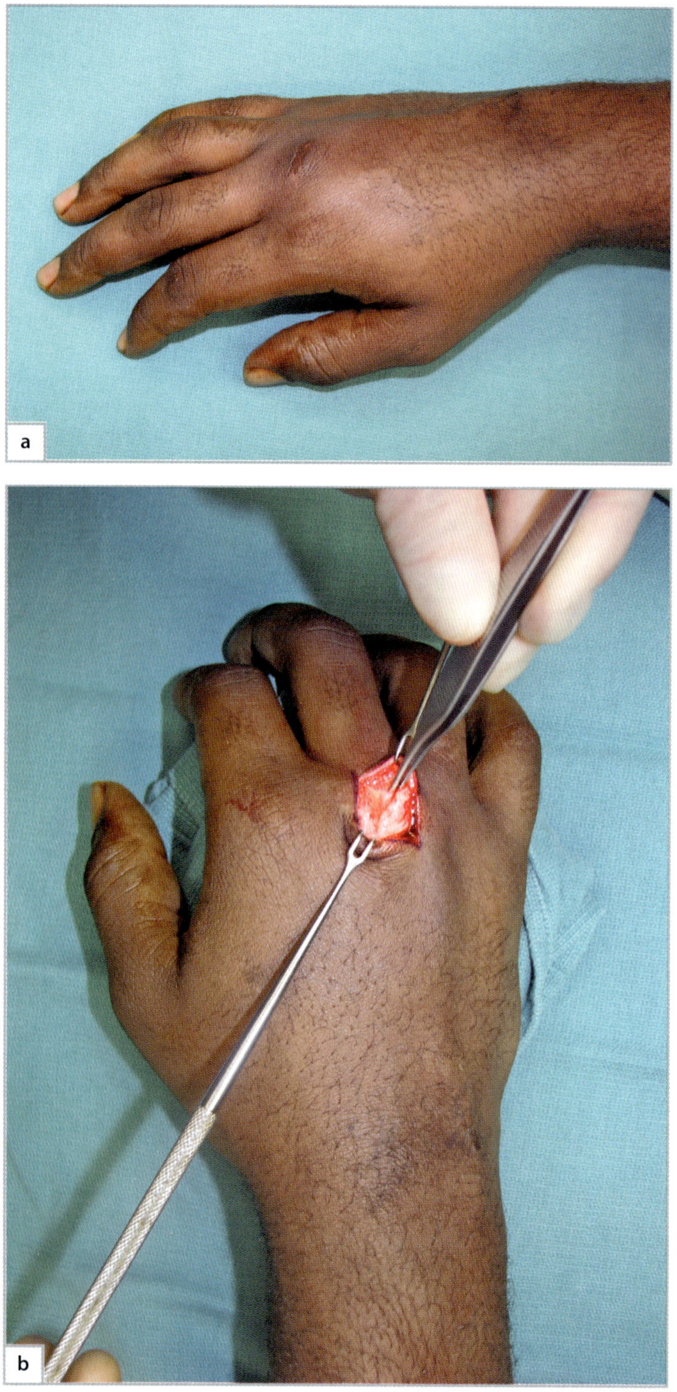

Figure 10.9 (a) Human bite injury over the dorsum of the metacarpophalangeal joint. (b) Exploration of human bite injury over the dorsum of the metacarpophalangeal joint.

Diagnosis

Depending on the attack, patients may present with large, traumatic degloving injuries, or with small puncture wounds accompanied by pain out of proportion to the physical examination. Patients in severe pain without overt clinical signs of infection should be presumed to have an infection and treated aggressively (**Figure 10.10a**). Laboratory values (CBC, ESR, CRP) are usually normal in acute injuries, but may be elevated in delayed presentations (e.g. cat bite several days ago with increasing swelling and pain).

Treatment

All patients should have their tetanus status reviewed and updated. The immunization status (e.g. rabies) of the animal should be confirmed if the animal was a household pet, and assumed to be unimmunized if it is unknown or wild. Pathogens commonly found in dog bite injuries include *S. aureus, Streptococcus viridans, Bacteroides* species, *Pasteurella multocida, and Capnocytophaga canimorsus.* Pathogens commonly found in cat bites include *S. aureus, Streptococcus viridans, Bacteroides* species, *P. multocida, Francisella tularensis,* and *Bartonella henselae. Streptobacillus moniliformis* is commonly isolated in rat bites, and may present with fever, blistering, polyarthritis, and desquamation.

Wounds should be explored, debrided of all necrotic and grossly infected debris, and copiously irrigated (**Figure 10.10b**). Smaller wounds may be dealt with under local anesthetic and oral antibiotics, but larger wounds may require surgical debridement in the operating room and intravenous antibiotics. All wound should be left open to heal by secondary intention, and delayed closure or reconstruction can be considered in several days if vital structures are exposed.

Prognosis

Similar to human bites, animal bites may result in complications including abscess, flexor tenosynovitis, osteomyelitis, and septic arthritis if misdiagnosed or treated inappropriately. Infections that fail to improve with standard measures should be reassessed immediately, and consideration should be given to the presence of atypical organisms, especially in bites caused by nondomesticated animals.

Aquatic organisms

Infections from aquatic organisms can result in both acute (*Staphylococcus, Streptococcus, Pseudomonas, Aeromonas,* and *Enterobacter*) and chronic infections (*Mycobacterium marinum*). Patients exposed to freshwater, brackish water, or leeches may present with *Aeromonas* infections, which have a high rate of necrotizing spread and mortality without treatment. Non-cholerae *Vibrio* infections may present after exposure in saltwater, and typically present as cellulitis. Although localized infections respond to surgical debridement and antibiotic therapy, immunocompromised patients may present with overwhelming systemic and necrotizing infections (**Figure 10.11**). In these rare cases, the rate of amputation and mortality is high.

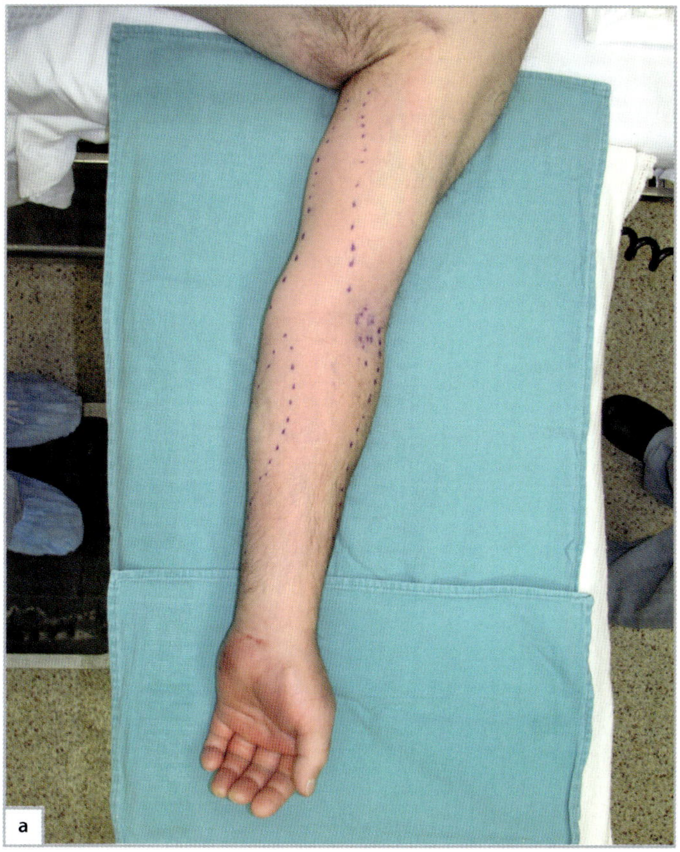

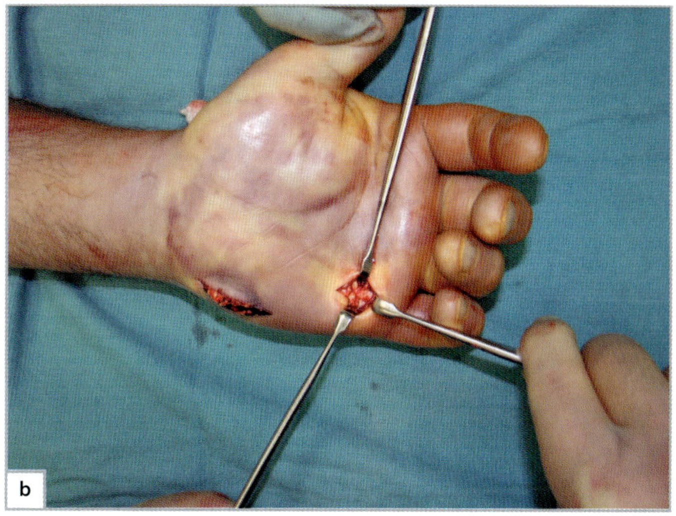

Figure 10.10 (a) Cellulitis caused by cat bite. (b) Exposure for washout of cat bite.

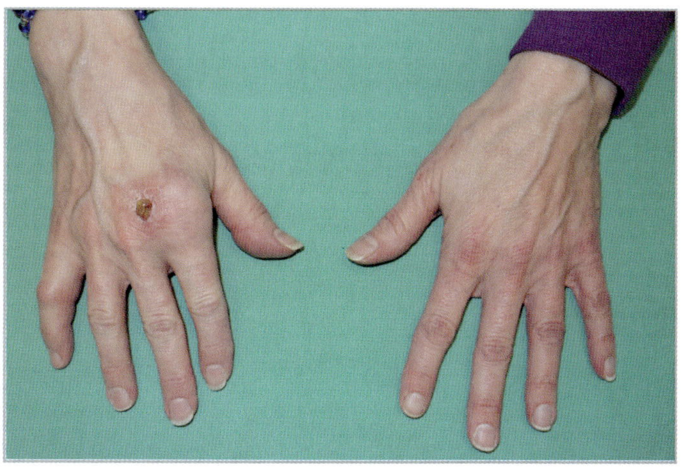

Figure 10.11 Mycobacterial infection of the right hand.

SUMMARY

Hand infections are prevalent in all patient populations, and have the potential to cause permanent hand disability if not treated early and appropriately. Although laboratory values and radiographic imaging can be useful adjuncts for specific infections, the patient's clinical presentation is the most important diagnostic tool. Patients who are immunocompromised (diabetes, steroid use, HIV, chemotherapy agents) present atypically and require aggressive management (e.g. inpatient administration of intravenous antibiotics and early surgical drainage). It is often difficult to obtain specific pathogen data, and infections should be treated based on either the most common pathogen or by using broad-spectrum antibiotics to ensure appropriate treatment. If treated correctly, hand infections should improve expeditiously. If the patient fails to improve within 24–48 hours, the surgeon must reassess the patient and consider an alternate course of therapy (e.g. surgical drainage, different antibiotic treatment, and additional studies).

SUGGESTED READING

Houshian S, Wedderkopp N. Epidemiology of bacterial hand infections. Int J Infect Dis 2006; 10:315–319.

The authors follow 418 patients with hand infections who required surgical intervention over a 9 year period. In this series, Staphylococcus aureus was the most common cause of hand infections, and typically resulted from minor wounds that were inadequately treated upon initial assessment.

LeBlanc D, Reece E, Horton J, Janis J. Increasing incidence of methicillin-resistant Staphylococcus aureus in hand infections: a 3-year county hospital experience. Plast Reconstr Surg 2007; 119:935–940.

This series examines the incidence of resistant organisms among 761 patients with hand infections over a 3-year period, and identified a substantial increase in the rate of methicillin-resistant Staphylococcus aureus.

McDonald LS, Bavaro MF, Hofmeister EP, Kroonen LT. Hand infections. J Hand Surg 2011; 36:1403–1412.

This article describes the many types of hand infections, with an emphasis on microbiology, and outlines the appropriate treatment plans for each anatomic location in the hand.

Talan DA, Citron DM, Abrahamian FM. et al. Bacteriologic analysis of infected dog and cat bites. N Engl J Med 1999; 340:85–92.

This prospective study examines the bacteriology of 100 patients who suffered dog and cat bites, and describes the polymicrobial nature of these common injuries.

Chapter 11 Nail bed injuries

Aviram M. Giladi, Sandeep Sebastin, Kevin C. Chung

The term nail bed injury refers to an injury to the nail complex, often associated with an injury to the adjoining structures, mainly the distal phalanx and the finger pulp. Trauma is the most common etiology of a nail bed injury. Crush and avulsion injuries can result in nail bed lacerations from pressure between nail plate and distal phalanx, whereas sharp injuries can damage the nail bed if enough force is applied to penetrate or lift up the nail plate. Nearly 50% of nail bed injuries have an associated fracture of the distal phalanx. The incidence of isolated finger injuries is highest in young boys, most often arising at home.

ANATOMY

The nail complex includes the nail plate, the nail bed, and the surrounding soft tissue structures (perionychium) (**Figure 11.1**). The nail plate, also known as the 'nail,' is the hard plate on the dorsum of each finger, composed of desiccated, keratinized squamous cells, referred to as onchyn. The white arc at the most proximal aspect of the nail plate is the lunula and it indicates the junction between the sterile and the germinal matrices of the underlying nail bed. The nail bed is a specialized soft tissue located deep to nail plate that provides a platform for nail growth and maturation. The deep surface of the nail bed lies directly on the dorsal surface of the distal phalanx in close proximity to the periosteum (**Figure 11.2**). The sterile matrix is the segment of the nail bed distal to the lunula and is adherent to the overlying nail plate. The segment proximal to the lunula is the germinal matrix, which extends proximally to within 2 mm of the extensor tendon insertion on the distal phalanx. The nail bed is innervated by terminal branches from the radial and ulnar proper digital nerves. The arterial inflow courses via multiple branches from the terminal radial and ulnar digital vessels, whereas venous outflow is regulated by random pattern fingertip veins.

The soft tissues surrounding the nail (perionychium) include the hyponychium, paronychium, and the eponychium. The hyponychium represents the junction of the distal end of the nail bed with the skin of the fingertip/pulp. The hyponychium also contains an increased concentration of immune modulating cells that help to prevent infection. The paronychium is the soft tissue fold on each side (radial and ulnar) of the nail plate. The eponychium is the skin overlying the dorsum of the nail plate proximal to the lunula and contributes to the sheen of the nail. The undersurface of the eponychium that is in contact with the nail plate forms the eponychial fold (dorsal nail fold) as it curves around the proximal end of the nail plate to become contiguous with the proximal end of the germinal matrix. The eponychial fold has fine filamentous attachments (nail vest) that connect it to the nail plate. The cells responsible for the nail sheen are concentrated in the proximal half of the underside of the eponychial fold.

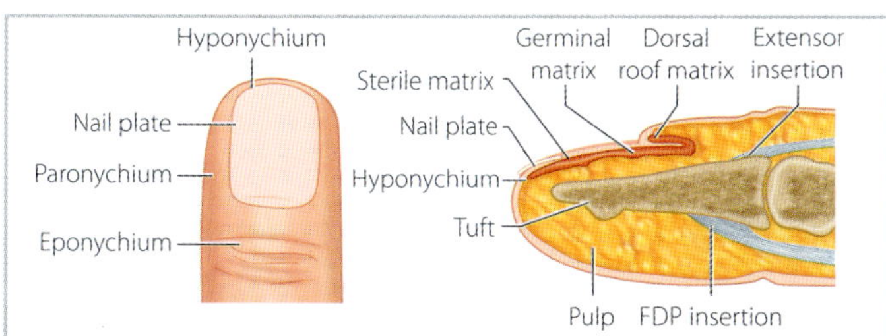

Figure 11.1 The nail complex.

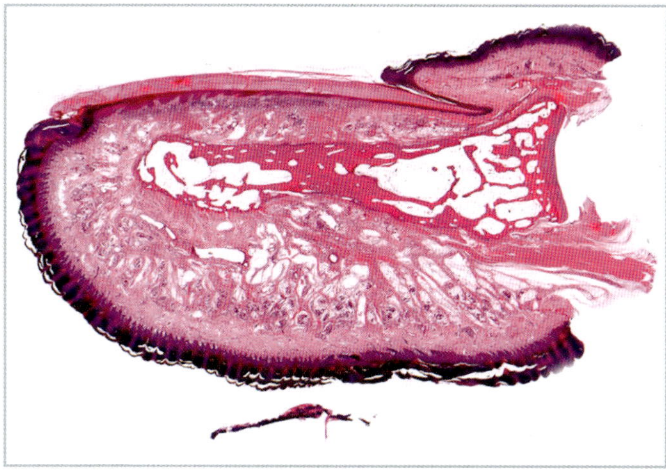

Figure 11.2 Cross-sectional anatomy of the fingertip.

PHYSIOLOGY

The nail complex forms in utero at approximately 10 weeks where the germinal matrix is responsible for 90% of nail growth. The sterile matrix produces the remaining 10% of the nail and is mainly responsible for adherence of the nail plate to the nail bed. The growth of the nail at the germinal matrix occurs via gradient perikaratosis, with the cells originating in the basal layer, near the periosteum. During nail growth, these cells duplicate, resulting in dorsal displacement of cell columns. At the nail plate, cells in each column are flattened by pressure against the plate, resulting in the formation of onchyn as cells die. The dying cells forming onchyn are forced to stream distally, supporting longitudinal nail growth. The cell nuclei die off distal to the lunula, making the nail translucent and allowing visualization of the pink nail bed. The nail grows at approximately 0.1 mm a day, propagating faster in young people, longer digits (e.g. long finger faster than small finger and fingers faster than toes), and in warmer weather conditions. As people age, the matrices produce less nail, decreasing overall nail strength and adherence.

FUNCTIONS

The functions of the nail complex include

- Sensory perception in the fingertip
- Assistance in manipulating small objects and other functions that require fine dexterity
- Providing stability and strength to the fingertip
- Playing an important role in aesthetics of the hand and finger

NAIL BED INJURIES

Injuries to the nail bed usually present acutely, and these acute injuries may be closed or open. Both closed and open injuries may be associated with fractures of the distal phalanx and/or wounds over the finger pulp. However, closed nail bed injuries often result in a subungual hematoma (hematoma between the nail plate and the nail bed) (**Figure 11.3**). The management of closed nail bed injuries depends on the extent of the subungual hematoma, the presence and stability of any associated fractures of the distal phalanx, as well as the nature of the finger pulp injury.

The injury to the nail bed and surrounding soft tissue structures is more severe in open injuries compared to closed injuries (**Figure 11.4**). The severity of nail bed lacerations range from simple linear lacerations to stellate lacerations, avulsions, and occasionally loss of the nail bed entirely. These injuries may also involve damage to the sterile matrix, the germinal matrix, or both. Varying degrees of injury to the surrounding soft tissues frequently accompany nail bed trauma, including damage to or loss of the eponychium and paronychium.

Occasionally patients present late with a deformity of the nail plate resulting from a traumatic event to the nail bed. Common deformities of the nail plate include onycholysis, nail ridging, split nail, and double nail. Onycholysis refers to a nonadherence of the nail plate to the nail bed, and can result from trauma, infection (often fungal), or periungual tumors such as mucous cysts and glomus tumors. Nail ridging results from scarring in or under the nail bed, usually due to malunited distal phalangeal fractures. A split nail occurs when the nail plate cannot grow properly due to a scar in the nail bed. A double nail is the result of a transverse scar in the germinal matrix.

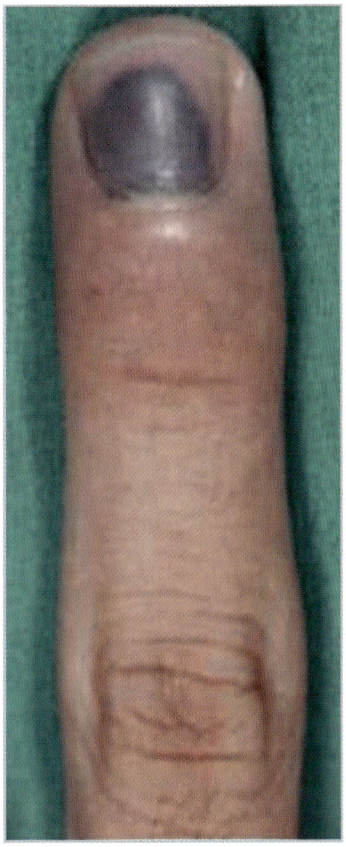

Figure 11.3 A closed nail bed injury with a subungual hematoma.

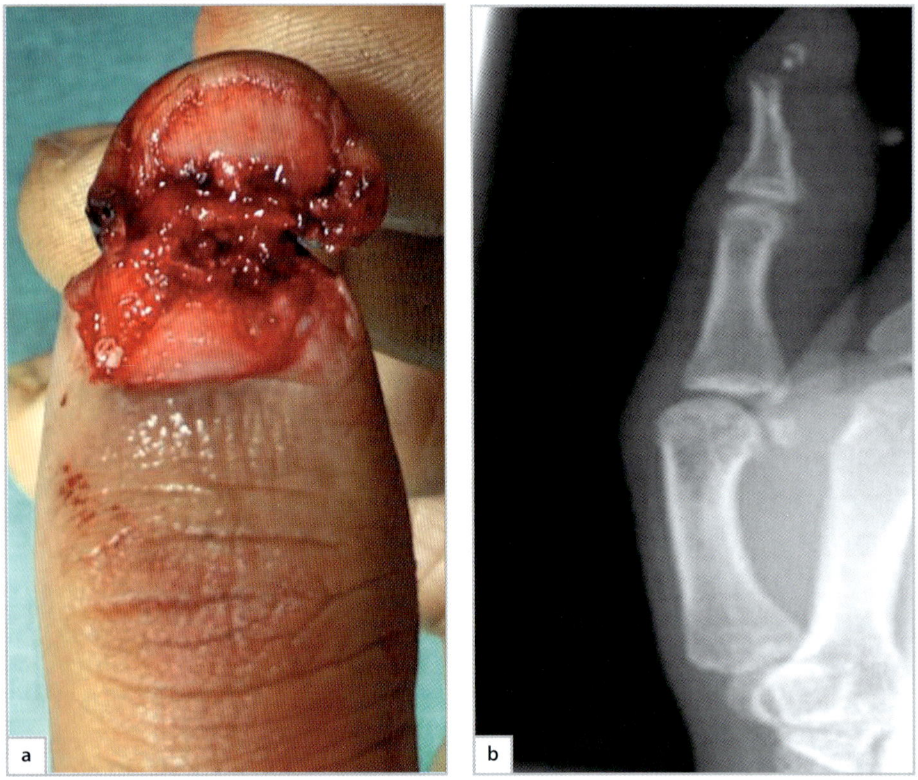

Figure 11.4 (a–b) An open nail bed injury with associated fracture of the distal phalanx.

EVALUATION

The following factors are important in determining the appropriate management of acute nail bed injuries:

- Is it a closed or an open nail bed injury?
- Is there an associated fracture of the distal phalanx? Is this fracture stable?
- Is there an associated injury to the pulp? Is the pulp sensate and viable?

Other factors that influence treatment include injury factors (mechanism of injury, time since injury, and environment of injury) and patient factors (age, handedness, occupation, smoking, comorbidities such as arthritis, diabetes, and Raynaud phenomenon).

The examination for viability (color, capillary refill, and pin-prick) and sensation must be completed before injection of local anesthesia. The extent and severity of a nail bed injury is often not apparent until the wounds are cleaned and examined under anesthesia. The presence of comminuted fractures and soft tissue injuries indicate a more severe nail bed injury. Plain radiographs with multiple views may be useful to identify associated fractures and retained foreign bodies.

TREATMENT

Closed nail bed injuries: The treatment of closed nail bed injuries depends on the degree of pain (related to extent of subungual hematoma), presence and stability of any associated fractures of the distal phalanx, and the nature of the finger pulp injury. Pain in a closed nail bed injury is usually due to the presence of a subungual hematoma. The hematoma results from a laceration to the nail bed, as blood collects in the limited space between the nail bed and the nail plate and elevates the nail plate causing pain. Tuft fractures and undisplaced or minimally displaced shaft or basal fractures of the distal phalanx can be considered as stable fractures. Displaced fractures that cannot be reduced or fractures whose reduction cannot be maintained by splints should be considered as unstable fractures. The Seymour fracture deserves special mention because this fracture is a juxtaepiphyseal fracture of the distal phalanx that is often associated with a nail bed injury, and because it mimics a mallet finger. However, the mallet deformity is at the fracture plane and not at the distal interphalangeal joint, and the nail bed is usually interposed at the fracture site, thus preventing closed reduction. This injury pattern was previously associated with a high incidence of osteomyelitis and should be managed as if it were an open nail bed injury.

Depending on the presence of pain, fracture, and pulp laceration, the treatment of closed nail bed injuries can be summarized as follows:

- No pain + no fracture/stable fracture + no pulp injury: No intervention required
- Pain + no fracture/stable fracture + no pulp injury: Trephination
- Unstable fracture: Nail elevation, nail bed repair, and reduction and fixation of fracture
- Pulp injury: Nail elevation, nail bed repair, and suture of pulp laceration

Trephination (**Figure 11.5**) involves drainage of the subungual hematoma through the nail plate. This can be performed using a hot wire or an 18-gauge needle to puncture the nail plate and allow drainage. During this procedure, one must take care not to injure the underlying nail bed. It is important to take all sterile precautions when this procedure is performed, especially in patients with an associated underlying fracture of the distal phalanx. In these patients, trephination converts a closed fracture into an open fracture. Nail plate elevation and nail bed repair are detailed in the next section on the treatment of open nail bed injuries.

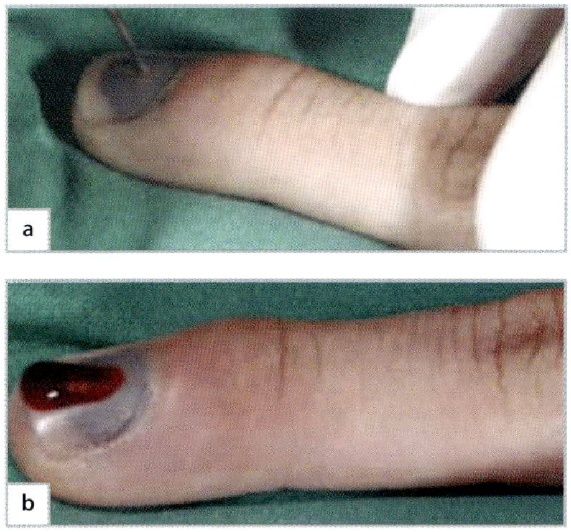

Figure 11.5 Trephination. (a) Trephination with heated blunt-tipped probe used to puncture nail plate. (b) Successful drainage of subungual hematoma.

Open nail bed injuries: The treatment of open nail bed injuries requires the following considerations:

- Anesthesia and tourniquet: A digital block and a finger tourniquet are sufficient in most cases. An arm or a forearm tourniquet can be used when multiple fingers are injured and general anesthesia may be indicated in children. One must remember to remove the finger tourniquet after surgery
- Elevation of nail plate: The nail plate may be partially adherent to the nail bed, and must be carefully elevated to prevent further damage to the nail bed. The nail plate must be cleansed and preserved for use as an eponychial splint following surgery. The undersurface of the nail plate must be examined for nail bed remnants that can be used as a free graft
- Debridement and washout: An aggressive debridement should not be carried out as nail bed tissue is precious and it is difficult to mobilize adjacent nail bed tissue
- Evaluation and stabilization of fractures: Small tuft fractures and undisplaced shaft fractures are adequately stabilized by nail bed repair and stenting of the eponychial fold. However, unstable fracture patterns require some form of fixation. This may include the use of Kirschner wires in minimally comminuted fractures (**Figure 11.6**) and absorbable 3-0/ 4-0 sutures as cerclage loops in comminuted 'bamboo' split type fractures
- Nail bed repair: Lacerations extending into the germinal matrix may require elevation of the eponychial fold. This is completed by making two oblique incisions at the corner of the eponychial fold and elevating it as a proximally based flap. A tension-free repair of the nail bed is performed using fine absorbable sutures (5-0/6-0 fast gut/vicryl rapid, etc.) (**Figure 11.7**). In severely comminuted stellate nail bed lacerations, a few strategically placed sutures are used to approximate the multiple nail bed flaps. The use of cyanoacrylate (Dermabond) or fibrin glue can be considered in such cases. In patients with an avulsion of the nail bed (tear at the junction of the germinal matrix and eponychial fold), the nail bed can be repositioned by horizontal mattress sutures passed from the dorsum of the nail fold to the proximal end of the germinal matrix
- Stenting the eponychial fold: The original nail plate (if available), an artificial nail, or a stent made from suture packing foil or

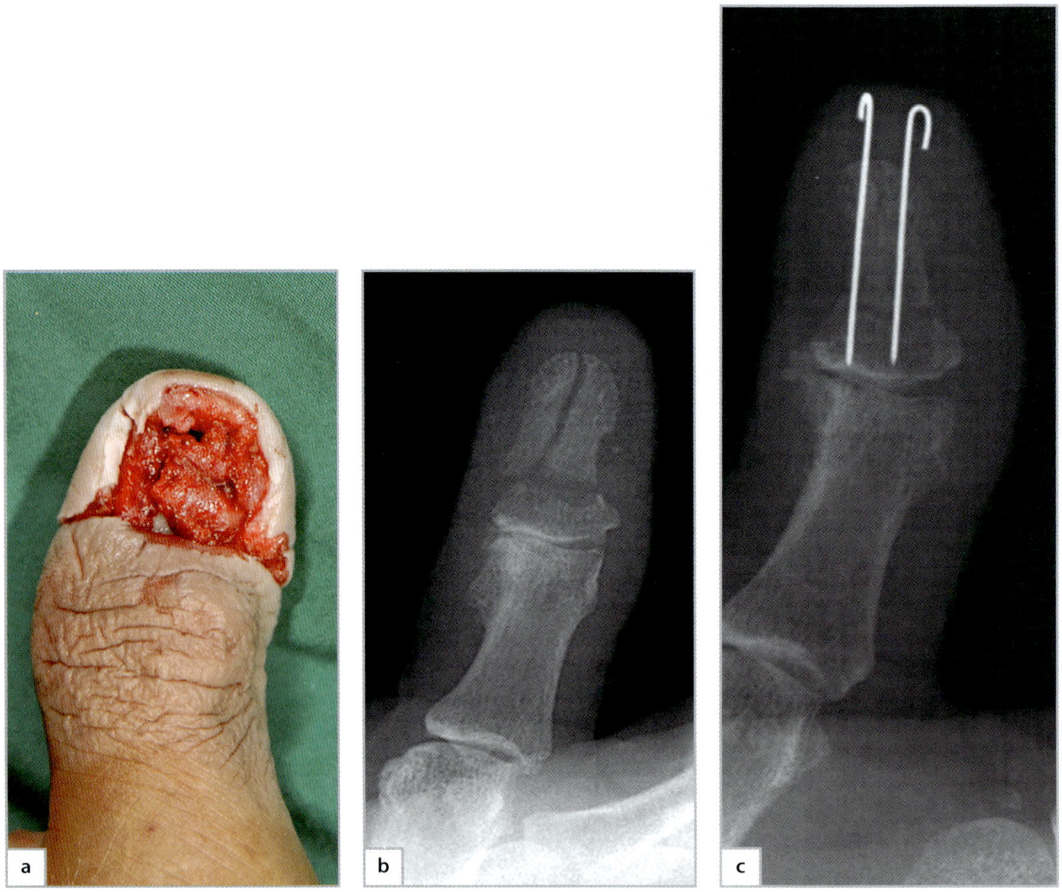

Figure 11.6 (a–c) Stabilization of a distal phalanx fracture with Kirschner wires.

other pliable sturdy material can be used as a temporary stent. This serves as a splint for tuft and undisplaced shaft fractures and prevents the dressing from adhering to the nail bed repair making dressing change less painful. It also prevents adhesion (synechia) formation between two adjacent injured epithelial surfaces in cases in which the nail bed laceration involves both the germinal matrix and the eponychial fold. The stent can be anchored to the nail bed and soft tissues using nonabsorbable sutures (**Figure 11.8**)

- Nail bed loss: A split thickness nail bed graft can be used in patients with a loss of the sterile matrix. This graft can be harvested from amputated digits (spare parts), uninjured segments of same nail bed (rarely available), or the great toe. A loss of the germinal matrix, on the other hand, is difficult to reconstruct, and it should be noted that a sterile matrix graft will not replace the function of the germinal matrix. A germinal matrix graft from the toes will cause loss of nail growth in the toes, and the result at the finger may not be successful. The options include excision of the nail bed and coverage with a local flap such as a reversed cross finger flap, or reconstruction of the nail bed with a free nail bed transfer from the toe. In patients with severe injury to the bone and soft tissues with loss of the nail bed, it may be reasonable to consider an amputation of the digit proximal to the germinal matrix

COMPLICATIONS

- Hypersensitivity/cold intolerance/dysesthesia: This can occur after relatively minor nail bed injuries and is difficult to predict or adequately treat, but many of these issues will improve with time. The patient may require desensitization therapy if function and use are limited
- Nail deformity: A scarred nail bed may result in poor adherence and deformities of the nail plate (**Figure 11.9**). This usually occurs after open nail bed injuries that did not receive any primary treatment or were not treated appropriately. Scarring or loss of the eponychial fold will result in surface irregularities and loss of nail sheen. Loss of the hyponychium (often with loss of distal sterile matrix) may result in a hook nail deformity (**Figure 11.9**). Nail bed scarring will require elevation of the nail plate, followed by excision of the scarred nail bed and linear repair, Z-plasty repair, or use of a split thickness nail bed graft. The correction of hook nail deformity and eponychial fold may require use of local flaps and local soft tissue rearrangement
- Distal phalanx fracture nonunion/malunion: Small tuft fractures often heal without intervention; however, pain with pulp pressure can persist for 3 months or more while healing. Fractures with larger distal segments that were not appropriately managed with fixation and splinting may result in a nonunion that may require bone grafting depending on the patient's symptoms

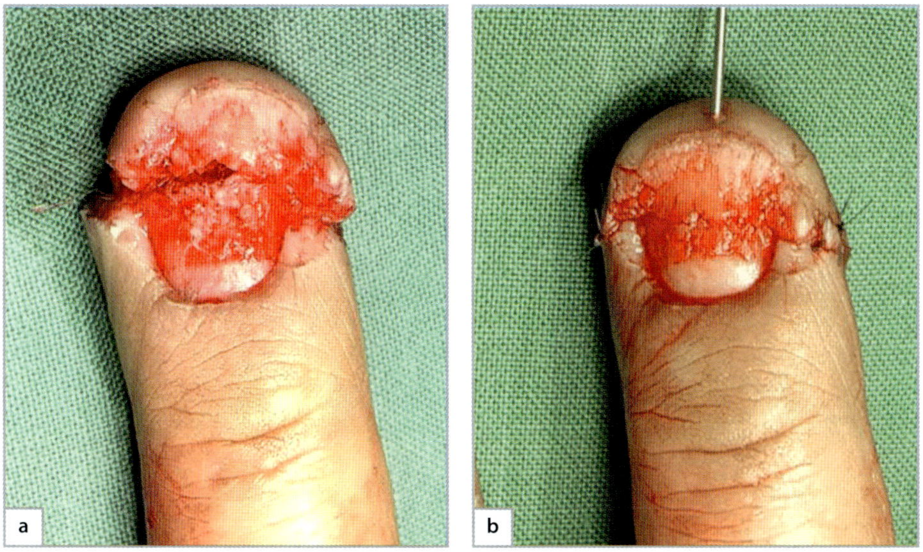

Figure 11.7 (a–b) Tension-free repair of nail bed with 6-0 vicryl rapid.

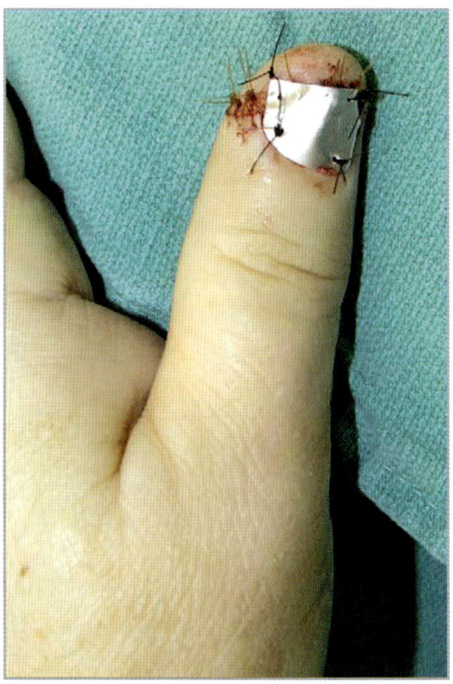

Figure 11.8 Stenting the eponychial fold with a foil from a suture pack.

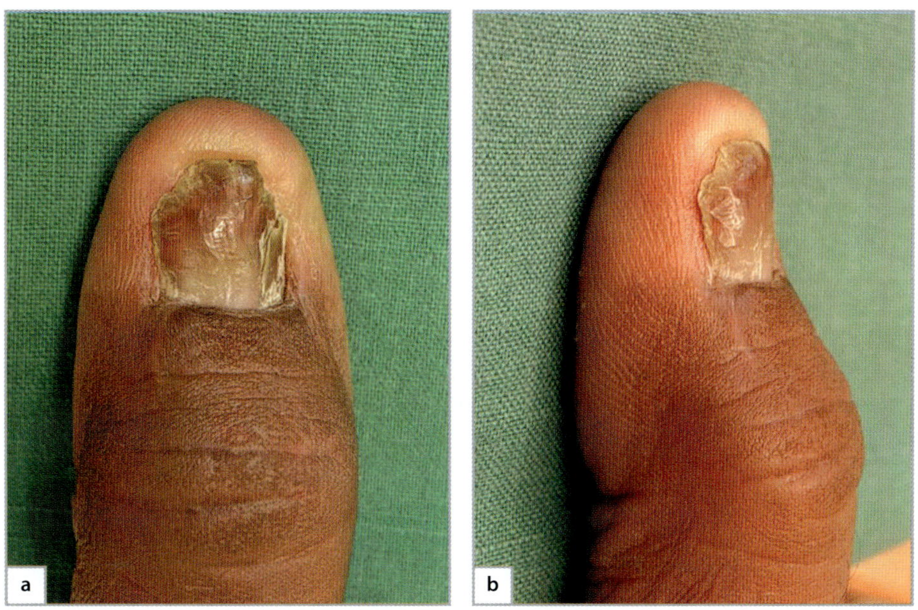

Figure 11.9 (a–b) Nail deformity following poor initial management.

SUGGESTED READING

Dean B, Becker G, Little C. The management of the acute traumatic subungual haematoma: a systematic review. Hand Surg 2012; 17:151–154.
It is a systematic review of the most current literature for evaluation and management of subungual hematoma. Guidelines on assessment, management, and treatment algorithm are included.

Yeo CJ, Sebastin SJ, Chong AK. Fingertip injuries. Singapore Med J 2010; 51:78–86.
It is an excellent review of fingertip and nail bed trauma. Includes up-to-date data on epidemiology and the social burden of these injuries, as well as comprehensive discussion of evaluation and management of the wide range of simple and complex fingertip injuries.

Zook EG. Reconstruction of a functional and aesthetic nail. Hand Clin 2002; 18:577–594.
It is a revision of the original Hand Clinics article (1990, Zook and Russell) covering the various nuances and management decisions in treating ungual and periungual pathology.

Chapter 12 Tendon injuries

Teemu Karjalainen (12.2), Alphonsus Chong (12.1), Erika D. Sears (12.3), Kevin C. Chung (12.3)

12.1 FLEXOR TENDON INJURIES

BACKGROUND AND EVALUATION

The flexor tendons lie in close relation to the skin, especially in the digits, and are frequently involved in hand trauma. The management of these injuries is challenging because it requires a strong repair that is not bulky, and that will also withstand the normal tensile forces and simultaneously allow gliding within the narrow confines of the tendon sheath. The postoperative management needs to be carefully considered to prevent adhesions and improve gliding.

Anatomy

The term flexor tendon refers to the tendinous portions of the wrist and digital flexors. The flexor tendons extend from the musculotendinous junction in the mid-forearm to their respective bony insertions. The three wrist flexors from radial to ulnar are the flexor carpi radialis (FCR), palmaris longus (PL), and the flexor carpi ulnaris (FCU). The digital flexors include the flexor tendon for the thumb, the flexor pollicis longus (FPL), and two flexor tendons for each of the fingers, the flexor digitorum superficialis (FDS) and flexor digitorum profundus (FDP). The flexor muscles are arranged in three distinct layers or compartments. The superficial compartment includes (radial to ulnar) the pronator teres (PT), FCR, PL, and FCU. The intermediate compartment includes the FDS, and the deep compartment includes the FPL, FDP, and the pronator quadratus (PQ).

The arrangement of the flexor tendons changes as they proceed from the distal forearm to the digits. The FPL and the FDP tendons lie in a deeper plane, superficial to the PQ, and the four tendons of the FDS lie superficial to the FDP. The FDS tendons to the ring and long fingers are superficial and central, whereas the tendons to the index and small fingers are deeper and located radially and ulnarly, respectively. This arrangement of tendons is maintained in the distal forearm and in the carpal tunnel. Once the tendons exit from the carpal tunnel, they diverge toward the respective fingers. A knowledge of the anatomical relationships between the tendons and other structures (**Figure 12.1**) is important when assessing and repairing flexor tendon injuries in the distal forearm and wrist. In the digit (**Figure 12.2**), the close relationship of the digital neurovascular bundle to the flexor tendons means that associated injuries to the bundle are common in flexor tendon injuries.

Flexor sheath and pulley system

The flexor sheath refers to the specialized tissue that covers the digital flexor tendons (FDS, FPL, and FDP). This sheath allows the tendon to glide and turn around a corner to produce smooth and efficient flexion of the digits. The flexor sheath has two major components, namely the synovial (membranous) component and the retinacular (pulley) component. The synovial layer is thin and begins at the level of the wrist, and is a double-walled synovial tube that is sealed at both ends. The inner layer of synovium is in close proximity to the surface of the flexor tendon and is known as the visceral layer, whereas the outer layer of synovium is related to the overlying retinacular layer and is known as the parietal layer.

The retinacular layer is thick, consisting of a series of fibrous tissue condensations also known as pulleys. It begins at the neck of the metacarpal (MC), lies superficial to the synovial component, and ends at the level of the distal interphalangeal (DIP) joint, or the interphalangeal (IP) joint for the thumb. It is segmental and not continuous, and each segment is represented by a pulley. The pulleys have been classified into four types based on their appearance, namely transverse, annular, cruciate, and oblique. The annular pulleys prevent bowstringing and maximize the angular rotation of the joints for the given tendon excursion, whereas the cruciate pulleys collapse to allow

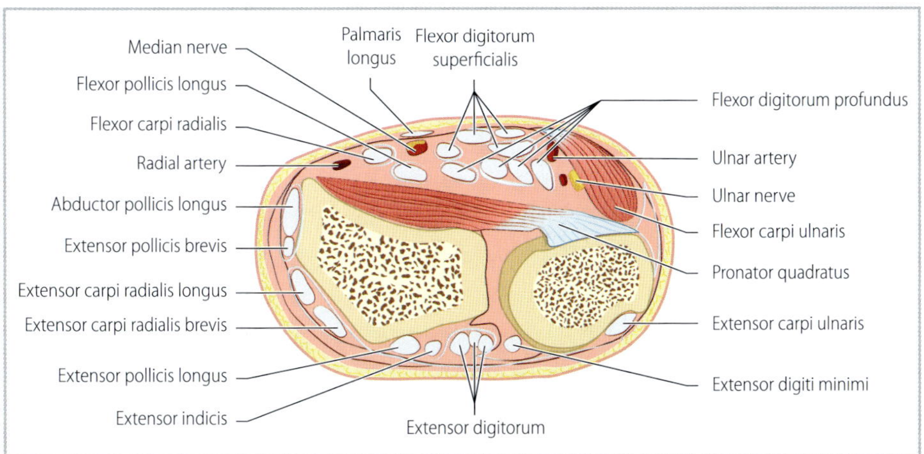

Figure 12.1 Transverse section at the distal end of the radius. Note the relationships of the various flexor tendons to the neurovascular bundles. The flexor digitorum superficialis tendons to the middle and ring finger lie palmar to that of the index and little.

full digital flexion. The retinacular component of the fingers includes one transverse pulley, five annular pulleys, and three cruciate pulleys. The transverse pulley is also known as the palmar aponeurosis pulley (PA). The annular and cruciate pulleys are numbered from proximal to distal as A1, A2, A3, A4, A5 and C1, C2, C3, respectively (**Figure 12.3**). The arrangement of the pulleys from proximal to distal for the fingers is PA, A1, A2, C1, A3, C2, A4, C3, and A5, respectively. The A1, A3, and A5 pulleys overlie the MP joint, PIP joint, and DIP joint respectively. The A2 and A4 pulleys over the proximal and middle phalanx are biomechanically the most important. The retinacular component of the thumb includes two annular pulleys and one oblique pulley, and the arrangement of the pulleys from proximal to distal for the thumb is A1, oblique pulley, and A2, respectively.

The combination of the synovial and retinacular components distal to the neck of the MCs results in the formation of a fibro-osseous tunnel for the passage of the flexor tendons. The floor of this fibro-osseous tunnel is formed by the transverse MC ligament, the volar plates of the metacarpophalangeal (MCP) joint, proximal interphalangeal (PIP) joint, and DIP joint, and the palmar surfaces of the proximal and middle phalanxes. This fibro-osseous tunnel is also known as the digital flexor sheath and has three important functions:

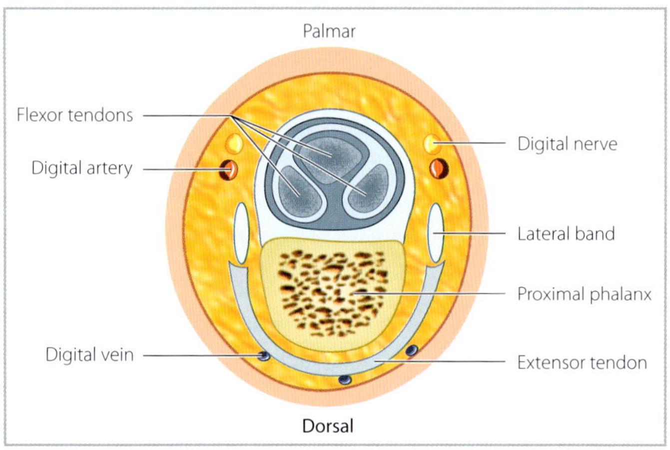

Figure 12.2 Cross section of a digit at the proximal phalanx. Note the two flexor tendons and the neurovascular bundle that is closely situated.

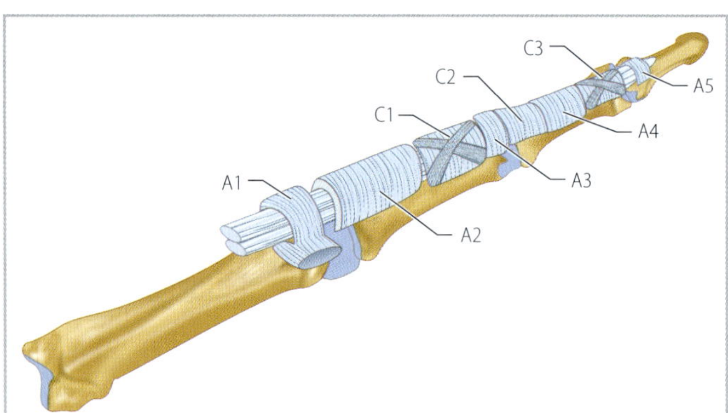

Figure 12.3 Flexor tendon pulley system.

1. It allows for smooth gliding of digital flexor tendons (FDS, FDP, and FPL) in flexion and extension
2. It provides a pulley that prevents bowstringing of the flexor tendon and improves the mechanical advantage during flexion
3. It plays a nutritive role by providing a contained bursa environment for synovial fluid

Zones of flexor tendon injury

The flexor tendons are divided into five zones (**Figure 12.4**). This is important, because there are anatomical differences in the tendons in the different zones (**Table 12.1**). Traditionally, the outcomes of tendon repair in zone II (commonly referred to as 'No man's land') are poorest as there are two tendons running in a tight fibro-osseous tunnel (**Figure 12.5**).

Evaluation

Most flexor tendon injuries, with the exception of FDP avulsion injuries, are open injuries. Any wound near the site of a flexor tendon should be evaluated for a possible tendon injury. The important steps in the examination include

- Note site and type of wound
- Look at finger cascade
- Test all digital flexor tendons individually
- Assess neurovascular status

The normal finger cascade is lost with a flexor tendon injury. The presence of a flexor tendon injury is confirmed by asking the patient to actively flex the digits (**Figure 12.6**). A partial tendon laceration should be suspected in patients in whom active motion is associated

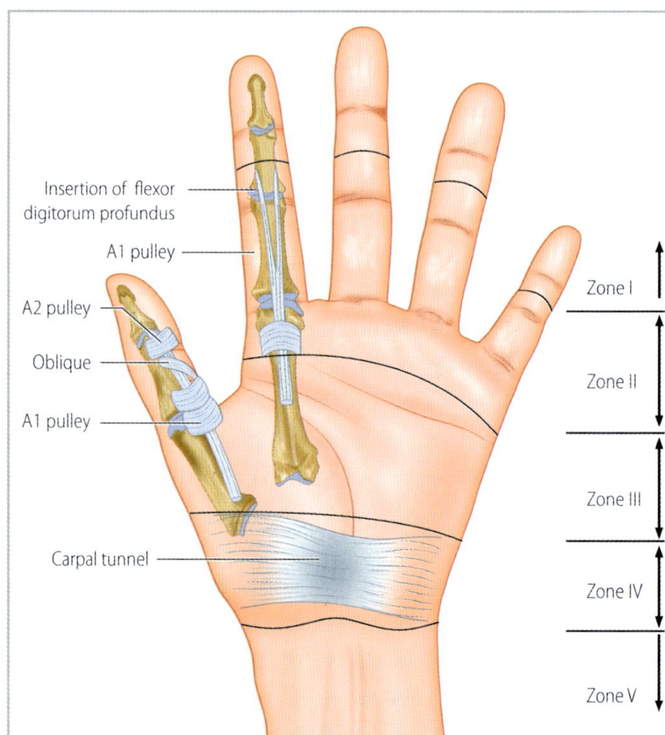

Figure 12.4 The zones of flexor tendon injury. There is a separate system for the thumb.

Table 12.1 Anatomic characteristic in different zones

Zone of injury	Extent	Unique characteristic
Zone I	Distal to FDS insertion	Only one tendon (FDP)
Zone II	A1 pulley till FDS insertion	Two tendons in a narrow fibro-osseous tunnel
Zone III	Distal edge of carpal tunnel till A1 pulley	Lumbricals origin
Zone IV	Within carpal tunnel	Nine tendons in a wide fibro-osseous tunnel
Zone V	Proximal to carpal tunnel	Musculotendinous junction

FDP, flexor digitorum profundus; FDS, flexor digitorum superficialis.

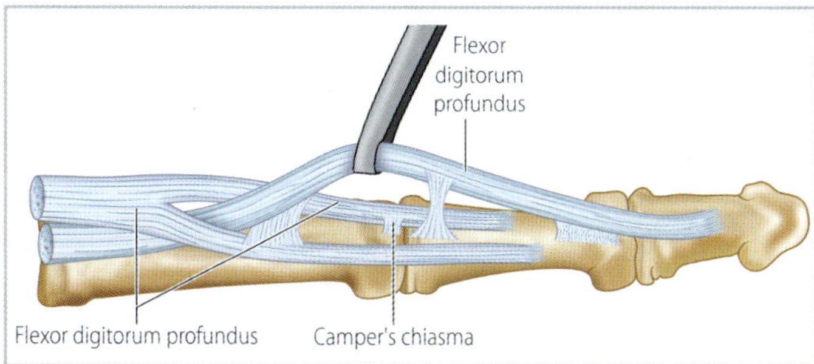

Figure 12.5 Relationship between the flexor digitorum profundus (FDP) and flexor digitorum superficialis (FDS) tendons. The FDS tendon divides into two slips at the proximal end of the tendon sheath. Each slip encircles one side of the FDP tendon and then unites dorsally to form Camper's chiasma. Pulleys are removed.

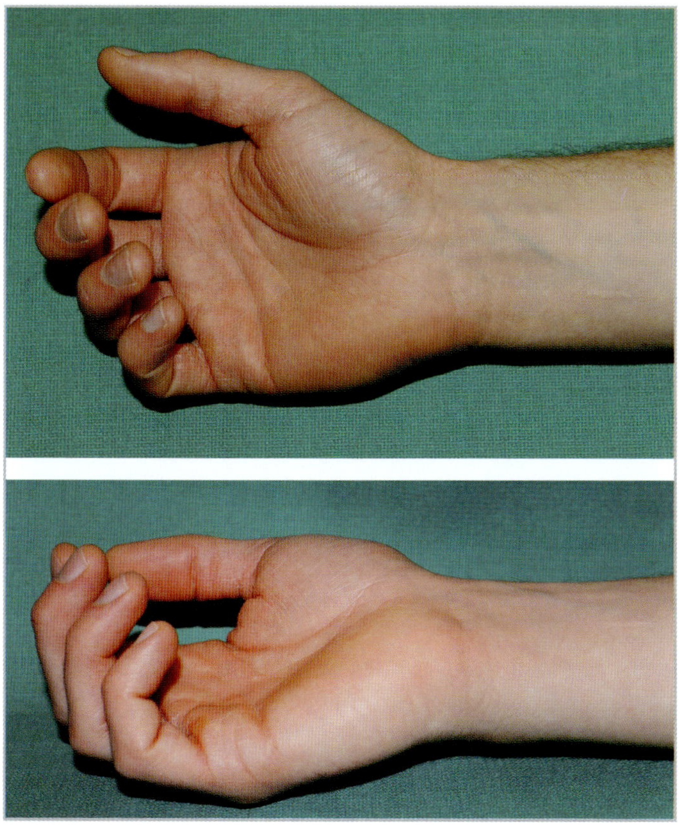

Figure 12.6 The normal cascade of fingers, with increasing flexion of the digits from radial to ulnar. This cascade is lost in complete flexor tendon injuries.

with pain or triggering. In patients who cannot cooperate (e.g. children, comatose, or intoxicated patients), one can look for passive movement of the fingers resulting from the wrist tenodesis effect or movement can be elicited by squeezing the forearm muscles.

The FDP, FPL, and FDS tendons should be tested individually. The FDP and FPL tendons are checked by asking the patient to flex the DIP joint of the fingers (**Figure 12.7**) and the IP joint of the thumb. Testing for injury to the FDS (**Figure 12.8**) is more complex than examination of the FDP because the PIP joint is flexed both by the FDS and by the FDP. Therefore, one needs to check the function of the FDS while blocking the action of the FDP. The standard test for the FDS takes advantage of the fact that the FDP tendons to the long, ring, and small fingers share a common muscle belly. The finger being tested is allowed to flex while the examiner blocks the action of the FDP tendon by preventing flexion of the DIP joint of the other two fingers. The standard test is not reliable for the index finger because the index finger FDP has an independent muscle belly. In addition, the action of the FDS to the small finger may either be absent or dependent on the FDS to the ring finger in about 20% of the population. The use of a modified test will reveal a normally functioning tendon in most of these cases (**Figure 12.9**). This is an important consideration when assessing the little finger for flexor tendon injuries.

The vascular status is assessed by observing color, capillary refill, turgor, temperature and if necessary a pin prick for bleeding.

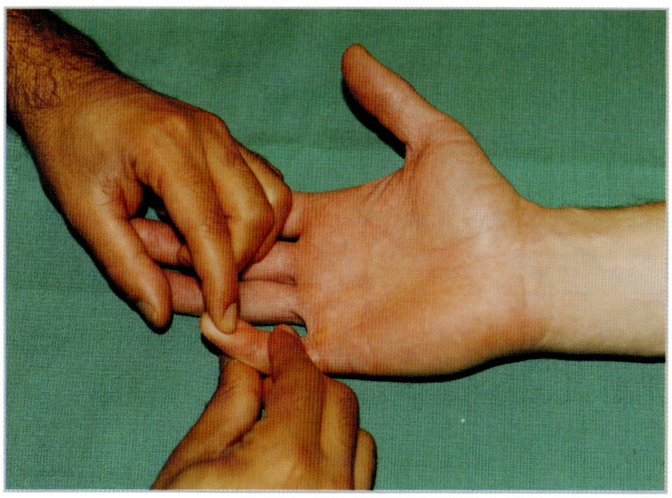

Figure 12.7 Test the flexor digitorum profundus tendon at the distal interphalangeal joint.

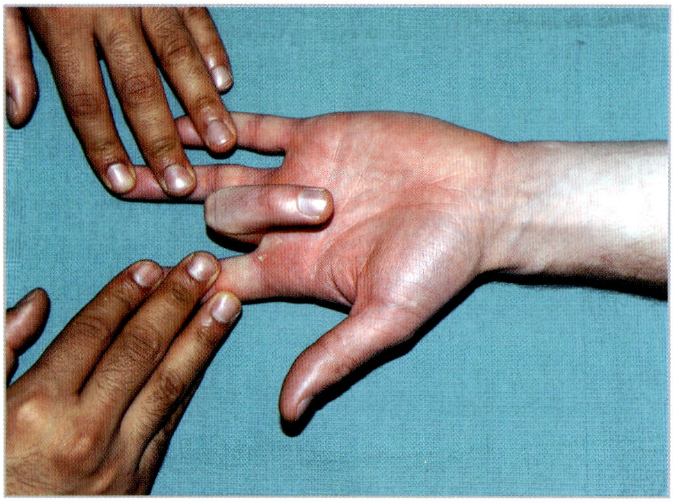

Figure 12.8 Test the flexor digitorum superficialis by passively keeping the other digits in extension.

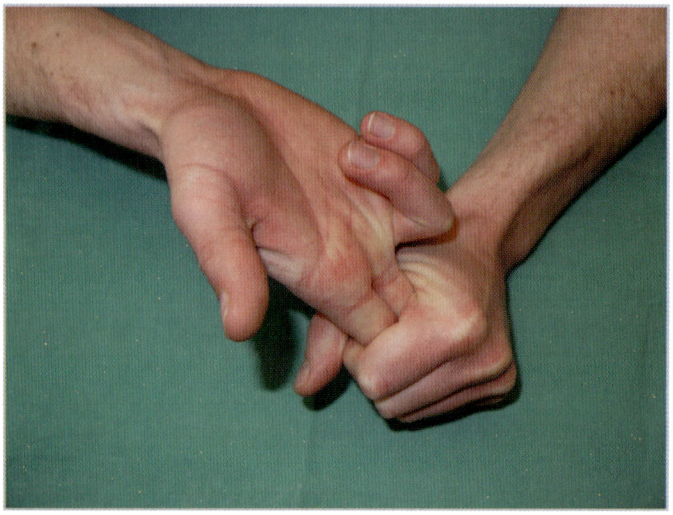

Figure 12.9 Modified test to assess flexor digitorum superficialis (FDS) if the standard test shows absent FDS function.

The sensory status is examined by measuring static two-point discrimination (2-PD). A 2-PD >10 mm indicates a high likelihood of digital nerve injury, and a bent paper clip is helpful for 2-PD assessment.

SURGICAL REPAIR

Timing of repair

Good surgical technique is necessary to achieve a strong and neat flexor tendon repair, ensuring the best functional recovery. This requires a surgeon properly trained in the repair techniques. Except where circulation of digit or hand is compromised, a flexor tendon repair does not need to be performed on the same day as presentation. Results of delayed repair up to 3 weeks are as good as primary repair. If there is no available properly trained surgeon to perform the flexor tendon repair at the primary setting, the wound can be cleaned and closed first, and the tendon repair can be performed at a later date.

Approach

A variety of incisions can be used, incorporating the original laceration while ensuring good exposure, extensibility, and no compromise of the skin flaps. Some forms of the Bruner incision (**Figure 12.10**) are commonly used.

Repair technique

Current flexor tendon repair techniques favor using a combination of a core suture repair with a circumferential suture. The circumferential suture smoothens the bunching up of the repaired tendon ends and augments the strength of the repair, and is placed 2 mm from the cut tendon edge and 2 mm from the tendon surface (**Figure 12.11**). There are several factors to consider when choosing the core suture technique:

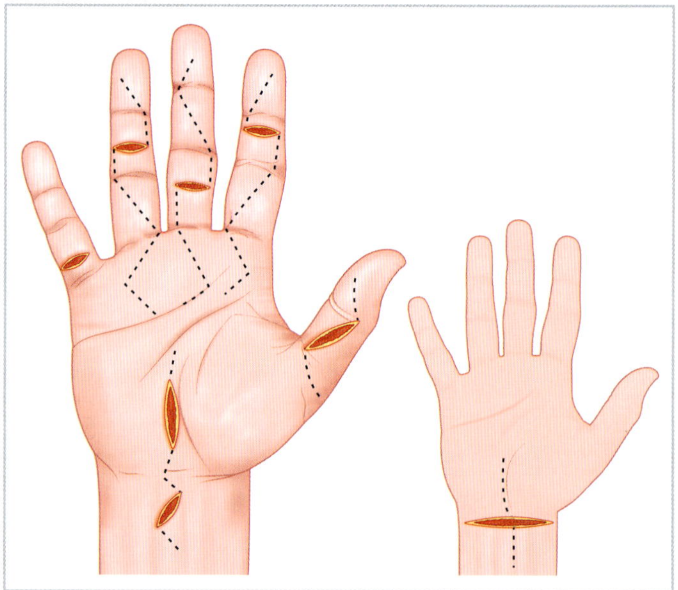

Figure 12.10 Brunner type incisions extending the original wound.

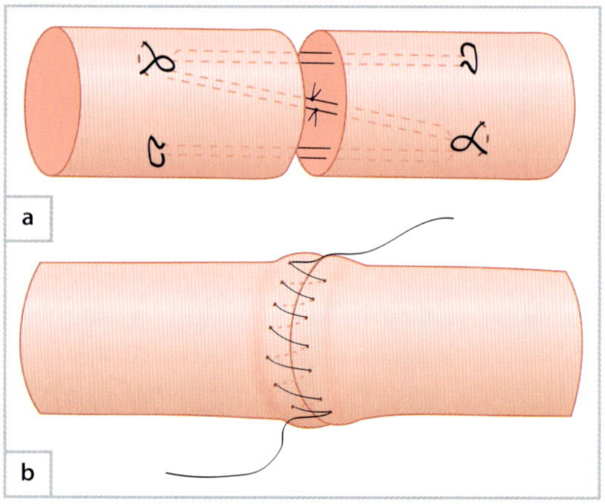

Figure 12.11 (a) Lim and Tsai technique using a loop suture (top). (b) Modified Kessler (bottom). Note the use of an epitendinous repair in both cases.

- Type of suture used: polypropylene (e.g. Prolene, Ethicon, USA) and braided polyester (e.g. Ethibond, Ethicon, USA) are common choices
- Size of the suture: 3/0 or 4/0 commonly
- Number of suture strands crossing the repair site

Tendon repairs should support early active or passive range of motion (ROM) therapy protocols. Active ROM can produce an average force of 10–35 Newtons (N), whereas passive protocols produce an average of 8–10 N of force. There is some loss of strength at the repair site in the first 5–7 days after the repair, and this should be considered in the strength of repair and the therapy protocol used. The current recommendation is to use at least a four strand core suture that is augmented with a circumferential suture technique. Some considerations in repair of flexor tendons specific to the individual zones are as follows:

- Zone I tendon repair: Zone I contains a portion of the A4, C3, and A5 pulley and contains only the FDP tendon. If at least 1 cm of distal tendon is available for repair, a direct suture repair of the tendon ends can be attempted. If <1 cm of the distal tendon is available for repair, it is preferable to advance the tendon and insert it directly into the bone. This can be done using bone anchors or a pull-through suture technique
- Zone II tendon repair: The three problems encountered in this zone are (1) difficulty in retrieval of the proximal end, (2) establishing the correct orientation of the FDS and FDP, and (3) limited space for repair. The application of gentle pressure in a proximal to distal direction on the forearm with the wrist and MCP joint in flexion may coax the tendon through the pulley system. If not, a single attempt with a fine-tipped mosquito forceps passed into the sheath from distal to proximal can be attempted. If both of these maneuvers do not work, an incision is made in the distal palm proximal to the A1 pulley. The flexor tendons are identified and a 5/6 French pediatric feeding tube is passed from retrograde through the flexor sheath to emerge at the distal incision. The feeding tube is sutured to the palmar surface of the flexor tendon and the tendon ends are delivered into the laceration, where they are transfixed using a hypodermic needle. It is important to preserve the orientation of the FDS chiasma around the FDP tendon. One can consider dividing the A3 pulley and venting up to 50% of the A2 and A4 pulleys to allow repair and prevent triggering after a repair
- Zone III, IV, and V tendon repair: The principles of these areas for tendon repair are similar to injuries in zone II. Zone III injuries are often associated with injury to the common digital nerves and vessels. In zone IV, one must consider release of the transverse carpal tunnel ligament for access and to prevent compression of the median nerve postoperatively. Zone V injury is also known as 'spaghetti wrist.' It can be difficult to identify and correctly match the proximal ends of the divided tendons. The oblique nature of the laceration and the depth of the tendon can help in matching the divided ends. Zone V injuries are often associated with injuries to the median and ulnar nerve and radial and ulnar arteries
- Partial tendon injuries: The problems associated with partial injuries include triggering, entrapment, and delayed rupture. After exploration, evaluate the amount of tendon intact and check for triggering or entrapment. Potential triggering and entrapment can be prevented by beveling the tendon edge. Partially injured flexor tendons with <50% cross-sectional area divided do not need to be repaired. For those >50%, the tendon can be reinforced with a core suture and epitendinous repair, followed by active rehabilitation

Complications

Early complications include infection, tendon rupture, and adhesions limiting tendon gliding. The rate of tendon rupture is reported variable, ranging from 3% to 9%. Late complications include joint stiffness or contracture, triggering, and tendon bowstringing.

Postoperative management

The aim of postoperative therapy is to allow the repaired tendon to heal, while simultaneously preventing adhesions to surrounding tissues. Although many different types of therapy protocols have been described in the literature, all involve one of three themes:

1. Immobilization
2. Early passive mobilization
3. Early active ROM

A long dorsal splint extending from the fingertip up to the proximal forearm is applied immediately after surgery. The splint maintains the wrist in 20° of flexion, MCP joint in 50–70° of flexion, and IP joints in extension. The patients are encouraged to begin immediate postoperative ROM exercises of all uninvolved joints, such as the shoulder and elbow. Passive/active motion exercises of the injured digits should be initiated 2–3 days after surgery under the supervision of a therapist, and gradually increased over a 4–6 weeks' period. After this period, the splint is removed and the patient started on strengthening exercises.

Tendon healing process

There are three overlapping phases during the tendon healing process. In the first 48–72 hours, the tendon healing is in the inflammatory stage, and then a proliferating stage occurs that lasts anywhere from 5 days to 4 weeks. The last stage of tendon healing is the remodeling stage, which takes place 6 weeks after tendon repair. The weakest point of tendon healing when the repaired tendon is most likely to rupture is 5–10 days postoperative, which needs to be taken into consideration during therapy. Surgical techniques, such as decreasing vascularity and gapping, as well as postoperative exercises, will all have an effect on tendon healing and adhesion formation.

Secondary tendon reconstruction

This may be required following a failed primary repair, or when a primary end-to-end flexor tendon repair was either not performed or not possible. This may be due to a loss of tendon substance or late situations when the tendon ends have retracted and cannot be apposed due to myostatic contracture. In more severe cases, the flexor sheath may have collapsed.

Secondary tendon reconstruction can be achieved using a tendon graft in a single stage or as a staged procedure. Single stage grafting can be performed only if there is supple skin and soft tissue, functioning muscle, and an intact flexor sheath with good passive ROM. A staged reconstruction must be considered if any of these conditions are not met. In a staged reconstruction, the first stage consists of addressing the problems in the skin, soft tissue, joints, and the flexor sheath. It usually involves creation of a flexor sheath using a silicone rod. This rod is then replaced with a tendon graft in the second stage. The PL is the most common source of tendon graft, but the plantaris can be used as an alternative. Salvage procedures, such as joint fusion and tenodesis, may also be considered when the patient suffers long-term disability from joint stiffness following a previous failed tendon reconstruction.

FDP avulsion also known as 'Jersey Finger' or 'Rugby Finger'

This is a closed injury due to avulsion of the FDP tendon from its insertion at the base of the distal phalanx. It may be a tendinous rupture or bony avulsion, and rarely a combination of both. The mechanism of injury is a forced hyperextension of the DIP joint when the FDP is contracting (**Figure 12.12**), and the ring finger is most commonly affected. The avulsed ends of the tendon and bone fragments may lie at different levels. Leddy and Packer proposed a classification based on the level of the proximal tendon end.

- Leddy-Packer classification:
  - Type 1: FDP tendon retracted to palm with rupture of short and long vinculae
  - Type 2: FDP retracted to level of PIP joint, only short vinculum ruptured. Often associated with small avulsion fragments
  - Type 3: FDP retracted to A4 pulley. Associated with large avulsion fragments

On examination, patients are unable to actively flex the DIP joint of the affected finger. The flexor sheath may feel empty on palpation and a mass may be palpable in the palm. In type 2 avulsions, patients may present with a flexion contracture of the PIP joint.

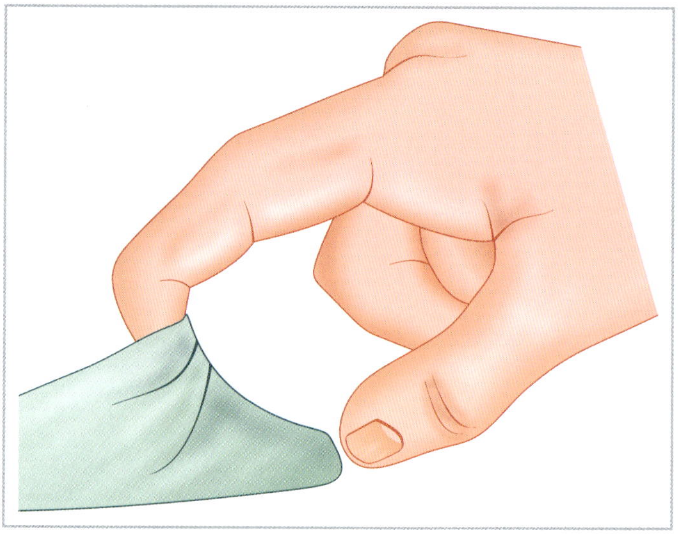

Figure 12.12 Mechanism of injury of flexor digitorum profundus avulsion.

Treatment

- Type 1 has the smallest window for tendon reinsertion
- It may be possible to repair type III injuries even up to 6 weeks
- The level of retraction determines the ability to reattach the distal tendon stump
- Reattachment can be achieved through bony fixation if the fragment is large or by a bone anchor, or by a pull-through technique if it is pure avulsion or if the fragment is small
- The options in late cases include no treatment, tendon grafting, DIP joint tenodesis, or DIP joint fusion

SUGGESTED READING

Lalonde DH. An evidence-based approach to flexor tendon laceration repair. Plast Reconstr Surg 2011; 127:885–890.
A recent case-based review of the literature to help decide the course of treatment in acute flexor tendon injury.

Momeni A, Grauel E, Chang J. After flexor tendon injuries. Hand Clin 2010; 26:179–189. doi: 10.1016/j.hcl.2009.11.004.
A practical overview of the complications following flexor tendon injuries and how to manage them.

Strickland JW. Flexor tendon injuries: foundations of treatment. J Am Acad Orthop Surg 1995; 3:44–54.
This article remains relevant today. It provides the scientific basis behind the clinical approach to flexor tendon surgery and rehabilitation.

Strickland JW. Development of flexor tendon surgery: Twenty-five years of progress. J Hand Surg (Am.) 2000; 25:214–235.
This article provides a useful perspective of modern flexor tendon surgery.

Viinikainen A, Göransson H, Ryhänen J. Primary flexor tendon repair techniques. Scand J Surg 2008; 97:333–340.
This article shows a good collection of repair techniques in use. It covers suture material, size, core repair techniques, and peripheral suture techniques.

12.2 EXTENSOR TENDON INJURIES

FUNCTIONAL ANATOMY

Extension of the fingers is achieved through the synergistic action of both the extrinsic and intrinsic muscles. Extrinsic muscles arise proximal to the hand, whereas intrinsic muscles originate from the hand. Several passive ligamentous structures also contribute to the extension of the finger (**Table 12.2**). The extrinsic and intrinsic tendons converge with the ligamentous structures to form an intricate extensor mechanism distal to the MCP joint (**Figure12.13a** and **b**).

- Extrinsic extensor tendons: The primary function of the extrinsic extensor tendons is MCP joint extension. The muscle bellies of these tendons are innervated by the radial nerve and lie in the forearm. There are two extrinsic extensors for the thumb, index, and small fingers, as well as one for the long and ring fingers (**Table 12.2**). Extrinsic extensor tendons traverse the six extensor compartments in the wrist level, and are connected with adjacent extensors by juncturae tendinae, centralized over the MCP joint by the sagittal bands. Extension of the proximal phalanx occurs primarily through the sagittal bands, which attach to the volar plate of the MCP joints and form a lasso mechanism that serves to extend the proximal phalanx
- Intrinsic extensor tendons: The intrinsic muscles (interossei and lumbricals) lie in the palm, and their primary function is extension of the PIP and DIP joint, but they also act as flexors of the MCP joint. The lumbricals originate from the FDP tendon in the palm and the tendons pass volar to the intermetacarpal ligament and radial to the MC head. The lumbricals then form the radial lateral band together with fibers from the interossei muscles, and also contribute fibers that extend over the proximal phalanx (extensor hood), which flexes the MCP joint and extends the PIP joint. On the ulnar side of the MCP joint, the interossei form the ulnar lateral band (**Figure 12.13b**).

In the finger, an intricate extensor mechanism is formed by fibers from both the extrinsic and intrinsic extensor tendons. The extensor mechanism moves not only along a longitudinal axis but also translation occurs in the coronal and sagittal plane. This translation is controlled by the triangular and transverse retinacular ligaments, and disturbance to this delicate balance of tension and translation results in deformity of the finger (**Figure 12.13**).

ZONES OF INJURY

Evaluation

The zones of extensor tendon injury have been depicted in **Figure 12.14**. Closed extensor injuries are relatively common and are often missed because they are considered as sprains. Wounds over the dorsum of the palm or the fingers should always arouse suspicion of a tendon injury due to the superficial location of the tendons. It is important to evaluate the function of the extensors systematically:

- Extrinsic extensors are evaluated by asking the patient to hold the palm flat on a table and then lift the fingertip up from the table. **Figure 12.15** demonstrates the test for the extensor pollicis longus
- If the finger can be lifted up (MCP joint hyperextension), the extrinsic extensor is intact. Some MCP joint extension can occur because of the action of the adjacent extrinsics through juncturae tendinae; however, hyperextension of the MCP joint cannot be achieved without intact extrinsic tendons
- PIP and DIP joint extension can be achieved by the intrinsic muscles

The integrity of the central slip is evaluated by Elson test (**Figure 12.16**):

- The PIP joint is held flexed and the patient is asked to extend the DIP joint
- In a normal hand, the conjoined lateral bands become loose when the PIP joint is flexed, and therefore, active extension of the DIP joint becomes impossible
- When the central slip is torn, conjoined lateral bands remain tight when the PIP joint is flexed and the DIP joint can still actively be fully extended
- The test is positive when there is active extension in the DIP joint when the PIP joint is held flexed

An avulsion of the terminal tendon (mallet finger) can be easily recognized because of the extension lag of the DIP joint. In these injuries, passive extension is normal but active extension is absent. X-rays should always be evaluated to rule out fractures/dislocations and identify possible avulsion fractures. A sagittal band injury is usually easily identified because the extensor tendon dislocates ulnarly in flexion and relocates in extension. An ulnar dislocation can usually be seen and palpated, as the MCP joint deviates ulnarly in flexion in the presence of this condition.

Table 12.2 The function and common pathologies of the digital extensor mechanism

Deformity	Anatomical structure			
	Central slip	Terminal tendon	Transverse retinacular ligament	Triangular ligament
Normal function	Extends PIP joint	Extends DIP joint	Prevents lateral band from displacing dorsally	Prevents lateral band from displacing palmarly
Mallet deformity	Intact with greater tension at PIP joint (PIP joint hyperextension)	Ruptured (DIP joint flexion)	Normal	Normal
Swan-neck deformity	Intact with greater tension at PIP joint (PIP joint hyperextension)	Intact and lax (DIP joint flexion)	Lax resulting in dorsal displacement of lateral bands	Normal
Boutonnière deformity	Ruptured or lax (PIP joint flexion)	Intact and tense (DIP joint hyperextension)	Normal or contracted	Lax resulting in palmar displacement of lateral bands

PIP, proximal interphalangeal; DIP, distal interphalangeal.

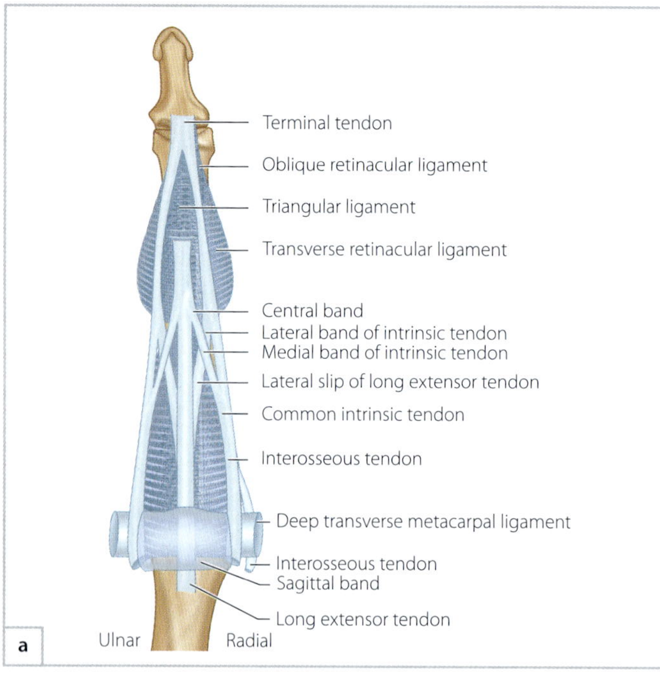

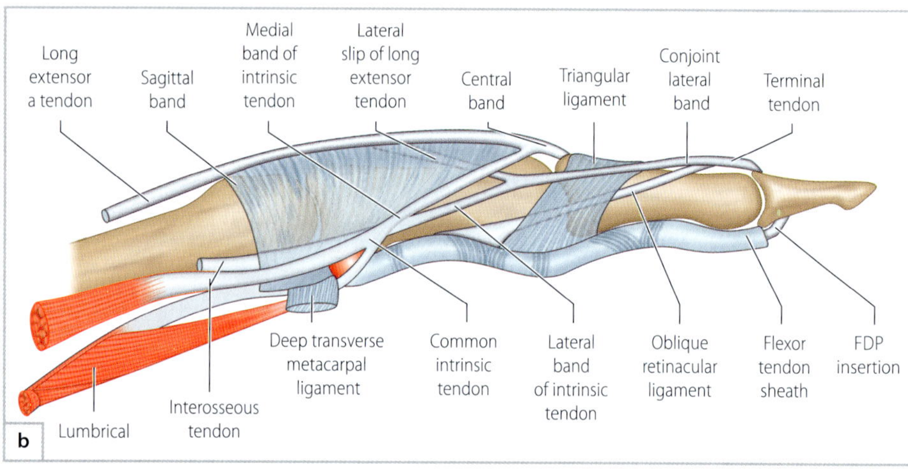

Figure 12.13 Anatomy of the extensor apparatus over the finger. (a) Dorsal view and (b) lateral view.

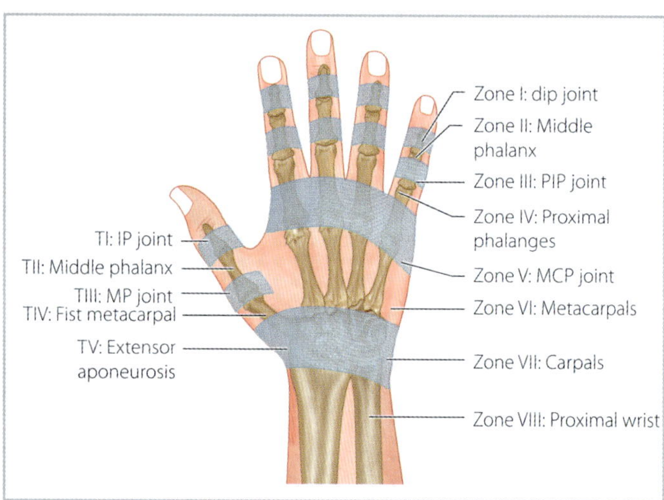

Figure 12.14 Zones of extensor tendon injury.

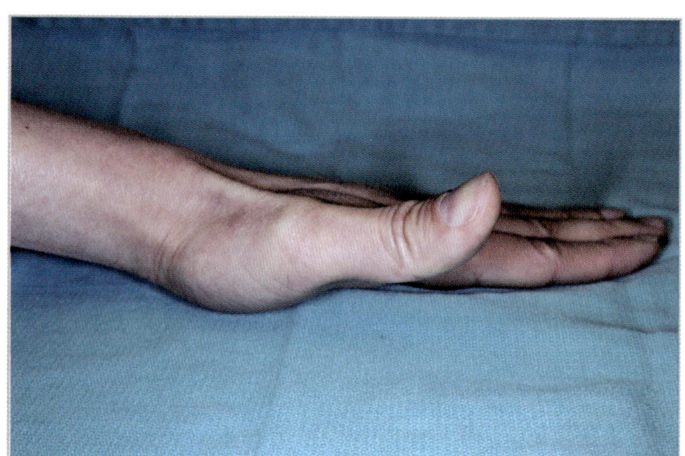

Figure 12.15 Testing integrity of the extensor pollicis longus by retropulsion of the thumb.

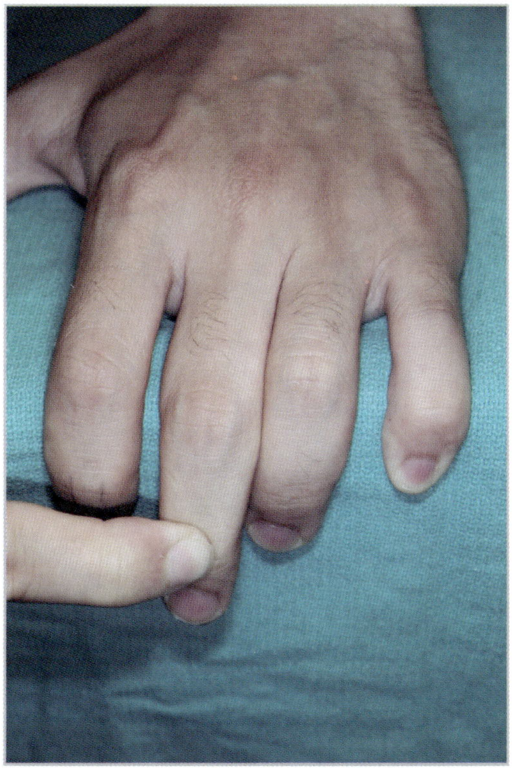

Figure 12.16 The Elson test for testing integrity of the central slip.

Primary repair of extensor tendon injuries

Zones I and II

- Acute mallet finger is immobilized for 6–8 weeks by a splint or an obliquely inserted k-wire. The method of immobilization is chosen according to the needs of the patient. The finger should be protected another 4–6 weeks from heavy manual action and during the night. Slight (5–10°) extension lag can be expected following repair of this injury
- In an open laceration, the skin and tendons can be closed in one layer using nonabsorbable 4-0 or 5-0 sutures. Alternatively, extensor tendons can be repaired with simple over and over running sutures followed by closure of the skin. The DIP joint is immobilized in full extension for 6 weeks either by k-wire or splint
- Any loss of a terminal tendon will severely restrict flexion of the DIP joint. In the event of tendon loss in zones I or II, the gap can be grafted with a proximal tendon flap, tendon, or extensor retinaculum graft, but good active ROM is seldom achieved. Splinting the finger in extension can also be attempted, and arthrodesis can be performed later if the extension lag is bothering the patient

Zones III and IV

- A partial laceration can be left unrepaired if extension of the PIP and DIP joints are normal
- To repair a laceration, one or two small core sutures (e.g. mattress or Kessler type) with 4-0 braided polyester are used. The core sutures are followed by continuous over and over, cross-stitch, or interlocking mattress type sutures, performed with either 5-0 or 6-0 polypropylene. Alternatively, tendons can be repaired by a double running technique: a simple over and over suture followed by a cross-stitch suture. If there is not enough tendon substance distal to the cut, bone tunnels or a bone anchor can be used
- Tendon loss can be reconstructed with a tendon graft or by a proximal tendon flap (**Figure 12.17**). Following reconstruction, the finger is immobilized in PIP joint extension for 4–6 weeks either by a splint or by a k-wire, and active ROM in the DIP joint is begun immediately

Zone V

A rupture of the radial sagittal band results in ulnar dislocation of the extensor tendon. Three types have been described:

Type I: A contusion without dislocation or instability

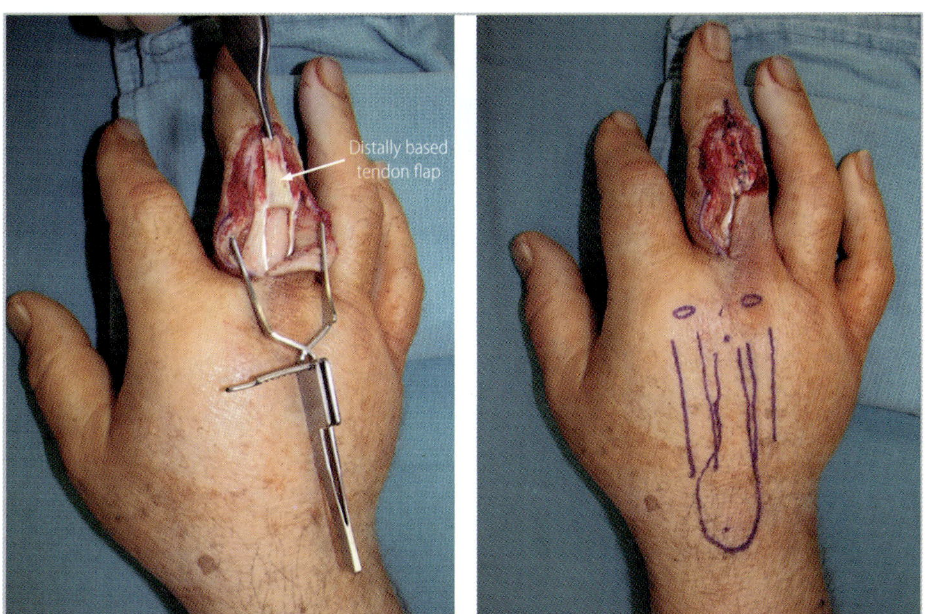

Figure 12.17 A distally based tendon flap used for reconstruction of the central slip. Photo by courtesy of Dr. Kevin C. Chung.

Type II: Partial tear with snapping but without complete dislocation
Type III: Complete tear with dislocation between the MC heads

- Treatment:
  - A type I injury is treated with 4 weeks of buddy taping. Pain and swelling may persist for several months
  - Type II and III injuries can be treated by a sagittal band bridge splint (MCP joint in extension and IP joints free) if they present within 2–3 weeks of injury. Splinting is continued for 8 weeks. Up to 30% of the patients have been reported to have persistent pain and instability after splinting. Patients failing conservative treatment or unwilling to tolerate 8 weeks of immobilization but are at risk of instability should be treated with operative intervention
- Sagittal band injuries in zone V are repaired using a cross-stitch type of continuous repair with 5-0 or 6-0 suture. In the event of late presentation, the sagittal band can be reconstructed with a proximally or distally based extensor tendon slip, or a pulley can be created with a free palmaris graft
- After surgical repair in zone V, the MCP joint should be immobilized in 40° of flexion for 4–6 weeks. Alternatively, a sagittal band bridge splint may be used. Active ROM exercises of the IP joints can be commenced immediately
- An open tendon laceration is repaired as in zones III–IV

Zones VI–VII

In these two zones, tendons are not so flat and repair techniques that are described in flexor tendon injuries can be used. A four-strand core repair with 3-0 or 4-0 suture followed by continuous running repair with 5-0 or 6-0 polypropylene is sufficient for controlled active motion (CAM) protocols.

Postoperative rehabilitation after extensor tendon repairs

Three different postoperative protocols have been used for rehabilitation following extensor tendon repair:

1. Static splinting
2. Dynamic splinting
3. CAM

CAM seems to yield better short-term results but none of these protocols have proven superior in long follow-up. The rehabilitation program should be tailored according to the patient's cooperation and local hand therapy resources.

CHRONIC EXTENSOR TENDON PATHOLOGIES

Chronic mallet deformity

This deformity occurs when acute mallet deformity is left untreated or the terminal tendon takes too long to heal despite treatment. It may result in a compensatory swan neck deformity as the tension in the central slip increases and the volar plate attenuates. Treatment of chronic mallet deformity is challenging due to the anatomy of the terminal tendon, although the functional deficit from this condition is relatively mild. In mild deformities, expectations should be discussed and no additional treatment may be prudent.

Treatment

- Splinting can be attempted if the deformity is <3–4 months old or the deformity is mild
- Tenodermodesis is aimed at shortening the terminal tendon
- Fowler tenotomy serves to increase the tension in the conjoined lateral bands by releasing the insertion of the central slip; i.e. creating a similar imbalance that is seen in boutonnière deformity (**Figure 12.18**). The net effect is correction of the mallet deformity without a swan neck deformity
- Superficial oblique retinacular ligament reconstruction functions to create a passive dynamic tenodesis link to improve the extension of the DIP joint when the PIP joint is extended
- An arthrodesis is reliable and functionally well tolerated, particularly in cases of mallet fractures. FDS tenodesis can be combined with arthrodesis if secondary swan neck deformity has developed

Chronic swan neck deformity

This deformity is characterized by hyperextension of the PIP joint and reciprocal flexion of the MCP and DIP joints. The hyperextension of the PIP joint is a result of insufficiency in the volar restraint of the PIP joint, namely the volar plate. In addition, there is over tension in the central slip, which extends the PIP joint and is frequently combined with insufficiency of the FDS. The insufficiency of the volar plate can be caused by a primary lesion or secondary attenuation.
Primary volar plate insufficiency can be caused by

- Chronic PIP joint synovitis, typically seen in rheumatoid patients
- Hyperextension injury of the PIP joint (volar plate avulsion)

Secondary attenuation of the volar plate can be caused by chronic tendon imbalance as a result of

- Chronic over tension in the central slip due to intrinsic tightness/spasticity or rupture of the terminal tendon (i.e. mallet finger)
- Loss of FDS function due to trauma or tendon transfer

Hyperextension of the PIP joint leads to a loss of tension in the conjoined lateral bands and stretching of the FDP, which results in a flexion deformity of the DIP joint. In addition, the oblique retinacular ligament loses its mechanical advantage in extending the DIP

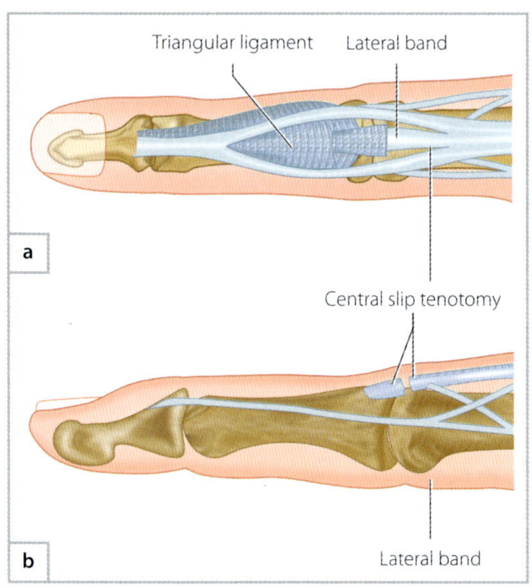

Figure 12.18 Dorsal (a) and lateral (b) views of Fowler central slip tenotomy. The central slip is transected immediately proximal to its insertion on the base of the middle phalanx. The lateral bands and triangular ligament are preserved.

joint. Over time, the conjoined lateral bands dislocate dorsally and adhesions develop between the central slip and lateral bands, which cause a fixed deformity of the PIP joint.

Assessment

- During evaluation of a patient's history, the following factors should be considered:
  - Trauma
  - Rheumatoid arthritis (RA)
  - Previous operations
- The condition of the PIP joint and passive ROM in the PIP joint dictate treatment of swan neck deformity:
  - Full passive ROM of the PIP joint
  - Limited passive ROM
  - No passive ROM
- Intrinsic muscle tightness should be determined because it contributes to swan neck deformity (see Chapter 25)
- X-rays will help rule out secondary osteoarthritis (OA)

Treatment (excluding RA)

- Full passive ROM, no intrinsic tightness/spasticity:
- FDS tenodesis: A radial slip of the FDS is cut proximal to the A2 pulley (suture anchor method) or proximal to the A1 pulley (bone tunnel method). The slip is then passed under the FDP to the ulnar side and fixed to the proximal phalanx with a suture anchor or through a bone tunnel. The tightness should be set to 5–10° of extension lag in the PIP joint. Four to five weeks of immobilization can be achieved with an extension block pin or a splint, and active flexion exercises can be initiated immediately

Limited passive ROM, no intrinsic tightness/spasticity:

- Passive manipulation of the PIP joint in flexion followed by FDS tenodesis
- The goal is to achieve 80–90° of flexion
- Passive manipulation is performed with local anesthesia to assess active flexion

No passive ROM:

- If there is secondary OA, arthrodesis should be considered
- If the joint is preserved, passive manipulation or open arthrolysis can be attempted to achieve flexion:
  - If an acceptable ROM is achieved, FDS tenodesis can be performed
  - If acceptable ROM is not achieved, arthrodesis should be considered

If swan neck deformity is caused by intrinsic tightness or spasticity, this must be addressed during the operation (see Chapter 25)

Chronic boutonnière deformity

This deformity is characterized by flexion of the PIP joint and reciprocal hyperextension of the DIP joint. It is always caused by disruption (trauma) or attenuation (synovitis of the PIP joint) of the central slip. In a chronic situation, the triangular ligament stretches and the lateral bands fall and remain volarly in respect to the PIP joint axis of rotation. Therefore, the lateral bands convert to flexors of the PIP joint. When the central slip is elongated, the pull in the extensor system is directed to the distal phalanx through the conjoined lateral bands, which causes hyperextension of the DIP joint. Eventually, the contracture of the volar plate and the collaterals of the PIP joint as well as the transverse retinacular ligament and oblique retinacular ligament cause a fixed boutonnière deformity.

Classification (Burton's)

- Stage I: Supple, passively correctable deformity
- Stage II: Fixed contracture, contracted lateral bands
- Stage III: Fixed contracture, joint fibrosis, collateral ligament, and VP contracture
- Stage IV: Fixed contracture and OA of the joint

Treatment of chronic boutonnière deformity

- Stages I can and II can usually be treated with splinting for 6–8 weeks. The PIP joint is splinted in extension and DIP joint flexion exercises are initiated, and a combination of dynamic and static splinting can be used. Operative treatment is usually based on the following principles or a combination of them:
  - Increasing the tension in the central slip by shortening or reconstructing the central slip or by transposition of one lateral band to the central slip
  - Decreasing tension in the conjoined lateral bands by tenotomy or lengthening
  - Relocation of the conjoined lateral bands by releasing the transverse retinacular ligament and re-enforcing the triangular ligament
- In stage III chronic boutonnière deformity, it is difficult to achieve good results. Dynamic and progressive static splinting can be attempted to relieve the contracture of the PIP joint. If the joint contracture does not respond to splinting, a PIP joint arthrolysis can be performed, followed by splinting and rehabilitation. If good passive ROM can be achieved but deformity persists, (converted to stage I-II) the previously mentioned operative strategies for stage I and II can be attempted
- In stage IV, PIP joint arthrodesis can be performed if the joint is painful or a contracture is functionally poorly aligned. Tenotomy or lengthening of the conjoined lateral bands can be performed at the same time to relieve DIP joint hyperextension deformity

The results of operative treatment are seldom excellent, mainly due to the complex anatomy and function of the extensor mechanism. Recreation of the normal tensional balance and multidirectional translational movement of the extensor mechanism is very difficult. Loss of flexion, joint fibrosis, and persistent boutonnière deformity are commonly seen. Therefore, accepting the deformity in cases with mild functional deficit after splinting may be preferable.

SUGGESTED READING

Bulstrode NW, Burr N, Pratt AL, Grobbelaar AO. Extensor tendon rehabilitation a prospective trial comparing three rehabilitation regimes. J Hand Surg Br 2005; 30:175–179.

The authors compare three different rehabilitation protocols for zone V and VI extensor tendon injuries. The authors found better total active range of motion in 4 weeks and better grip strength in 12 weeks in dynamic and controlled active motion protocols compared with static splinting.

Houpt P, Dijkstra R, Storm van Leeuwen JB. Fowler's tenotomy for mallet deformity. J Hand Surg Br 1993; 18:499–500.

The authors present a series of 30 patients with chronic mallet deformity treated by Fowler's tenotomy. Twenty six of the patents regained full range of motion of the DIP joint after the tenotomy procedure.

Lee S, Dubey A, Kim B, Zingman A, et al. A biomechanical study of extensor tendon repair methods: introduction to the running-interlocking horizontal mattress extensor tendon repair technique. J Hand Surg Am 2010; 35:19–23.

The authors compare the modified Bunnell repair, Augmented Becker, and running interlocking mattress repairs in zone 6 of human cadaveric extensor tendons. Running interlocking mattress repair was the fastest to perform and stiffest of the repairs, resulting in the least amount of tendon shortening. Furthermore, it had equal mean ultimate strength compared with the other repair techniques. All of the repairs carried the loads that are present in controlled active motion. The running interlocking mattress procedure therefore seems to be an easy yet reliable repair technique for zone 6 extensor tendon injuries.

Smith RJ. Balance and kinetics of the fingers under normal and pathological conditions. Clin Orthop Relat Res 1974; (104):92–111.

The functional anatomy of the finger extensor system as well as the kinetics of Boutonnière deformity, swan neck deformity, and mallet deformity are described in detail in this paper.

Souter WA. The problem of boutonnière deformity. Clin Orthop Relat Res 1974; (104):116–133.

In this paper, the author describes the pathology of the boutonnière defect and summarizes the different treatment strategies for this difficult imbalance. He also presents the results of 54 cases and concludes that conservative treatment (splinting) yields superior results even when the condition is diagnosed >6 weeks after the initial injury or in severe imbalance (extension lag >40 degrees). The superior results of splinting prevail in the long-term follow-up. In the authors' opinion, the only indication of primarily surgical treatment is an avulsion fracture or open injury; particularly when there is a loss of skin/tendon substance.

12.3 REHABILITATION OF TENDON INJURIES

INTRODUCTION

Proper rehabilitation techniques are vital for optimal outcomes after repair of tendon injury. Neglect of this critical component of the treatment plan can lead to poor outcomes, even in the setting of a meticulous surgical repair. No protocol has been universally accepted for all types of flexor or extensor tendon injuries; rather, selection of the appropriate program depends on the patient, injury characteristics, and strength of surgical repair. The goal of rehabilitation after tendon repair is to promote healing, optimize tendon gliding, and avoid rupture or gapping of the repair that will lead to scar formation at the repair site rather than strong tendon structure. This chapter will outline the scientific basis for tendon rehabilitation protocols, commonly used protocols in practice, and considerations for selection of rehabilitation programs for tendon repairs.

SCIENTIFIC BASIS FOR REHABILITATION PROTOCOLS

Surgeons and hand therapists must have a thorough understanding of the scientific basis from which rehabilitation protocols have been developed, including principles of tendon healing, strength of tendon repair techniques, and forces generated across tendon repairs with various maneuvers of the involved digits. Greater understanding of these principles will help to guide selection of appropriate protocols for individual patients.

Tendons heal by a process of intrinsic and extrinsic healing. With extrinsic healing, fibrous tissue is laid down from a fibroblastic response from the tendon sheath and surrounding tissues to achieve repair strength, at the same time forming adhesions between the tendon and surrounding tissues. Intrinsic healing occurs within the tendon itself and is mediated by diffusion of nutrients from synovial fluid. Adhesions do not form from intrinsic healing. Repair strength and intrinsic healing increases in response to controlled stress across the tendon repair. Thus, to optimize tendon gliding and strength, intrinsic healing should be maximized while minimizing extrinsic healing. Controlled mobilization of tendons during the healing phase promotes intrinsic healing, results in faster return of tensile strength, and reduces adhesion formation compared to immobilized tendons. The minimum movement required to prevent adhesions is approximately 3–5 mm, which can be achieved with passive motion of the joints. However, tendon excursion is greater with active range of motion. In addition, when both flexor digitorum superficialis (FDS) and flexor digitorum profundus (FDP) tendons are both injured, differential gliding must occur to prevent adhesions between the two tendons and is greater with active motion compared to passive motion.

The therapist must also have a thorough understanding of the forces generated across the repair with various movements of flexor and extensor tendons and determine whether the strength of repair is sufficient to avoid rupture with these maneuvers. Controlled movement and stress, whether active or passive, help to improve tendon gliding and the strength of repair. However, these movements and stress must be matched with the amount of force that the repair can withstand to prevent gapping and rupture across the repair site. Proper positioning of the wrist, metacarpophalangeal (MCP) joints, and interphalangeal (IP) joints during these movements is also critical to reduce stresses across the repair.

The surgeon should be in close communication with the therapist immediately after surgery because details of the surgical repair will determine tolerance for different therapy protocols. The caliber of suture, suture technique (number of strands, use of epitendinous suture), quality of repair, associated injuries, and zone of injury will help to determine the strength of repair and tolerance for early motion. Extensor tendons are thinner, weaker, and flatter, compared to flexor tendons. These factors make it difficult to place many core sutures and achieve strong repairs, particularly at distal zones. The strength of flexor and extensor tendon repair decreases over the first week after repair up to 50%, with the weakest point of repair at 5-10 days postoperatively, and strength increases gradually over several months. Active extension forces are estimated to be approximately 30N across the index finger and 20N across the small finger with the wrist in 40 degrees of extension.

Flexion forces have been studied more thoroughly and forces have been estimated with various passive and active maneuvers. There is an estimated 2–5 N of force generated with passive flexion, 10 N with active flexion of mild resistance, 20 N with active flexion of moderate resistance, 120 N with index tip pinch, and up to 200 N with power grip. Forces increase up to 50% in the setting of resistance due to edema and inflammation after injury and surgical repair. Four and six-strand repairs with epitendinous suture are typically strong enough to permit active flexion with mild resistance through all phases of tendon healing. An understanding of these biomechanical parameters will ensure that therapists are cognizant that forces applied during rehabilitation programs are less than the tensile strength of tendon repairs to prevent gapping or rupture (**Figure 12.19**). These studies are the basis of safely performing early controlled mobilization beginning in the immediate days following tendon repair.

FLEXOR TENDON REHABILITATION

All flexor tendon rehabilitation programs fall into one of three main types despite many variations: 1) immobilization, 2) early passive motion, and 3) early active motion. Early passive motion is popularly used, but early active motion has been increasingly advocated to improve range of motion outcomes. However, immobilization is still indicated in select patients who are not able to comply with rehabilitation regimens. It is common for therapists to use components of different protocols to fit individual patient needs.

Immobilization

- Indications: young children (generally infant to 10 years) and adults who are not able to comply with early motion rehabilitation protocols and in patients who have associated injuries that prevent mobilization of the injured digits
- 0–4 weeks: cast or dorsal blocking splint immobilization with wrist and MCP joints in flexion and IP joints in extension
- 4–5 weeks: dorsal splint modified with wrist neutral, passive flexion and extension exercises with wrist in 10 degrees extension and active differential tendon gliding exercises (**Figure 12.20**) initiated
- 5–6 weeks: dorsal blocking splint discontinued, gentle active blocking exercises (**Figure 12.21**) initiated
- 6–8 weeks: gentle resistive exercises initiated and progress gradually

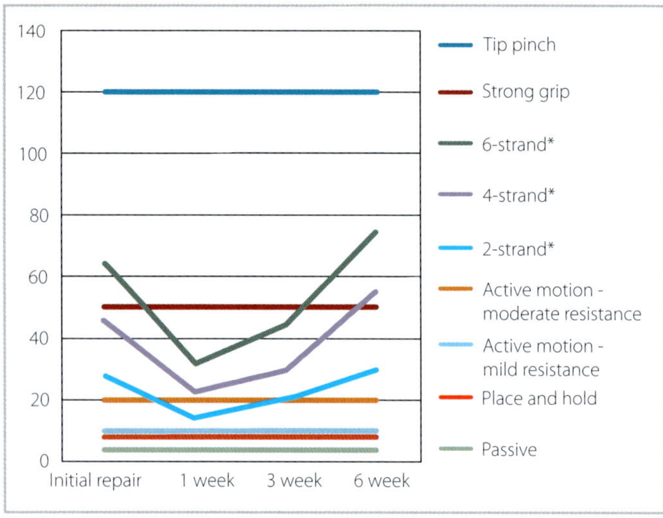

Figure 12.19 (a) An example of a dorsal splint that can facilitate extensor mechanism tendon gliding. (b and c) This same splint can be used for flexor digitorum profundus and flexor digitorum superficialis gliding exercises.

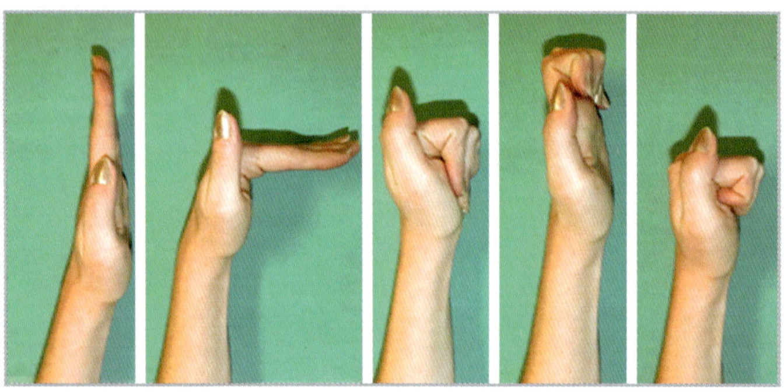

Figure 12.20 Differential gliding exercises.

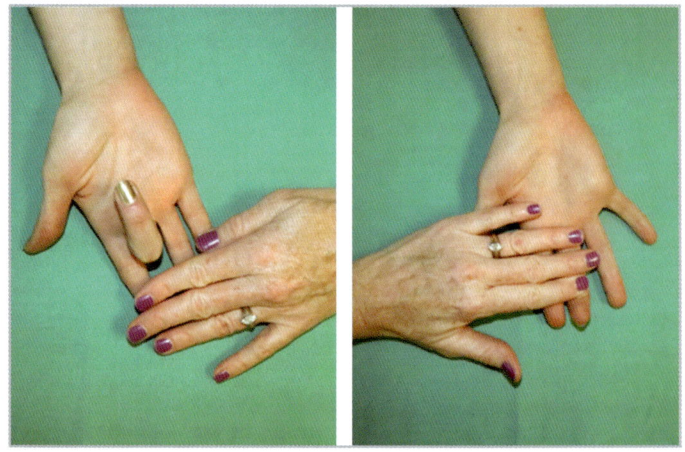

Figure 12.21 Active blocking exercises.

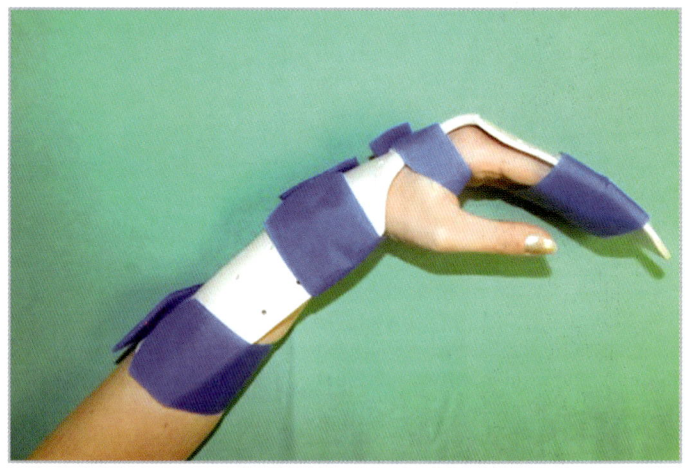

Figure 12.22 Standard dorsal blocking orthosis used in Duran protocol.

- If patients are unable to perform the above exercises due to age, the splint is removed after 4 weeks and the patient is allowed to return to usual activities as tolerated

Early passive motion

- **Duran and Houser protocol** is the most popular early passive motion protocol, with many modifications developed. The protocol was designed based on theory that approximately 3–5 mm of tendon excursion is needed to decrease adhesion formation, which can be achieved with passive motion. Passive motion protocols continue to be popular due to less risk of tendon rupture compared to early active motion protocols.
  - Initial orthosis: splint wrist in 20 degrees flexion, MCP joints in 50–70 degrees flexion, and IP joints fully extended (**Figure12.22**)
  - 0–3.5 weeks: proximal interphalangeal (PIP) and distal interphalangeal (DIP) joint noncomposite and composite passive flexion and extension exercises initiated within confines of splint
  - 3.5 weeks: active composite flexion and extension exercises within confines of splint initiated
  - 4.5 weeks: composite wrist and digital flexion and extension exercises started outside of splint
  - 5.5–6 weeks: splint weaned. Passive extension stretching and blocking active flexion exercises started
  - 8–12 weeks: progressive resistive exercises started with gradual increase to allow unrestricted activities
- **Kleinert protocol** is another early passive motion protocol, less commonly used, which allows active extension and passive flexion motion within a dynamic traction splint in addition to Duran protocol activities.
  - Initial orthosis: splint with wrist in approximately 20–30 degrees flexion and MCP joints in 50–70 degrees of flexion, with rubber band traction from fingertips to volar forearm with palmar pulley, passively flexing PIP and DIP joints (**Figure 12.23**)
  - 0–3 weeks: passive finger motion activities (composite and noncomposite), plus active extension against rubber bands with passive flexion within splint; IP joints are immobilized in extension when not performing exercises to reduce IP joint flexion contracture
  - 3 weeks: place and hold exercises initiated, in which joints are individually flexed passively but active contraction performed to hold fingers in position for approximately 5 seconds
  - 4 weeks: splint adjusted with wrist in neutral position. Differential gliding and passive IP joint extension stretches started
  - 6 weeks: patient weaned from splint. Composite wrist and digital motion started with blocking active range of motion exercises
  - 8–12 weeks: progressive resistive exercises are started with gradual increase to unrestricted activities

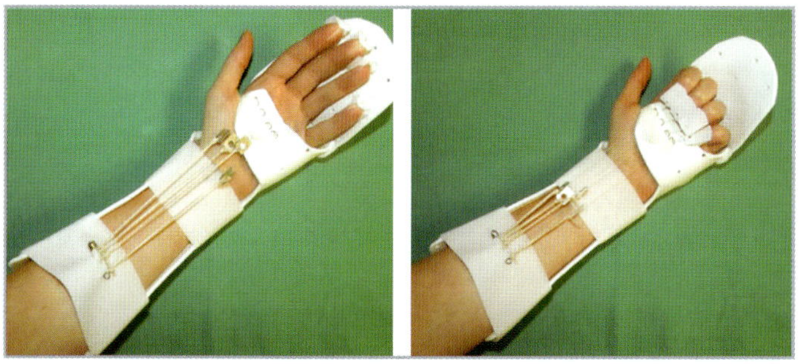

Figure 12.23 Kleinert traction splint with palmar pulley.

- Passive motion protocols should be started within the first postoperative week.

Early active motion

- Absolute and differential excursion of tendons is greater with active motion compared to passive motion. Thus, early active range of motion may have greater reduction in adhesion formation compared to passive range of motion protocols
- Active range of motion rehabilitation protocols are less commonly used, but recent studies have shown better outcomes with greater range of motion compared to passive range of motion protocols. However, there is concern that these programs may be associated with higher rupture rates
- Indications: must have strong repair with at least 4 core strands, a reliable patient, and minimal associated trauma to the surrounding tissues
- Several variations exist, but any movement other than passive flexion of the digit is considered an active motion protocol. Two popular protocols are briefly described below, with active contraction exercises performed in addition the passive activities described above. The protocols differ in their progression of controlled stress, method of achieving active motion, and wrist position during activities. Studies have demonstrated the least amount of tension across the repair when active motion activities are performed with the wrist in extension
- Active protocols typically begin in the first 3–5 days postoperatively, before the repair reaches its lowest tensile strength
- **Indiana protocol**
    - An exercise orthosis is used with a wrist hinge to allow for 30 degrees of wrist extension and MCP joints in 50 degrees flexion. Alternatively, two splints can be used, one for exercise with the wrist in 30 degrees extension and another static splint for use with the wrist in flexion when not performing exercises. Patient performs place and hold exercises within the splint with the wrist extended during the first few weeks (**Figure 12.24**). These activities are performed in addition to Duran protocol exercises
    - Active composite fist formation is initiated at 4 weeks. As therapy progresses the patient continues with progressive active motion and resistive exercises similar to the Duran protocol above
- **Mass protocol**
    - Orthosis places the wrist in 20 degrees of extension, MCP joints in 70 degrees of flexion, and IP joints neutral
    - Utilizes Duran protocol exercises plus active composite fist exercises within the splint early on (**Figure 12.25**)

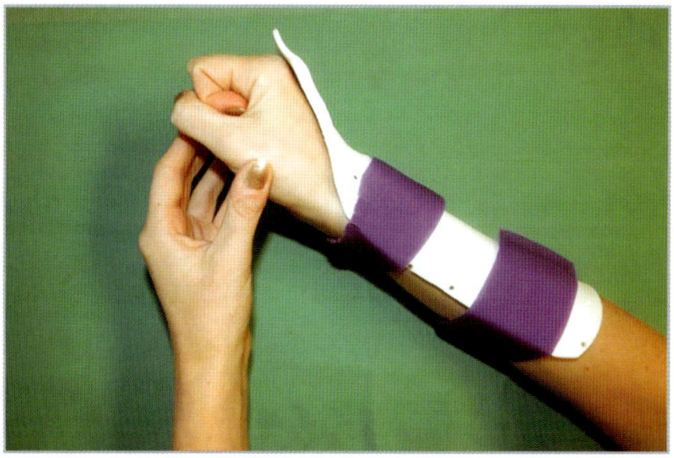

Figure 12.24 Indiana early active motion splint with wrist extended to 30 degrees wrist extension while performing place and hold exercises within the splint. Wrist placed in different splint with wrist flexion when not performing exercises to reduce tension on repair while at rest. Alternatively can use a single splint used that has hinge at wrist to change wrist position for exercises.

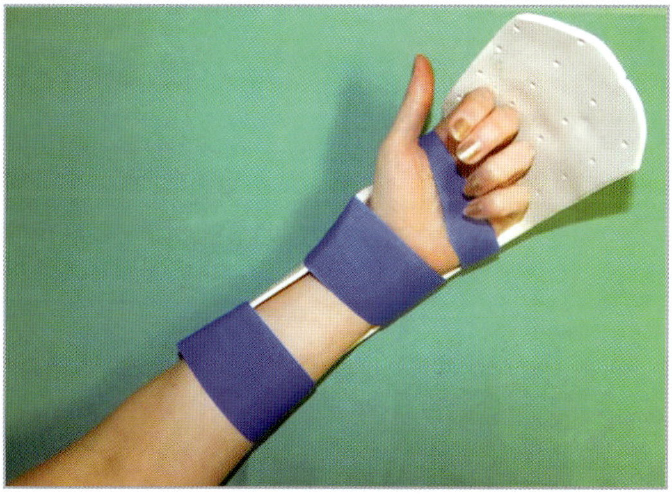

Figure 12.25 Active composite flexion exercises within dorsal blocking splint.

EXTENSOR TENDON REHABILITATION

Similar to flexor tendon injuries, extensor tendon rehabilitation protocols are classified into immobilization and early motion categories. Therapists and surgeons must determine if the repair has sufficient strength to safely allow for early mobilization protocols, as extensor tendon repairs tend to be weaker with cross-sectional anatomy not always allowing for placement of 4 or more strands of core sutures. Similar to flexor tendon injuries, patients may have improved outcomes with earlier mobilization of tendons. Studies suggest that early mobilization of extensor tendon injuries achieves better range of motion in the short-term. However, it is inconclusive whether patients achieve similar range of motion with early motion and static splinting protocols in the long run, particularly with injuries distal to the MCP joint.

Immobilization

- Injuries to zones I and II, whether treated conservatively or surgically, are splinted for 6–8 weeks in extension before initiating motion exercises. The mallet finger splint includes only the DIP joint while leaving the PIP joint and wrist free (**Figure 12.26**). Patients are weaned from the splint at 6–8 weeks where activity progresses with few restrictions. Patients are monitored for signs of extension lag, where if present the patient is returned to extension splinting
- Due to the often delicate nature of extensor tendon repairs, most extensor tendon primary repairs involving zones III–VIII are classically splinted in extension for 4–6 weeks before starting range of motion exercises. The wrist is placed in approximately 30 degrees of extension, with the MCP joints in approximately 15 degrees of flexion and the IP joints neutral (**Figure 12.27**)
- Indications: all zone I–II injuries, pediatric patients and adults who are unable to comply with early motion rehabilitation protocols, and patients with tendon repairs that are tenuous or have less than 4–6 core strands
- Immobilization protocols for extensor tendon repair are less costly and require less patient effort early on postoperatively

Early motion protocols

- Indications: repair has to have at least 4 core strands and be strong enough to tolerate forces generated with active motion. Zones I, II, and VIII are not strong enough to tolerate early motion protocols
- Early motion should be started within the first week postoperatively
- The therapist must monitor for loss of active extension with all early motion protocols, which signals gapping across the repair site, and requires discontinuation of progression of motion for at least 1 week
- **Dynamic extension splinting (reverse Kleinert protocol)**
  - Used more often for repairs of zone V to VII, but has also been reported for use in zone III and IV injuries
  - 0–3.5 weeks: orthosis similar to the Kleinert splint used for flexor tendon repair, but traction bands keep digits in extension, allowing for active flexion and passive extension within the splint (**Figure 12.28**). The wrist is extended 30 degrees, MCP joints are flexed 0 to 30 degrees, and the IP joints are free
  - 3.5 weeks: MCP joints are gradually flexed from 50–70 degrees, and place and hold and hook fist exercises are initiated
  - 5–6 weeks: active flexion and extension of individual fingers and composite fist exercises are initiated

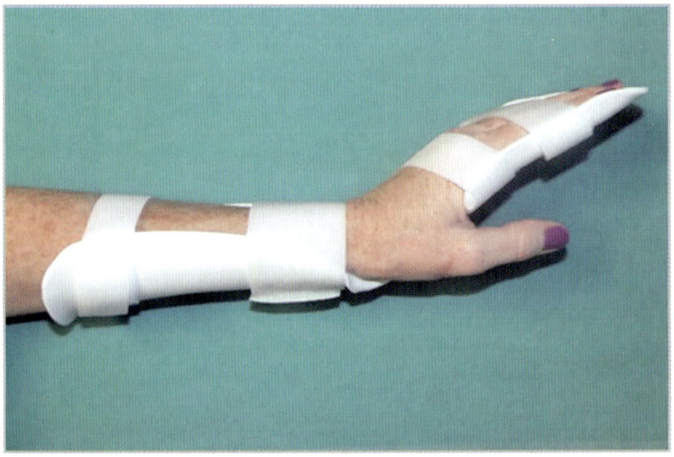

Figure 12.27 Static extension splint.

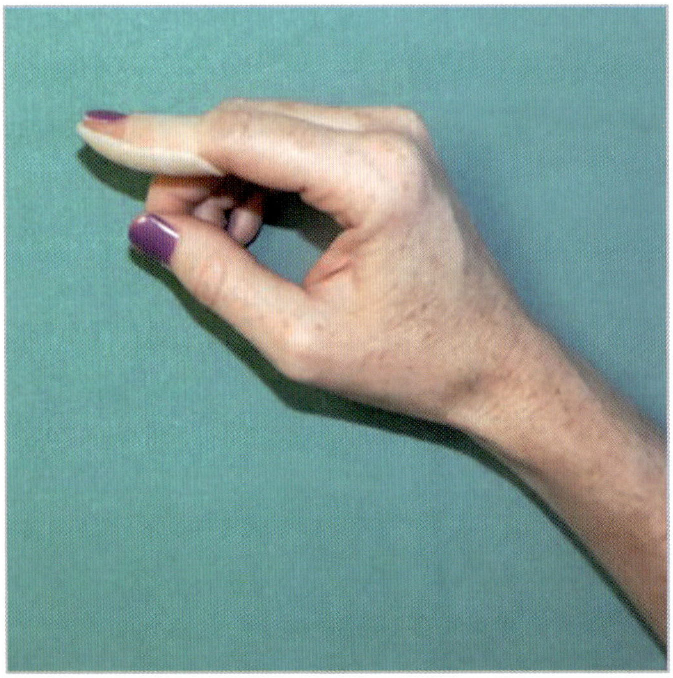

Figure 12.26 Mallet finger (DIP joint extension) splint.

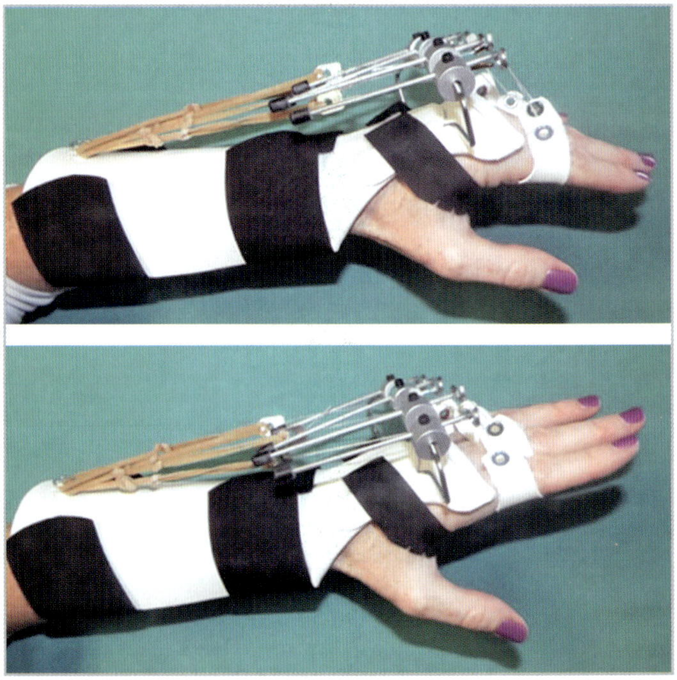

Figure 12.28 Dynamic traction splint for extensor tendon repair.

- 6 weeks: dynamic splint is discontinued, and active composite wrist and digit range of motion through full range with progressive resistive exercises are begun
- 10 weeks: unrestricted activities are initiated

- Short arc motion (SAM) protocol
  - Used for repairs of zone III and IV
  - 3 custom fabricated orthoses are required:
  - Static splint used with PIP and DIP joints in extension when patient not performing exercises (**Figure 12.29A**)
  - PIP joint exercise splint allows PIP joint motion within short confines of splint (**Figure 12.29B**), initially up to 30 degrees, and progressing to greater angles at later stages
  - DIP joint exercise splint immobilizes the PIP joint in full extension while allowing range of motion of the DIP joint (**Figure 12.29C**)
  - 0–2 weeks: exercises performed with wrist in 30 degrees extension, MCPs neutral and supported by opposite hand, with patient performing active range of motion exercises within the PIP and DIP joint exercise splints
  - The PIP blocking orthosis is adjusted gradually to allow more flexion ranging from 40 degrees at 2 weeks, 60–70 degrees at 5 weeks, and 90 degrees at 6 weeks
- Immediate controlled active motion (ICAM) protocol
  - Also called relative motion protocol
  - Best if started within 1 week after repair
  - Used for repairs of zones IV–VII, cannot be used when more than 3 tendons are injured
  - Easier to implement compared to SAM protocol
  - 0–3 weeks: initial splint fabricated with wrist in 30 degrees extension, repaired digit(s) MCP joint blocked at 45 degrees of flexion and IP joints free. The injured finger(s) are in 15–20 degrees greater MCP joint extension than the adjacent digits to shield the repair from excess tension; the reason it is also called a relative motion splint (**Figure 12.30**). Active composite flexion and extension are performed within the splint
  - 3–5 weeks: wrist component of splint removed and active wrist motion is introduced
  - 6–8 weeks: splint removed for active range of motion exercises; patient is weaned from splint when full composite wrist and finger range of motion are achieved

OUTCOME EVALUATION

- Outcome measures vary across studies for evaluation of flexor and extensor tendon repair results:

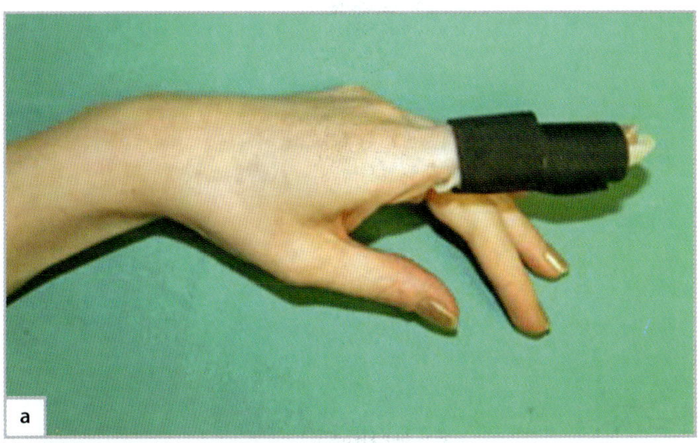

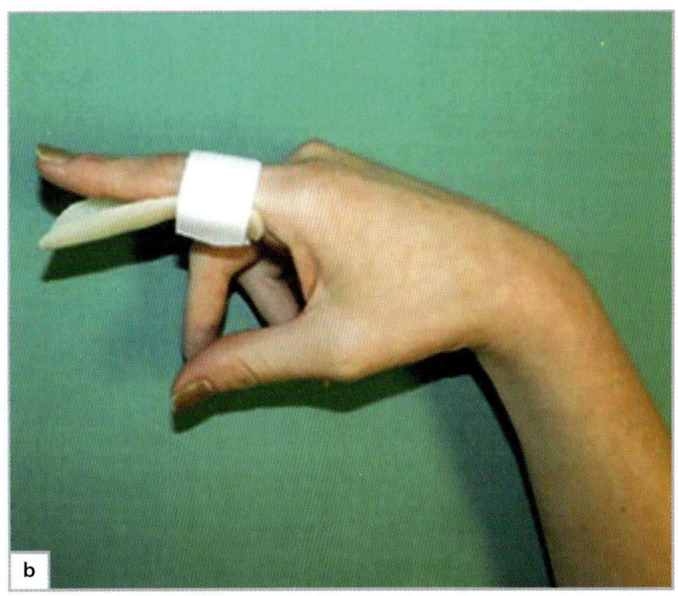

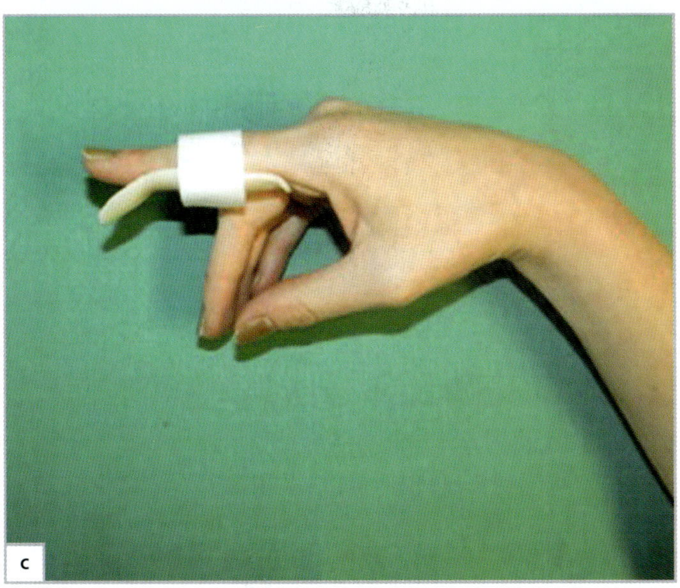

Figure 12.29 Splints used for short arc motion (SAM) protocol. (a) Static splint for use when not performing exercises. (b) PIP joint exercise splint, where limited active flexion and extension of the PIP and DIP joints is performed within splint. (c) DIP joint exercise splint, where limited active flexion and extension of the DIP joint is performed within splint, while keeping the PIP joint extended.

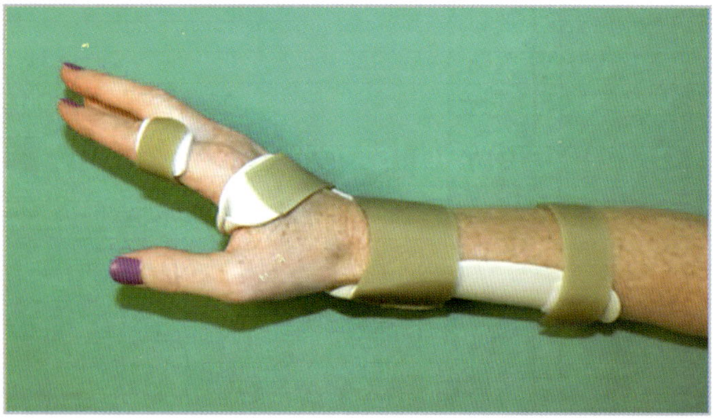

Figure 12.30 Relative motion splint for immediate controlled active motion (ICAM) protocol.

- **Range of motion:** classically measured in total arc of motion (TAM) for each involved digit and are compared to the uninjured contralateral digit. American Society for Surgery of the Hand (ASSH) grading for TAM after tendon repair include excellent (100%), good (75–99%), fair (50–74%), and poor results (<50% TAM compared to contralateral side). For example, the normal flexion arc of motion of the MCP (90 degrees) + PIP (110 degrees) + DIP (80 degrees) = 280 degrees. TAM equals the flexion arc of motion minus extension lag at the respective joints. TAM greater near normal is considered excellent, whereas 210 to 279 degrees is good, 209 to 160 degrees is fair and less than 160 degrees is considered poor. The Strickland criteria is also commonly used and includes excellent (85–100%), good (70–84%), fair (50–69%), and fair (0–49%) categories for return of range of motion of IP joints
- **Secondary procedures:** adhesion formation and rupture can lead to need for tenolysis, joint contracture release, and secondary tendon reconstruction. Tendon rupture is the worst complication following primary tendon repair, with published rates from 2–10%, with higher rupture rates reported in the thumb and with early active motion protocols. Ruptures occur most commonly 1–2 weeks postoperatively, followed by around 6 weeks postoperatively as therapy progresses to allow more active motion exercises. Up to 33% of patients require tenolysis or secondary tendon reconstruction
- **Patient-based outcome measures:** Michigan Hand Outcomes Questionnaire (MHQ), and Disabilities of the Arm, Shoulder and Hand (DASH) are commonly used to assess patient-reported outcomes after primary tendon repair

- Prognosis is related to zone of injury and associated injuries. Zone II injuries fare worse in flexor tendon injuries and distal zones fare worse in extensor tendon injuries

SUGGESTED READING

Clancy SP, Mass DP. Current flexor and extensor tendon motion regimens: a summary. Hand Clin 2013; 29:295–309.

An up-to-date review of popular flexor and extensor tendon repair rehabilitation protocols, discussing mechanics of protocols in detail.

Havenhill TG, Birnie R. Pediatric flexor tendon injuries. Hand Clin 2005; 21:253–256.

Discusses management, including rehabilitation of pediatric flexor tendon injuries.

Matarrese MR, Hammert WC. Flexor tendon rehabilitation. J Hand Surg Am 2012; 37:2386–2388.

Summarizes outcome studies in the literature relating to selection of flexor tendon rehabilitation protocols, with highlights of shortcomings in the current evidence and directions for future research.

Newport ML, Tucker RL. New perspectives on extensor tendon rehabilitation and implications for rehabilitation. J Hand Ther 2005; 18:175–181.

Summarizes current biomechanical studies to date for extensor tendon repair in order to discuss implications for selection of rehabilitation protocols and support for early immobilization protocols.

Strickland JW. Flexor tendon injuries: I. foundations of treatment. J Am Acad Orthop Surg 1995; 3:44–54.

An excellent review of biomechanical studies and parameters that serve as basis for early motion protocols after flexor tendon repair.

Trumble TE, Vedder NB, Seiler JG, et al. Zone-II flexor tendon repair: a randomized prospective trial of active place-and-hold therapy compared with passive motion therapy. J Bone Joint Surg Am 2010; 92:1381–1389.

Study demonstrating superior range of motion outcomes without increased tendon rupture rates with active place and hold protocol compared to passive motion therapy after zone II flexor tendon repair.

Chapter 13 Fractures and dislocations

Maneesh Singhal (13.2), Keming Wang (13.3), Evan J. Kowalski (13.3), Yeong-Pin Peng (13.4, 13.5), Kevin C. Chung (13.2, 13.3), Amitabha Lahiri (13.1), Kris Tong DL (13.6)

13.1 PRINCIPLES OF SKELETAL FIXATION FOR THE HAND

INTRODUCTION

A stable skeleton forms the foundation for the motor function of the hand and is essential for the force transmission from the extrinsic and intrinsic muscular system. As discussed elsewhere, it is also fundamental to the functional reconstruction of the hand in complex trauma. A stable skeletal fixation allows fracture healing with commencement of early mobilization, which prevents tendon adhesions as well as joint stiffness. At the same time, injudicious skeletal fixation with surgical damage to surrounding tissue and devascularization of the bone may add to the insult and result in poor outcomes due to the resultant scarring, adhesions, and avascular necrosis (AVN) of the bone, especially in smaller condylar fragments. Therefore, fracture exposure with the least amount of 'collateral' damage (i.e. careful dissection of surrounding soft tissue to avoid disruption of tenuous blood supply to the fracture site) is equally as important as the skill of fracture fixation.

This chapter is written as a practical guide to fracture fixation, and therefore detailed biomechanical discussion is omitted. The reader should consult the suggested reading text for an in-depth understanding of these concepts. The surgical approach to hand fractures is usually dorsal, with some exceptions. The reader should familiarize themselves with the anatomy and various surgical approaches before commencing any fracture fixation.

TECHNICAL OPTIONS

According to the site and individual fracture patterns, a wide variety of fixation devices are available. This includes Kirschner (K) wires, screw and plate combinations, cannulated screws, and headless compression screws, which are extremely useful to achieve an adequate fracture fixation. Other fracture fixation modalities, such as the use of small size external fixators designed for the use in the hand bones, are also readily available and can be used in complex trauma or for distraction lengthening.

INDICATIONS AND GOALS OF FRACTURE FIXATION

There are two independent indications when fracture fixation is needed, although, when surgical fixation is performed, both of these aspects are addressed simultaneously:

- To restore the anatomical parameters of the bone (i.e. prefracture position).
- To provide stability to the bone against the deforming forces of muscles

Restoration of anatomical parameters

There are specific parameters for each bone, but these parameters can be generalized into:

1. Articular congruence
2. Alignment
   - Alignment of the bone segments to the anatomical axis of the bone
   - Alignment of the axis of the bone itself to the limb
3. The length of the bone (shortening or lengthening as a result of the fracture or the fixation)

Restoration of stability

This refers to the ability of the fixation to counteract the deforming forces created by the fracture pattern and the muscle attachments on the bone at rest, and during active mobilization, and to the external forces applied during passive mobilization. In general, both the aims of anatomical reduction and stability are achieved simultaneously. In complex situations, different techniques may be combined (e.g. external fixators with K-wires) to address different issues.

Techniques for anatomical restoration

Factors that dictate the choice of technique:

- Configuration of the fracture
- Size of the fracture fragments
- Degree of fragmentation
- Bone comminution resulting in loss of structure or 'bone loss.'
- The nature of the soft tissue injury in the proximity of the fracture

Restoring articular congruence

Intra-articular fractures require realignment of the fractured articular surface through bone fixation, with the elimination of any step or gap. The techniques that are commonly used are K-wire fixation of the fragments and interfragment screws. These techniques are illustrated in **Figure 13.1**.

Restoring bone alignment

This involves the correction of angular or rotational deformities in the diaphyseal segment of the long bones. The technique of fixation is selected based on the configuration of the fracture.

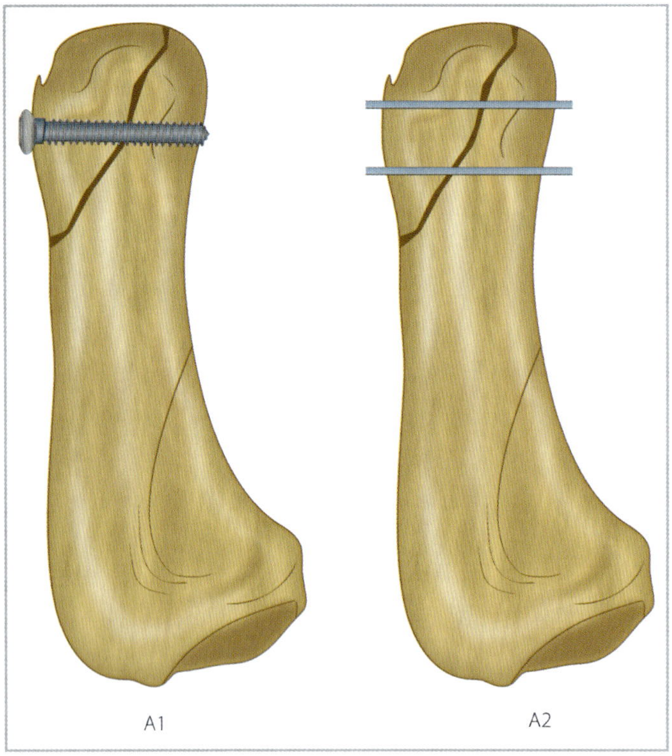

Figure 13.1 Realignment of articular congruence using screws (left) and pins (right).

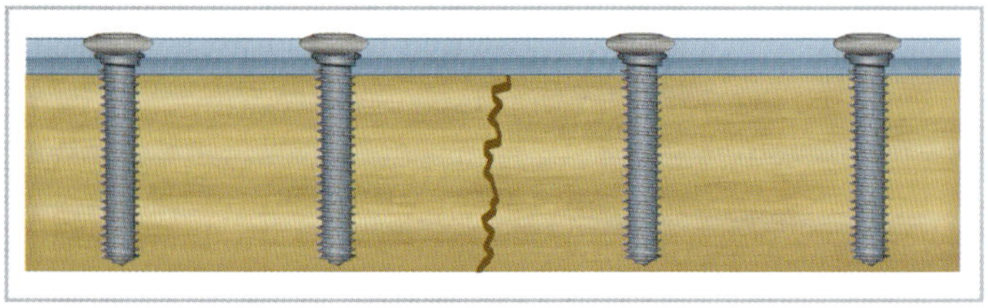

Figure 13.2 Demonstrating the principles of compression plating. The lockup hole moves the screw head toward the fracture line as the screw is tightened.

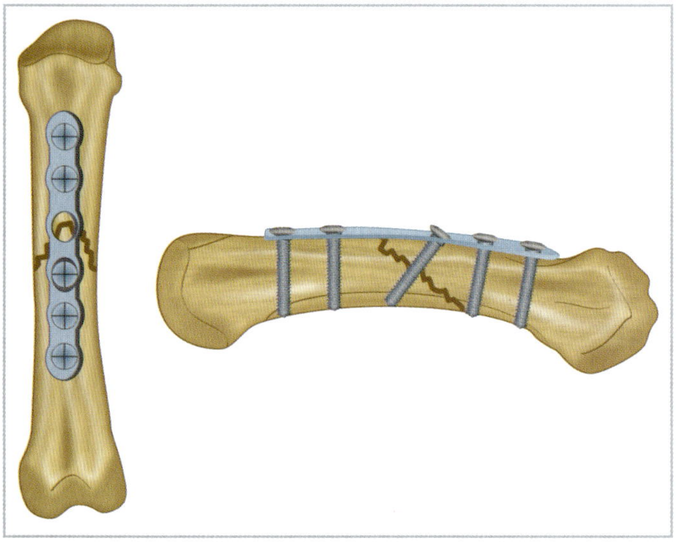

Figure 13.3 Short oblique fracture fixed with a combination of a neutralizing plate and a lag screw.

Transverse fractures

Compression can be obtained by using specially designed compression plates (**Figure 13.2**). All plates should be contoured to the normal shape of the bone after reduction. The plate consists of specially designed screw holes that create an axial compression as the screws are tightened.

Short oblique fracture

In these fractures, the fracture line is less than twice the diameter of the bone. Such fractures require the use of neutralization or a protection plate (i.e. the plate is used for the internal fixation of a long bone fracture to neutralize the forces producing displacement). It does not provide compression and is usually combined with a lag screw (**Figure 13.3**).

Spiral fracture

Lag screws (explained in more detail below) are placed equidistant and perpendicular to the fracture plane. Ideally, the fracture should accommodate a minimum of two screws for stability, which is possible when the length of the fracture is at least twice the diameter of the bone. Placement of three screws offers an even higher degree of stability (**Figure 13.4**).

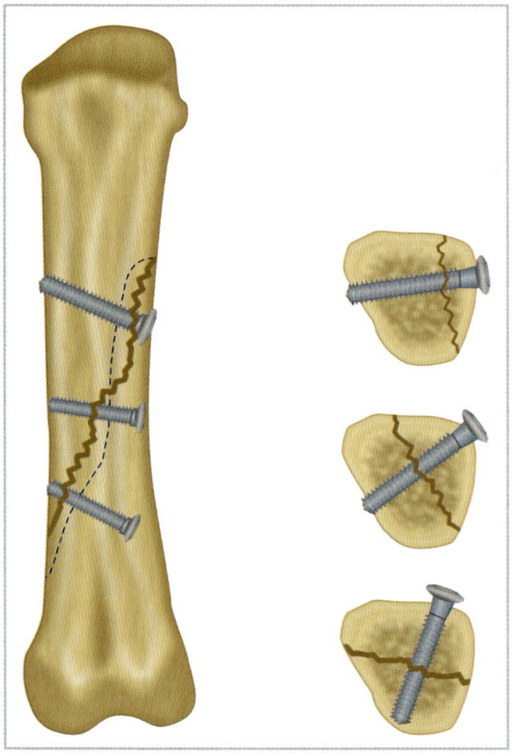

Figure 13.4 Lag screw fixation of a spiral fracture.

Shear fractures involving the epiphyseal and the metaphyseal region

These fractures are treated with buttress plating. The plate provides axial loading forces that are acting perpendicular to the deformity (**Figure 13.5**).

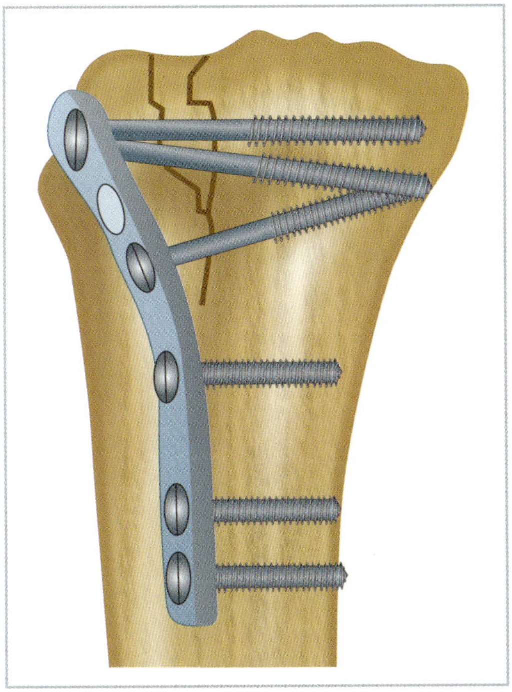

Figure 13.5 This demonstrates a buttress plate preventing the displacement of a fractured segment after axial compression.

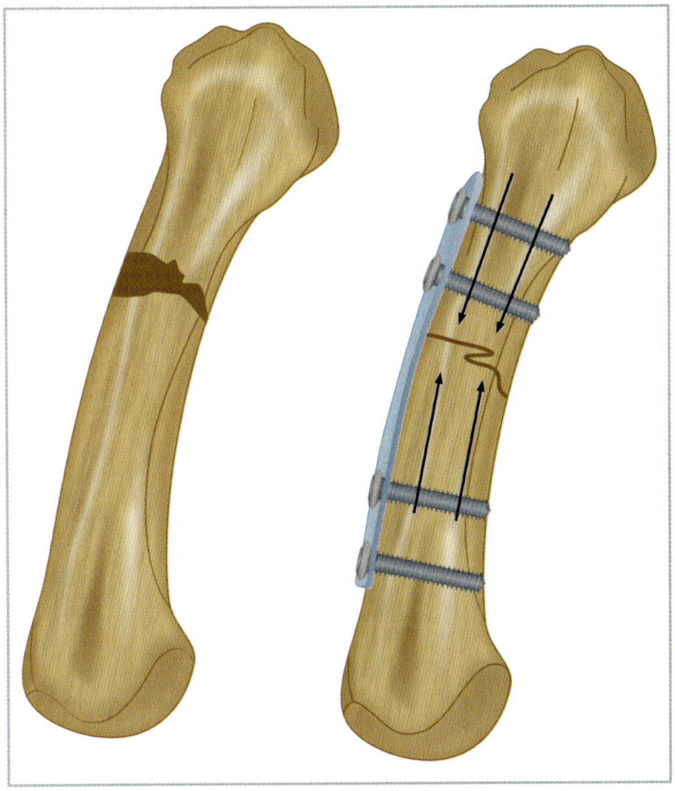

Figure 13.6 Fixation techniques to reduce a curved bone fracture by using tension band plating.

Transverse fractures in curved bones

Tension band plating/wiring

This technique is used in curved bones (olecranon, or metacarpal neck fractures) that are loaded eccentrically (**Figure 13.6**). The plate or a figure of eight wires is applied on the tension side of the fracture. In the hand, the flexor tendons tend to displace the fracture in the apex dorsal posture. In other words, the dorsal fracture gaps and the tension band principle is to stabilize the dorsal gapping and distribute the tension evenly at the fracture site. The opposite cortex should be intact to provide a buttress. In the absence of a rigid buttress, the plate undergoes cyclical loading and fractures.

Restoring length

In simple fractures, length is restored upon restoring the alignment of the bone. In situations of severe comminution or bone loss in open fractures, the length is restored by using either plates or external fixators ± bone grafting.

Bridging plate

The plate bridges the bone gap or a zone of severe comminution. The plate is fixed to the two end fragments of the bone without interfering with the fractured fragments (**Figure 13.7**).

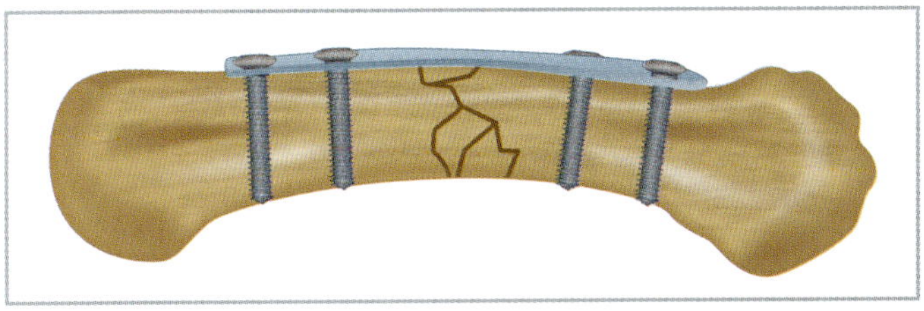

Figure 13.7 A bridging plate across a comminuted fracture segment.

External fixator

These are useful in open fractures with bone gap. The pins are placed into the proximal and distal bone segments. The bones of the hand are relatively small, and thus, appropriately sized pins that are designed specifically for application in the hand should be used.

Guide to the size of plates for the hand

- Distal phalanx: Generally small K wires (0.6–1.1 mm are used)
- Middle phalanx: 1.2- to 1.5-mm screws and plates
- Proximal phalanx: 1.5- to 2-mm screws and plates
- Metacarpals: 2- to 2.4-mm screws and plates

Application and principles of lag screw fixation

Lag screw fixation (Figure 13.8)

Lag screw fixation is achieved by allowing the screw threads to slide into the near cortex but tap into the far cortex, resulting in a relative traction force on the far cortex when the screw is tightened. The technique required the following steps:

1. The glide hole: A drill hole wider than the thread diameter of the screw is drilled perpendicular to the fracture so as to prevent engagement and allow the fully threaded screw to slide freely.

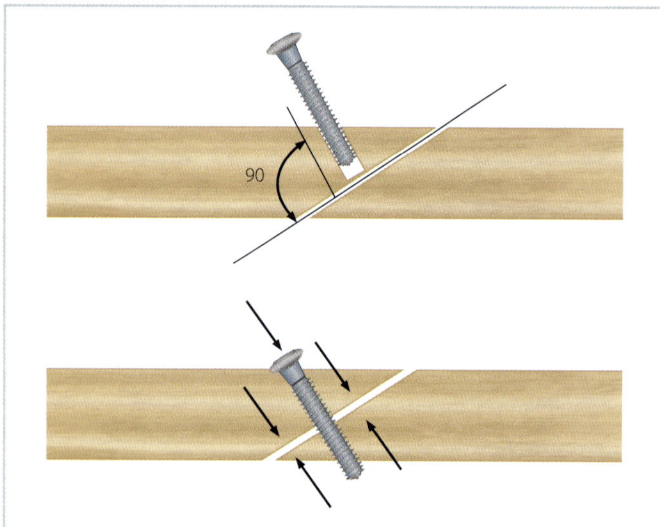

Figure 13.8 This demonstrates the steps of lag screw insertion. Note that as the lag screw is tightened, compression is created between the bone fragments, bringing them together.

2. Pilot hole: The pilot hole is the diameter of the core of the screw, and it is drilled by passing the correct drill guide through the glide hole to maintain the correct direction and alignment of the two holes.
3. The head of the screw engages the cortical surface while advancement of the screw through the pilot hole creates a compression at the fracture line, pulling the bone segments together.

SUMMARY

There a number of fracture fixation devices available for fixation of hand fractures, and these devices can be used in different ways depending on the fracture pattern and associated injuries. Similar to all other surgical techniques, there is a learning curve with using these fixation devices, and the surgeon should gradually develop the skills adhering to the standards and principles of bone healing and fixation.

SUGGESTED READING

Bernstein ML, Chung KC. Hand fractures and their management: an international view. Injury 2006; 37:1043–1048.

The authors discuss the differences in management of hand fractures around the world and the differences created by economical factors, resource availability, and availability of expertise in various geographic regions.

Gaston RG, Chadderdon C. Phalangeal fractures: displaced/nondisplaced. Hand Clin 2012; 28:395–401.

The authors discuss the role of conservative treatment in the fractures of the hand as well as techniques of fracture fixation in athletes that can provide early return to function.

Jupiter J, Ring DC. AO manual of fracture management—hand and wrist. New York: Theime, 2004.

This is a comprehensive manual that provides a guide to principles and techniques of fracture management by each bone and fracture pattern with well-illustrated examples.

Kawamura K, Chung KC. Fixation choices for closed simple unstable oblique phalangeal and metacarpal fractures Hand Clin 2006; 22:287–295.

The authors compare all the treatment techniques for the surgical fixation of simple oblique unstable metacarpal fractures and provide the pros and cons of each technique with the aim of helping the surgeon to tailor a specific technique to a particular patient's needs.

Ruchelsman DE, Mudgal CS, Jupiter JB. The role of locking technology in the hand. Hand Clin 2010; 26:307–319.

In this article, the authors discuss the role of locking systems in the treatment of fractures of the hand and wrist and also emphasize the rational use of the technology available.

Teoh LC. Operative fixation of fractures of the hand in surgery of the injured hand. In: Venkataswami R, ed. Delhi; Jaypee Brothers, 2009.

A very well-written chapter, where the author Prof. Teoh through his extensive surgical experience provides a rational understanding of fractures of the hand and the application of various techniques for stable fixation. A must read for all hand surgeons.

13.2 PHALANGEAL FRACTURES AND INTERPHALANGEAL JOINT DISLOCATIONS

INTRODUCTION

Phalangeal fractures and dislocations are among the most commonly encountered fractures. Although not life threatening, they represent considerable burden in terms of loss of work and quality of life, with the potential for causing major social problems, such as when the patient is the sole breadwinner for the family. All phalangeal fractures will heal with time, but with proper, cost-effective, and timely intervention one can avoid long-term complications such as malunion and stiffness. The best results are obtained when hand fractures are managed as quickly as possible, followed by effective rehabilitation. Although the majority of these injuries can be managed nonoperatively, it is vital to understand the surgical decision-making process for the instances when surgery is the appropriate treatment option.

SURGICAL ANATOMY

Phalanges, unlike metacarpals, are isolated skeletal units. The length of the proximal phalanx is roughly equal to the sum of the distal and middle phalanx, making the proximal interphalangeal (PIP) joint the nucleus of digital anatomy and function. The normal skeletal and muscle–tendon relationship, along with alignment, keep the digit in equilibrium. Any alteration in length or rotational misalignment can cause a loss of function. The proximal and middle phalanges can be divided into base, shaft, neck, and condyles. In a similar fashion, the distal phalanx is structurally divided into the base, shaft, and tuft. Compared with the metacarpals, the phalanges have a thick cortex dorsally. The phalanges also lack overlying muscles and have minimal subcutaneous fat, and thus, tendon dysfunction is more common.

Because of the proximity of the nail bed, fractures of the distal phalanx are almost always associated with a nail bed injury. The stability of a shaft fracture depends on the configuration of the fracture along with the integrity of the soft tissue and nail bed. In proximal phalangeal fractures, the flexion attitude of the proximal fragment causes volar apex angulation, aided by the extension attitude of the distal fragment due to the action of the interossei and extensor tendons. The more distal the fracture, the more angulation is present.

The displacement in middle phalangeal fracture depends on the site of the fracture and generally has dorsal apex angulation if the fracture is proximal to the insertion of the flexor digitorum superficialis (FDS). If the fracture is distal to its insertion, then volar angulation is seen. The distal interphalangeal (DIP) joint is a bicondylar hinge joint stabilized by articular congruity and stout capsular ligaments, which permit flexion and extension. The PIP joint is similar but with asymmetric condyles and proper collateral ligaments as its main stabilizers.

Fractures of the phalanges can be classified by various methods as shown in **Table 13.1**. Dislocations are classified as simple or complex and are mostly dorsal, volar, or lateral. The mechanism of dislocation can be hyperextension, hyperflexion, lateral deviation, or a shear. A simple dislocation has no associated fracture, whereas a complex dislocation is associated with a fracture of the involved bones and thus cannot be reduced easily. A dorsal PIP dislocation means that the middle phalanx is dislocated dorsal to the line bisecting the proximal phalanx.

CLINICAL FEATURES

Age, occupation, hand dominance, mechanism of injury, the specific needs of a patient, and medical comorbidities should all be considered in the decision-making process. In open fractures, it is important to ascertain the nature of the environment in which the injury was sustained, as this can foretell contamination and the likelihood of foreign bodies. This becomes more important with industrial workers and patients with sugarcane machine injuries. All items such as rings, jewelry, and clothing from the entire limb should be removed before examination. Both open and closed skeletal injuries can have associated injury to the tendons, nerves, or blood vessels. Examination of the digit distal to the site of injury should be performed to assess tendon function, capillary refill, and sensory function. Missed injuries always lead to long-term complications, and therefore a thorough clinical examination is essential. The examination of the contralateral hand is an important tool in making the correct diagnosis.

The common features of fracture dislocations include pain, swelling, deformity, crepitus, bruising, instability, or restricted motion. Deformity, shortening, and overriding can be further confirmed with a thorough examination under a local anesthetic, which can simultaneously help with the irrigation and management of open fractures. Subtle injuries or injuries in a victim of polytrauma are easily missed, and the treating physician must take care to look for a rotational deformity. Rotation is best appreciated with 90° flexion of the intervening joint (**Figure 13.9**).

Table 13.1 Fracture terminology and characteristics

Location	Pattern of fracture	Skeletal involvement	Deformity	Soft tissue involvement	Associated structures injured	Stability
Base	Transverse	Simple	Angulation (dorsal or Palmar)	Open	Skin	Stable
Shaft	Oblique	Comminuted	Shortening	Closed	Nerve	Unstable
Neck	Spiral	Bone loss	Rotation		Tendon	
Head (condyle or tuft)	Avulsion				Joint	
Epiphysis					Ligament	
					Blood vessel	

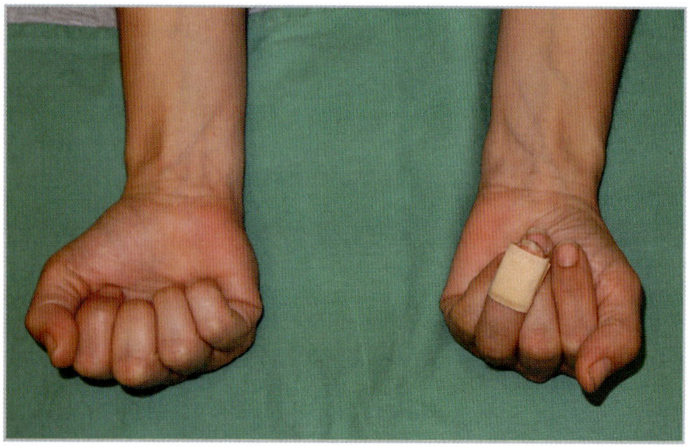

Figure 13.9 Rotation in left hand during flexion of digits

IMAGING

Plain posteroanterior (PA) and lateral view radiographs should be supplemented by additional oblique views and cross-sectional imaging whenever required. An injured digit should be radiographed in isolation to avoid superimposition by other digits. Ultrasound expertise, if available, can supplement the assessment of ligament and tendon integrity. Computed tomographic (CT) scan or magnetic resonance imaging (MRI) is rarely used in the acute setting to diagnose phalangeal fractures and interphalangeal (IP) dislocations.

EMERGENCY DEPARTMENT MANAGEMENT

Immediate treatment includes rest, ice, elevation, and splinting. Bleeding can almost always be controlled by direct pressure and limb elevation. Any blind attempt to clamp bleeders in the emergency department should be avoided. Open fractures are initially treated by irrigation, debridement, and splinting, along with tetanus prophylaxis. Definitive treatment includes anatomic reduction and stabilization with care taken to minimize soft tissue injury, followed by early range of motion (ROM).

Definitive management

Treatment is dependent upon fracture location and pattern, the surgeon's resources, and the patient's motivation. The goals of treatment in management of phalangeal fractures and general treatment of diaphyseal fractures are mentioned in **Tables 13.2** and **13.3.** A stable fracture maintains acceptable position at rest and early mobilization, unlike an unstable fracture.

Factors that influence stability include:

- External forces
- Muscle imbalance
- Fracture configuration
- Integrity of soft tissue

Stable fractures include impacted shaft fractures, fractures with minimal or no displacement, and most distal phalangeal fractures, and they can be managed nonoperatively. With instability, the best treatment option involves the least invasive surgical procedure and the restoration of skeletal mobility. Some fractures that require operative intervention are compound fractures, fractures that fail to achieve acceptable reduction by closed reduction, rotational deformity, fractures with bone loss or shortening, neck fractures, malunion, nonunion, and some intra-articular fractures.

Table 13.2 Goals of treatment for phalangeal fractures

Restoration of function
Acceptable skin cover
Early mobilization
Correction of angulation and rotation

Nonoperative treatment

Most phalangeal fractures can be treated through a nonoperative approach. Splint mobilization still remains the standard for simple injuries, whereas operative techniques are used for more complex injuries. Digital fractures unite without any intervention, so the primary goal in hand fractures remains the restoration of complete hand function. Union of a fracture into the perfect anatomical position does not always correlate with a restoration of hand function. The restoration of bony anatomy should never be attempted at the expense of soft tissue scarring and loss of motion. Emphasis should be given on proper clinical examination, results of radiological investigations, and early intervention.

For fractures that can be reduced with stability include:

- Closed reduction can be performed via axial traction under adequate anesthesia, which leads to a reversal of the deformity
- The intrinsic muscles can be relaxed by flexion of the metacarpophalangeal (MCP) joints

To promote protected motion of the injured finger, secure it to an adjacent noninjured finger. The index and ring fingers can be taped with the long finger, the long finger can be taped with the index finger, and the small finger can be taped with the ring finger. This is known as buddy taping and is the method of choice for the management of undisplaced phalangeal fractures.

In the absence of perfect reduction, rigid fixation does not usually benefit the patient. Phalangeal shaft fractures can tolerate up to 6 mm of shortening and 10 degrees of angulation, provided there is no rotational deformity. Even articular fractures can be satisfactorily treated by closed reduction techniques. All patients managed nonoperatively should be followed up early in the outpatient clinic to reassess reduction, otherwise operative reduction becomes inevitable.

Fracture location can be an important determining factor in the selection of technique. Although displaced fractures at the head of the phalanx should be treated by open reduction and internal fixation (ORIF), a similar displaced fracture at the base of the phalanx should be treated by closed reduction techniques. Surgical options should be considered if conservative management is not suitable.

Operative treatment

Surgical fixation should be rigid and performed with the least amount of soft tissue disruption (**Table 13.4**). This allows early active motion, which helps avoid iatrogenic stiffness. There is very little data that compares the different treatment options in a scientific way, and therefore, no consensus has been reached for the treatment of even the most simple fractures. In this context, the surgeon should perform operative procedures that are easily available rather than more complex techniques that are relatively new. Sometimes a patient benefits more by a less than perfect position as compared with a more rigorous fracture reduction. However, if

Table 13.3 Treatment of diaphyseal fractures

Fracture type	Treatment
Stable fractures that are closed and aligned	Buddy strapping
Stable fractures that are closed but misaligned after reduction	Cast
Unstable fractures that are closed and misaligned after reduction	Percutaneous fixation
Unstable fractures that are closed, misaligned, and comminuted after reduction	Open reduction and internal fixation

Table 13.4 Fractures that may require operative intervention

Impacted fractures of the proximal portion of proximal phalanx of the finger
Intra-articular fractures when >25% of the joint surface is involved
Fracture dislocation of the proximal interphalangeal joint, in general chip fractures around any joint represent ligamentous injury and are potentially serious
Open fractures
Fractures with associated tendon, vascular, or nerve injury

a patient so desires or the occupation of a patient requires a more complex procedure, a properly trained surgeon should perform the procedure.

Screws and plates (**Figure 13.10**) have expanded the options in fracture fixation but have not substituted for plaster splints or K-wires (**Figure 13.11a** and **b**). If closed reduction of a phalangeal fracture is not suitable, percutaneous pinning may be the mainstay of treatment. Although pinning has complications such as pin loosening, pin tract infections, osteomyelitis, nerve or tendon injury, nonunion, and malunion, it can still address most of the shortcomings of splinting and casting techniques. Percutaneous fixation can treat nearly all fractures of the hand skeleton that are without segmental bone loss and are not significantly comminuted. It can be used for shaft fractures; however, articular fractures and fracture dislocations should ideally be addressed by screw and plate fixation. Improvement in intraoperative imaging techniques has made percutaneous pin fixation a very useful tool.

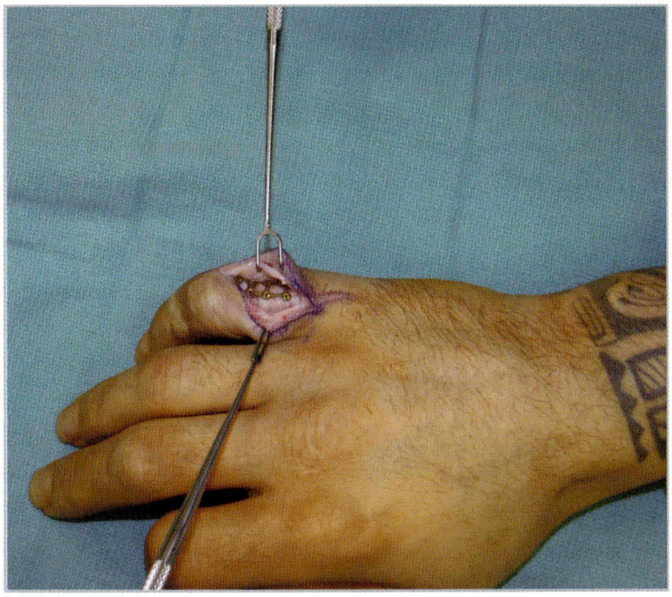

Figure 13.10 Use of screws and plates for fracture management.

Minimally invasive techniques guided by fluoroscopy and arthroscopy allow rigid fixation while simultaneously preserving the soft tissue envelope. Dynamic external fixators have been developed that aid in treating difficult articular fractures. In addition, highly specialized headless cannulated compression screws and biodegradable plates may change the practice of fracture management in the future.

Surgical technique

Operative management is performed under appropriate anesthesia using tourniquet control. In the percutaneous technique, the wires are inserted through the skin with the help of a motorized hand held drill. In open fixation, the fracture is exposed from the dorsal side, and the extensor tendons in the way are either retracted or carefully incised vertically. Although general or regional anesthesia is used, local blocks may facilitate intraoperative movements to confirm rotational alignment. The various types of implants used in phalangeal fractures include K-wires, interosseous wiring, screws and plates, compression screws, and external fixators.

K-wires

K-wires are cheap, versatile, and easily available implants that can be inserted both by closed and open methods. They are also a very useful tool for reduction during internal fixation. Almost any fracture can be managed by K-wires; however, they have the limitation of being nonrigid, and immobilization by additional plaster is required to maintain reduction.

The K-wire fixation is still the standard for many fractures, and most of the new techniques are compared with this method of fixation. K-wires can be inserted as crossed, longitudinal intramedullary wire, multiple parallel wires (**Figure 13.12**) across the fracture site, or in combination with interosseous wiring (**Table 13. 5**). Exposed implants can impale the extensor tendons. In transverse fractures of the shaft, intramedullary fixation gives an advantage of avoiding removal of the implant. Rotatory instability, however, needs the additional use of stainless steel wires.

Insertion of K-wires can be accomplished through an antegrade or retrograde approach. The middle phalanx is approached antegrade, extraarticularly through the base, whereas the proximal phalanx can be approached either antegrade through a flexed MCP joint or retrograde at the PIP joint.

Interosseous wiring

In this technique, a small stainless steel (26 G) wire is passed across the fracture line. This technique is used in transverse fractures associated with soft tissue injury or for arthrodesis. The advantages of this technique are that it is technically straightforward, requires minimum instrumentation, and offers early mobilization. It is also a safe substitute for screw fixation and can be used in isolation for fractures of the head or base of the phalanx, or supplemented with K-wires (tension band wiring) to interlock the fracture fragments.

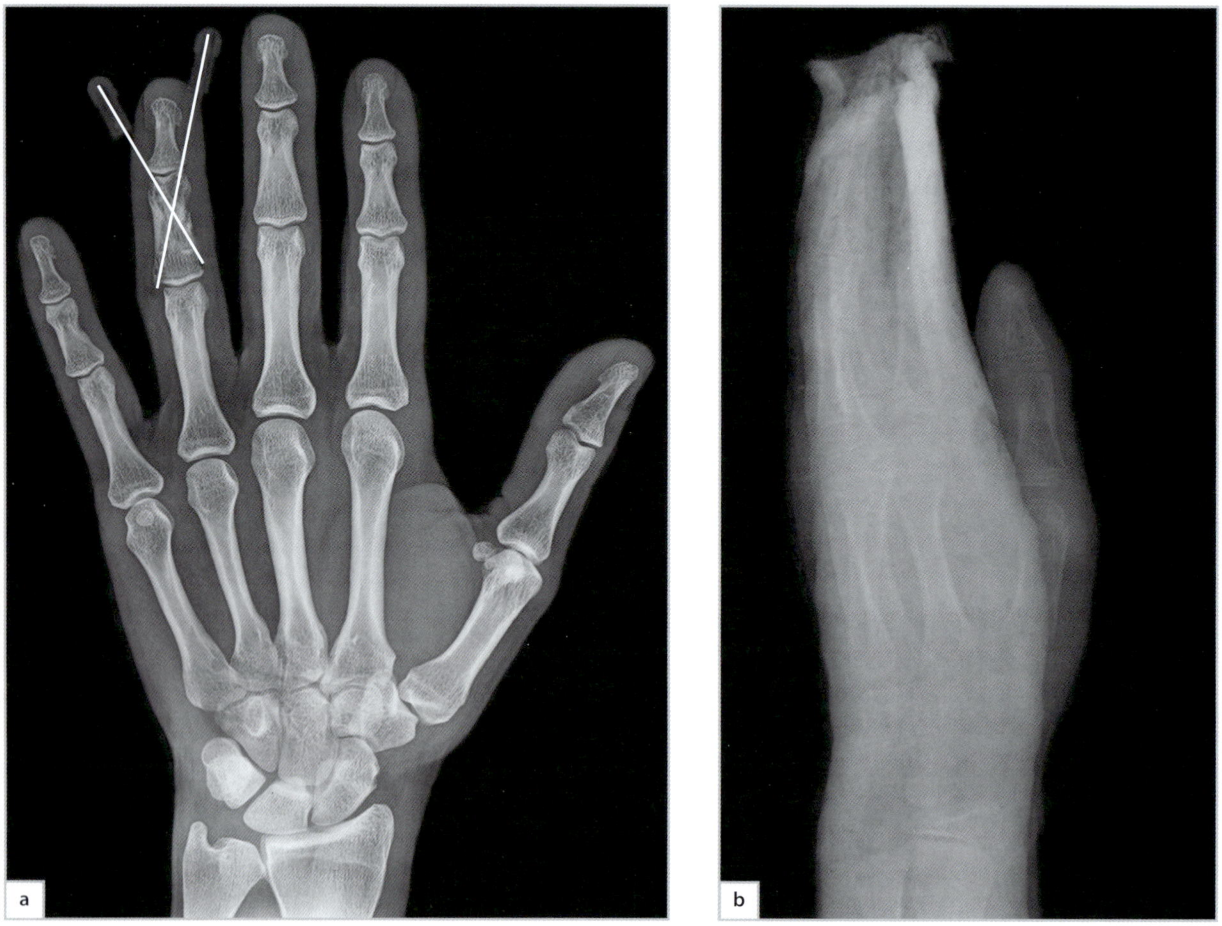

Figure 13.11 (a) Use of cross K-wires for management of fracture. (b) Management of fracture by plaster of Paris slab.

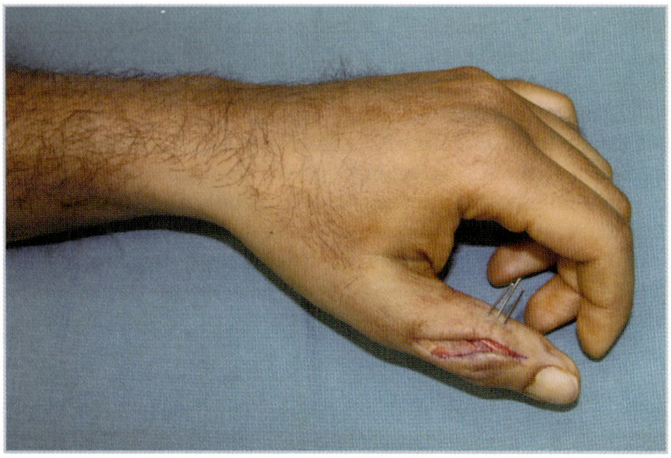

Figure 13.12 Placement of multiple parallel K-wires for management of fracture.

Table 13.5 Various methods of stabilizing by K-wires

Intramedullary
Crossed
Transarticular intramedullary
Direct and intramedullary combined
Along with interosseous wires

Screws and plates

This remains the most stable method of internal fixation, with strength as good as intact bone. It is a costly and technically demanding method of fracture fixation, useful in oblique unstable fractures, fractures with bone loss, and some intracondylar fractures. A minimum of two screws are required on either side to obtain a rigid fixation. Plates using 1.5- and 2.0-mm screws are preferable in the phalanges. These devices should not be prominent as they may require additional surgery for removal and therefore should only be reserved for highly complex fracture patterns. Whenever screws and plates are used, protected motion should be initiated immediately to prevent the development of soft tissue adhesions. Bioabsorbable screws have not gained much importance until recently, although they appear to be promising for the future.

Compression screws

Unicondylar and large avulsion fractures can be treated by single interfragmentary screw fixation. Compression screws have the advantage of allowing early functional rehabilitation. Microscrews of 1.5-mm size are preferable in phalanges.

External fixator

Traditionally, external fixators are used for the management of fractures with severe soft tissue injuries in fractures throughout the body. Sometimes these fixators are applied temporarily until soft tissue coverage is obtained, but they may also be used as a definitive fixation device. Recent improvements in the design of external fixators have made them suitable for PIP dislocations and even comminuted diaphyseal fractures.

CLASSIFICATION AND SPECIFIC FRACTURES

Distal phalanx

Tuft fractures

- Tuft fractures can be simple or comminuted, but nearly all fractures of the tuft are associated with some degree of nail bed injury
- Trephination of the nail bed can be performed in symptomatic nail bed hematomas
- Nail bed lacerations require repair of the nail bed itself, and irreducible fractures with interposition of the nail will require reduction and K-wire fixation

Shaft fractures

- Shaft fractures can be transverse or longitudinal
- The soft tissue envelope in nondisplaced fractures provides adequate stability
- Open fractures need irrigation, debridement, antibiotics, and nail bed repair along with percutaneous K-wire fixation
- Fractures of the base of the distal phalanx are unstable and angulate with the apex pointing dorsally

Distal articular fractures

- Can be dorsal (mallet) or volar due to an avulsion of the flexor digitorum profundus (FDP) tendon
- A mallet fracture is usually treated by 6–8 weeks of extension splinting of the DIP joint fracture followed by 1 month of night splinting
- Percutaneous K-wire fixation is performed in cases of volar subluxation of the distal phalanx

Pilon fractures

- These fractures result from an impaction injury of the volar base of the distal phalanx. All attempts should be made for closed reduction. FDP avulsions can occur with or without bony avulsion. Patients often complain of an inability to flex while passive motion is normal. This injury is frequently missed as sprained finger
- Anatomic repair by tendon insertion into the bone is the treatment of choice. If large bony fragments are present, small screw fixation should be performed.

Middle and proximal phalangeal shaft fractures

- They can be transverse, oblique, spiral, or comminuted. A simple technique such as buddy taping with closed monitoring is usually adequate
  - Occasionally, displaced fractures, even if reduced, are difficult to maintain in reduction
  - Transverse fractures tend to be stable, whereas oblique, spiral, or comminuted fractures and fractures near the base of the phalanges tend toward instability.
  - Intra-articular fractures are treated by buddy strapping (**Table 13.6**)
- Axial traction, increasing the deformity, and reversal of the deformity are the three steps for closed reduction. Relaxing the tension on intrinsic musculature by MCP joint flexion is sometimes required for successful reduction of shaft fractures. After reduction, rotational alignment is confirmed clinically, the hand is splinted in a functional position with flexion of the MCP joints and extension of the IP joints, and check radiographs are obtained. If minimum tissue disruption is present in displaced fractures, percutaneous fixation is the most suitable technique. **Table 13.7** mentions the approaches and surgical steps required for fixation of proximal phalanx.

Base fracture

- Closed fractures usually tend toward a hyperextension deformity of the distal fragment and should be rigidly fixed either with crossed K-wires through the base or transmetacarpal head pins
- Long oblique and spiral oblique fractures are technically more challenging and are repaired by lag screws

Condylar fractures

- Torsional or lateral bending injuries to DIP or PIP joints can lead to condylar fractures of the head of the middle or proximal phalanx. These fractures may be misdiagnosed as sprains
- In addition to PA and lateral views, oblique views are also required
- If left untreated treated, these fractures can lead to significant disability. The best fixation is obtained by more than one K-wire

DISLOCATIONS

DIP dislocations

- Because of the thin skin at the DIP joint, these injuries are mostly open
- Closed injuries are treated with longitudinal traction, and the digit is held in flexion
- Open injuries are treated by open reduction
- Post reduction radiographs must demonstrate concentric reduction

Proximal interphalangeal joint dislocations

- Dorsal dislocations of the PIP joint are commonly encountered dislocations of the hand

Table 13.6 Intra-articular fractures of the base of the proximal phalanx

Collateral ligament avulsion
Compression
Vertical shear
Treatment: Buddy strap (if minimal displacement)

Table 13.7 Steps and surgical approaches to proximal phalanx function

Mid axial or dorsal longitudinal incision
Diaphysis is approached by extensor splitting incision or by creating space between common extensor and lateral band
Long flap of periosteum is raised to cover back implants

- To reduce PIP dislocations, apply distal tension on the injured finger while using the thumb to apply counter pressure to the middle phalanx on the volar aspect

Overview of treatment options for dislocations

- Options include skeletal traction, static or dynamic external fixation, dynamic traction with active or passive motion, volar plate arthroplasty, closed reduction with transarticular K-wire fixation, and ORIF with or without bone grafting
- ORIF is possible only if fracture fragments are large enough to accept a screw
- External fixation along with closed reduction provides an advantage over internal fixation as it preserves the blood supply and gives an opportunity to start early motion of the PIP joint

Complications

Phalangeal fractures can be complicated by deformity from no treatment, stiffness from overtreatment, and both deformity and stiffness from poor treatment. Complications of fracture dislocations include flexion contractures, joint stiffness, or redisplacement. Pin tract infections can be present in fractures treated by external fixators.

Distal phalangeal fractures

Fingertip and nail injuries are commonly associated with this fracture. If not managed properly, long-term pain, cold intolerance, altered sensation, nail bed deformity, malunion, or nonunion may occur.

Loss of motion

This is the most common complication of any phalangeal injury. Early mobilization within 3–4 weeks helps in preventing long-term loss of motion. Loss of motion usually results from intra-articular adhesions, capsular contracture, and tendon adhesions. Intra-articular adhesions and stiffness can be prevented by immobilization in a 'safe position.' Once loss of motion develops, it is treated by aggressive physiotherapy. Occasionally, surgical release of the contracted joints is required. Tendon adhesions are formed by adhesions of the tendons with an injured tendon sheath. Tenolysis is required if aggressive therapy is not effective.

Malunion

Malunion results from a loss of closed reduction, inadequate initial reduction, or failure of internal fixation. Muscular imbalance due to resultant angular and rotational imbalance leads to a deviation of the digits and loss of grip and pinch function. Established malunions require corrective osteotomies, and early detection is essential, as any revision beyond 3–4 weeks is extremely challenging.

Infection

The hand has an excellent blood supply, and therefore, infection is much less likely than in other body sites. Inadequate debridement of devitalized tissue in open fractures, pin tract infections, and internal fixation devices are the most common causes. Pin site infections can be minimized by proper cleaning of pins and antibiotics. Removal of hardware is usually required in cases of frank osteomyelitis, loose hardware, or overlying cellulitis.

Nonunion

This usually only responds to operative correction and is functionally disabling.

Special considerations

Athletes

In athletes, stable fixation is recommended in view of their career and recurrent injuries. Athlete's coaches frequently perform closed reduction of fractures sustained during play, so the presentation for these patients is typically subacute or when they start having pain again. A comminuted fracture in an athlete who is in the playing season and wants to play immediately will require plate fixation. Plates should be placed on the radial or ulnar border instead of the dorsum. Dorsal dislocation of the PIP joints is common in athletes playing games in which a ball frequently hits the tip of the digit.

Children

Clinical examination and radiological investigation in children is sometimes not possible without sedation. In addition, radiographs are difficult to interpret because of nonossified cartilage in a child's hand (**Figure 13.13**). Usually, misdiagnosis is due to a wrong interpretation of normal epiphyses. If the clinician is unsure about ossification, it is helpful to have X-rays of the opposite hand for comparison. Children remove the dressings quite often, and therefore, all casts should be applied above the elbow to prevent this occurrence. Operative intervention is rarely (**Figure 13.14**) required; however, the location of the growth plate must be kept in mind during fixation (**Figure 13.14**). Plate fixation, if required in extremely rare circumstances, will subject the child to another surgery for removal of the plate.

Salter–Harris (**Table 13.8**) type I and II fractures are more common in pediatric distal phalanx fractures. Complications of the pediatric phalangeal fracture include nonunion, malunion, osteonecrosis, and growth disturbance. Although bone remodeling is very good in children, osteotomy is occasionally required.

Rehabilitation

Early mobilization prevents adhesions of the soft tissue and gliding tendons, along with contracture of the joint capsule. Ideally, mobilization should be initiated as soon as possible (**Figures 13.15–13.16b**). Splints should be small to permit motion in uninvolved joints.

SUMMARY

Social and economic factors influence treatment decisions. Surgeons dealing with phalangeal fractures should be able to decide that anatomic reduction is almost always necessary in malrotated and intra-articular fractures, whereas some other types of phalangeal fractures can be allowed to malunite without any significant loss of function. Fortunately, most hand fractures benefit without operative intervention, and the application of the most appropriate method of fracture immobilization and fixation should be followed by proper rehabilitation.

Low-energy trauma leading to closed, minimally displaced fractures with acceptable alignment and intact supporting tissue, can be managed with protected mobilization. Even fractures with rotational or angular misalignment can be treated with closed reduction and splinting in the intrinsic plus position. The goal of treatment in dislocations is the restoration of a congruous articular surface along with full ROM.

Open techniques provide the surgeon with the opportunity for anatomic reduction and stable fixation. They are generally indicated for irreducible fractures, fractures with segmental bone loss requiring grafting, and inadequate fixation by percutaneous methods. The choice of technique depends upon fracture pattern, soft tissue injury, and the available resources and experience of the surgeon.

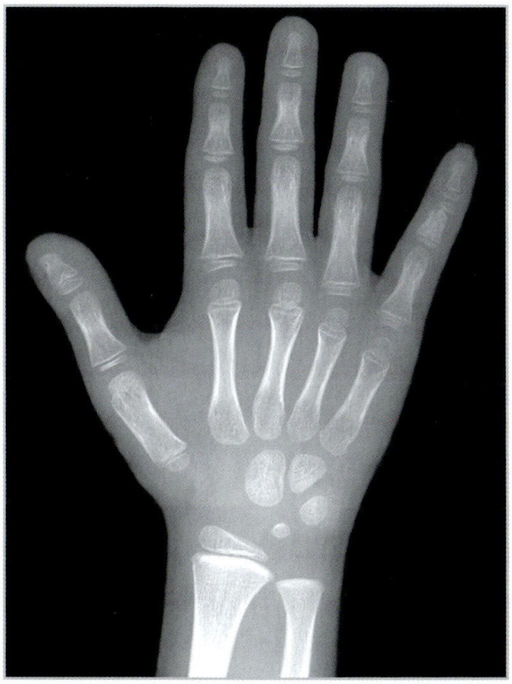

Figure 13.13 Growth centers in the pediatric hand.

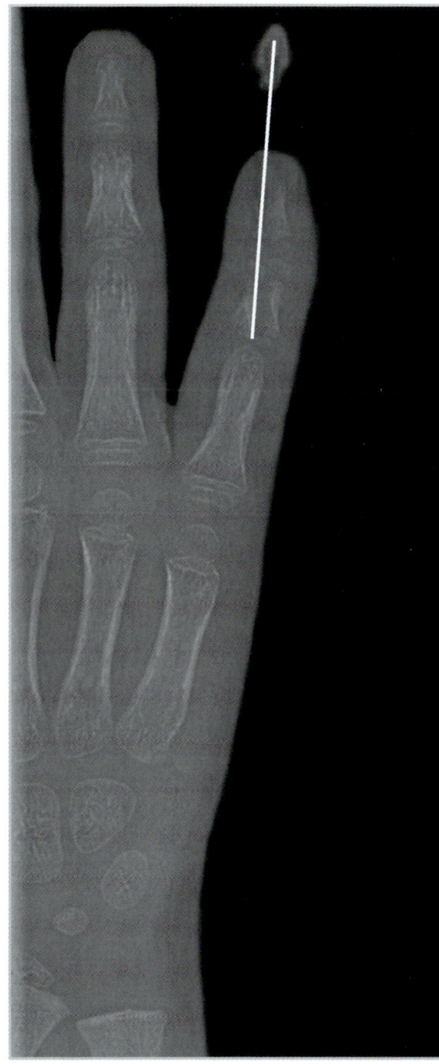

Figure 13.14 Careful insertion of K-wires avoiding growth plates.

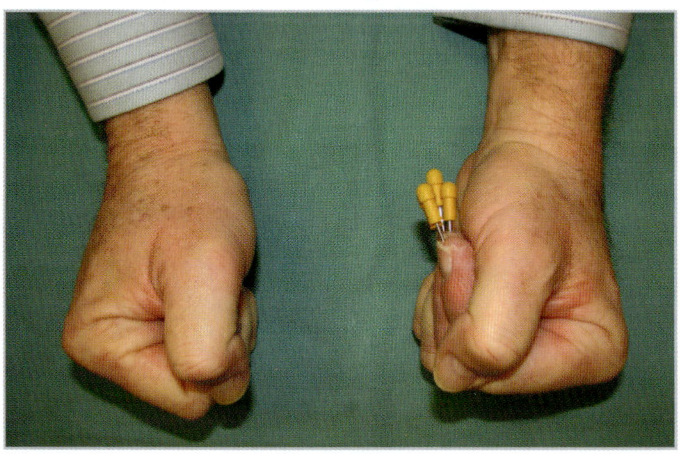

Figure 13.15 Early physiotherapy (before removal of implants).

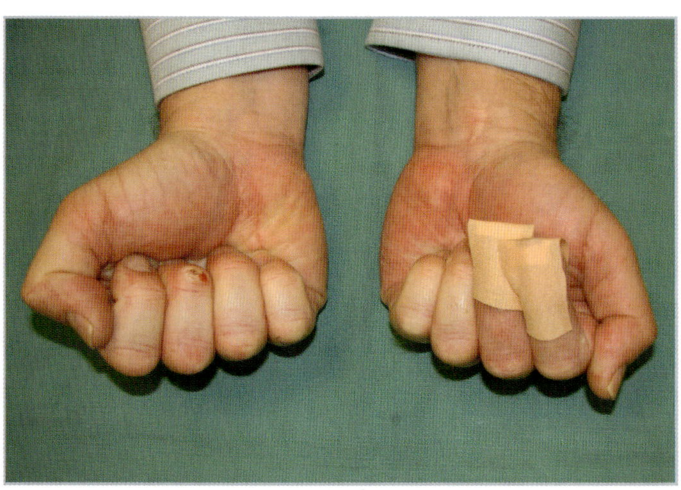

Figure 13.16a Good hand function due to early physiotherapy.

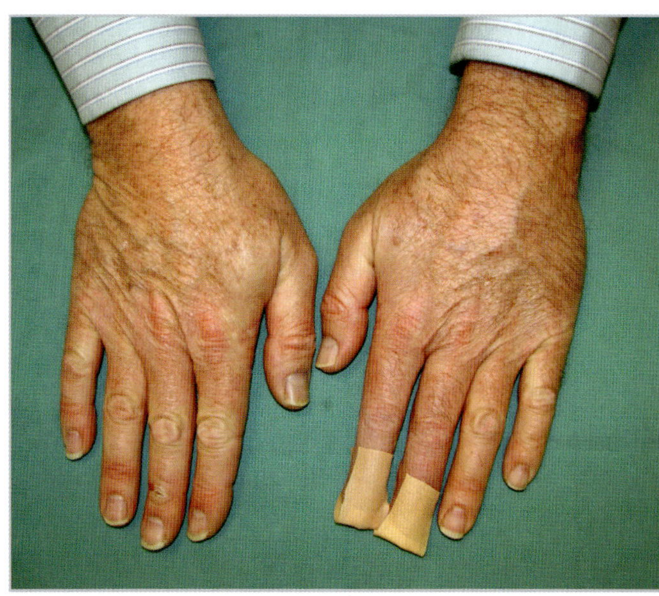

Figure 13.16b Good hand function due to early physiotherapy.

Table 13.8 Salter–Harris classification of pediatric fractures

Type I	Widening of epiphyseal plate
Type II	Fracture through the metaphysis
Type III	Fracture through the growth plate
Type IV	Fracture through the epiphysis and metaphysic
Type V	Compression of epiphysis

SUGGESTED READING

Calfee RP, Sommerkamp TG. Fracture-dislocation about the finger joints. J Hand Surg Am 2009; 34:1140–1147.

The authors describe treatment options and planning of interphalangeal dislocations with special focus on residual pain and stiffness.

Dean BJF, Little C. Fractures of metacarpal and phalanges. Orthop Trauma 2011; 25:43–56.

This article summarizes the key concepts in management of phalangeal fractures and also explains the rationale behind the treatment planning process.

Kamath JB, Harshvardhan, Naik DM, Bansal A. Current concepts in managing fractures of metacarpal and phalanges. Indian J Plast Surg 2011; 44:203–211.

The article reviews the current concepts in management of phalangeal fractures along with incorporating tips and indications for fixation of these fractures.

Smita A, Hooper G. Fractures in the child's hand. Curr Orthop 2006; 20: 461–466.

This article gives good overview of pediatric phalangeal fractures and interphalangeal dislocations.

Tuncer S, Aksu N, Dilek H, Ozkan T, Hamzaoglu A. Fractures of the fingers missed or misdiagnosed on poorly positioned or poorly taken radiographs: a retrospective study. J Trauma. 2011; 71:649–655.

This study describes the importance of proper positioning during radiography in diagnosis and treatment of phalangeal injuries.

13.3 METACARPAL FRACTURES

INTRODUCTION

Hand fractures account for 19% of all fractures in the body and can reach a prevalence as high as 30% for manual laborers. Metacarpal fractures account for 30–40% of all fractures in the hand, and 18% of fractures below the elbow, with a lifetime incidence of approximately 2.5% for an individual. The border metacarpals of the hand (i.e. thumb and little metacarpals) are more frequently involved than the other metacarpals. Metacarpal fractures can be categorized as head, shaft, neck, and base fractures. The loss of function that occurs due to these injuries not only reduces patient's productivity but also is a considerable burden upon society.

RELEVANT ANATOMY

A good understanding of the skeletal anatomy of the metacarpal bones and the supporting structures (i.e. tendons and ligaments) will help guide the management of different fractures. The metacarpals are the long bones in the hand and serve to support the structure of the palm, articulating proximally to the carpus and distally to the phalanx. The strong supporting interosseous and deep transverse intercarpal ligaments stabilize the relationship of the base of the metacarpal with the carpus. The index and middle carpometacarpal (CMC) joints are very stable because of the strong ligamentous support and the congruent articulations of the trapezoid and capitate, and therefore, fractures in this area are rare. In contrast, the ring and small metacarpals are more frequently injured because they have a limited support structure, making them more susceptible to trauma. In addition, the lack of flexibility in the index and middle finger CMC joint compared with the ring and little finger is an important factor regarding treatment. The ring and little finger CMC joint can compensate for dorsal apex angulation to a greater degree than the index and middle finger due to the mobility of the ring and little finger CMC joints.

The pull at the tendon insertion in the bone is the main deforming force after a fracture, and this can cause deformities at the fracture site. Understanding the tendon insertions is critical to successfully reduce a metacarpal fracture.

- The abductor pollicis longus (APL) inserts onto the dorsal base of the thumb metacarpal bone, abducting the thumb in the frontal plane and extending the thumb at the CMC joint. It is the main deforming force of metacarpal fractures at the base of the thumb (Bennett fracture)
- The extensor carpi radialis longus inserts onto the base of the index metacarpal bone and functions to extend and radially extend the wrist. The extensor carpi radialis brevis (ECRB) inserts onto the base of the middle metacarpal bone, where it facilitates extension of the wrist. The extensor carpi ulnaris (ECU) inserts onto the base of the little metacarpal bone, extending and assisting with ulnar extension of the wrist. These muscles act as the main deforming forces after a metacarpal base fracture
- Three palmar and four dorsal interossei muscles arise from the metacarpal shaft. Shaft and neck fractures have apex dorsal angulation due to the deforming pull of these interossei. As a result, compensatory MCP hyperextension and PIP joint flexion known as 'pseudoclawing' may also occur

EVALUATION

- A comprehensive evaluation is critical to determine the type of fracture and the appropriate treatment, because the treatment of metacarpal fractures depends on many factors, including the fracture pattern, location of fracture, any deformity of the fracture, and whether it is an open or closed fracture. Additional factors include patient age, occupation, and the surgeon's skill. It is important to obtain this information before any decision making regarding treatment is initiated
- Both the surgeon and patient should have a clear idea of and agree upon the treatment objectives before treatment begins. The overall aim is to restore function of the hand by maintaining joint mobility and stability. It is not always possible to reduce fractures back to perfect anatomical alignment, but treatment should aim to provide acceptable functional outcomes

HISTORY

A pertinent patient history helps the treating physician assess the fracture and any associated injuries. The details regarding the mechanism of injury are critical to understand the pattern of the fracture, as this will dictate treatment. The precise mechanism of injury (e.g. high-energy injury), symptoms (e.g. compartment syndrome), neurovascular compromise, and time from injury to presentation can significantly influence the available treatment options. Information such as patient age and occupation are also key components of a pertinent history and are useful to tailor treatment according to the specific needs of the patient.

Patient age

- In pediatric patients, involvement of the physeal plate (located in the distal end of the finger metacarpals and proximal end of the thumb metacarpals) should be considered. The growth plate in a child may appear to be a fracture, or a fracture may be hidden within the physis itself. Comparison with the child's normal hand is usually adequate to make a correct diagnosis
- Fractures in young adults are frequently associated with high-energy trauma, and therefore often have increased comminution, making these fractures inherently unstable. In addition, young patients typically have a high requirement for functional outcomes and cosmetic appearance, which needs to be taken into consideration during the decision-making process
- Fractures in elderly patients are typically caused by low-energy trauma, and they are commonly the result of a fall from standing height. Late fracture displacement is common because osteoporotic bone tends to displace after fracture fixation. In addition, elderly patients have less resilient soft tissue in the hand, which makes it more difficult to splint metacarpal fractures, as there is less available padding to hold the fracture in place

Occupation

- A patient who requires an early return to work time should be treated with a technique that permits rapid mobilization and minimizes adhesions
- Athletes need special consideration in regards to recovery time and function, and they may require more aggressive treatment methods than other patients

IMAGING

Plain radiographs should be obtained, consisting of PA, lateral, and oblique views in all patients with hand fractures. The normal neck to shaft angle is 15°, which should be kept in mind during radiological evaluation. Unlike the phalanges, individual radiological views of each metacarpal are not possible; however, angulation is best seen with a true lateral view. Certain fractures or dislocations may require special views for appropriate evaluation, such as the Brewerton view (see Chapter 3) to evaluate the metacarpal head. If a fracture is suspected, but plain radiographs appear normal, CT scans or MRI may be helpful to determine intra-articular fractures not seen due to overlapping bone shadows.

CLINICAL SYMPTOMS AND DECISION MAKING

Typically, patients with metacarpal fractures present with pain, shortening deformities, and limited ROM. These fractures are usually easy to diagnose, except in patients who are unconscious or have multiple injuries, and under such circumstances fractures may not be diagnosed early. In a patient with complex hand trauma, the entire limb should be inspected for the presence of more proximal injuries. When examining for fractures of the metacarpal bone, the following points should be considered:

- The main deformities encountered with metacarpal fractures are rotational, angulation, and shortening deformities, and generally the more proximal the fracture, the greater the deformity. Usually in a normal hand, the fingertips point toward the scaphoid tuberosity when flexed. The alignment of the digits in a metacarpal fracture can be determined by flexion of the digits, and a rotational deformity (**Figure 13.17**) or shortening will change the finger alignment. Malalignment of the fingers will help indicate the site of the fracture
- A rotational deformity will deviate the affected finger from the normal alignment when the hand is flexed into a fist position. It is crucial to correct any rotational deformity, as the deformity gets amplified by finger flexion. Five degrees of rotational error in a finger metacarpal result in almost 1.5 cm of crossing when the fingers are fully flexed
- Metacarpal fractures typically deform with apex dorsal angulation of 10°–15° (**Figure 13.18**), and this is acceptable because it does not substantially interfere with hand function. However, more than 30° of apex dorsal angulation can cause serious functional deficits and requires treatment
- Shortening deformities are caused by an overlap of the proximal and distal fracture fragments, comminution, or angulation, all of which can decrease the length of the bone
- Sensation can be assessed by two-point discrimination to determine any associated injury to the nerves. Circulation can be evaluated by timed capillary refill, with the contralateral hand as a reference for examination

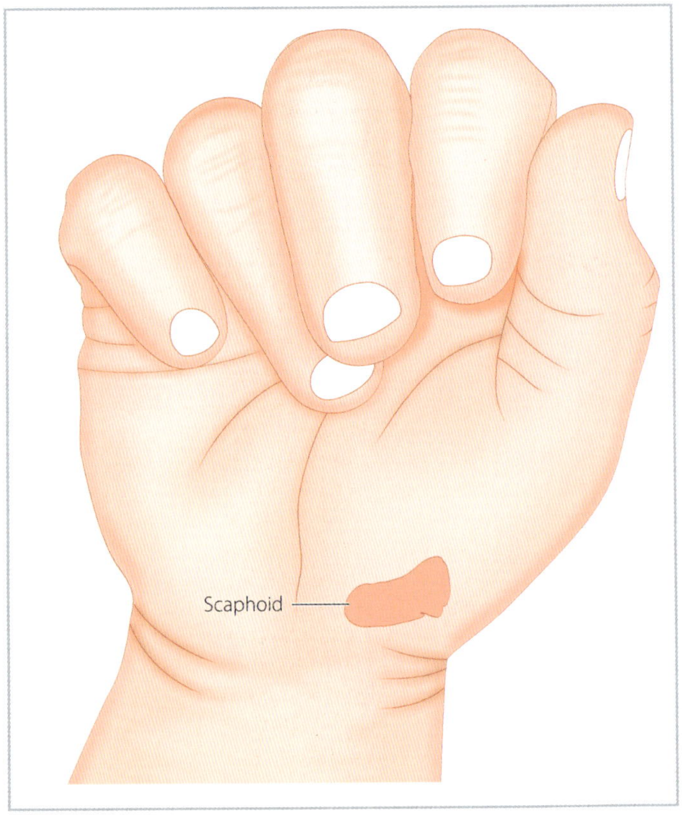

Figure 13.17 The index and middle fingers are normal and aligned toward the scaphoid, whereas the ring and little fingers are pointing away from the scaphoid, indicating a rotational deformity.

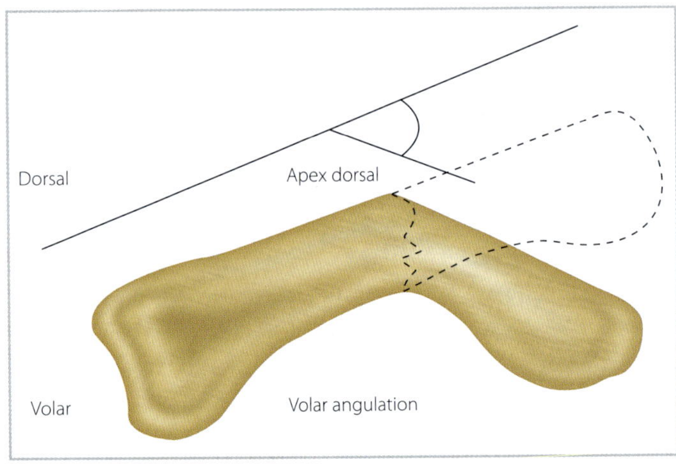

Figure 13.18 Apex dorsal angulation occurs when the distal fracture fragment points dorsally, which is the most common presentation of angulation in metacarpal fractures.

Closed fractures

- For closed fractures, the fracture pattern and location largely determine the available treatment options
- For stable fractures in the middle and ring metacarpal bones, conservative treatment with a volar splint is recommended. The transverse metacarpal ligament coupled with the location of these bones in the center of the hand renders them particularly stable compared to the index and little metacarpal bones, and therefore, splinting is adequate. The little metacarpal bone can be splinted in an ulnar gutter splint. If the fracture is stable after 1 week, splinting can continue until the bone is fully healed, but the hand should not be splinted for than 3 weeks to avoid stiffness. If the fracture is displaced after 1 week of splinting, surgical correction is indicated

- For unstable fractures, such as transverse fractures, K-wire fixation or plating will provide adequate support for the bone to heal
- If the fracture is severely comminuted, K-wires and plating will not hold the fragments in place, and therefore, external fixation may be indicated
- If there are multiple metacarpal fractures simultaneously, ORIF with plates is indicated

Open fractures

- With open hand fractures, it is recommended to inspect the hand, examine for any wounds or associated injuries, and determine the degree of contamination. The initial step in treatment is debridement of all nonviable tissue or contaminated tissue, followed by the decision-making process. Associated soft tissue injuries, the fracture pattern, and extensive comminution must all be taken into consideration when determining treatment methods.
- For simple open fractures that are clean and can be closed primarily, K-wire fixation or plating is the recommended treatment option, depending upon the treating surgeon's skill, available resources, and patient preference in regards to recovery time.
- Simple open fractures with extensive soft tissue damage that do not allow primary closure should be treated with external fixation. Plates and K-wires are not suitable for this type of injury because they would remain exposed after fixation.
- For open severely comminuted fractures, external fixation is the optimal treatment option. It is difficult to stabilize the bone fragments using plates or K-wires, whereas the external fixator is able to span the length of the fracture fragments and anchor to healthy bone on both sides of the fracture.

TREATMENT

The mainstay of treatment for hand fractures is anatomical reduction and full functional restoration of hand function. Hand therapy is critical whether fractures are treated conservatively or surgically, and early mobilization of the injured finger is preferred to prevent post-traumatic stiffness. Although no technique is perfect, overall results of metacarpal fractures are good whether fractures are treated nonoperatively with splinting and traction or operatively.

Indications of nonoperative and surgical management

Indications of nonoperative treatment

Nonsurgical management can be used to treat the majority of the metacarpal shaft or neck fractures, as long as suitable reduction can be applied. This is particularly true for the isolated metacarpal fracture, which can be supported by the adjacent bone and the transverse metacarpal ligament. The following are indications of nonoperative management:

- Undisplaced isolated metacarpal shaft fractures
- Minimally displaced metacarpal shaft fractures
- Rotational deformity:
  - <10°
- Angulation deformity:
  - Index and middle metacarpal: <10°
  - Ring metacarpal: <20°
  - Little metacarpal: <30°
- Shortening deformity:
  - <5 mm as long as it does not interfere with function
  - Surgical management is indicated for shortening < 5 mm that causes functional impairment

Indications of surgical management

- Closed isolated fractures with failed conservative treatment
- Open fractures
  - Debridement and irrigation along with antibiotic coverage should be performed with reduction of an open fracture
- Intra-articular fractures
- Angulation deformity:
  - Index and middle metacarpal: >10°
  - Ring metacarpal: >20°
  - Little metacarpal: >30°
- Rotation deformity:
  - Greater than 10°
- Shortening deformity: >5 mm
  - Irreducible or unstable fractures

METACARPAL HEAD FRACTURES

- Metacarpal head fractures are uncommon and are usually intra-articular, and the index finger is frequently involved
- Radiographic views include the three standard views (PA, lateral, oblique), in addition to the Brewerton view
- Fractures should be treated on an individual basis. For fractures with displacement, fixation can be performed with K-wires (**Figure 13.19a** and **b**). Headless screws allow early ROM and are suitable for patients who require an early return to work
- A comminuted intra-articular fracture is one of the most complicated fractures, necessitating ORIF (**Figure 13.20a** and **b**) or implant arthroplasty. Whatever the mode of treatment, the most common postoperative complication is stiffness of the MCP joint. A delayed tenolysis and capsulotomy procedure will help improve the functional outcome

METACARPAL NECK FRACTURES

- Metacarpal neck fractures are common, generally caused by the direct impact of a clenched fist onto a solid object. The ring and small finger metacarpal have the least amount of support from the surrounding ligaments and tendons and hence are often involved
- Asking the patient make a grip maneuver while palpating the metacarpal head in the palm will elicit a pain response
- Apex dorsal angulation occurs due to a combination of the axial load and the deforming forces of the lumbricals and interossei muscles. These fractures are characterized by MCP joint hyperextension and PIP joint flexion on attempted extension of the finger due to an imbalance between the forces of the extensor and interosseous muscles
- Radiographs include PA and lateral views of the hand, in addition to 30–45° supinated and pronated views

Conservative treatment

- Warranted for fractures without significant angulation deformities. The reduction may be difficult to maintain because of the deforming forces of the intrinsic muscles
  - Reduction by the Jahss reduction maneuver is indicated for closed, fresh metacarpal neck fractures

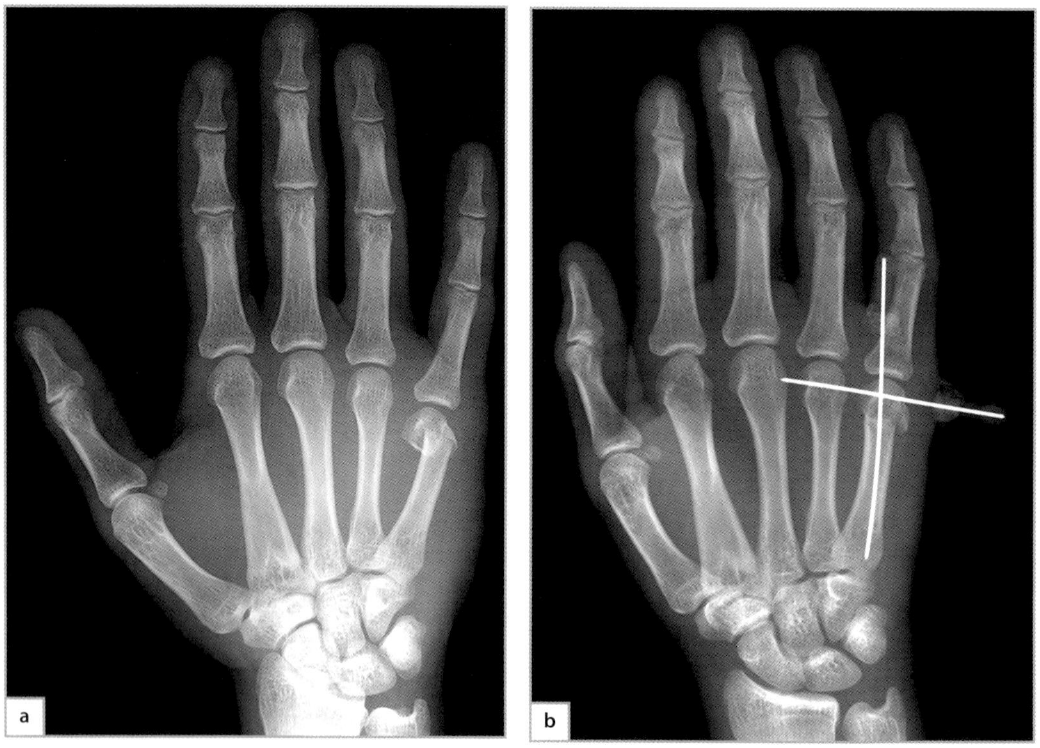

Figure 13.19 (a) Metacarpal head fracture of the little metacarpal. (b) Metacarpal head fracture fixed with crossed K-wires.

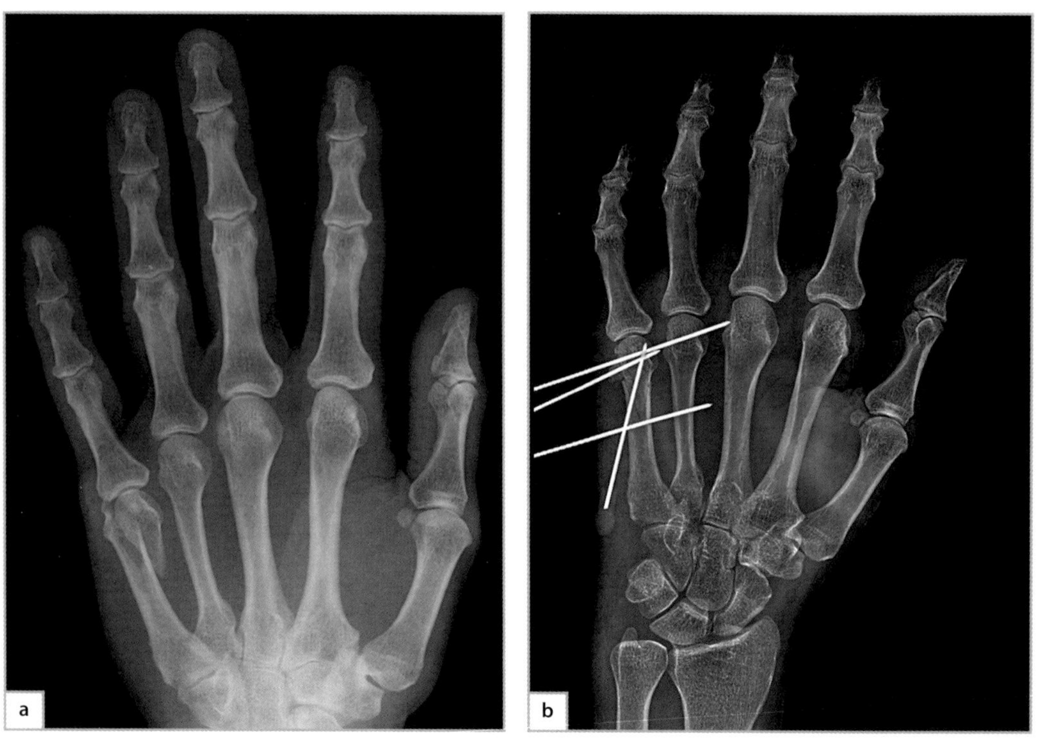

Figure 13.20 (a) Comminuted intra-articular metacarpal head fracture of the little metacarpal. (b) Treatment with open reduction and internal fixation using K-wires.

  - In this maneuver, the proximal fragment is compressed in a palmar direction while the metacarpal head is pushed dorsally (**Figure 13.21a**)
- After reduction, examine finger alignment to confirm that any rotational deformity has been corrected. The hand should then be immobilized with a splint or cast for 3–4 weeks, with the MCP joint in 70–90° of flexion and the wrist in 20–30° of extension. The PIP and DIP joints can be left unrestricted so that finger alignment can be assessed when needed (**Figure 13.21b**)

Surgical treatment

- For fractures with unacceptable angulation deformities, or those unstable in a splint, closed reduction and percutaneously crossed K-wires is the recommended (**Figure 13.22a** and **b**) surgical treatment

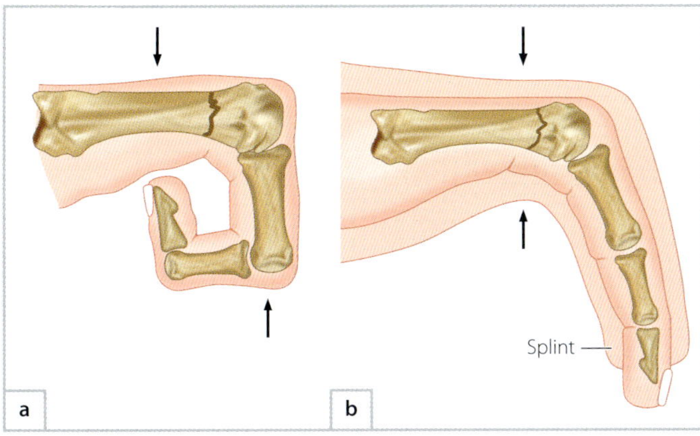

Figure 13.21 (a) Reduction using the Jahss maneuver. With the metacarpophalangeal (MCP) and proximal interphalangeal (PIP) joints in full flexion, simultaneously apply downward pressure on the dorsal side of the fracture and upward pressure along the proximal phalanx to the MCP joint. (b) The finger is splinted with the MCP joint in 70°–90° of flexion, and the PIP and distal interphalangeal joints free to check finger alignment.

- For unstable fractures, compression screws (**Figure 13.23a** and **b**) or a locked T plate will provide stable fixation and allow early motion

Metacarpal shaft fractures

These are common fractures that can be categorized into transverse, oblique, spiral, and comminuted fracture patterns. Most of these fractures can be treated with closed reduction and plaster immobilization, and the hand should maintain the interossei muscles in a relaxed position. Displaced metacarpal shaft fractures result in apex dorsal angulation due to the deforming forces of the interossei muscles. Oblique fractures tend to rotate and cause shortening deformities.

- Transverse fractures can be treated with conservative methods if stable (splinting), or if unstable by K-wires or plates (see previous section on phalangeal fractures for more on K-wires, plates, screws, interosseous wiring, and external fixation)
- Oblique fractures can be treated with screws, K-wires, or plating
- Spiral fractures are very unstable and therefore require internal fixation
- Comminuted fractures may be treated with K-wires, plate, or external fixation, depending upon the degree of comminution and soft tissue involvement

Open reduction internal fixation

- For many displaced metacarpal fractures, especially oblique (**Figure 13.24a**), spiral, and comminuted fractures, ORIF is required. Internal fixation includes K-wires, interosseous wires, lag screws, or a plate and screws. The choice of technique usually depends on the degree of deformity and expertise available
  - For long oblique fractures, we prefer compression screws (**Figure 13.24a** and **b**)
  - For displaced short oblique fracture (**Figure 13.25a** and **b**) or unstable transverse fracture (**Figure 13.26a and b**), plating is recommended
- Percutaneous crossed K-wire fixation provides good resistance to torsion in cases of transverse metacarpal fractures, and perpendicular or transverse pins can be used for border index and little metacarpal shaft fractures
- When performing internal fixation, one should avoid damaging the extensor tendons
- Postoperatively, early motion after any of the fixation techniques is important to prevent tendon adhesion and stiffness. However,

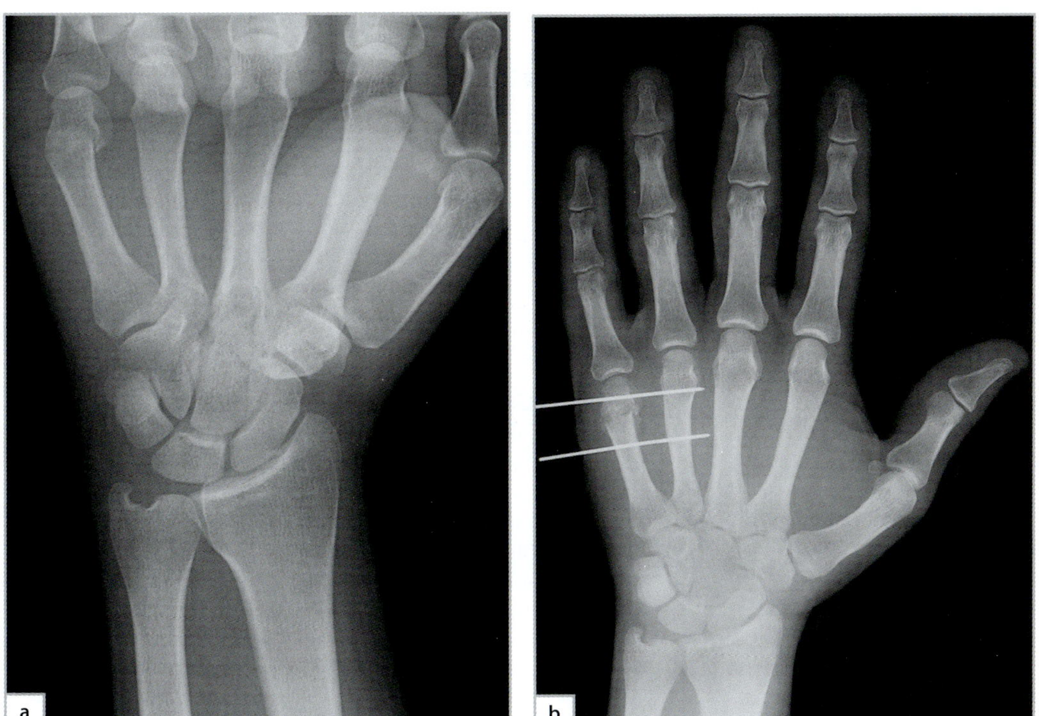

Figure 13.22 (a) Unstable metacarpal head fracture of the little metacarpal causing an angulation deformity. (b) After failed conservative treatment (closed reduction and splinting), percutaneous crossed K-wires are used to reduce the fracture.

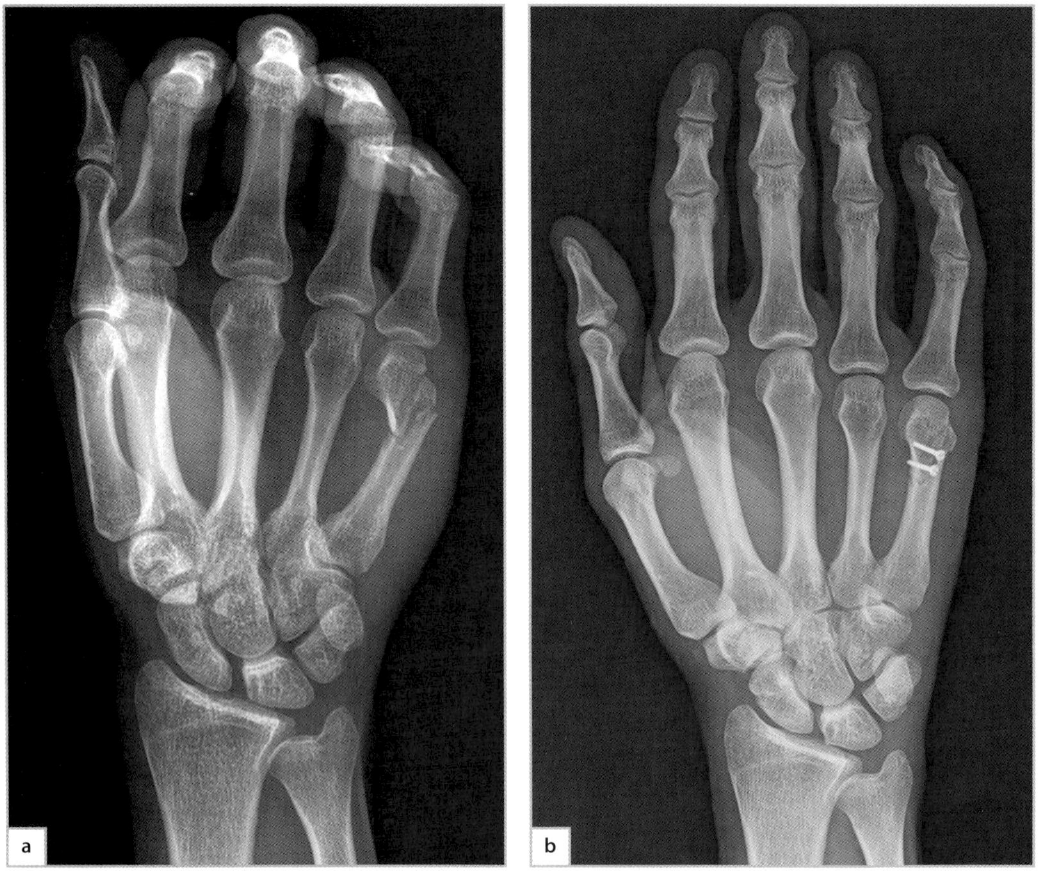

Figure 13.23 (a) Unstable metacarpal neck fracture of the little metacarpal. (b) Fracture treated with compression screws.

immobilization should not be continues longer than 3 weeks due to the potential for stiffness.

Metacarpal base fractures

The metacarpal base fracture is commonly seen in the thumb and small finger, but it is rare in the index and middle metacarpal base due to a lack of motion in the joint. Thumb metacarpal base fractures occur when the thumb metacarpal is axially loaded and partially flexed. Because of the presence of surrounding ligaments, these are the most stable of all hand fractures. Metacarpal base fractures can severely compromise hand function because they cause a loss of CMC joint integrity.

- Little metacarpal base fractures are usually the result of a hammering motion onto a stationary object. Pain and swelling can be found at the base of the metacarpal and along the dorsoulnar aspect of the hand
- Insertion of the flexor and extensor carpi muscles can lead to deformity. When marked displacement, comminution, or complete avulsion of a tendinous insertion is present, closed reduction with percutaneous pinning (**Figure 13.27a** and **b**) or open reduction is recommended
- The fractures can be subdivided into intra-articular and extra-articular fractures.
  - Intra-articular fractures can be subdivided into Bennett and Rolando fractures
  - The fracture pattern of extra-articular fractures is apex dorsal, with the distal fragment in an adducted, flexed, and supinated position. Nonsurgical management is indicated for stable extra-articular fractures, whereas surgical reduction and fixation is required for unstable extra-articular fractures

Fractures of the thumb metacarpal

Fractures of the thumb can be classified as

1. Involving the joint
   a. Bennett fracture
   b. Rolando fracture
2. Extra-articular fractures

Bennett fractures

- The Bennett fracture is characterized as a two-part fracture dislocation at the base of the thumb metacarpal bone. The proximal part remains attached to the trapezium bone while the distal part is dislocated (**Figure 13.28a**)
- The oblique ligament is inset onto the base of the metacarpal bone in the volar side, and the APL is inserted into the dorsal base of the metacarpal bone. When a fracture occurs at the base of the metacarpal bone of thumb, the thumb will be subluxed dorsally, radially, and proximally due to the pull of the APL. The fragment of the fracture is a single, variable-sized volar ulnar fracture
- Proper reduction of the fracture requires axial traction, palmar abduction, and pronation of the metacarpal base. It is difficult to maintain the reduction position with a cast alone, but closed reduction can be accomplished by percutaneous K-wires. The K-wires pin through the base of metacarpal, across the joint, and into the trapezium to hold the bone in place (**Figure 13.28b**). The K-wires should remain in place for 4 weeks, after which time the K-wires can be removed and a rehabilitation program initiated
- If the fracture is irreducible, ORIF is preferred. The large fragment of the fracture can be secured by a 1.5- or 2-mm lag screw. For small fragments, 0.9-mm (0.035 inch) K-wires can be pinned across the

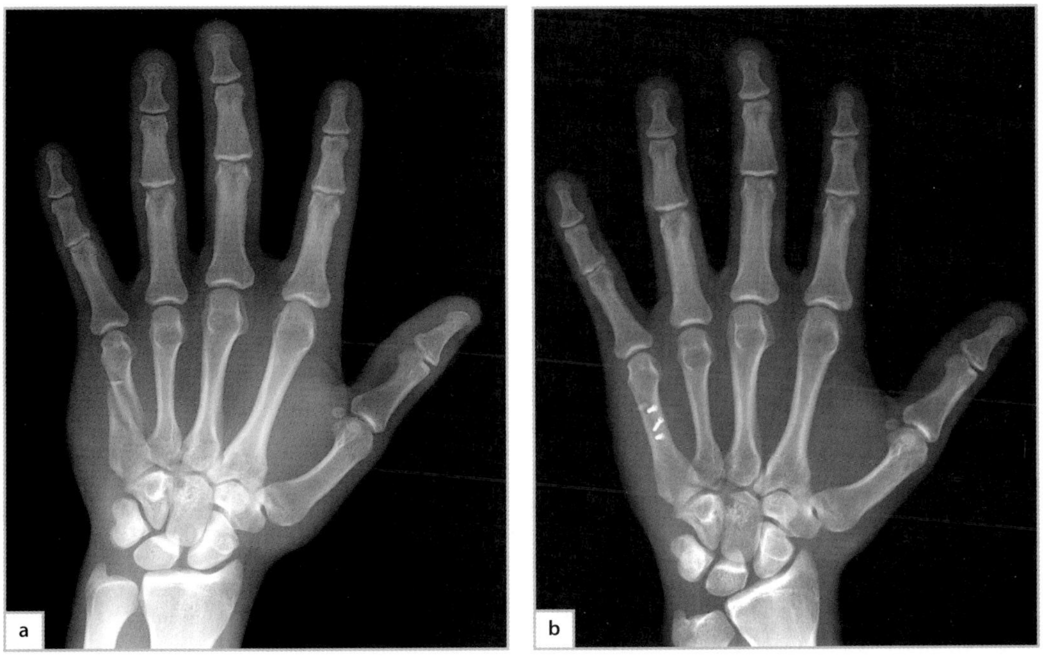

Figure 13.24 (a) Long oblique fracture of the little metacarpal. (b) Compression screws used to fix long oblique fracture.

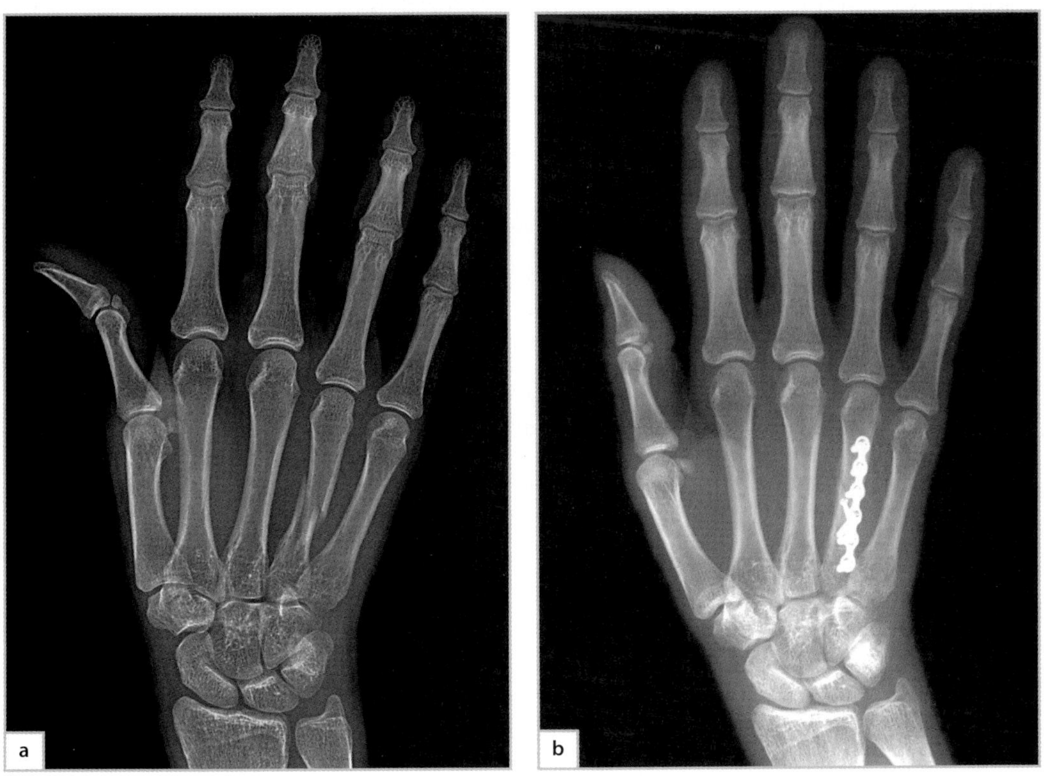

Figure 13.25 (a) Displaced short oblique fracture of the ring metacarpal. (b) Plate used to fix short oblique fracture.

fracture. After screw fixation, ROM exercises can be initiated 5 to 10 days postoperatively

Rolando fractures

Rolando fractures include any type of comminuted intra-articular metacarpal base fracture of the thumb (also known as a comminuted Bennett fracture). The proximal part can be fractured in either a T or Y pattern. This fracture is relatively difficult to treat and typically has worse outcomes than that of the Bennett fracture.

- For fractures with two large fragments, ORIF can be achieved by K-wire fixation, tension banding, or screw fixation
- For markedly comminuted fractures, it is difficult to reduce the fractures by closed percutaneous pinning. L-shaped or T-shaped plates, or external fixation can be applied for fracture fixation

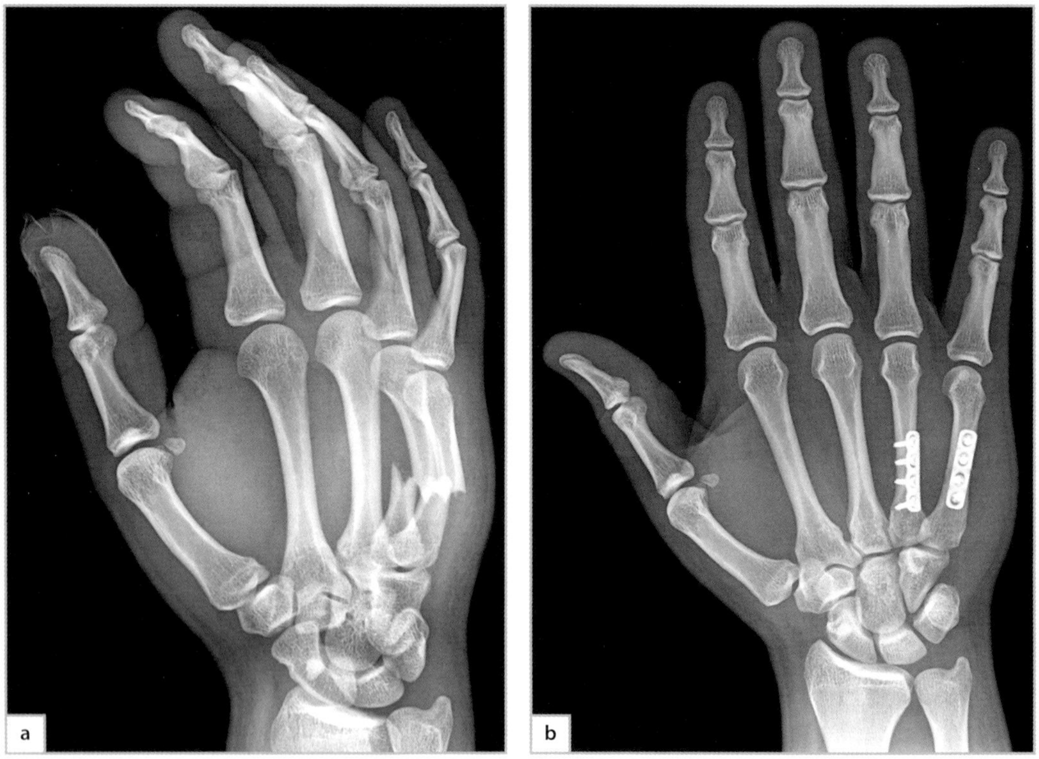

Figure 13.26 (a) Unstable transverse fractures of the ring and little metacarpals. (b) Plating used to restore alignment of the ring and little metacarpals.

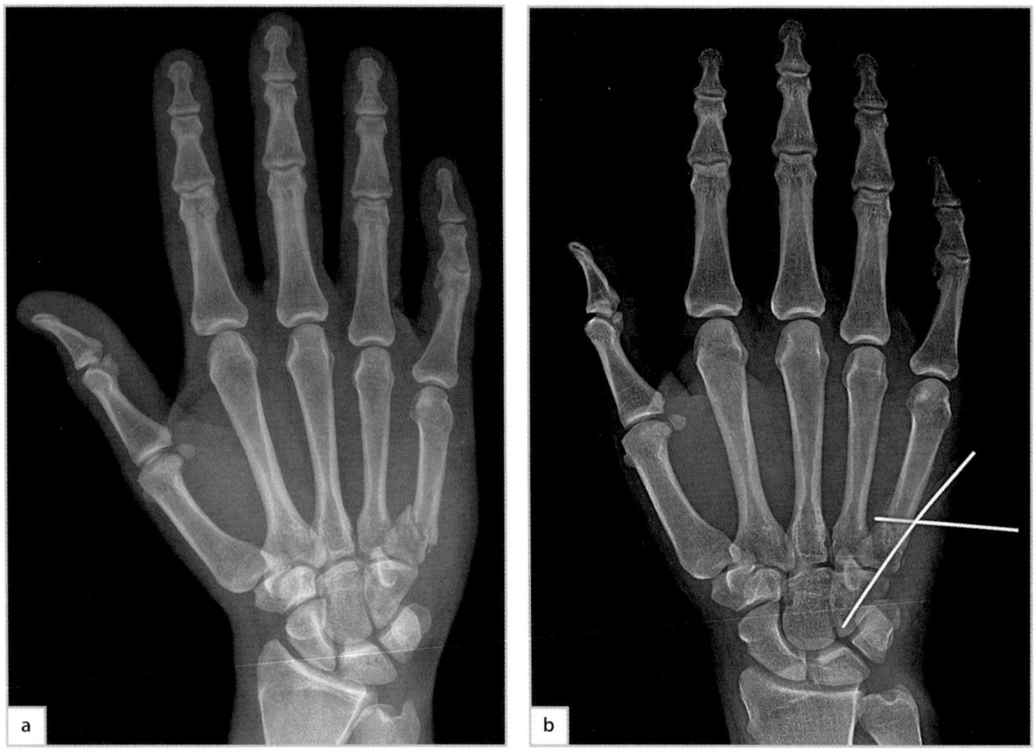

Figure 13.27 (a) Displaced metacarpal base fracture of the little metacarpal. (b) Displaced metacarpal base fracture repaired with closed reduction and percutaneous K-wires.

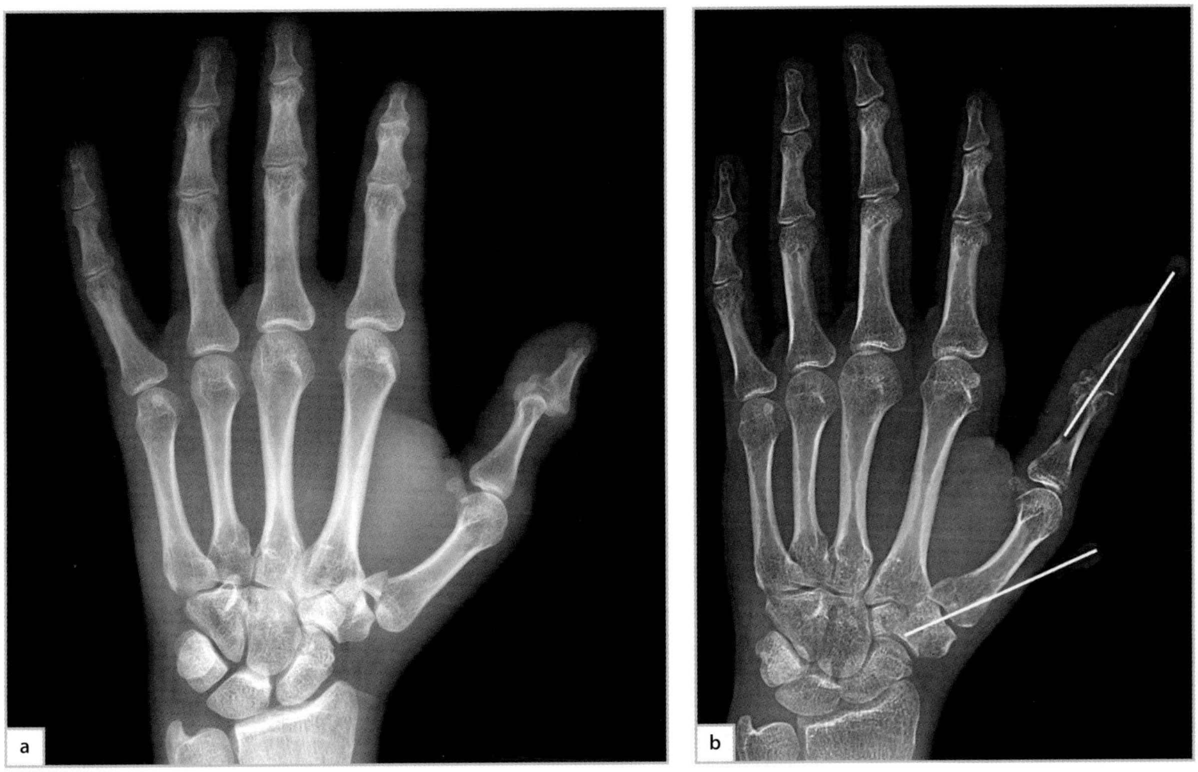

Figure 13.28
(a) Polytrauma patient with Bennett and thumb interphalangeal (IP) joint fracture. Note that a small proximal fragment remains attached to the trapezium while the remaining portion of the thumb is dislocated. (b) Percutaneous K-wires are pinned through the metacarpal base and into the trapezium to hold the fracture in place. The IP joint of the thumb was also treated with K-wire fixation.

SUGGESTED READING

Jones NF, Jupiter JB, Lalonde DH. Common fractures and dislocation of the hand. Plast Reconstr Surg 2012; 130:722e–736e.
The paper reviewed the literatures and described the main points in treating with metacarpal fractures. They described the indications for conservative treatment, closed reduction, and open treatment for metacarpal fractures. Any apex dorsal angulations of middle and small finger > 20°–30°, and index finger and middle finger > 10°–15° need to be fixed with surgical treatment. Because the CMC joints can compensate for the angulation, which is 10°–15° at the index and middle fingers, 20°–30° at the ring and small fingers. In patients managed with conservative treatment, immobilization should not be continued > 3 weeks due to the potential stiffness may occur.

Kelsch G, Ulrich C. Intramedullary K-wire fixation of metacarpal fractures. Arch Orthop Trauma Sur 2004; 124:523–526. Epub 24 July 2004.
This article reported the indications for surgical treatment of metacarpal fractures, which include palmar dislocation > 30° and shortening of >5 mm. The authors described the intramedullary K-wires fixation in 34 patients. The operation was performed within 24 hours after admission, and the operating time was averaged 30 minutes. Most cases started the range of motion 2 weeks postoperatively.

Sletten IN, Nordsletten L, Hjorthaug GA, et al. Assessment of volar angulation and shortening in 5th metacarpal neck fractures: an inter- and intra-observer validity and reliability study. J Hand Surg Eur Vol 2013; 38:658–666.
This paper described how to measure the angulation and shortening when the fracture occurred at the small metacarpal bone, and the relationship between the angulation and shortening. One millimeter of increased shortening corresponded to 2.4° of increased volar angulation. They concluded that the medullary canal-lateral method is the most reliable and accurate for measurement of the volar angulation. Regarding to the measurement of shortening, they recommended the Shortening Stipulated (SH-Stip) method. A line was drawn through the distal end of the ring and small metacarpal heads on the PA view, the shortening of the fracture was defined as the distance from the line to the distal point of the small finger metacarpal head.

Stahl S, Schwartz O. Complications of K-wire fixation of fractures and dislocations in the hand and wrist. Arch Orthop Trauma Surg 2001; 121:527–530.
The authors reported the complications occurrence after K-wire fixation for hand wrist in 238 patients and analyzed the reasons, as well as the recommended treatment. Overall, there were 15% patients experienced complications. In these patients who were involved the complications. The most common complication is pin loosing (42% of 15%) due to poor pin placement not recognized initially. The second common complication is pin tract infection (36% of 15%), which can be treated by oral antibiotics and early removal of the loose pins.

Winter M, Balaguer T, Bessiere C. Surgical treatment of the boxer's fracture: transverse pinning versus intramedullary pinning. J Hand Surg Eur Vol 2007; 32:709–713.
The authors described the treatments for boxer fractures. They compared the transverse pinning with intramedullary pinning in 36 patients, with a period of 12-month follow-up. Both treatments achieved good results, and patients treated with intramedullary pinning experienced better outcomes regarding to the active range of motion at the MCP joint at final follow-up period. They mentioned the disadvantages of the transverse K-wire that included the potentially damage of the MCP joints, and the involvement of the ring metacarpal may reduce the mobility of the hand. Also, complications of the intramedullary pinning included the articular surface damage and the potential injury of the dorsal branch of the ulnar nerve.

13.4 LIGAMENTOUS INSTABILITY AND CARPAL FRACTURES

ANATOMY

The distal radius and ulna, the proximal carpal row (scaphoid, lunate, triquetrum, and pisiform), distal carpal row (trapezium, trapezoid, capitate, and hamate), and the bases of the five metacarpals make up the osseous components of the wrist (**Figure 13.29**). These structures together form the radiocarpal joint, midcarpal joint, and CMC joint. When viewed on X-rays, the concentric outlines are known as Gilula lines, as described in Chapter 3 (**Figure 13.30**). In the horizontal plane, the bones of the carpus are situated in an arciform manner with a palmar concavity. This arch is closed palmarly by the transverse carpal ligament (flexor retinaculum) constituting the carpal tunnel, the narrowest portion of which is located at the level of the distal carpal row.

EXTRINSIC AND INTRINSIC LIGAMENTS

The ligaments of the wrist are divided into extrinsic (those that connect the distal radius–ulna to the carpus) and intrinsic (those that connect carpus to carpus) (**Figure 13.31**).

- Extrinsic ligaments: The extrinsic ligaments [radioscaphocapitate (RSC), ulnocarpal, long and short radiolunate, and dorsal ligaments] are stiffer but possess a lower yield strength, making them more susceptible to failure from a midsubstance rupture. The long and short radiolunate ligaments originate from the anterior edge of the radius and insert into the palmar aspect of the lunate, becoming an important stabilizing structure that prevents this bone from dislocating dorsally in hyperextension injuries. The RSC ligament courses around the palmar concavity of the scaphoid, forming a fulcrum over which the scaphoid rotates. The ulnocarpal ligaments complete the ulnar limb of this V-shaped arrangement. The broad dorsal radiotriquetral ligament spans the radiocarpal joint and plays a significant role in the stabilization of the proximal carpal row
- Intrinsic ligaments: The intrinsic ligaments (scapholunate, SL, and lunotriquetral, LT) have large cartilage areas of insertion and less elastic fibers and are consequently more likely to fail due to an avulsion

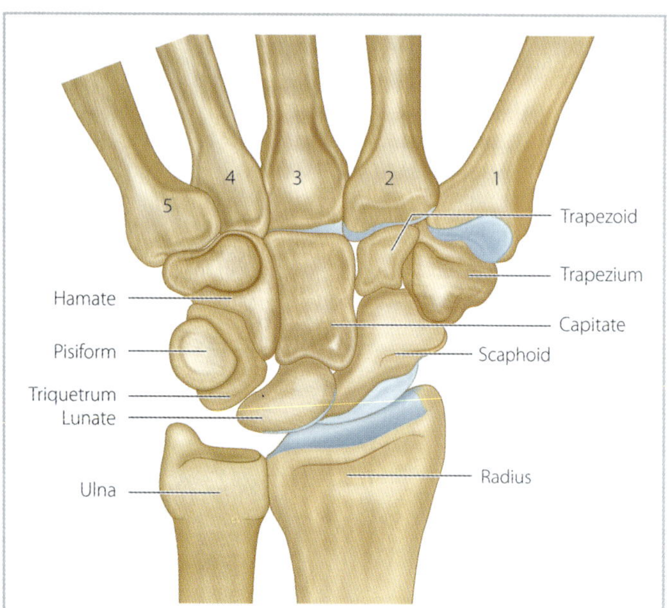

Figure 13.29 The osseous components of the wrist joint.

BIOMECHANICS

To facilitate positioning of the hand to manipulate objects and lift loads, the wrist needs to be highly mobile and yet able to sustain substantial forces and torques without yielding.

Wrist kinematics (carpal motion)

- Distal carpal row: In a normal wrist, the distal carpal row is rigid and works as one functional unit. During flexion of the wrist, the distal row rotates into flexion and ulnar deviation. During wrist extension, the distal carpal bones rotate into extension and a slight radial deviation. This 'dart throwing motion' mostly occurs at the midcarpal joint
- Proximal carpal row: It is more mobile, although there is synergistic movement as a row and in between carpal bones. During radioulnar deviation of the wrist, the three proximal carpal bones move synergistically from a flexed position in radial deviation to an extended position in ulnar deviation. During flexion in the sagittal plane, the scaphoid flexes to a greater extent than the lunate when the wrist flexes

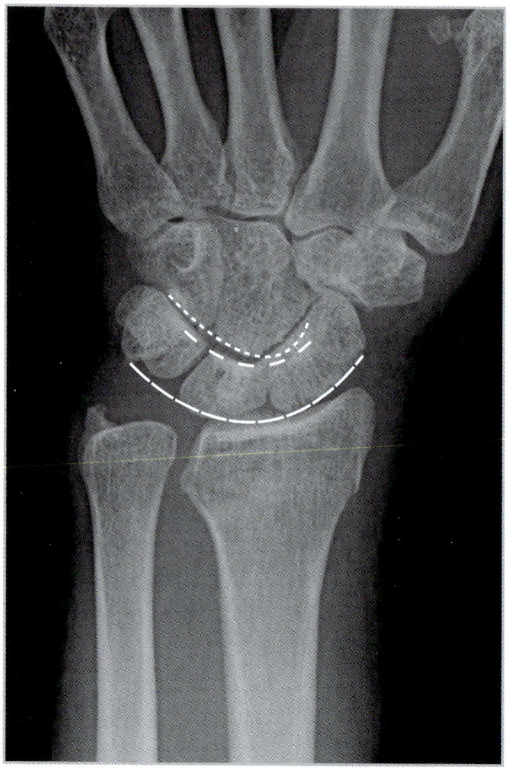

Figure 13.30 The three arcs described by Gilula.

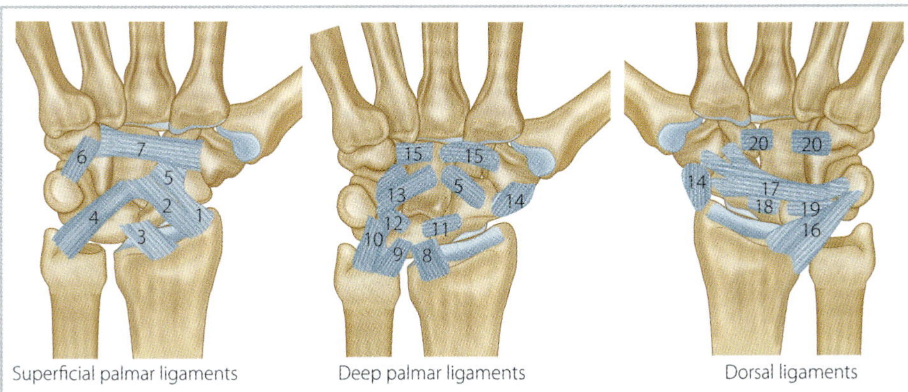

Figure 13.31 Extrinsic and intrinsic ligaments of the carpus.
(a) Superficial palmar ligaments
1. Radioscaphocapitate
2. Long radiolunate
3. Ulnocarpal
4. Pisohamate
5. Flexor retinaculum
(b) Deep palmar ligaments
6. Scaphocapitate
7. Short radiolunate
8. Ulnolunate
9. Ulnotriquetral
10. Palmar scapholunate
11. Palmar lunotriquetral
12. Triquetral-hamate-capitate (Ulnar limg of arcuate)
13. Dorsolateral scaphotrapezial
14. Palmar transverse interosseous
(c) Dorsal ligaments
15. Radiotriquetral
16. Dorsal intercarpal
17. Dorsal scapholunate
18. Dorsal lunotriquetral
19. Dorsal transverse interosseous

Wrist kinetics (force transmission)

During prehensile motion of the hand, the wrist needs to be stable to sustain the compressive forces derived from the contraction of muscles that activate the fingers. The magnitude of these forces can range anywhere from 400–500 kgf (880–1100 lbf). Approximately 50% of the force is transmitted through radioscaphoid joint, 30% through the radiolunate joint, and 20% through the ulnocarpal joint. Stabilization of the wrist under loading depends on bone geometry, proprioception of the joint, integrity of key ligaments under load, and coordinated contraction of the muscles across the joint.

- Radiocarpal joint stabilization: The extrinsic radiocarpal ligaments are vital to resist the carpus from sliding volarly and ulnarly, as the proximal carpal row sits on the scaphoid and lunate fossa of the distal radius and the triangular fibrocartilage complex (TFCC), which is angulated volarly and ulnarly
- Proximal carpal row stabilization: When axially loaded, the scaphoid is allowed larger rotation into flexion and pronation than the lunate, and the triquetrum is tightly constrained. The intrinsic SL and LT ligaments provide the restrains for the proximal carpal row to move in a synchronous motion
- Midcarpal joint stabilization: Under axial load, the distal carpal row exerts an axial compressive force onto the proximal row bones. The flexion and pronation moment produced by the scaphoid is transmitted to the lunate and the triquetrum. If not for the presence of midcarpal stabilizers, namely, the palmar triquetral-hamate-capitate ligament (the so-called ulnar leg of the arcuate ligament), the scaphocapitate (SC) ligaments (radial leg of arcuate ligament), and the dorsal intercarpal ligament, the unconstrained proximal row would rotate into flexion and pronation [volar intercalated segment instability (VISI) deformity]

Mechanism of carpal ligament injuries

Two mechanisms of injury may result in a carpal ligament injury, a direct force or an indirect force.

1. Direct force: A direct force from the injury-causing object to the dislocating bone will result in axial dissociation of the carpus. In all these cases, the dislocating force is applied over a wide surface area of the wrist creating a global dislocation.
2. Indirect force: The deforming load is initially applied at a distance from the injured joint. The tensile forces are usually transmitted by ligaments and compressive forces are transferred by the adjacent articular surfaces. This is well described in Mayfield's progressive perilunate instability, which describes a radial to ulnar progression of perilunate injuries.

Clinical examination and imaging

Direct palpation of the underlying wrist structures in search of tenderness serves as a vital technique for diagnosing wrist pathology. The surface anatomy and landmarks of the wrist need to be familiarized for this to be fruitful. Other useful diagnostic criteria include persistent swelling, decreased motion, joint instability during ballottement, and decreased grip strength. The initial routine radiographic examination in a patient with a suspected carpal injury should include at least four views of the wrist: PA, lateral, scaphoid (PA in ulnar deviation), 45° semipronated oblique, and 45° semisupinated oblique (**Figure 13.32**).

- PA view: Three fairly smooth radiographic arcs (Gilula lines) can be drawn to define normal carpal relationships. A step off in the continuity of any of these arcs indicates displaced intercarpal derangement at the site where the arc is broken
- True lateral of the wrist: The palmar surface of the pisiform should lie between the palmar surfaces of the distal scaphoid tuberosity and the capitate head
- PA in ulnar deviation: Should be centered over the scaphoid, allowing appreciation of the long axis of the scaphoid
- Semipronated oblique views: Enables evaluation of the dorsoulnar and radiopalmar aspects of the wrist.

Dynamic fluoroscopy of the carpal movements will help in the appreciation of the kinematics of carpal instability. This is especially so for instabilities that are dynamic and not static. MRI has shown a sensitivity and specificity of 63 and 86% in the evaluation of liga-

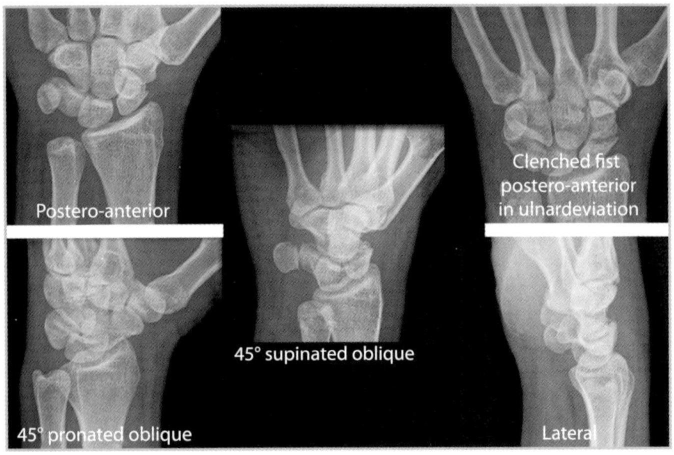

Figure 13.32 Standard wrist views.

ment injuries of the wrist compared with the gold standard of wrist arthroscopy.

CARPAL INSTABILITY

A wrist joint should be considered unstable when it is not capable of preserving a normal kinematic and kinetic relationship between the radius, carpal bones, and metacarpals. Hence, stability implies both the ability to transfer functional loads without yielding or losing its internal joint congruency and the capacity to maintain motion throughout its range without sudden alterations of intercarpal alignment.

Classification

An analytical approach developed by Larsen helps in the understanding and management of these conditions. This is based on six features: chronicity, severity, etiology, location, direction, and pattern.

1. Chronicity
   a. Injuries < 1 week old (acute) have the best healing potential
   b. At 1–6 weeks (subacute), the deformity can still be reduced, but the healing potential of the ligament is decreased
   c. After 6 weeks (chronic), it is unlikely that the ligament can heal in its original state, with the exception of avulsion injuries, whereby the ligament can be reattached
2. Severity
   a. Predynamic instabilities (partial ligament tears with no malalignment under stress)
   b. Dynamic instabilities (complete ruptures exhibiting carpal malalignment only under certain loading conditions)
   c. Static instabilities (complete ruptures with permanent alteration of the carpal alignment)
3. Etiology
   a. Besides trauma, inflammatory conditions such as rheumatoid arthritis can cause carpal instability, whereby the prognosis will be less optimistic
4. Location
   a. The identification of the pain generator and the affected joint is vital to the management of this problem. This can be achieved with a detailed clinical examination and radiography
5. Direction
   a. Dorsal intercalated segment instability (DISI), when the lunate is abnormally extended relative to its proximal and distal links
   b. VISI, when the lunate is abnormally flexed
   c. Ulnar translocation, when the proximal row is displaced ulnarly beyond normal limits
   d. Radial translocation, when the proximal row is displaced radially beyond normal
   e. Dorsal translocation, when the carpal condyle, often as a result of a dorsally malunited fracture of the radius, is subluxed or dislocated in a dorsal direction
6. Pattern
   a. Carpal instability dissociative (CID), when there is a major derangement within or between bones of the same carpal row, e.g. SL dissociation (SLD)
   b. Carpal instability nondissociative (CIND), when there is dysfunction between the carpus rows, e.g. midcarpal instability
   c. Carpal instability complex (CIC), when there are features of both CID and CIND types, e.g. perilunate dislocations
   d. Carpal instability adaptive, where the reason for the malalignment is not located within the wrist but proximal or distal to it, e.g. malunited distal radius fractures causing adaptive carpal instability

Scapholunate dissociation

Scapholunate dissociation is the most common form of carpal instability, typically resulting from a fall on an outstretched hand or with a concomitant distal radius fracture. Clinical symptoms include weakness in grip and dorsal SL pain. Arthroscopy is considered the standard for direct visualization of the intracarpal ligaments, with increasing degrees of SL incongruency, as described by Geissler. X-ray evidence of SLD (**Figure 13.33**) includes the following:

- Increased SL gap (Terry Thomas sign)
- Scaphoid ring sign (scaphoid flexion) – a sign of rotatory subluxation of scaphoid
- Increased SL angle

The SLD presents with a wide clinical spectrum, and the progressive clinical stages have been recognized as follows:

1. Predynamic – Dorsal synovitis, no rotatory subluxation scaphoid, static X-rays and stress films normal, Geissler 1 or 2 on arthroscopy
2. Dynamic – Wrist gives way under stress, no rotatory subluxation of scaphoid, static X-rays normal, stress films reveal SL gap, Geissler 2, 3, or 4 on arthroscopy, no arthritis
3. Static – Failure of secondary stabilizers giving rise to rotatory subluxation of scaphoid, SL gap on normal X-ray, deformity reducible, no arthritis, high Geissler grade
4. Static fixed – SL gap not reducible due to capsular fibrosis
5. SLAC – Radial styloid-scaphoid impingement (stage 1) to complete radioscaphoid (RS) osteoarthritis (stage 2) or even midcarpal arthritis (stage 3).

Permanent carpal malalignment occurs when there is a concomitant failure of the secondary scaphoid stabilizers, (scaphotrapeziotrapezoid and SC ligaments) together with complete rupture of the SL ligament, of which the dorsal component is the most important. The loaded lunate and triquetrum rotate into an abnormal extension (DISI), supination, and radial deviation, whereas the scaphoid rotates around the RSC ligament into an abnormal flexion, ulnar deviation, and pronation posture. As SLD progresses, the proximal pole of the scaphoid subluxes

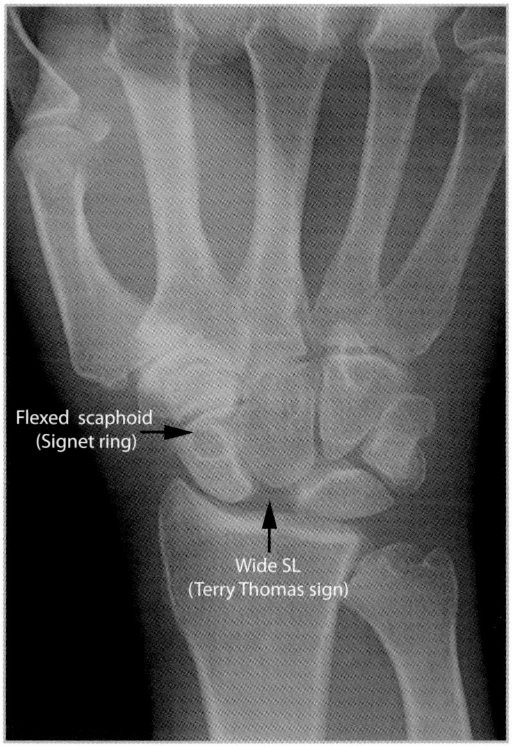

Figure 13.33 Radiographic features of scapholunate dissociation.

dorsoradially, and an increased compressive and shear stress appears on the dorsal and lateral aspect of the RS fossa, increasing peripheral contact and the development of long-term degenerative changes at the dorsolateral edge of the RS joint.

Treatment

Treatment for SLD is often difficult and unpredictable. The late presentation of many patients and the inability to observe the early signs of SLD on plain X-rays add to the difficult nature of this injury. Principles of treatment include:

1. In acute SL injuries, the SLD has good healing potential and can be repaired with K-wire fixation and splinting of the joint for 6 weeks to facilitate healing
2. Avulsions at the insertion of SLD can be reanchored with good results as the quality of the ligament is preserved
3. In subacute injuries (after 6 weeks) with midsubstance tears of the SL ligament, repair is not possible as the ligament degenerates. When the SL joint is reducible, reconstruction or augmentation of the SL ligament is often performed and the ligament protected for 6 weeks after surgery.
4. In chronic injuries where the SLD is not reducible (static), or with SLAC, a salvage operation such as a partial fusion can be carried out

Lunotriquetral dissociation

Lunotriquetral dissociation can present as part of perilunate instability (stage 3), as an isolated injury from a fall resulting in injury on the ulnar side of the wrist, or as a long-term consequence of ulnar abutment syndrome in an ulnar-plus wrist, resulting in wear of the LT ligament. The strongest part of the LT ligament has been determined to be the palmar aspect. When only the palmar and dorsal LT ligaments are sectioned, increased mobility of the LT joint is detected (dynamic instability), but not a complete destabilization of the carpus, with no significant change to the force transmission across the wrist. This explains why there is little observed degenerative arthritis in static LT dissociation. When both the LTq and dorsal radiotriquetral ligaments were experimentally sectioned in axially loaded cadaver wrists, the flexion moment of the scaphoid became unconstrained, inducing a conjoint rotation in flexion of the scaphoid and lunate, with subsequent anterior subluxation of the capitate. This results in a static VISI pattern of instability.

Clinical presentation ranges from:

1. Asymptomatic partial tears with occasional pain under stress
2. Painful complete dissociation with static collapse, causing a fork-like deformity and prominence of the distal ulna
3. Some patients describe painful crepitus as they ulnarly deviate the hand
4. Point tenderness directly over the dorsal aspect of the LT joint. Pain is usually aggravated with ulnar deviation and supination (turning a screwdriver under torque)
5. Wrist motion is seldom diminished except in the more advanced cases with static carpal collapse. A frequent complaint is weakness or a sensation of instability or giving way

   Radiological features include:

- Static VISI pattern of malalignment: The lunate has a triangular (moonlike) appearance, and there is abnormal flexion of the SL complex, which does not extend with ulnar deviation of the wrist (fixed)
- The disruption of the normal convex arc of the proximal carpal row. This is visualized as a step off between the lunate and the triquetrum on a PA radiograph

Arthroscopy remains the standard for diagnosis of an LT dissociation. Principles of treatment include:

- Anatomical repair of the volar LT ligament in acute injuries when possible, supplemented by K-wire transfixation for 6 weeks
- Limited LT fusions in painful instability cases
- Radiolunate fusions for static painful VISI deformity – deformity cannot be corrected
- Ulnar shortening for ulnar abutment syndrome

Perilunate injuries

Perilunate injuries are classified as a CIC – a combination of carpal instabilities between bones in the same row and between bones from different rows. These injuries are a result of high impact trauma to an outstretched wrist and occur due to a zone of weakness around the lunate. This area is commonly recognized as the cornerstone of the wrist, for its strong attachments to the distal radius by the volar radiolunate ligaments.

Five distinct patterns are recognized:

1. Dorsal perilunate dislocations (lesser arc – ligamentous injuries with no fractures)
2. Dorsal perilunate fracture-dislocations (greater arc – with carpal bones fractures)
3. Palmar perilunate dislocations (lesser or greater arc) – rare
4. Axial dislocations
5. Isolated carpal bone dislocations

The pathomechanics of perilunate injuries have been described by Mayfield into four stages (**Figure 13.34**)

- Stage 1 – SL ligament disruption or scaphoid fracture
- Stage 2 – capitolunate dislocation or capitate fracture
- Stage 3 – lunocapitate ligament disruption or triquetral fractures
- Stage 4 – lunate dislocation

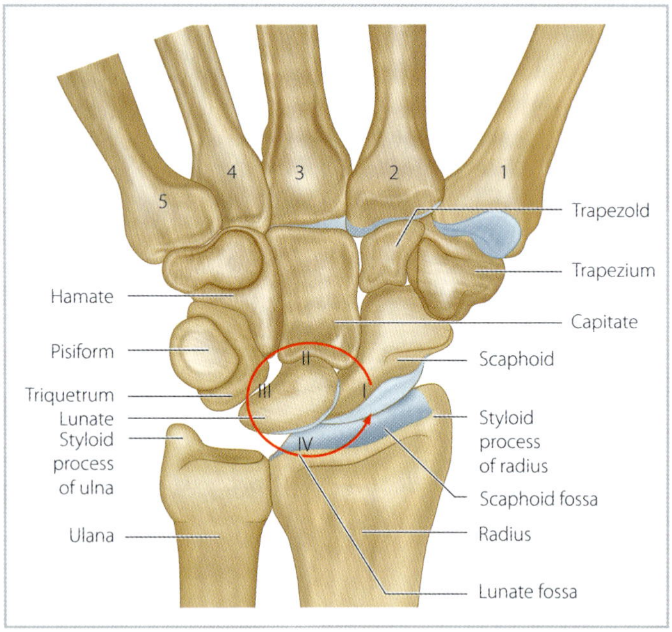

Figure 13.34 Stages of perilunate injury as described by Mayfield. Stage 1 – scapholunate ligament disruption or scaphoid fracture. Stage 2 – capitolunate dislocation or capitate fracture. Stage 3 – lunocapitate ligament disruption or triquetral fractures. Stage 4 – lunate dislocation.

Management should focus on recognition of this injury with a high degree of suspicion. A lateral wrist X-ray with lunocapitate dislocation is pathognomonic, with the corresponding PA X-ray showing signs of carpus crowding or disruption of Gilula lines. Patients will present with wrist pain with varying degrees of swelling and limited motion, accompanied by acute carpal tunnel syndrome in cases of median nerve compression.

Treatment

Reduction of the dislocation should be performed as an emergency procedure, under regional/general anesthesia, with adequate longitudinal traction for 10 minutes and Tavernier's maneuver.

- Tavernier's Maneuver: The physician's thumb is positioned on the volar side of the patient's lunate to prevent volarlunate dislocation while longitudinal traction is maintained, and the capitate is pulled to overcome the edge of the lunate

Definitive treatment includes accurate reduction of the carpal bone relationships and either percutaneous pinning of the joints for 6 weeks (optimal reduction) or open reduction and acute ligament repair (if reduction is less than perfect). Anatomical reduction and fixation of carpal fractures constitute the treatment for greater arc injuries. Management for neglected cases with missed early diagnosis will depend on whether the dissociated joints can be reduced, whereby joint preservation and ligament reconstruction can be performed. If the deformity is static and irreducible, a salvage surgery based on carpal fusions or proximal row carpectomy is the preferred option.

Axial carpal fracture dislocations

These dislocations are often the result of high-energy dorsopalmar compressions that disrupt the palmar arch in a transverse and longitudinal fashion.

There are two axial patterns

1. Axial ulnar – Where the radial column of the carpus is stable with respect to the radius and the ulnar column dislocates (**Figure 13.35a**)
2. Axial radial – Where the ulnar column carpus is stable and the radial column dislocates (**Figure 13.35b**)

Management includes radical debridement of nonviable muscles, an extended volar approach to explore neurovascular structures, and an extended dorsal approach for open reduction and fixation. The flexor retinaculum is often ruptured in axial carpal fracture dislocations and the function of the hand is frequently compromised.

CARPAL FRACTURES

Carpal bone fractures account for anywhere from 8 to 19% of all hand injuries. Because of this high frequency of occurrence, it is critical that a surgeon have a basic understanding of the principles behind diagnosis and treatment of these injuries. The carpus is a complex set of eight bones supported by stout, intrinsic ligaments that link the forearm to the hand. The proximal row consists of the scaphoid, lunate, pisiform, and triquetrum, and the distal row consists of the

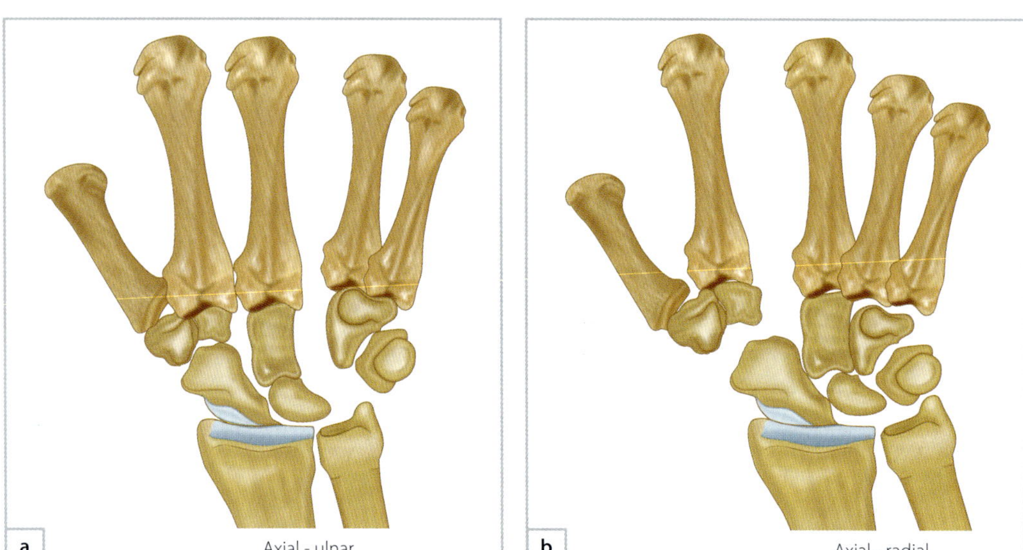

Figure 13.35 Axial carpal dislocation.

trapezium, trapezoid, capitate, and hamate. The intrinsic ligaments are intracapsular and function to link adjacent carpal bones, but a disruption of these ligaments can lead to carpal instability. These complex relations make radiological interpretation difficult and confusing, and therefore, missed injuries are very common, leading to inadequate and delayed treatment.

Physical examination and clinical findings are not adequate for most surgeons to make a definitive diagnosis. The complex three-dimensional relationships of the carpal bones make plain radiographs difficult to use. Adequate knowledge and experience, along with special radiographic views and CT scans are required for accurate diagnosis and effective treatment. Nondisplaced fractures should be treated nonoperatively, whereas displaced fractures require surgical intervention. Treatment should not only be directed to the fracture, as surrounding structures are frequently injured. Appropriate treatment for these injuries is essential, as inadequately treated injuries frequently lead to nonunion, malunion, AVN, osteoarthritis, and tendon ruptures. Accurate assessment of displacement and the severity of symptoms are key factors in determining overall outcomes, and prompt diagnosis and treatment lead to better recovery.

Carpal fractures consist of three main groups:

1. Perilunate – Scaphoid, capitate, lunate, triquetrum
2. Axial pattern injuries – Covered in previous section
3. Carpal avulsion – Dorsal triquetral avulsion, pisiform, hook of hamate

Scaphoid fractures

Scaphoid fractures have the highest incidence of all carpal injuries, accounting for approximately 11% of hand fractures and almost 80% of all carpal bone fractures The scaphoid is a bean-shaped bone serves as a stabilizer of the mid-metacarpal bone and contributes to the mechanical integrity of the wrist. It is the largest bone of the proximal carpal row and forms a stable link between the proximal and distal row. The bone is 80% covered by cartilage, and articulates with the radioscaphoid fossa laterally, the lunate medially, and the capitate, trapezium, and trapezoid distally. It is subjected to continuous shearing and bending forces during recovery, which makes the bone-healing process slow.

The nonarticular scaphoid waist is where 80% of the vascular elements of the scaphoid enter the bone. The blood vessels enter the scaphoid mainly through the distal half of its blood supply, often leading to AVN of the proximal pole of the scaphoid after a proximal pole fracture. The proximal palmar surface of the scaphoid is supplied by branches from the palmar carpal artery. The blood supply of the middle third and distal third originates from the superficial palmar artery, and the distal vessels supply the region of tuberosity.

Mechanism of injury

Scaphoid fractures often result from a fall on an outstretched wrist in full extension and radial deviation (which locks the scaphoid in the scaphoid fossa of the distal radius), with load concentrated on the radial side of the palm. These fractures often result from a compressive force on the volar side and a tension force on the dorsal side of the bone. With fractures that are proximal to the waist of scaphoid, the distal pole tends to flex when loaded by the thumb ray, whereas the proximal pole extends with the lunate, resulting in the commonly seen humpback deformity.

Clinical diagnosis

Patients typically present with radial-sided wrist pain after a fall. Examine for tenderness over the scaphoid tubercle, in the snuffbox and at the proximal pole of the scaphoid. Radiography confirms the diagnosis, and the five-recommended X-ray views include the PA, lateral, two obliques, and PA in ulnar deviation (**Figure 13.33**). When the X-rays are equivocal and the patient has scaphoid tenderness, the patient can be splinted and the X-rays repeated in 2 weeks, to wait for the fracture line to show up. However, this has been associated with a false-negative rate of up to 25% and will delay diagnosis. The current recommendation for equivocal cases with strong clinical suspicion is to perform an MRI of the wrist, with 100% sensitivity and specificity. Healing time is related to the location of the fracture, with healing time increasing for more proximal fractures.

Classification and prognosis

The Herbert's classification takes into account the anatomy of the fracture, stability, and chronicity as a prognostic tool (**Figure 13.36**). Undisplaced fractures have a good prognosis for union with conservative management. On the other hand, displaced fractures, comminuted fractures, and fractures associated with carpal instability (DISI or VISI deformity) are classified as unstable. Fractures neglected for > 4 weeks of duration and proximal pole fractures have a poorer prognosis for union and are best managed with surgical stabilization.

Treatment

- Undisplaced fractures can be managed by casting for 6–12 weeks. The wrist position should be such that the fracture is coapted and the carpus shows normal alignment. There is little evidence to support thumb, forearm, and elbow immobilization. Fracture union is confirmed by CT evidence of trabecular bridging, because clinical assessment can be unreliable.
- Surgical management of scaphoid fractures is based on the principles of stable fixation, with a preference for minimally invasive methods (to preserve ligamentous integrity), and bone grafting for comminuted fractures with carpal instability. The preferred method involves cannulated compression screws inserted under fluoroscopic guidance into the central axis of the scaphoid.

Nonunion of scaphoid fractures

Long-term nonunion of scaphoid fractures will lead to degenerative arthrosis of the wrist and loss of motion. Management is surgical to achieve union in prearthritic cases but will become salvage cases in the presence of arthritis, limited to carpal arthrodesis. Surgical principles include resection of the fibrous nonunion margins to healthy bone, corticocancellous bone grafting to bridge the defect and restore scaphoid and carpal alignment, and stable fixation for bone healing. This treatment is difficult and requires open surgery. Proximal pole fractures have a higher risk of AVN, and because of the blood supply of the scaphoid, management is surgical. MRI evidence of proximal pole necrosis and direct observation of the absence of punctate bleeding of the proximal pole are diagnostic of AVN. Vascularized bone grafts to replace the necrotic proximal pole have achieved union in two thirds of the AVN cases. Scaphoid nonunion advanced collapse is covered in another section.

Preiser disease

In 1910, Preiser described a rarefying osteitis of the scaphoid. Both entire scaphoid and proximal pole necrosis have been described. The possible etiology is related to collagen vascular disease, steroid therapy, and repetitive stress, but this disease is largely idiopathic. Clinically, there is a presence of scaphoid tenderness with sclerosis,

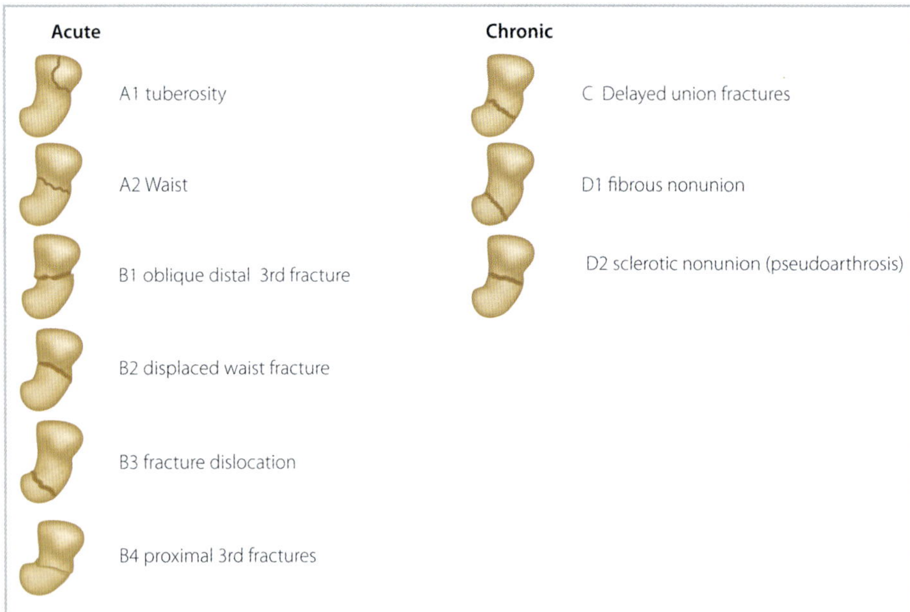

Figure 13.36 Herbert's classification of scaphoid fractures. Type A: stable fractures. Type B: unstable fractures. Type C: delayed union fractures. Type D: established nonunion fractures.

and possible fragmentation of the proximal pole observed on X-rays. In the absence of severe pain and disability, management is conservative. Attempts at revascularization of the scaphoid have not been successful, and a limited carpal fusion with scaphoid excision is the salvage procedure of choice.

Kienböck disease (lunatomalacia) – AVN of the lunate

The lunate occupies a central position in the wrist and is the keystone of the wrist. Laterally, it is moon shaped and larger palmarly than dorsally. The blood supply of the lunate arises both volarly and dorsally with intraosseous anastomosis.

Proposed etiology of Kienböck's disease:

1. Includes factors that increase mechanical pressure on the lunate, resulting in a nutcracker effect between a prominent radius and the head of the capitate on the lunate
   a. Increased intraosseous pressure on repeated loaded extension of the wrist
   b. Significant association between an ulnar minus wrist and Kienböck's disease
   c. Type 1 lunate, which leaves more of the bone uncovered by the radius, theoretically increasing mechanical pressure on the bone. This is usually related to an ulnar minus wrist
   d. Radial inclination is decreased in patients with Kienböck's disease. This may have increased pressure loading on the lunate
2. Associated with patients with collagen vascular disease and chronic use of steroids

Diagnosis

The typical patient with Kienböck's disease is young and presents with an insidious onset of pain and stiffness in the wrist, with swelling and tenderness over the lunate. There is usually no history of trauma. The patient's grip is often weak and associated with a limited range of wrist motion. Radiographs may show an ulnar minus wrist and type 1 lunate. MRI is useful to study the vascularity of the lunate and differentiate this from an ulnocarpal impaction, whereby the ulnar side of the lunate shows edematous change in an ulnar-plus wrist. The lunate shows up hot on a bone scan in its initial stages. Late deformities include sclerosis and loss of lunate height, and eventual fragmentation of the lunate, with a collapse of carpal height and arthrosis, forcing the wrist into a DISI deformity (**Figure 13.37**).

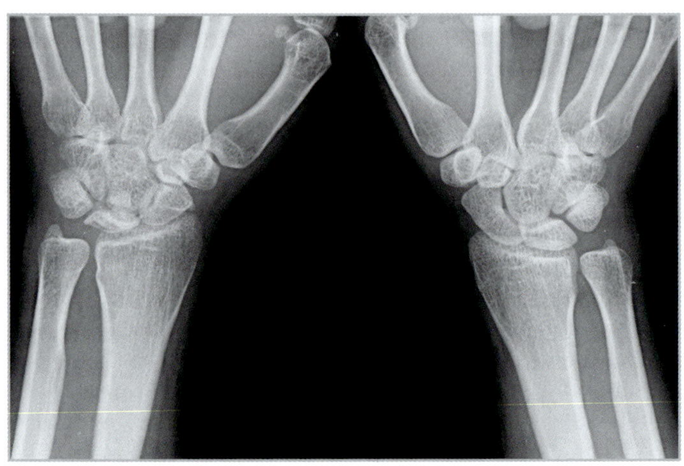

Figure 13.37 Kienböck's disease of left wrist showing collapse of the lunate.

Staging of Kienböck's disease has been described by Lichtman, based on X-ray appearance of the lunate:

- Stage 1 – Linear lunate fracture, but normal bone density and architecture
- Stage 2 – Lunate becomes dense, but without collapse
- Stage 3 – Lunate collapses, no arthritis
- Stage 4 – Perilunate arthritis

Treatment

Many treatments for Kienböck's disease have been described, but results have varied widely.

- Conservative treatment: It has been observed that patients managed conservatively rarely changed their job, whereas 50% of surgically managed patients are unable to continue with their original job. Tajima surveyed 80 Kienböck's disease patients of > 42 years and noticed no difference in the outcome between conservative and surgical management. Kristensen monitored 46 nonsurgical patients over a mean of 20 years and found that although two thirds developed arthritis of the wrist, only one fourth were symptomatic. Most patients had satisfactory hand function despite the radiographic arthritis.
- Surgical treatment: Based on a few principles
  - Intracarpal fusions – A scaphotrapezial trapezoid or capitohamate fusion will help unload pressure off the lunate
  - Joint leveling procedures – Radial shortening to improve the ulnolunate relationship in an ulnar minus wrist has become the mainstay of surgical treatment. This works on the principle of unloading the lunate, and many studies have reported reduced pain, improved grip strength, and improved symptoms with this procedure
  - Metaphyseal decompression of the radius and ulnar – This is based on the theory that increased vascularity and enforced immobilization of the distal radius region after a surgical procedure improve clinical symptoms
  - Vascularized bone grafting – Replace the necrotic lunate while retaining the cartilage shell and outline of the lunate. Early results have been impressive, with good pain relief and improved grip strength, and evidence of successful lunate revascularization. However, long-term outcomes have not been sustainably satisfactory
- Salvage operations: Indicated for advanced Kienböck's disease with arthritis. Radiocarpal fusion and proximal row carpectomy are viable surgical options

Triquetral fractures

Second most common group of carpal fractures often seen with other carpal fractures or as part of perilunate injuries. The mechanism of injury involves trauma due to twisting or rotation, or from direct blow from the ulnar styloid. Tenderness to palpation along with localized edema is present just distal to the ulnar styloid with the hand in radial deviation. In patients with wrist injuries and ulnar-sided pain, triquetral fractures are relatively common and should be considered in the differential diagnosis. Standard PA, lateral, and oblique views of radiographs should be obtained, and a CT scan may be required to confirm the diagnosis. Three types of triquetral fractures:

1. Dorsal cortical fracture – Related to avulsions or impaction, often leads to little morbidity and can be treated conservatively
2. Body fracture – Often related to perilunate injuries. A nonunion of this fracture is rare and treatment is predicated by a combination of bone and ligament injury
3. Volar avulsion fracture – Often overlooked and can be associated with an LT ligament injury. Treatment recommendations not definitive

Treatment

- Treatment involves cast immobilization for 4–6 weeks
- Painful nonunion fragments can be excised if necessary

Capitate fractures

These fractures are uncommon and can be part of SC syndrome in which there is a concomitant fracture of the scaphoid waist and neck of the capitate, a variant of the perilunate injury. The capitate has a retrograde blood flow and the proximal pole of the bone is intra-articular, and as a consequence, waist fractures can result in AVN. Because of the anatomical position of this bone, the capitate is protected by the surrounding carpal bones. As a result, capitate fractures are often nondisplaced because of the stability provided by the surrounding intercarpal ligaments. A high degree of suspicion is necessary when evaluating possible capitate fractures, and a clinical examination that reveals capitate tenderness requires further radiological imaging. A CT scan or MRI can be used to confirm the diagnosis.

Treatment

- Nonunion and AVN is common if left untreated
- Conservative management is indicated for nondisplaced capitate fractures, and immobilization is recommended with a short-arm thumb spica cast for 6–8 weeks
- Displaced fractures are treated with K-wire or headless compression screws
- Nonunion is diagnosed late (around 1.5 years), and treatment involves bone grafting with or without screw fixation

Hamate fractures

The two most common types of hamate fractures recognized are body of hamate fractures and hook of hamate fractures. Clinical presentation is similar in both of these etiologies, with ulnar-sided wrist pain over the hamate, and pain is present with palpation in the hypothenar area. Pain with resisted small and ring finger flexion, and axial loading of the ring or little metacarpal should also be tested. The ulnar nerve and artery can be injured when the hamate is fractured, and symptoms such as delayed capillary refill and paresthesia may accompany these injuries. The standard radiography views should be obtained, including PA, lateral, and oblique views. A high degree of suspicion is required when evaluating possible hamate fractures, and the carpal tunnel view or a CT scan in the praying position will both useful to diagnose hamate fractures.

- Body of hamate fractures
  - Fractures of the body of the hamate are relatively stable and can be treated conservatively
- Hook of hamate fractures
  - These are commonly associated with racquet sports, typically resulting from a contusion by the butt of a golf club/racquet

- Finger flexion accentuates the pain, because the hook of hamate functions as a pulley for the flexor tendons with the wrist in ulnar deviation
- Hook of hamate nonunion is common because of the tenuous blood supply and the displacement of the fracture fragment by the flexor tendons
- Excision of the hook of hamate is recommended for nonunion as the outcome has been found to be satisfactory

Pisiform fractures

The pisiform is a sesamoid bone into which tendons of flexor carpi ulnaris (FCU) insert, and fracture of this carpal bone is uncommon. It is the last bone to ossify (8–12 years), and multiple centers of ossification give it a fragmented appearance, making it difficult to differentiate a normal from a fractured pisiform bone. Patients who have suffered acute pisiform fractures typically present with ulnar-sided wrist pain. A CT scan of the wrist is recommended because adjacent bones make the diagnosis difficult on standard radiographs.

Treatment

- Most acute pisiform fractures are treated by immobilization with a cast for 6 weeks for minimally displaced fractures and by pisiform excision with FCU repair if the fracture is displaced with a concomitant FCU injury
- The pisiform forms one of the boundaries of the Guyon's tunnel through which the ulnar nerve passes, thus an ulnar nerve injury can be associated with this fracture. Nerve exploration is indicated if a sensory deficit persists or sensation deteriorates
- For a patient who has persistent problems resulting from a comminuted or chronic pisiform fracture, early excision is essential to promote recovery with no complications and should provide reliable pain relief and an early return to work

Trapezium fractures

Fractures of the trapezium account for only about 3% of all carpal fractures and are usually associated with a fracture of the thumb metacarpal. These fractures are significant because they are associated with injuries of the trapeziometacarpal joint. Standard PA and lateral views do not provide complete information regarding the status of the trapezium, because the trapezium is obscured by a superimposition of the trapezoid and base of the index metacarpal in the PA view, and it is obscured by a superimposition of the hook of hamate in the lateral view. However, oblique radiographs (Bett view) are able to provide a clear representation of the status of the trapezium and is therefore the best view to diagnose this type of fracture. Oblique views are obtained by lifting the elbow off the table, with the hypothenar eminence on a wedge, the thumb abducted and extended, the hand semipronated, and the X-ray beam at the scaphoid-trapezium-trapezoid joint. A CT scan may still be required for diagnosis and treatment planning in patients whom a fracture is suspected but not adequately diagnosed on plain radiographs.

Treatment

- Fractures are classified into two main types, palmer ridge fractures and body fractures, depending upon the location of the injury
- Nondisplaced body fractures are treated by a short-thumb spica cast, whereas displaced and comminuted fractures are treated by closed or open reduction methods
- Palmer ridge fractures are managed by a short-thumb spica cast for 4–6 weeks. Pinch and grip impairment is a consequence of inadequate treatment

Lunate fractures

Lunate fractures are the fourth most fractures carpal bone after the scaphoid, triquetrum, and trapezium. The mechanism of the fracture is a fall onto a stretched hand with hyperextended wrist. Patients present with palpation tenderness over the volar wrist. The standard radiographic lateral view shows the capitate, lunate, and distal radius collinear with the wrist in a natural position. A CT scan is often needed to properly diagnose subtle injuries.

Treatment

- Nondisplaced fractures or small avulsions are treated with a cast for 4–6 weeks
- Displaced fractures require ORIF

Trapezoid fractures

The trapezoid bone is situated in a protected position between the trapezium, scaphoid, capitate, and second metacarpal bone, articulates distally with the index metacarpal base. The main blood supply originates from the dorsal side, so dorsal displacement may lead to injury to the vasculature and AVN. Fractures of the trapezoid are the least common carpal fracture of the wrist, accounting for < 1% of all carpal bone fractures. The mechanism of injury is axial loading of the index metacarpal or direct dorsal trauma to the hand. Patients present with some degree of swelling over the dorsum of the hand, and palpation shows tenderness just proximal to the index metacarpal base.

Treatment

- Nondisplaced fractures are managed with a cast for 4–6 weeks
- Displaced fractures are treated by reduction and fixation

SUGGESTED READING

Berger RA. The ligaments of the wrist: a current overview of anatomy with considerations of their potential functions. Hand Clin 1997; 13:63–82.
Carpal instability cannot be fully understood without a thorough knowledge of the functional anatomy of the different carpal ligaments. This is one of the most complete reviews of carpal ligaments published.

Cohen MS, Taleisnik J. Direct ligamentous repair of scapholunate dissociation with capsulodesis augmentation. Tech Hand Upper Extrem Surg 1998; 2:18–24.
The best way to prevent carpal instability is to repair all acute ruptures of the dorsal SL ligament, the most important SL joint stabilizer.

Dobyns JH, Linscheid RL. A short history of the wrist joint. Hand Clin 1997; 13:1–12.
This paper reviews the history of our understanding of wrist problems. It offers an excellent review of the contributions made in the past by a number of hand experts.

Geissler WB, Freeland AE, Savoie FH, et al. Intracarpal soft-tissue lesions associated with an intra-articular fracture of the distal end of the radius. J Bone Joint Surg Am 1996; 78:357–365.
With the introduction of arthroscopy in the diagnosis of wrist problems, the true incidence of carpal derangements in association with distal radial fractures was investigated. This paper, later validated by other similar studies, established a basis to the understanding of this important aspect of wrist instability.

Kauer JMG. The mechanism of the carpal joint. Clin Orthop 1986; 202:16–26.
This paper, written by a renowned professor of anatomy and world expert in wrist biomechanics, is one of the best analyses of carpal mechanics ever published. In a very didactic way, the interactions between the different bone structures in the wrist are explained both in terms of ability to move as well as capacity to bear loads.

Linscheid RL, Dobyns JH, Beabout JW, Bryan RS. Traumatic instability of the wrist: diagnosis, classification, and pathomechanics. J Bone Joint Surg Am 1972; 54:1612–1632.
Despite being published more than 30 years ago, most statements made in this paper are still valid; most uncertainties then still remain controversial or unsolved today.

Mayfield JK, Johnson RP, Kilcoyne RK. Carpal dislocations: pathomechanics and progressive perilunar instability. J Hand Surg [Am] 1980; 5:226–241.
Dr. Mayfield and associates conclusively demonstrated that there is a pattern of progressive perilunar destabilization when the wrist is exposed to a particular type of hyperextension/ulnar-deviation stress. From that study, we learned that entities as dissimilar as palmar lunate dislocations and dorsal perilunate dislocations are to be treated following the same principles. This classic study still remains unchallenged.

Short WH, Werner FW, Green JK, Masaoka S. Biomechanical evaluation of ligamentous stabilizers of the scaphoid and lunate. J Hand Surg [Am] 2002; 27:991–1002.
This publication is one of the many examples of the excellent work done during the past 20 years by the group of investigators led by Drs. Palmer and Werner, from Syracuse, New York, in the field of wrist mechanics. A sophisticated experimental cadaver model allowing real-time detection of force transmission and carpal kinematic analysis during simulated physiologic motion is presented. This elegant study allowed the authors to demonstrate the stabilizing role of the dorsal SL ligament and that of the secondary constraints, the distal STT and SC ligaments. Truly, this is a great contribution to the understanding of wrist instabilities.

13.5 FRACTURES AND DISLOCATIONS OF THE DISTAL RADIUS AND THE DISTAL RADIOULNAR JOINT

DISTAL RADIUS FRACTURES AND DISLOCATIONS

Distal radius fracture is a common fracture worldwide, and one of the most common fractures seen in the emergency department. It has a bimodal age distribution, with peaks of incidence occurring in the youth and in the elderly. In young patients, distal radius fractures typically occur due to high-energy trauma (motor vehicle accidents, fall from heights), predominantly in males. Most elderly fractures are related to low energy trauma (slipped and fall) in osteoporotic wrists and occur predominantly in females.

Anatomy of the distal radius and ulna

The radius (with the associated carpus and hand) rotates around the ulna by virtue of the proximal and distal radioulnar joints (DRUJ) (**Figure 13.38**). The metaphyseal flare of the distal radius consists of the distal 25.4 mm (1 inch) of the radius. The volar surface of the distal radius is thicker and relatively flat, with the flexor tendons only coming into close contact at the volar rim of the distal radial lip. In contrast, the dorsal surface is convex and closely related to the overlying extensor tendons. The dorsal cortex is thin and is typically comminuted in an osteoporotic fracture.

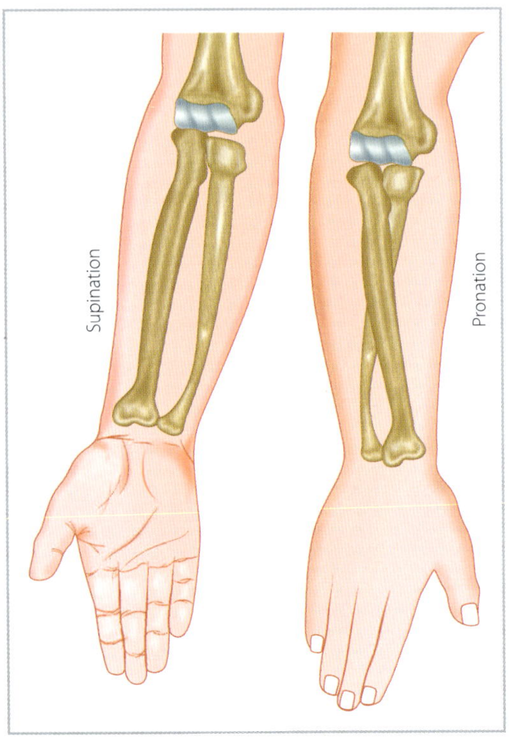

Figure 13.38 Rotation of the radius and the hand around the ulna.

The distal ends of the radius and ulna articulate with the proximal carpal row and the distal margin of the radius on the volar and dorsal side mark the insertion of the extrinsic ligaments that stabilize the carpus and provide radiocarpal motion. An anteroposterior ridge (interfacet ridge) separates the RS fossa from the more ulnar lunate fossa. The sigmoid fossa is located along the distal ulnar surface of the radius and articulates with the ulnar head. The carpus is separated from the distal end of the ulna by the TFCC. The TFCC originates on the ulnar border of the lunate fossa and inserts onto the base of the ulnar styloid.

Classification and pathomechanics of the fracture

Approximately 80% of the axial load across the wrist is transmitted through the distal end of the radius and 20% across the TFCC and the distal end of the ulna. Most fractures of the radius occur at the metaphysis, which consists of cancellous bone that lacks the strength and density of cortical bone. These fractures are frequently comminuted dorsally, resulting in the classic dinner fork deformity (dorsal displacement with dorsal tilt, radial tilt, and shortening) (**Figure 13.39**). A significant deforming force of this fracture is due to the brachioradialis tendon insertion into the radial styloid, which causes radial shortening and displacement.

There are three main classification systems for distal radius fractures:

1. The Melone classification
2. The AO classification
3. The Fernandez classification

The Melone classification

The Melone classification identifies the main fracture fragments, and a multifragmentary intra-articular fracture pattern with four large fracture fragments is described. These fragments are the radial styloid, the radial shaft, and the medial complex consisting of the volar and dorsal lunate fossa fragments. The displacement, involvement, and comminution of the medial complex have prognostic values (**Figure 13.40**).

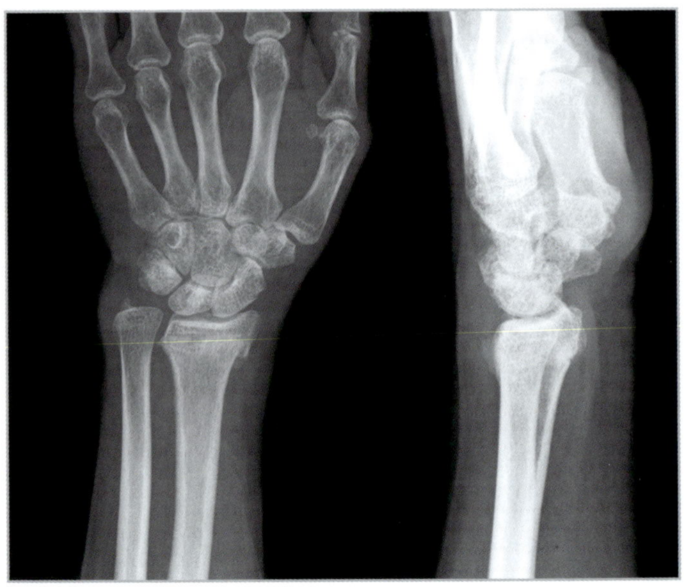

Figure 13.39 A Colles fracture showing the classic dinner fork deformity.

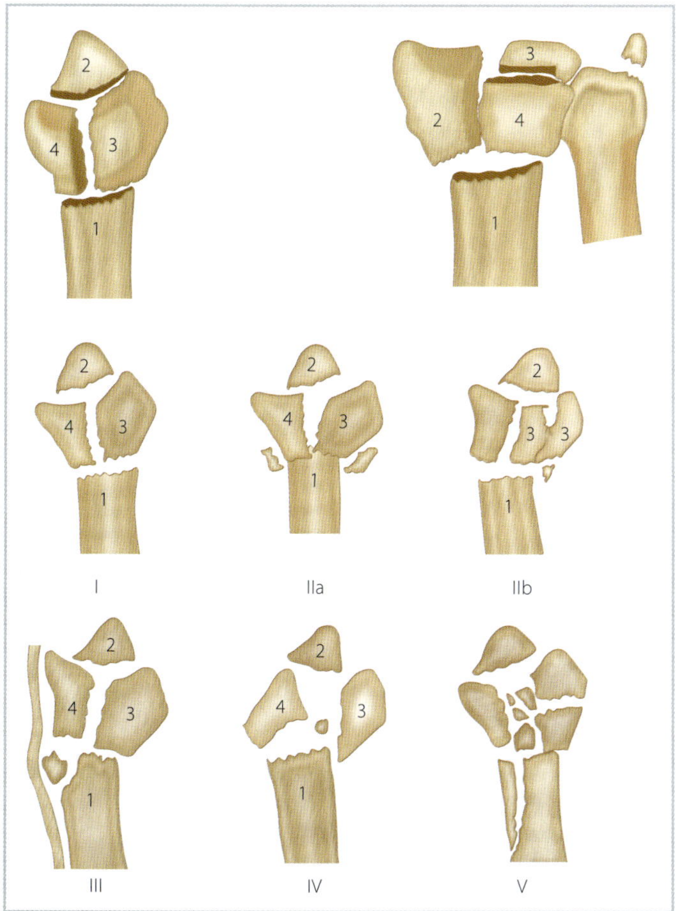

Figure 13.40 Melone classification of distal radius fractures.

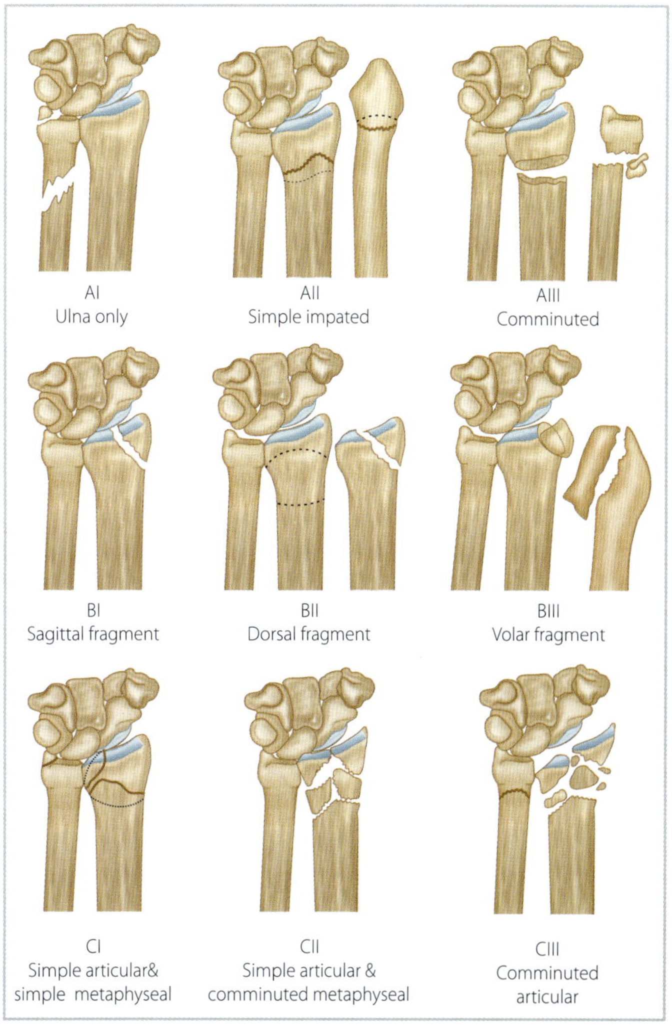

Figure 13.41 AO classification of distal radius fractures.

The AO classification

The AO classification is descriptive and comprehensive, dividing the fracture into extra-articular, simple intra-articular, and complex intra-articular fractures. This is then further divided into a total of 27 subgroups, with increasing severity of fracture that theoretically correlates with a poorer prognosis (**Figure 13.41**).

The Fernandez classification

The Fernandez classification is based on the mechanism of injury and divides the fractures in categories of bending, articular shearing, intra-articular compression, avulsion fractures, and combination fractures (**Figure 13.42**). This system also attempts to relate associated soft tissue injuries with the fracture pattern, which can help in the understanding of the fractures and to rationalize the various treatment options. This is one of the most comprehensive and practical classification systems developed.

- Type I fractures: Bending fractures of the metaphysis in which one cortex fails due to tensile stresses and the opposite cortex undergoes a certain degree of comminution (extra-articular Colles or Smith fractures)
- Type II fractures: Shearing fractures of the joint surface (Barton's, reversed Barton's, and radial styloid fractures)

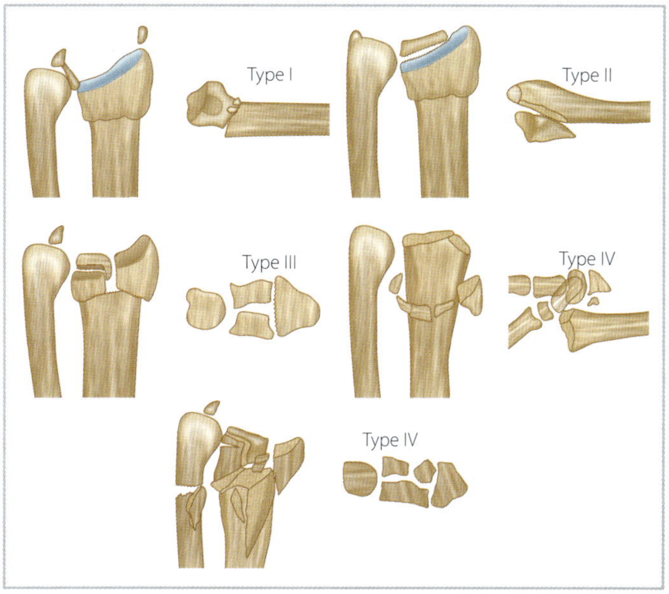

Figure 13.42 Fernandez classification of distal radius fractures.

- Type III fractures: Compression fractures of the joint surface with impaction of the subchondral and metaphyseal cancellous bone. Current terms used for this fracture type are intra-articular comminuted fractures, complex articular fractures, and pilon radial fractures
- Type IV fractures: Avulsion fractures of ligament attachments, including ulnar and radial styloid fractures associated with radiocarpal fracture dislocations
- Type V fractures are high-velocity injuries that involve combinations of bending, compression, shearing, and avulsion mechanisms or bone loss

History and clinical examination

A careful history is essential to establish the circumstances surrounding the accident and to determine any neurological or cardiac causes for the fall/injury. The mechanism of injury is important to understand the energy of the injury and to alert the treating physician to associated nerve and ligament injuries. If there are concomitant injuries to the head or spine, the remainder of the upper limb should be carefully evaluated to look for other injuries. Determining a patient's functional status and social support structure is critical to help map treatment. Physical examination should focus on the wrist, searching for any breach of the soft tissue envelop (open fractures), median nerve compression, or tendon injuries, and also including a vascular assessment of the radial and ulnar pulse, as well as assessment of the proximal joints including the elbow and shoulder.

Radiological evaluation

X-rays centered on the wrist should be obtained with the shoulder in 90° abduction, the elbow in 90° flexion, and the wrist and forearm in neutral rotation. In a true standard PA view, the groove for the tendon of the ECU should be at the level or radial to the base of the ulnar styloid (**Figure 13.43**). In a true lateral view, the palmar cortex of the pisiform should overlie the central third of the interval between the palmar cortices of the distal scaphoid and the head of the capitate (**Figure 13.44**). The three radiographic measurements performed on standard PA and lateral views that correlate with patient outcomes are the radial height, radial inclination, and the volar tilt (**Figure 13.45**). Radial height averages 11 mm (10–14 mm), radial inclination averages 22° (20°–25°), and volar tilt averages 11° (5°–15°). As a result of the radial inclination at the wrist, a 22° proximally angled view provides better visualization of the articular surface.

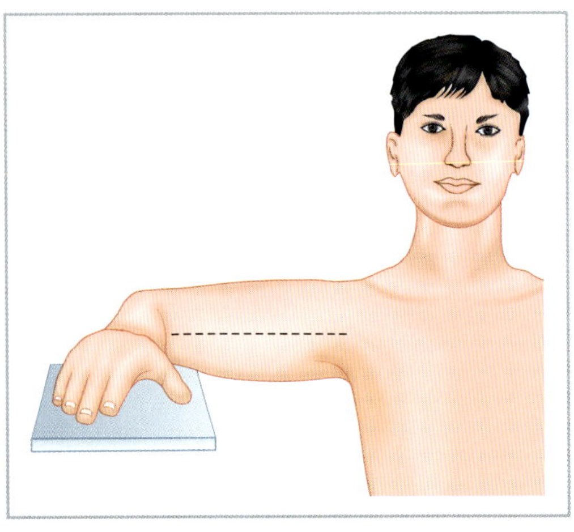

Figure 13.43 Patient positioning for a true posteroanterior radiograph of the wrist.

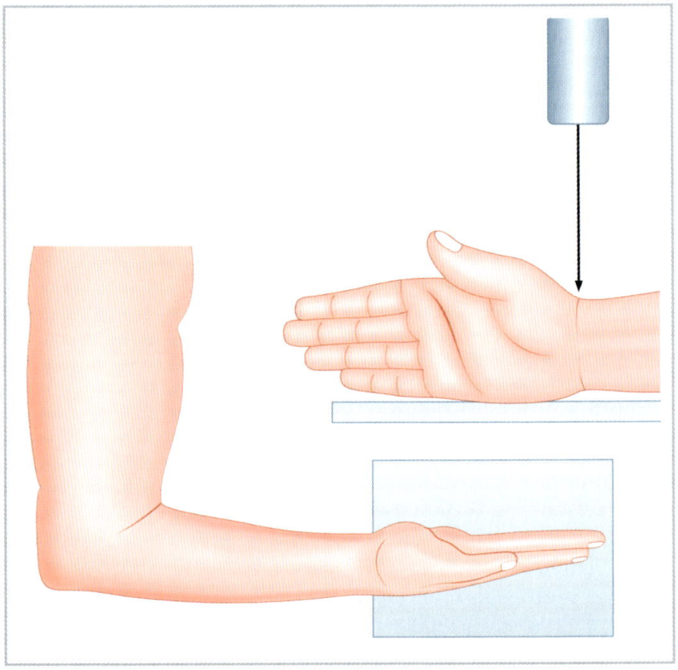

Figure 13.44 Patient positioning for a true lateral radiograph of the wrist.

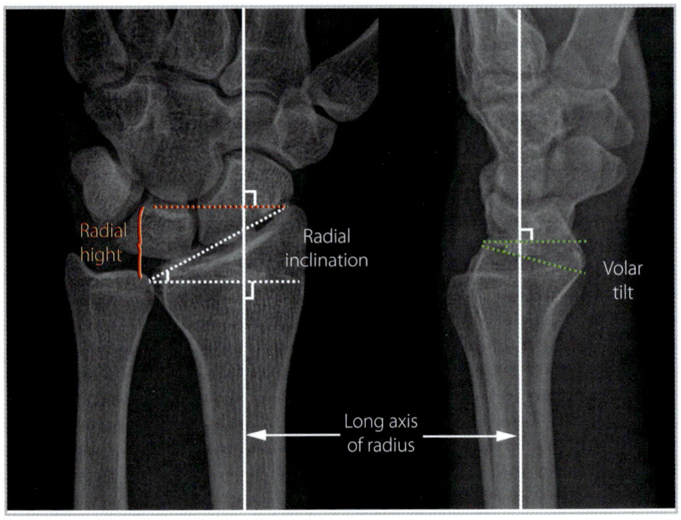

Figure 13.45 The three important radiographic parameters used to assess distal radius fractures.

Computed tomographic scans improve the ability to evaluate intra-articular displacement and degree of comminution, helping treatment planning. MRI is useful for assessing SL ligament tears and TFCC injuries, which are associated with 50% of distal radius fractures. However, neither one of these modalities have been evaluated with respect to patient outcome, hence, they should be ordered only when it is anticipated that their findings would help plan treatment. A CT scan or MRI will not replace the diagnostic value of a standard X-ray, and therefore should only be used to supplement the standard X-ray views during evaluation of a distal radius fracture.

Outcomes

In younger patients, the aim of treatment of distal radius fractures is to restore articular congruity and normal extra-articular anatomy. Fractures that heal with >20° of dorsal angulation, axial shortening of

>6 mm, >2 mm articular step off, associated injuries of the TFCC and SL ligament, instability of the DRUJ, and work-related injuries had less favorable outcomes. In older patients > 60 years old, malunion of the distal radius is not always correlated with poor functional outcome. Patients have normal health-related quality of life with high levels of satisfaction and little self-reported disability despite the presence of significant deformities.

Treatment

In a prospective analysis of 4000 distal radius fractures, age and comminution were found to be the most significant predictors of fracture instability. The stability of the fracture is a determining factor in the type of treatment that will provide the best outcomes for the patient.

Stability of fractures

- Stable fractures: These fractures are minimally displaced at presentation and do not displace after manipulative reduction. The deformity will have a dorsal angulation < 5° and radial shortening < 2 mm. This type of fracture can be managed with cast immobilization.
- Unstable fractures: These fractures cannot be reduced or the reduction cannot be maintained. The factors that have been associated with instability after closed reduction have been listed in **Table 13.9**. Unstable distal radius fractures require surgical intervention to maintain reduction. There is no consensus regarding the optimal treatment of unstable distal radius fractures; however, the current trend is toward internal fixation. Multiple surgical options are available that include percutaneous pin fixation, external fixation, open reduction and plate fixation, and arthroscopically assisted fixation. There is currently insufficient data to provide evidence-based support for any particular treatment method in terms of the long-term functional benefits.
- Displaced fractures: A displaced fractures should undergo manipulation and reduction as an emergency procedure under a hematoma block or regional intravenous anesthesia. Under adequate anesthesia, the deformity is accentuated to disimpact the fracture and regain radial height and inclination under traction, using the principles of ligamentotaxis (**Figure 13.46**). A semicircular cast is initially applied to secure the reduction, with anticipation of swelling in the limb due to the trauma (**Figure 13.47**). The cast should allow free MCP and finger joint movements and the patient advised to maintain a strict elevation of the limb. The wrist must not be immobilized in >15° of flexion, because this increases the risk of carpal tunnel syndrome, digital stiffness, and complex regional pain syndrome (CRPS).

Table 13.9 Factors associated with instability after closed reduction of distal radius fractures

Injury factors (radiographic findings)
More than 5 mm shortening
Dorsal tilt > 20°
Articular displacement > 2 mm
Displacement more than two thirds of the width of the shaft in any direction
Dorsal metaphyseal comminution
Associated ulnar fracture
Patient factors
Age > 60 years (osteoporosis)

Treatment options

- Conservative management: This type of treatment involves close follow-up and may require remanipulation if the fracture displaces and the deformity is deemed unacceptable. The patient should be put in a long-arm cast when the swelling subsides. Understanding

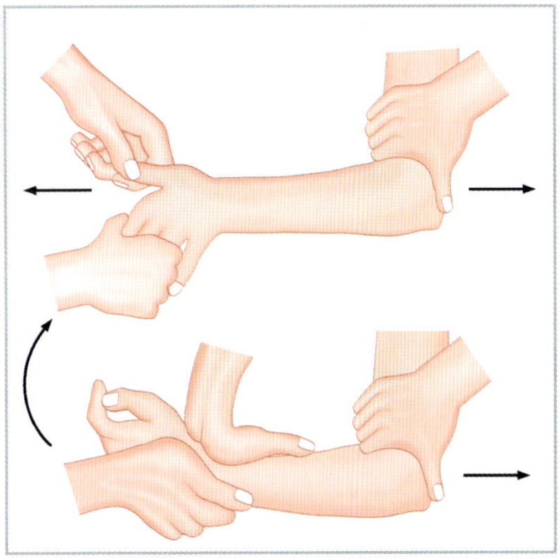

Figure 13.46 The procedure for closed reduction of distal radius fracture.

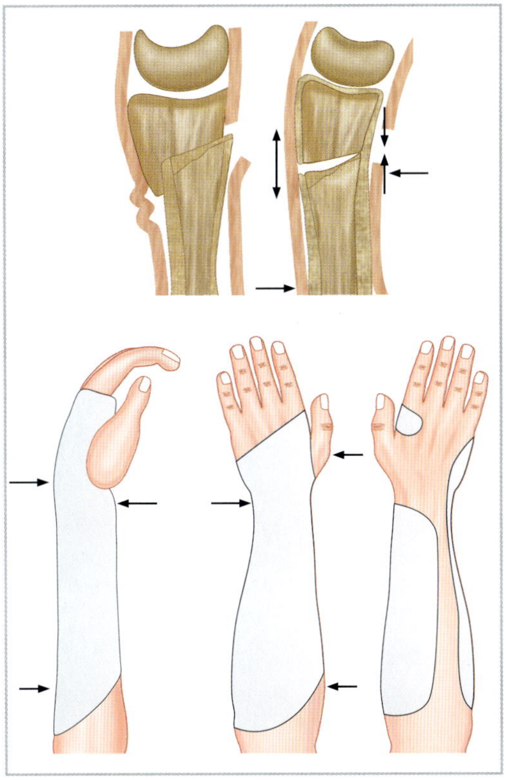

Figure 13.47 The technique of three point splinting for maintaining reduction after closed manipulation of distal radius fractures.

the functional status and social support of the patient is important in determining the acceptable level of deformity, as many of these fractures are unstable in the elderly who have osteoporosis. Fortunately, many of the older patients with this injury have good functional outcomes and high patient satisfaction despite significant malunion, mainly due to the fact that their functional demands are low

- Percutaneous pinning: Intrafocal (Kapandji) (**Figure 13.48**) pinning places pins within the fracture, using them to lever large fracture fragments into reduction and support. This type of treatment is indicated for noncomminuted extra-articular fractures with no osteoporosis (i.e. in younger patients). In patients with significant comminution, additional external fixation is required to unload the joint and prevent fracture collapse. Kapandji pinning should not be used alone in osteoporotic bone without the addition of trans-styloid pinning or external fixation to maintain alignment
- External fixation: Bridging external fixation (across the radiocarpal joint) utilizes ligamentotaxis to indirectly reduce and maintain stability of the fracture fragments. External fixators function by holding the fracture out to length and neutralizing compressive, bending, and torsional forces across the fracture site. They are useful in patients that have suffered highly unstable fractures with significant metaphyseal comminution as they allow alignment of the articular surface with the shaft of the radius. These devices are uniplanar, with half pins placed into the second metacarpal and radial shaft across the radiocarpal joint, connected by a bar that maintains a distracting force (**Figure 13.49**). Excessive traction, flexion, and ulnar deviation must be avoided when attempting reduction, because this leads to complications of stiffness, nerve compression, and nonunion with prolonged immobilization. The addition of supplemental K-wires provides a direct effort at reduction of the fracture fragments and may lead to better outcomes. This technique is not indicated as the definitive treatment for displaced intra-articular fractures because good articular reduction cannot be achieved
- Open reduction and internal fixation: Dorsal plate fixation was popular in the 1980s because it offers the opportunity to visualize the joint and reduce intra-articular fractures. However, there were common complications with extensor tendon irritations and ruptures. The recent introduction of volar locking plates has enabled surgeons to produce predictable fixation results. This is because the volar plating system is designed to reside in the concave surface of the distal radius proximal to the watershed line of volar ligament insertion, hence avoiding flexor tendon irritation, and utilizes fixed angle screws as cantilevers to provide subchondral support of the articular surface after fracture reduction. This is gaining popularity in the treatment of this common fracture (**Figure 13.50**)

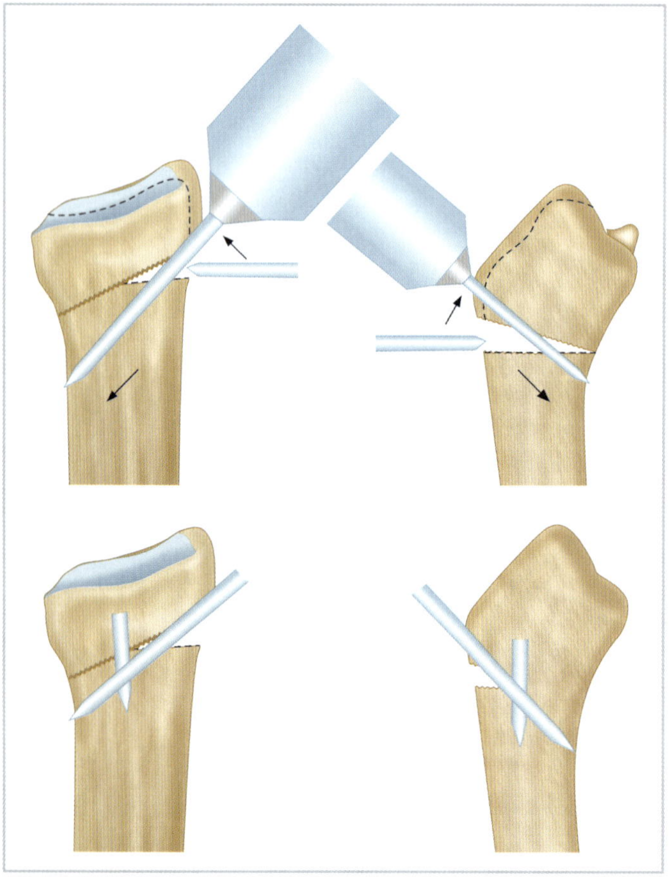

Figure 13.48 Kapandji intrafocal technique for reduction and pinning of distal radius fracture.

Associated injuries

Ulnar styloid fractures

A concomitant ulnar styloid fracture is seen in >50% of distal radius fractures, but not all ulnar styloid fractures need to be fixed. The

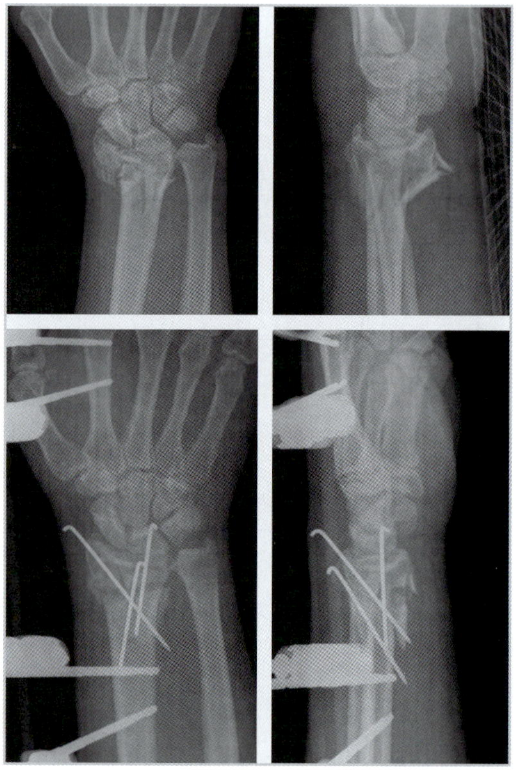

Figure 13.49 External fixation combined with pinning for distal radius fracture.

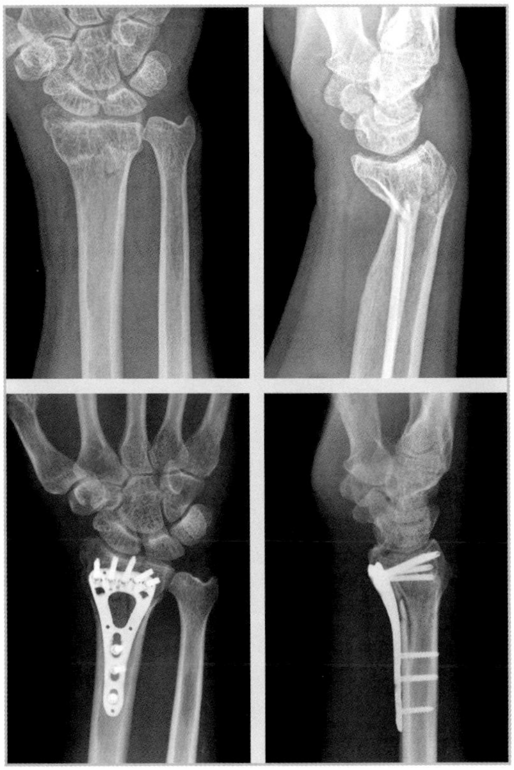

Figure 13.50 Volar plate fixation of distal radius fracture.

decision to fix the styloid depends on the stability of the DRUJ. The opposite uninjured DRUJ should be examined to establish the patient's natural degree of laxity, and the injured DRUJ examined after the distal radius has been stabilized to ascertain its stability. The ulnar styloid can be easily fixed using the tension band technique, and the forearm then immobilized in neutral rotation for 6 weeks using a Muenster type splint. The recovery of mobility is often slower in these cases.

DRUJ instability

Distal radioulnar joints instability may result from an intra-articular fracture involving the sigmoid fossa or a tear of the TFCC, and therefore, the stability of the DRUJ should be reassessed after fixation of these types of fractures. If the DRUJ is stable in full supination or pronation, one may consider one of the following two options:

1. Immobilizing the forearm in supination
2. Reducing the DRUJ in neutral position and maintaining the reduction using two parallel 1.6 mm (0.062 inch) K-wires passed below the ulnar head into the radius

If the DRUJ is unstable in all positions, there is probably an avulsion of the radioulnar ligament at the foveal insertion. This will require direct bone anchor repair of the radioulnar ligament and pinning of the radius and ulna for 6 weeks.

Ligament injury

Arthroscopic studies have shown a 30% incidence of SL ligament injury and 15% incidence of LT ligament injury after a distal radius fracture. After fixation of the distal radius, a fluoroscopic assessment of the carpus in radial and ulnar deviation and flexion and extension should be performed, and ligament injury can be confirmed with an arthroscopic assessment of the ligaments. Complete interosseous ligament injuries in young and active individuals will need exploration and repair, whereas partial ligament injuries can be managed by pinning the respective joints under fluoroscopy for 6 weeks.

Carpal tunnel syndrome

If nerve symptoms of paresthesia and numbness do not improve or worsen within 24–48 hours after satisfactory closed reduction, one must perform early carpal tunnel release and surgical stabilization of the fracture. However, there is no evidence to support routine release of the carpal tunnel at the time of operative fixation in patients without preoperative evidence of median nerve dysfunction.

Complications

Stiffness

The most common complication after a distal radius fracture is finger and wrist joint stiffness and often simultaneous frozen shoulder. This complication can be minimized from the onset by edema control and arm elevation, proper placement of plaster casts so that finger joint movements are not restricted and early mobilization of the unaffected shoulder joint. It is often prudent to allow edema to subside for 1 week after the acute fracture before surgical intervention so that the wound closure will not be under tension.

Malunion

Only symptomatic malunion requires operative intervention. Elderly low-demand patients who are pain free and function well despite significant radiographic deformity do not need any intervention. Malunion in young adults with higher functional demands can result in pain, loss of motion, and deformity. If there is >25°–30° of dorsal tilt or 6 mm of discrepancy between the radius and ulna, surgical intervention is required. This may include a corrective osteotomy (lengthening) of the distal radius or a shortening osteotomy of the ulna (**Figure 13.51**). The distal radius osteotomy aims to restore radial height, volar tilt, and radial inclination and improves the flexion/extension arc of motion.

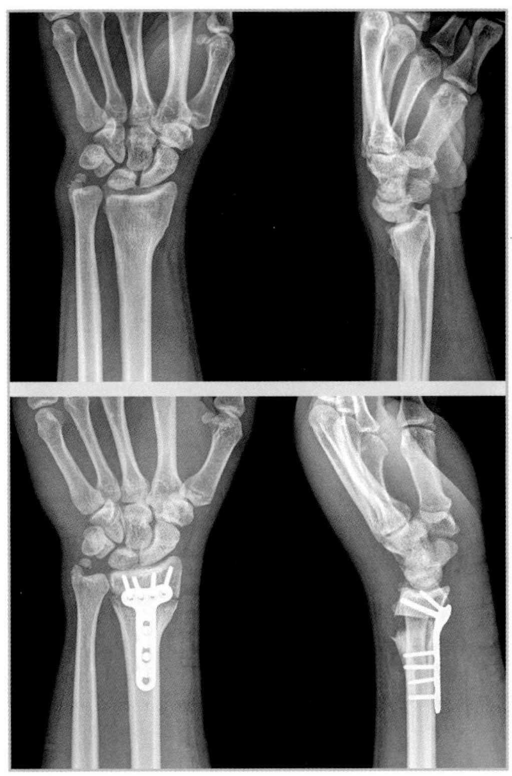

Figure 13.51 Corrective osteotomy of the distal radius via a volar approach.

Tendon rupture

It is common for a tendon rupture to occur due to implant irritation, but this can be minimized by avoiding protruding screw tips and placing the volar implants proximal to the watershed line. Spontaneous rupture of the extensor pollicis longus is an uncommon complication after distal radius fractures. It is believed to result from ischemia of the tendon as a result of compression by a fracture hematoma within the third extensor compartment, usually associated with a minimally displaced extra-articular fracture. The treatment of choice is a transfer of the extensor indicis proprius to restore thumb extension.

Chronic regional pain syndrome

Patients with increasing pain, joint stiffness, and paresthesia will need early attention and referral to a pain management service. The use of supplemental vitamin C after distal radius fractures was found to significantly reduce the incidence of chronic regional pain syndrome.

DRUJ INJURIES

Anatomy and biomechanics

The DRUJ is an incongruent joint of the distal radius and ulna that functions as a pivot for forearm pronosupination. Translation of the joint occurs during forearm rotation because the sigmoid notch is shallow and its radius of curvature is larger than the ulnar head. At the extremes of pronosupination, there is as little as 2 mm of articular contact. The dorsal and palmar rims of the sigmoid notch, together with the radioulnar ligaments, provide the major constraining mechanism. The palmar and dorsal radioulnar ligaments, together with the triangular fibrocartilage, are the main components of the TFCC that stabilize DRUJ. The superficial fibers of the DRUL insert into the ulnar styloid, and the substantial deep fibers inserting into the fovea (**Figure 13.52**).

The ECU subsheath is a stout structure that attaches its groove in the ulnar head to the dorsal carpus and contributes to the DRUJ and ulnocarpal stability. Stability of the mobile DRUJ is a topic of much debate, but the latest understanding is that the joint is the most stable in the extremes of pronosupination, where the compressive forces of the radius and ulna are resisted by the reciprocal tensile forces in the opposite radioulnar ligament.

Acute DRUJ injuries

Clinical presentation

Dislocations and instability at the DRUJ can result when there is a significant disruption of the bony anatomy, such as a comminuted ulnar head fracture or a fracture through the sigmoid notch; but most commonly, injuries occur within the TFCC.

- Palmer classified TFCC injuries based on location and chronicity [acute (**Figure 13.53**) versus degenerative (**Table 13.10**)]
- Injury to the TFCC can occur in the central portion of the disc itself, at its radial attachment to the radius, at the foveal attachment to the ulna or at its periphery
- Peripheral lesions and injuries to the foveal insertion tend to produce pain and instability, whereas those occurring in the central portion of the disc or at its radial insertion tend to produce pain alone
- Dorsal dislocation is more common than volar dislocations
  - Dorsal dislocations are believed to result from a hyperpronation force
  - Volar dislocations thought to result from a hypersupination force

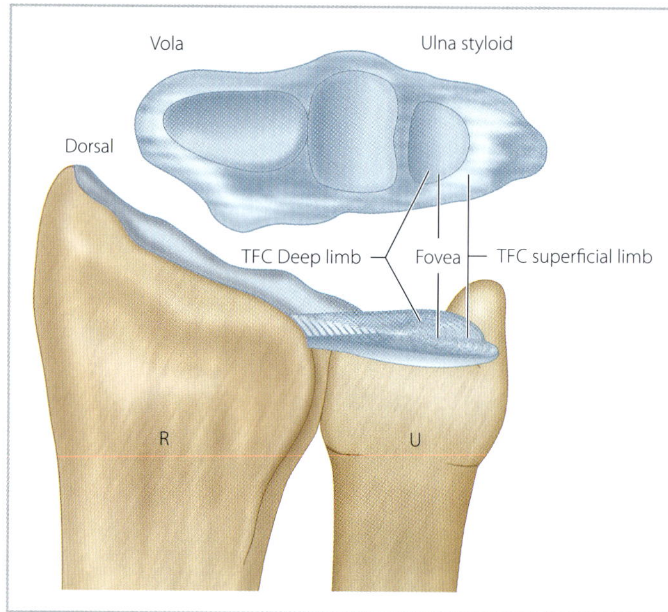

Figure 13.52 The anatomy of the triangular fibrocartilage complex.

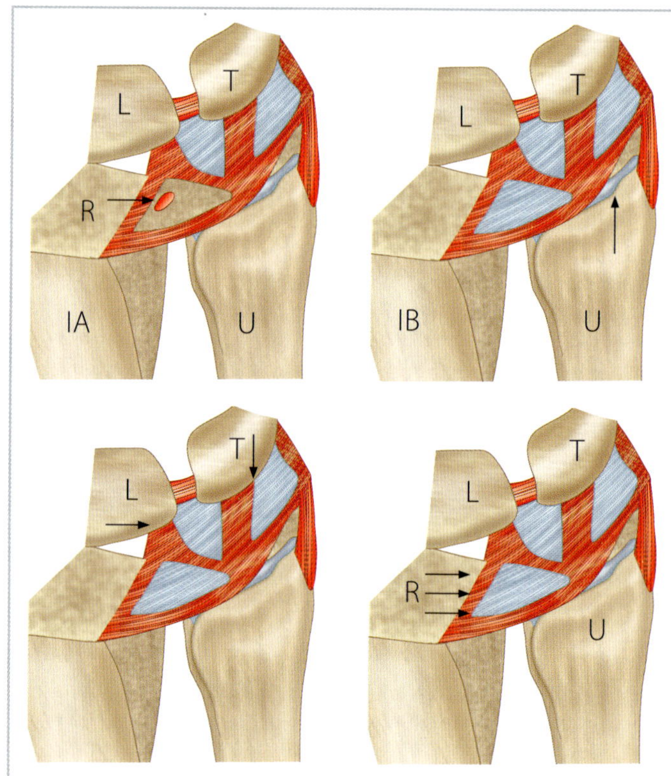

Figure 13.53 Palmer classification of traumatic tears of the triangular fibrocartilage complex.

- Acute pain and swelling of the joint without antecedent trauma may be related to an inflammatory process, for which an accurate history is crucial in terms of management

Table 13.10 Palmer classification of triangular fibrocartilage complex (TFCC) injuries

Classification	Description
Class 1	Traumatic
1A	Central perforation or tear
1B	Ulnar avulsion (with or without distal ulnar fracture)
1C	Distal avulsion
1D	Radial avulsion with or without sigmoid notch fracture
Class 2	Degenerative
2A	TFCC wear and thinning
2B	TFCC wear with lunate and/or ulnar chondromalacia
2C	TFCC perforation with lunate and/or ulnar chondromalacia
2D	TFFCC perforation with lunate and/or ulnar chondromalacia and LT ligament perforation
2E	TFCC perforation with lunate and/or ulnar chondromalacia, LT ligament perforation, and ulnocarpal arthritis

Radiological evaluation

- The ulnar styloid changes position on the PA X-ray when the forearm goes through pronosupination. With the forearm in mid rotation (neutral), the ulnar styloid can be seen to be at the ulnar most corner of the wrist, which shifts to be in the center of the ulnar head in full pronation or supination
- The AP view in a dorsal dislocation will typically demonstrate a widened DRUJ with divergence of the radius and ulna when compared with the contralateral normal DRUJ. A volar dislocation will show an overlap of the radius and ulna on AP view due to the convergent pull of the pronator quadratus

Treatment

Treatment of acute dislocation without fracture begins with closed reduction under anesthesia.

- With dorsal dislocation of the ulna, reduction is accomplished with gentle traction, dorsal pressure over the ulnar head, and supination. The joint must be assessed for instability and typically is most stable in supination
- With volar dislocation, reduction is usually more difficult due to the pull of the pronator quadratus muscle, and therefore regional or general anesthesia may be necessary. Closed treatment is frequently successful in restoration of a stable construct
- Complex DRUJ dislocations occur when there is interposed soft tissue that blocks closed reduction; such dislocations require operative intervention to remove the interposed structures and reduce the joint
- If the joint is unstable and has a tendency to dislocate or subluxate, the stabilizing structures of the DRUJ must be repaired. Direct repair of the TFCC to the foveal insertion is preferred using suture anchors or heavy suture through bone tunnels

Chronic DRUJ injuries

Clinical presentation

Chronic DRUJ injuries often result from a fall on an outstretched hand that damages the TFCC, compromising the integrity of the radioulnar ligaments. Patients commonly complain of pain when carrying heavy loads or a painful clunking sensation that is exacerbated with forearm rotation due to subluxation of the ulnar head under stress (instability). Malunion after distal radius fracture or significant ulnar head fractures are also associated with DRUJ instability. In particular, significant loss of the volar tilt of the distal radius is associated with altered DRUJ kinematics. Chronic DRUJ instability may also be found after Galeazzi or Essex–Lopresti injury patterns.

Ulnar-sided wrist pain is not always a result of DRUJ instability, and other diagnoses must be considered and ruled out, such as ulnar styloid nonunion, ECU tenosynovitis, ulnocarpal impaction, LT ligament injury, nondestabilizing TFCC tears, dorsal ulna sensory nerve injury, and inflammatory arthritides. Instability of the DRUJ is a subjective evaluation, and therefore, the DRUJ should be assessed with the wrist in neutral, pronated, and supinated positions and compared with the contralateral normal side. DRUJ pathology will typically produce pain in the fovea region of the ulnar head on palpation.

Imaging

- If X-rays demonstrate a widened DRUJ space and ulnar head displacement in DRUJ instability, there is evidence of distal radius malunion and DRUJ arthritis
- CT scans that demonstrate sigmoid notch incongruity may be indicative of DRUJ arthritis
- MRI is the most useful tool for assessing TFCC injury, as well as LT ligament injuries and ECU tendinitis

Treatment

- Arthroscopy of the wrist is the standard for assessment of the TFCC, and it can simultaneously assess the status of the other ligaments and joint surface. Arthroscopic debridement and repair of the TFCC has been determined to be an effective treatment
- Conservative treatment with functional bracing can be used as initial treatment for instability, with wrist strengthening programs directed at the dynamic stabilizers of the DRUJ
  - In particular, the programs designed to strengthen the pronator quadratus and ECU may also prove beneficial
- Surgery is indicated for patients presenting with pain and gross instability. Peripheral tears and volar tears (Palmar class IB and IC) of the TFCC may be repaired arthroscopically or with open repair
- In chronic cases in which the TFCC cannot be repaired primarily, DRUJ reconstruction focused on reconstruction of the dorsal and volar radioulnar ligaments has been found to be successful by using tendon grafts through drill holes to stabilize the DRUJ

- Distal radius malunion should be treated with corrective osteotomy of the radius prior to any attempts at DRUJ reconstruction
- Patients with instability and ulnar impaction are best treated with ulnar shortening
- Patients presenting with instability and DRUJ arthritis are best managed with DRUJ salvage procedures such as the Sauve-Kapanji procedure, the Darrach procedure, or the DRUJ arthroplasty

SUGGESTED READING

Knirk JL, Jupiter JB. Intra-articular fractures of the distal end of the radius in young adults. J Bone Joint Surg [Am] 1986; 68:647–659.

This paper brings to attention the importance of anatomical restoration for intra-articular distal radius fractures to reduce the risk of radiological post-traumatic arthritis in young adults.

Orbay JL, Fernandez DL. Volar fixation for dorsally displaced fractures of the distal radius: A preliminary report. J Hand Surg [Am] 2002; 27:205–215.

This paper challenges conventional wisdom by demonstrating excellent results in 31 dorsally displaced fractures treated with a fixed angle device applied through a volar approach to the distal radius. For articular comminution, the authors describe an extended volar incision that reflects the proximal radius to allow articular restitution prior to placement of the volar plate.

Palmer AK, Werner FW. The triangular fibrocartilage complex of the wrist – anatomy and function. J Hand Surg [Am] 1981; 6:153–162.

This now classic work describes the anatomy and function of the TFCC through anatomic dissections and biomechanical testing of cadavers. The TFCC is a confluence of several structures including the articular disc, dorsal and volar radioulnar ligaments, meniscus homologue, and ECU sheath. Signs of ulnocarpal impaction syndrome are described. Biomechanical studies demonstrated its role in ulnocarpal joint load transmission and DRUJ stability.

Prommersberger KJ, van Schoonhoven J, Lanz UB. Outcome after corrective osteotomy for malunited fractures of the distal end of the radius. J Hand Surg [Br] 2002; 27:1:55–60.

A large series of corrective osteotomy for dorsal ($n = 29$) and palmar ($n = 20$) malunited distal radius fractures is presented, together with objective follow-up data at 18 months. The authors conclude that function is correlated with restoration of alignment, and patients with multiplanar preoperative deformities fare less well after surgical correction.

Stuart PR, Berger RA, et al. The dorsopalmar stability of the distal radioulnar joint. J Hand Surg [Am] 2000; 25:689–699.

A specialized testing machine analyzed the stabilizing structures of the DRUJ in a cadaveric study. The major constraint to dorsal translation of the ulna was the palmar radioulnar ligament, whereas palmar translation was constrained primarily by the dorsal radioulnar ligament, with secondary constraint provided by the palmar radioulnar ligament and interosseous membrane. The ulnocarpal ligaments and ECU subsheath did not contribute significantly. Twenty per cent of DRUJ constraint is provided by the articular contact of DRUJ.

13.6 THERAPY FOR FRACTURES AND DISLOCATIONS IN THE HAND

Fractures and joint dislocations in the hand are very common throughout the world. These injuries can be complicated by deformity and stiffness, severely restricting functional use of the hand in activities of daily living such as self-care, productive work, and leisure. It is essential to involve hand therapists when providing rehabilitation after hand fractures and IP dislocations to maximize the functional outcomes for the patient. Teamwork and communication among the therapist and physician/surgeon are crucial in developing an effective rehabilitation plan. A referral should always be written to the hand therapist with detailed fracture information, including the following:

- Location and nature of the fracture (e.g. undisplaced or displaced, simple or comminuted, transverse or oblique)
- Type of reduction and fixation
- The alignment post reduction and fixation
- Nature of additional soft tissue injury

KEY THERAPY TECHNIQUES/ EXERCISES FOR HAND INJURIES

Although the management of each injury is different, healing can be broken down into three main phases:

1. The early protective phase
2. The mobilization phase
3. The functional/strengthening phase

Table 13.11 describes the therapy process throughout the different phases of fracture and tissue healing.

Distal radius fractures

Early protective phase

Splinting is critical in this phase of therapy. A wrist cock-up splint with the wrist in 20°–30° extension is recommended for distal radius fractures. Mobilize the shoulder, elbow and fingers, and include forearm supination/pronation if the DRUJ is stable. Hand edema can limit active composite finger flexion leading to adaptive shortening of intrinsic muscles; therefore, it is important to introduce blocked active hook exercises to stretch the intrinsic muscles.

Mobilization phase

During the mobilization phase, encourage tenodesis motion by extending the wrist with the fingers flexed and flex the wrist with the fingers extended. Be sure the patient avoids a substitution pattern of extending the wrist with the finger extensors or flexing the wrist during attempted grasp. Progress to passive stretching exercises for the wrist at 4–6 weeks post injury or operation, and consider manual joint mobilization to stretch the tight joint capsular ligaments. Design dynamic, serial static, or progressive splinting when a gain in ROM plateaus before an acceptable functional level is achieved.

Functional/strengthening phase

Improve endurance for daily activities of living with wrist and grip strengthening exercise using resistive exercise bands, free weights, or a spring-loaded gripper. Promote weight bearing at the wrist with closed kinetic chain activities such as wall push-ups and pulling or pushing activities.

Table 13.11 Therapy process during the different phases of fracture or tissue healing

	Early protective phase	Mobilization phase	Functional/strengthening phase
Time line	1–6 weeks post injury or operation (varies with fracture stability)	Starts immediately after immobilization or after stable fixation	Initiated when there is evident healing/ bone fixation (usually at 8 weeks post injury or surgery)
Goals and relevant therapy activities	Control swelling and pain. • Elevation, retrograde massage, pressure garment, Coban wrapping, and/or contrast bath Facilitate wound healing and prevent infections. • Regular wound inspections and dressing Restore mobility of noninvolved joints. • Provide patient education on the importance of doing home exercises regularly Promote fracture/tissue healing through maintaining alignment with splinting.	Regain functional ROM. • Begin mobilization at the involved joints as early as possible • Use of different mobilization techniques such as blocking exercises, place and hold, passive stretching, and manual joint mobilization as healing progresses • Apply physical agent modalities (e.g. superfical thermal heating agent, electrical stimulation device, or ultrasound) as an adjunct to reduce pain and facilitate motion Minimise stiffness and scar adhesions. • Scar management with scar massage, topical scar compression, or desensitization for hypersensitive, hypertrophic, or adhered scarring • Consider dynamic, serial static, or progressive splinting Prevent pain and swelling by avoiding excessive vigorous ROM exercises and splinting	Restore/maximize strength and endurance for activities of daily living • Prescribe conditioning exercises: resisted exercises with weights, exercise bands, and spring-loaded devices. • Work conditioning or return-to-work program

ROM, range of motion.

Carpal fractures

Early protective phase

For most carpal fractures, 6–8 weeks of conservative management is sufficient, with up to 2 weeks post open reduction internal fixation.

Splinting

- Scaphoid fractures
  - Circumferential thumb spica splint after initial cast immobilization. Up to 24 weeks for fracture at proximal pole
- Other carpal fractures
  - Wrist cock-up splint with wrist in 20°–30° extension

Mobilization phase

During this phase, instruct on regular gentle wrist and fingers ROM and educate the patient against substitution motion. For associated carpal fracture-dislocation injuries, avoid wrist deviation for 4–6 weeks. For associated SL ligament dissociation injury, it is safe to start a dart thrower's motion early, because this motion moves the wrist without much lunate and scaphoid motion.

Functional/strengthening phase

The aim at this phase is to regain dynamic stability of the wrist, especially for fractures with associated carpal ligament injuries.

- Proprioception re-education with isometric strengthening of the flexor carpi radialis, FCU, ECRB, and APL for SL injuries
  - FCU tendon and hypothenar muscles for LT injuries
- Reactive muscle activation to promote cocontraction of the appropriate muscles for wrist stability, e.g. weight-bearing on a soft ball

Metacarpal fractures

Early protective phase

Early protective motion can be initiated with buddy strapping for stable, nondisplaced metacarpal fractures. When splinting is required, the type of splint used is dependent upon the location of the bone that is fractured:

- Thumb metacarpal fracture – long-thumb spica with thumb in opposition to prevent first web space contracture
- Second to fifth metacarpal fracture – intrinsic-plus splint to protect the involved metacarpal with the adjacent ones; position MCP joints in 70°–90° flexion, IP joints in full extension, and wrist in 20° extension

Mobilization phase

In this phase, buddy strapping can be used to guide motion at the involved digit from the adjacent digit. If further treatment is required:

- Remediate extensor lag at the MCP joints with:
  - Isolated extensor digitorum communis (EDC) exercises – actively extend the MCP joint with the PIP joint taped in flexion
  - Scar massage/ultrasound for scar adherence on extensor mechanism
- Improve MCP joint motion with:
  - Blocking exercises – wrist and CMC joint of the involved finger held in neutral to isolate the MCP joint in flexion. This is especially important for fourth and fifth metacarpal fracture to prevent substitution motion at the relatively mobile CMC joint
  - A splint to place the PIP joint and DIP joint in extension to exercise the lumbricals in directing motion at the involved MCP joint
  - Flexor, extensor, and intrinsic stretching to reduce muscle tendon unit tightness or tendon adherence – from week 4–6 onwards
  - Static progressive splinting with flexion strapping for low load and prolonged stretch at the involved MCP joint – from week 6 onwards

Functional/strengthening phase

Resistive and progressive strengthening of the intrinsic muscles and grip should be initiated at this phase with resistive putty, or spring-loaded gadgets.

Proximal phalanx (P1) fractures

Early protective phase

Splinting should be initiated with a hand-based intrinsic plus splint, with the MCP joints of the affected digit and its adjacent digit in at least 70° of flexion and the PIP joints in full extension. Buddy strapping can be utilized for a stable fracture.

Mobilization phase

- Remediate extensor lag at the PIP joints with:
  - Blocking exercises – block the MCP joint in flexion to direct action of the EDC to extend the PIP joint
  - An exercise splint can be made for wear during the day to actively extend the PIP joints with the MCP joint blocked in flexion (**Figure 13.54a–c**)
- Minimize a PIP joint flexion contracture with:
  - A gutter splint for night wear as early as possible if there is extensor lag
  - Regular intermittent PIP joint passive extension stretching at week 4–6
  - Progressive static splinting with a belly gutter during the night or dynamic extension splint such as a ready-made capener splint (passively extends the PIP joint while allowing active flexion)
- Improve PIP joint flexion with:
  - Differential FDS and FDP tendon gliding exercises – active initiation of DIP joint flexion followed by PIP joint flexion with the MCP joint blocked in extension (active hook exercise) (**Figure 13.55a** and **b**)
  - An exercise splint to hold the MCP joint in extension while the IP joints are free to actively flex (**Figure 13.56a–c**)
  - Intermittent PIP joint passive stretching at week 4–6
  - A PIP-DIP joint elastic flexion loop can be fitted for night wear

Functional/strengthening phase

At this stage, initiate resistive and progressive strengthening of intrinsic muscles and grip using resistive putty, or spring-loaded gadgets.

Middle phalanx (P2) fractures

Early protective phase

Splinting for middle phalanx fractures is completely dependent upon the type and location of the fracture:

- Stable P2 shaft fracture – Gutter splint
- Intra-articular P2 base fracture – a dorsal extension block splint to place the PIP joint in 10°–20° less of full extension or a traction splint

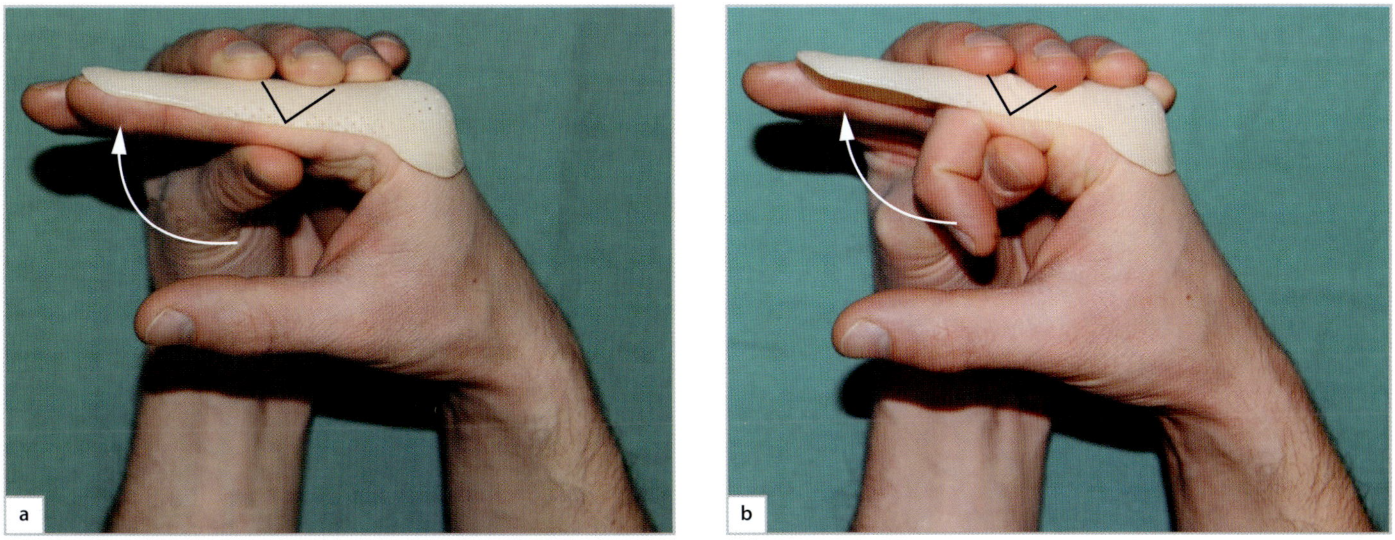

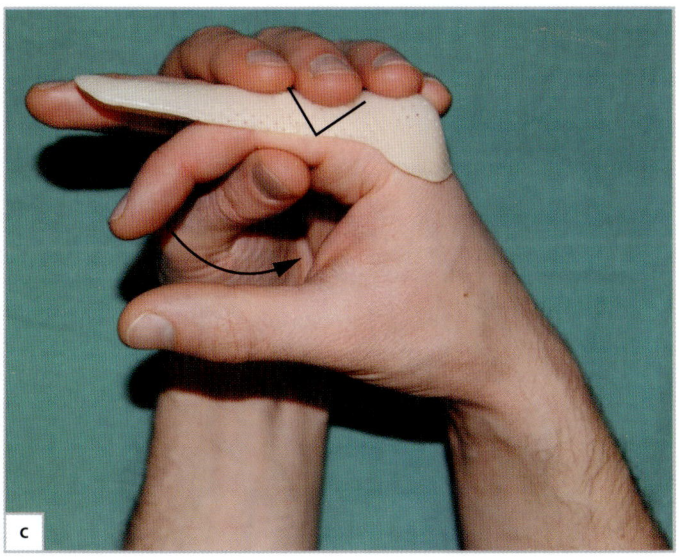

Figure 13.54 (a) An example of a dorsal splint that can facilitate extensor mechanism tendon gliding. (b and c) This same splint can be used for flexor digitorum profundus and flexor digitorum superficialis gliding exercises.

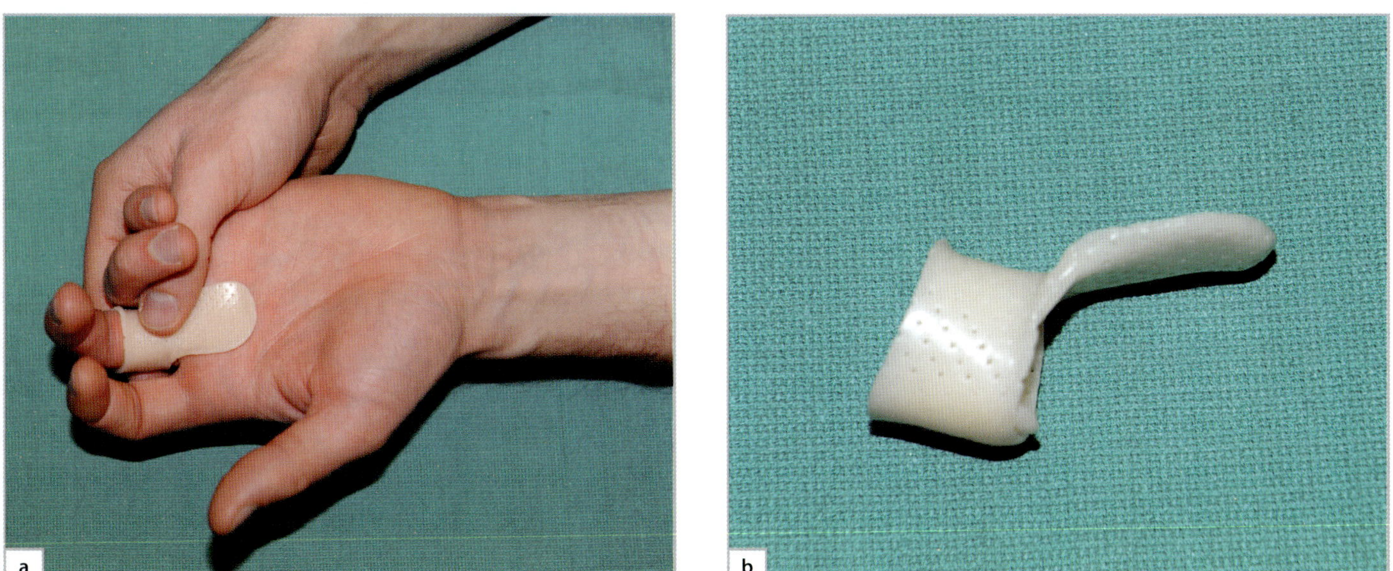

Figure 13.55a and b An exercise splint for effective single-finger active hook exercises.

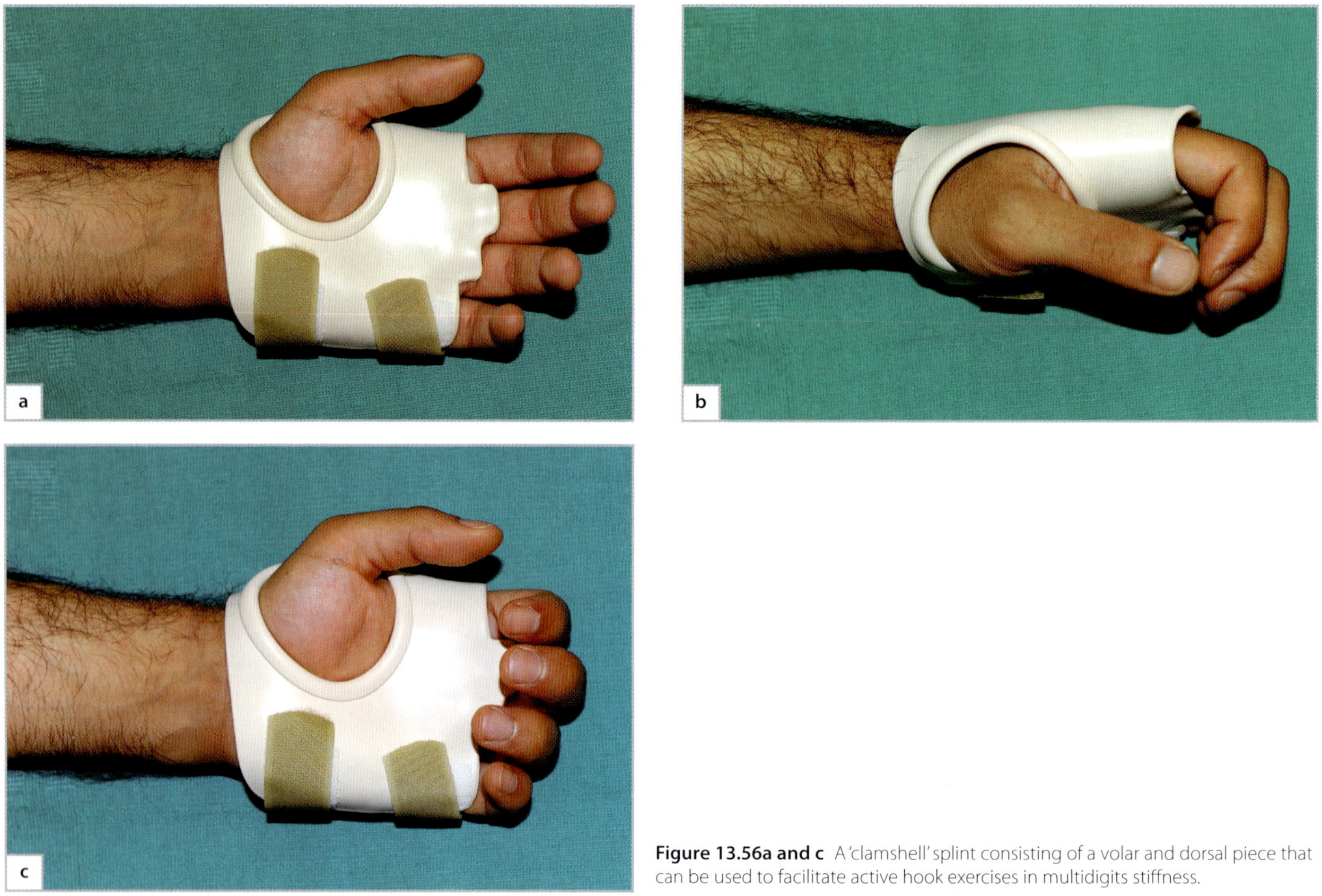

Figure 13.56a and c A 'clamshell' splint consisting of a volar and dorsal piece that can be used to facilitate active hook exercises in multidigits stiffness.

Mobilization phase and functional/strengthening phase

This is similar to the management for a P1 fracture.

Distal phalanx (P3) fractures

Early protective phase

A mallet or short gutter splint can be used for protection of tuft, shaft, and base P3 fractures. The therapist should begin desensitization and scar management at the involved fingertip/pulp as soon as the wound has healed. In addition, encourage intermittent active motion every hour the patient is out of the splint at the involved DIP joint for tuft or stable P3 shaft fractures. For a P3 base avulsion fracture, 6 weeks of immobilization in a mallet splint is recommended.

Mobilization phase

- Improve DIP joint flexion or reduce oblique retinacular ligament tightness with:
  - Blocking exercises with the PIP joint held in maximum extension for active DIP joint flexion
  - An exercise splint to allow blocking exercises as described above
- Manage extensor lag at the DIP joint:
  - For extensor lag < 30°: intermittent resting of the DIP joint in a mallet splint during the day
  - For extensor lag > 30°: full time in mallet splint for a period of time.
  - Blocking exercises to actively redirect extensor force to the DIP joint with the MCP joint and PIP joint held in slight flexion
- Incorporate desensitization with sensory stimulation from various textures, vibration, tapping, and deep pressure

Functional/strengthening phase

Resistive and progressive strengthening exercises should be utilized in this phase, especially for pinch and grip.

Interphalangeal joint dislocations and collateral ligament injuries

Early protective phase

Early protective motion can be initiated with buddy strapping for stable injuries at the fingers. As with other injuries, splinting is largely dependent upon the location of the injury:

- Ulnar collateral ligament (UCL)/radial collateral ligament (RCL) tears of the thumb – short-thumb spica for injury at the MCP joint; gutter splint for injury at the IP joint
- UCL/RCL tears at the MCP joints of the digits – hand-based intrinsic plus splint with the injured and adjacent MCP joints in 70° of flexion; free IP joints

- Volar dislocation of PIP joints – finger gutter splint with the PIP joint in extension; the DIP joint can be free for full motion and can also consider exercise gutter splint to allow PIP joint flexion to 30° and DIP joint flexion to 25° during the day
- Dorsal dislocation of the PIP joints – extension block splint that prevents full PIP joint extension while allowing full active flexion when the distal strap is removed

Mobilization and functional/ strengthening phase

A figure-of-eight splint at the PIP joint can be fitted to control deviation motion during the day (**Figure 13.57a–c**). It is important to help the patient regain motion at the involved joints with the various exercise or splinting techniques described earlier. Resume the functional use of the hand and grip/pinch strength with the strengthening exercises mentioned above.

THERAPY MANAGEMENT OF COMPLICATIONS AFTER A FRACTURE/SOFT TISSUE INJURY

Stiffness

Stiffness is commonly used to describe joints that are rigid and lacking full motion. Injuries at the hand can lead to stiffness when edema is not well managed, mobilization is delayed, or there is extensive tissue adherence over the joints. Stiffness in the hand can have a substantial impact on a patient's functional performance.

Therapy management for stiffness

- Edema control
- Adjunct use of physical agent modalities (e.g. superfical thermal heating agents, electrical stimulation devices, or ultrasound) to reduce pain and facilitate motion
- Exercise programs
  - Start active ROM as early as indicated
  - Provide instruction on home exercises for the patient to ensure frequent intermittent ROM exercise
  - Avoid aggressive exercises that can lead to more tissue damage, pain, and swelling.
  - Focus on improving functional motion such as flexion at the MCP joints and PIP joints, as well as thumb opposition at the CMC joint.
- Patient education on the use of the hand in functional activities
- Splinting
  - Most effective when splints can offer low load, and prolonged stretch
  - Serial static and dynamic splinting for slightly or moderately stiff joint
  - Serial progressive splinting or casting for very stiff joints
  - Exercise splints to block proximal joints to facilitate active redirection of forces towards the stiff joints

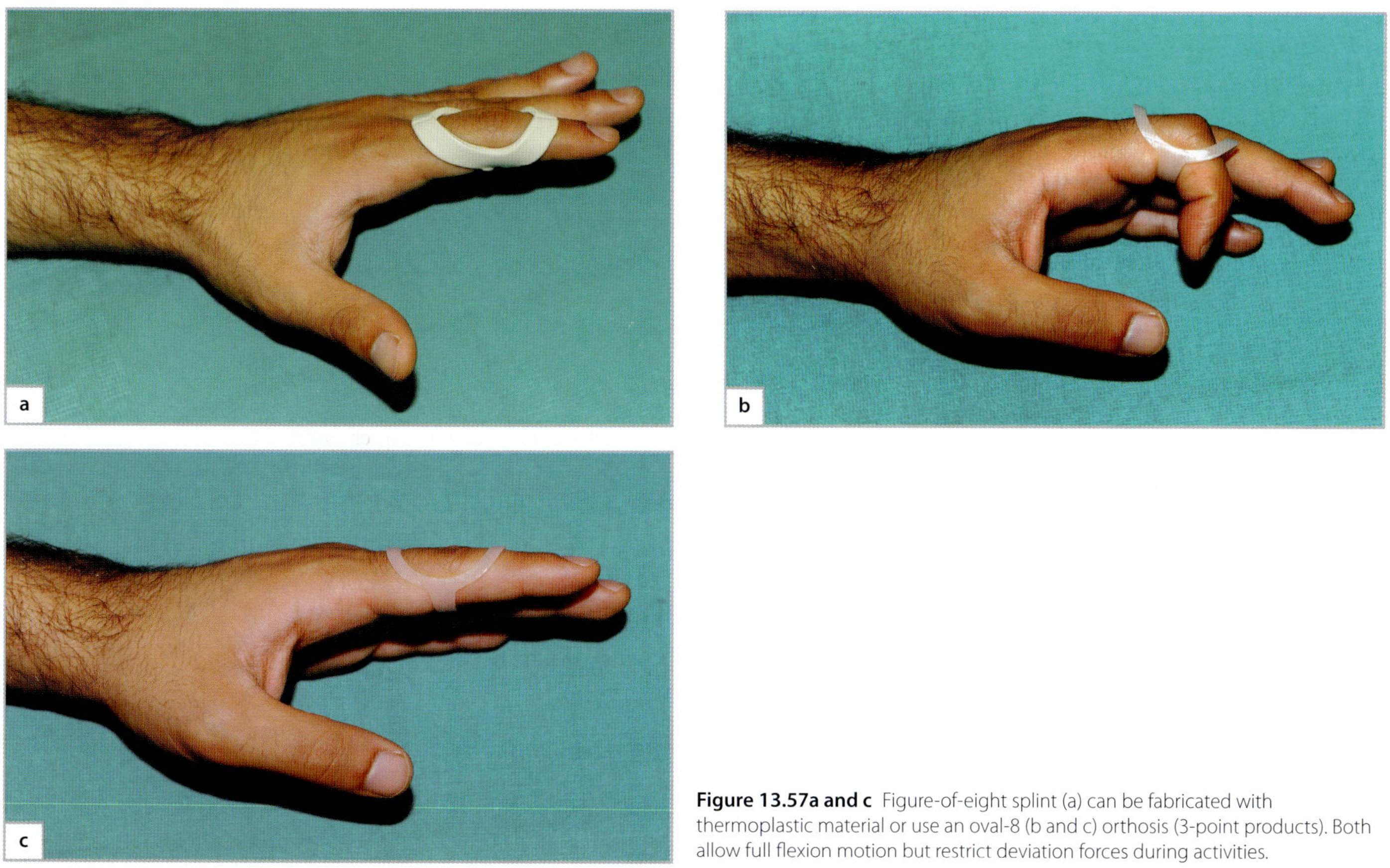

Figure 13.57a and c Figure-of-eight splint (a) can be fabricated with thermoplastic material or use an oval-8 (b and c) orthosis (3-point products). Both allow full flexion motion but restrict deviation forces during activities.

Complex regional pain syndrome

Patients with CRPS often experience substantial pain, sensory disturbances, and autonomic and motor dysfunction that typically limit the functional use of the affected hand. Hand therapy is usually the main conservative treatment for CRPS.

Therapy management for CRPS

- Pain control
  - Heat therapy
  - Transcutaneous electrical nerve stimulation machine treatment
  - Desensitization
  - Splints to allow intermittent rest of the affected digits or joints
- Edema control
- Exercise
  - Encourage gentle active or active assisted exercises within the patient's tolerance
  - Avoid aggressive exercises that cause more pain and swelling
  - Instruct on ways to normalize the pattern of motion to prevent repatterning of the motor cortex by using substitution motions
- Functional restoration
  - Encourage use of the affected limb in light activities
  - Introduce the use of adapted equipment or devices
  - Work simulation or hardening program
- Graded motor imagery (GMI)

Recent studies have implied that there are cortical changes in people with CRPS. GMI works to sequentially activate cortical reorganization without initially involved motion at the affected extremity. This technique consists of three stages that the patient progresses through as the pain improves (as described by Priganc & Stralka, 2011):

- Stage 1: Recognition of limb laterality
  - Patient learning to identify right or left hand from picture cards showing the hand in various positions
  - Aim to activate premotor cortices and re-establish body schema by discriminating between right and left
- Stage 2: Imagined hand movements
  - Patient to deliberately imagine moving the affected hand to adopt the posture shown in the picture cards
  - Aim to activate cortical mechanisms similar to executed movements without evoking pain
- Stage 3: Mirror therapy
  - Patient to slowly and smoothly adopt the posture in each picture card with the unaffected hand (and gradually together with the affected hand) while observing mirror reflection
  - Aim to correct sensorimotor incongruence, improve attention to the affected limb and reduce guarding motion

SUGGESTED READING

Ahearn D, Colditz JC. Exercise splint for effective single-finger active hook exercises. J Hand Ther 2005; 18:372–374.
Active hook exercises can facilitate efficient interphalangeal joint flexion and intrinsic muscles stretching. This article described the steps to fabricate an exercise splint to promote effective blocked active hook position.

Flowers KR, LaStayo PC. Effect of total end range time on improving passive range of motion. J Hand Ther 1994; 7:150–157.
The increase in passive range of motion of PIP joint contractures was found to be directly proportional to the length of time the joint is positioned at its total end range time (TERT). This theory complements a 'low-load prolonged stretch' protocol whereby the stiff joints should be stretched under low stress and for extended duration.

Flowers KR. A proposed decision hierarchy for splinting the stiff joint, with an emphasis on force application parameters. J Hand Ther 2002; 15:158–162.
This paper proposed a method to assess joint stiffness (called a Modified Weeks test, MWT) and to assist with the selection of an appropriate splint to remediate stiffness.

Feehan M, Bassett K. Is there evidence for early mobilization following an extraarticular hand fracture? J Hand Ther 2004; 17:300–308.
This systematic review found six level III studies that consistently suggested the potential of early mobilization in promoting earlier recovery of mobility and strength and earlier return to work, and also refuted that early mobilization affects fracture alignment.

Jones AR. A custom brace for treatment of angulated fifth metacarpal fractures. J Hand Surg 1996; 21:319–320.
This study has demonstrated that a custom metacarpal brace is similarly effective and safe in reducing and immobilizing angulated fifth metacarpal neck and shaft fractures as conventional closed reduction in an ulnar gutter cast.

Priganc VW, Stralka SW. Graded motor imagery. J Hand Ther 2011; 24:164–168.

Chapter 14 Burns

Keming Wang, Evan J. Kowalski, Kevin C. Chung

SURGICAL CARE AND MANAGEMENT OF HAND BURNS

EPIDEMIOLOGY

The hand functions to grasp and contact objects, making it the most commonly injured aspect of the body. According to a 2001–2011 report compiled by the American Burn Association, approximately 450,000 people in the United States each year sustain burns with sufficient severity to require medical treatment, causing about 3500 burn-related deaths. Forty-four per cent of burns are the result of fire or open flame, 32% are due to scalding incidents, 8.8% result from contact with a hot object, 4% are from an electrical injury, and 3.2% of burns are from chemical materials. Overall, males between 20 and 50 years of age are at the highest risk for burns.

Worldwide, an estimated 6 million people suffer from burn injuries annually. In the developing country of Sri Lanka, the overall mortality rate was 27% from burn injuries. In China, scalds constitute the majority of injuries (80.5%), whereas electrical burns account for 7.8%, followed by chemical burns comprising 6.9% of burn injuries. The highest risk group was found to be patients between 16 and 35 years of age, and in the pediatric population, preschool children sustained the majority of burns accounting for 29.4% of all burn victims. In Angola, the mortality rate of hospitalized burn patients was 21.3%, and all patients with 40% total body surface area (TBSA) burn died. It has been previously documented that approximately 39% of all burn injures involve the hands or upper extremity and that nearly 90% of all advanced burns affect one or both hands. The high incidence of hand burns demonstrates the importance of efficient and effective treatment for these injuries.

THERMAL BURNS

Hand burns occur quite commonly because the hands are exposed, leaving them vulnerable to burn injury. Burns in the hand and upper extremity have been shown to account for 50% of burn injuries in North America. Fadaak reported that hand burn injuries accounted for 49% of all burns in the Republic of Yemen.

PATHOLOGY

The temperature and duration of exposure determine the extent of tissue destruction hand burn injuries. Burns cause local tissue destruction in three specific zones, described by Jackson in 1947 (**Figure 14.1**):

- Zone of coagulation: The tissue of this zone experiences the maximum amount of damage. Excessively high temperature results in coagulation of constituent proteins and irreversible tissue loss
- Zone of stasis: Tissues in this zone are faced with decreased perfusion. This zone is salvageable, if adequate intervention such as local wound care is initiated to increase the tissue perfusion. Without appropriate intervention, circulation will cease, leading to tissue loss
- Zone of hyperemia: This zone is found below the zone of stasis and experiences increased perfusion due to nearby inflammation-induced mediators

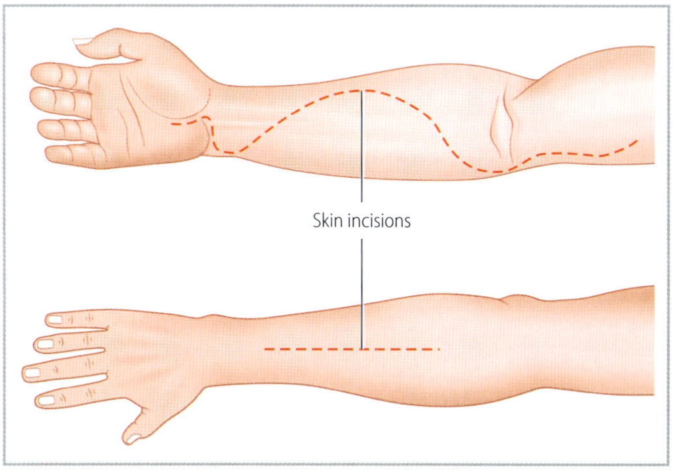

Figure 14.1 Jackson burn zones and the result of effective and ineffective treatment.

CLASSIFICATION

The depth of tissue destruction determines the degree of the burn and long-term hand functional outcome. According to the depth of the burn, hand burns are categorized as follows (**Figure 14.2**):

- First degree:
  - The burns involve only the superficial epidermis, with pain and erythema
  - The skin is dry and red, without blistering, and the epidermis barrier is intact
  - By about 1–4 days, the epidermis sloughs off, replaced by a new, healthy epidermis
- Second degree (superficial thickness burns):
  - The epidermis and superficial dermis are involved
  - The skin is red with the possibility of blister formation
  - Re-epithelialization occurs at approximately 10–14 days after injury
  - With proper care, these wounds heal without incident and ordinarily do not impair hand function
- Second degree (deep thickness burns):
  - The burns extend into the deep layers of the dermis
  - It may take 3 weeks to completely heal, with great risk of hypertrophic scar formation
- Third degree (full thickness burns):
  - The burns destroy all layers of dermis and skin appendages
  - The tissue is pale, contracted, insensate, and leathery
- Fourth degree:
  - Deep structures such as muscle, tendon, and bones are involved

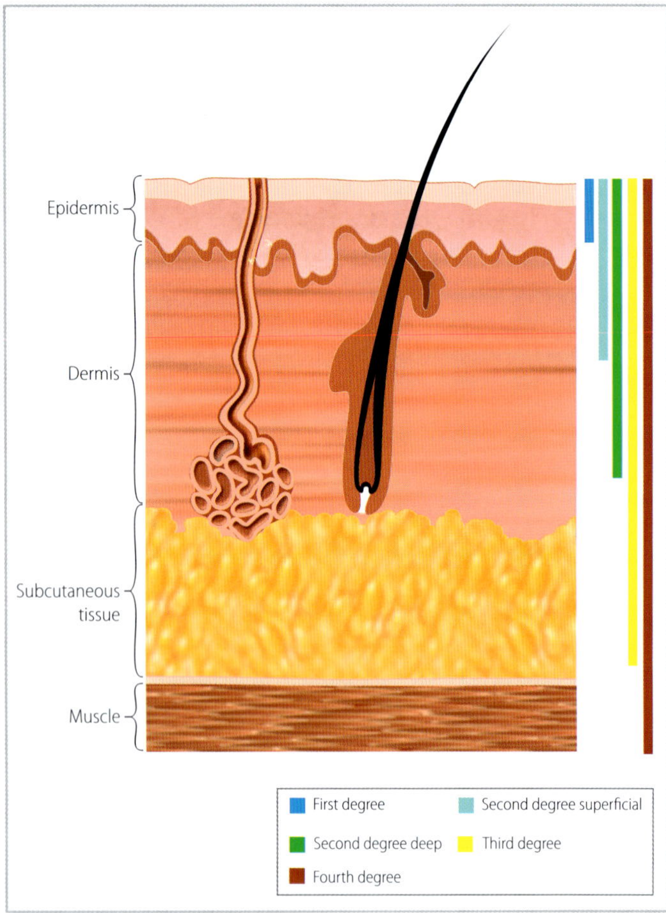

Figure 14.2 Burns are classified according to the layers of skin damaged.

INITIAL MANAGEMENT

A detailed history of the burn injury should be obtained. It is crucial to make a comprehensive trauma evaluation of the patient and determine the percentage of TBSA affected. The surface area of bilateral hand burns has been calculated to be 5% of TBSA (**Figure 14.3**). The decision must then be made whether to manage the patient as an inpatient or outpatient. Burns to the hand are an indication to move the patient into a burn unit for treatment.

The American Burn Association recommended that a burn victim be treated as an inpatient if the following criteria are met:

- Partial-thickness burns greater than 10% TBSA
- Burns involve the hand, face, feet, genitalia, perineum, or major joints
- Third-degree or fourth-degree burn injury
- Concomitant trauma such as a fracture

Nonoperative treatment

Adequate fluid administration and nutritional support is critical for severe hand burn injuries. Charles Baxter proposed the Parkland formula in 1964 for the total fluid requirement in 24 hours as follows:

1. 4 mL × TBSA (%)× body weight (kg)
2. 50% given in first 8 hours
3. 50% given in next 16 hours of the first day

Children should receive maintenance fluid in addition to the above fluid requirement, at an hourly rate of:

1. 4 mL/kg for the first 10 kg of body weight plus
2. 2 mL/kg for the second 10 kg of body weight plus
3. 1 mL/kg for >20 kg of body weight

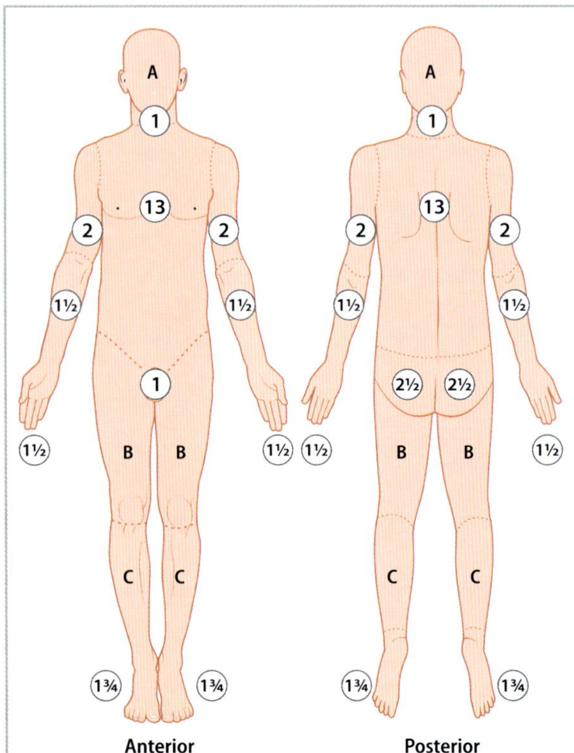

Relative percentage of body surface area (% BSA) affected by growth

	(A) Half of head	(B) Half of thigh	(C) Half of one lower leg
0 year	9½	2¾	2½
1 year	8½	3¼	2½
5 years	6½	4	2¾
10 years	5½	4¼	3
15 years	4½	4½	3¼

Tip: Patient's palm size is approximately 1% BSA

Figure 14.3 Relative percentage of body surface area (% BSA) affected by growth.

The infusion rate is determined by the urine output, not by the Parkland formula, and output of the urine should be maintained at a rate of:

- Adult 0.5–1 mL/kg/h
- Children 0.5–2 mL/kg/h

Local wound care

- One per cent silver sulfadiazine (SSD) cream maintains antibacterial properties for 8–10 hours and is commonly used twice per day (**Table 14.1**).
  - Transient leukopenia may present secondary to SSD use on a large burn wound, but it is self-limiting and has not been shown to be a major health concern
  - Choban reported that transient leukopenia presented in 60% of patients treated with SSD, predominately in patients with more than 15% TBSA. The white blood cell count returned to normal 24 hours after discontinuation of the drug
  - It is recommended to stop treatment with SSD in the event of transient leukopenia, and to switch to a different cream indicated for burn treatment, such as mafenide acetate
- Mafenide acetate (Sulfamylon) is an alternative agent with excellent burn eschar penetration and bacteriostatic action (**Table 14.1**).
  - Absorption of mafenide acetate may produce metabolic acidosis by inhibiting carbonic anhydrase activity, usually occurring after 3–5 days of use
  - Hyperventilation compensates for the acidosis in normal patients
  - Close monitoring of the acid-base balance is recommended during therapy
- Wound care should be initiated immediately after the burn event and continued until healing has occurred for the first and superficial second burn degree or excision and skin grafting for full-thickness injuries
- The local wound treatment for hand burns largely depends on the depth of a burn injury, making it crucial to quickly and accurately make this distinction. Generally, a rapid burn assessment and patient resuscitation begin simultaneously after occurrence of a burn injury. In addition, timely intervention can help to control the pathogenic factor, minimizes adverse consequences, prevents the zone of stasis from becoming coagulated, and obtains optimal functional outcomes.

TREATMENT OF VARIOUS DEGREES OF BURN INJURY

Treatment of first-degree and superficial thickness second-degree hand burns

- The burn wound should be washed with chlorhexidine gluconate, followed by the use of SSD to minimize infection rates
- Dressings should be changed twice per day, and each finger should be wrapped separately with the appropriate dressing
- Full passive range of motion exercises should be initiated twice daily for each joint approximately 24–48 hours after the burn event
- These wounds tend to heal within 2–3 weeks with no surgical intervention required

Treatment of deep thickness second-degree and third-degree hand burns

- Similar to a superficial burn injury, initial wound cleaning, and SSD use should be performed ahead of the surgical treatment, along with dressing changes twice per day
- If the hand or forearm is affected by a circumferential injury and edema continues to progress after the first 24 hours, circulatory compromise to the hand is an indication of escharotomy during the first 24–48 hours after injury. Delayed escharotomy can lead to a Volkmann contracture
- Timely removal of dead tissue and skin grafting minimize the risk of hypertrophic scarring and contracture formation
  - The principle behind excision is to preserve as much hand tissue as possible
  - A tourniquet should be used to minimize blood loss during debridement
  - Tissue viability should be verified after deflation of the tourniquet, and tissue with dubious viability should be preserved for possible recovery
- Skin grafts for the volar surface of the hand and fingers as well as for the release of burn contractures

Table 14.1 Topical antimicrobial agents

Agent	Indications	Dosage	Nursing implications
Silver sulfadiazine 1% (Silvadene)	• Most commonly used • Gram positive bacteria • Most gram negative bacteria • Minimal penetration of eschar	Apply approximately 11/6-inch thickness layer of cream twice daily	Leukopenia occurs within 2–4 days of initiation of therapy (rebound to normal leukopenia levels following onset within 2–3 days)
Mafenide acetate 5–10% (Sulfamylon) hydrophilic-based cream	• Effective against gram-negative and gram-positive organisms • Good penetration through the eschar • Dirty burn wounds • Infected burn wounds	Apply thin layer with sterile glove twice a day and leave open as prescribed; if the wound is dressed, change the dressing every 6 hours as prescribed	• Monitor arterial blood gas levels and discontinue as prescribed, if acidosis occurs • Premeditate the patient with an analgesic before applying mafenide acetate because this agent causes severe burning pain for up to 20 minutes after application

- The nonweight bearing aspect of the instep of the foot is an appropriate donor site for the palm that is superior to other skin donor sites
- Skin grafts for the dorsum of the hand
  - An adequate size skin graft is required to resurface the damaged area and restore normal hand function
  - Split-thickness grafts are more likely to survive in defects with less vascularity but are less robust in the presence of a severe contracture. Split-thickness skin grafts contract to as much as 30–50% of the original size as a result of secondary contraction
  - Full-thickness skin grafts undergo less contraction but require a better vascular bed for survival and are not commonly used for large wounds
  - Chandrasegaram compared full-thickness skin grafting versus split-skin grafting and found that the incidence of contractures with split-skin grafting was 26 versus 11% with full-thickness skin grafting
  - Burns JS and Chung CH compared the results of a hand splinted in a fist position and in a functional position after skin grafting. They found that the fist position improved the skin graft length of the dorsal surface of hand from 11–20% and the dorsal surface of the fingers 12–17%. The hand obtained good joint range of motion with immobilization for 7–9 days after skin grafting. In the fist position, all of the metacarpophalangeal (MCP) and proximal interphalangeal joint (PIP) joints of the fingers are flexed to 90° and the distal interphalangeal (DIP) joints to 30° of flexion. The thumb is at 90° of flexion and the wrist is placed at 20° flexion after skin grafting (**Figure 14.4**)
- The hands should be immobilized in a functional position 1 week before initiation of passive and active therapy. This position serves to protect hand function from contracture after skin grafting

Treatment of fourth-degree hand burns

- Deep hand burns with exposed tendons, joint capsules, or bones are difficult to manage
- Timely removal of dead tissue through debridement is critical
- Typically, skin grafting is not suitable to cover defects with tendon exposure, bone without periosteum, open joints, or exposed nerves
- Options for soft tissue coverage depend on the wound location, and pedicled flaps from the chest, abdomen, or groin can be used if available. The hand should be immobilized at the donor site for 2–3 weeks, after which time the hand can be divided from the pedicle
  - A groin flap can be used for a soft tissue defect of the digits or defects that encompass the entire palm or dorsum of the hand, with a maximum defect size of 10 × 25 cm
  - Urushidate reported that an abdominal wall flap (glove flap) was very useful for burns on the dorsal surface of the hand and fingers. This flap can provide functionally and aesthetically pleasing results, especially for the treatment of severe and extensive burns of the hand
  - Gao et al. obtained good functional and aesthetic results with a pedicled intercostal cutaneous flap at an average size of 9 × 12 cm for hands with extensive burns or burn scar contractures
- Passive and active hand therapy as well as scar management can be initiated early
  - It can be initiated at 1 week after skin grafting
  - Hand therapy can be initiated 2–3 weeks after pedicle flap reconstruction
- For patients with unstable IP or MCP joints, Kirschner-wire fixation should be considered to ensure proper joint positioning during the healing process to minimize the risk of joint contracture. The Kirschner wire is fixed within 2–3 days after injury and maintained for no more than 2–3 weeks.

Hand therapy

- Burn hands should be kept elevated at 45° to minimize edema
- Hands should be splinted in a position opposite to the anticipated deformity, mainly depending upon the phase of wound healing and the location of the injury
  - Typically, during the initial management of a patient, the hand should be splinted in a functional position as follows:
    - Interphalangeal joints in extension and MCP joints in 70–90° of flexion (**Figure 14.5**)
    - The thumb in abduction with the first web space maximally open
    - The wrist in 20–30° of extension
  - When a burn injury affects the extensor tendon of the PIP joint, splinting the PIP joint at full extension with 6 weeks of immobilization is required for sufficient healing
  - For skin grafts on the dorsal surface of hand, the fist position is preferred during splinting to minimize the incidence of skin contractures

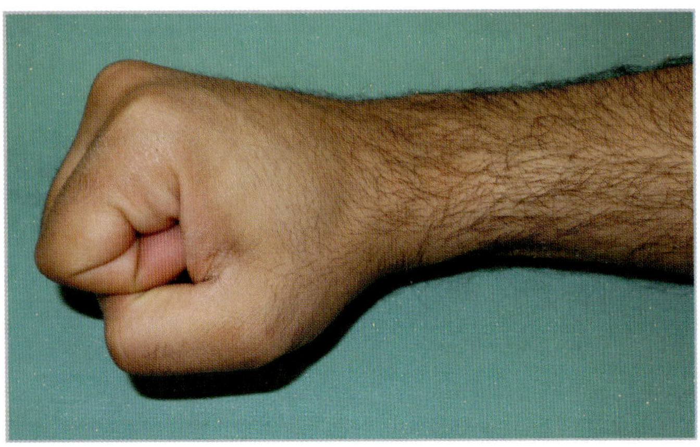

Figure 14.4 Full fist position, in which all the joints are flexed maximally.

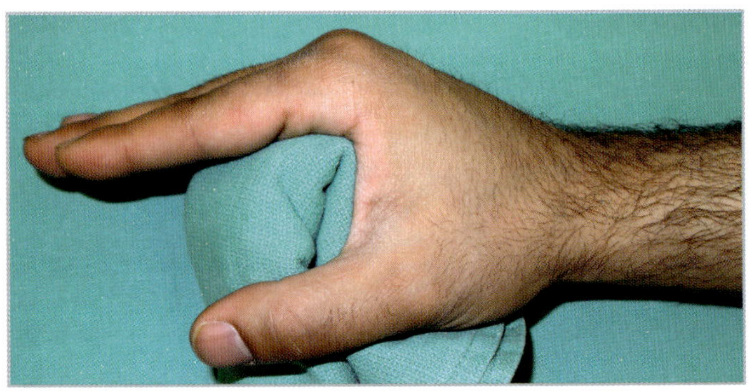

Figure 14.5 Functional position, in which the interphalangeal joints are held in extension and the metacarpophalangeal joints are held in 70–90° flexion.

- For a fourth-degree burn, splinting the hand in an anticlaw position is recommended
  - Kirschner wires can be used to fix the joints in extension if required

Hand function measurements

Total active motion (TAM) is measured using a dorsal goniometer with the wrist in a neutral position and the forearm in pronation. Calculate the TAM for each digit, including the MCP joint, PIP joint, and DIP joint. The TAM for the thumb MCP and IP joints should also be calculated.

COMPLICATIONS

Infection

Patients with large surface area burns have a higher risk of infection, and therefore, local wound care and daily observation of wounds is crucial. Early removal of any necrotic tissue and coverage with a skin graft decreases the incidence of infection.

Skin and soft tissue contractures

Contractures may result from inadequate size or thickness of skin grafts, hypertrophic scar and keloid formation, inadequate splinting, and inadequate physical therapy. After contracture formation, surgical release and split-thickness skin grafting should be considered to restore function.

Hypertrophic burn scars

Hypertrophic burn scars limit hand function and damage the cosmetic appearance of the hand. These scars most likely occur in hand burns that have not healed within 3 weeks. Many factors contribute to the development of hypertrophic burn scars, such as skin color and age, depth of burn, mechanical tension of the wound, and extended healing time owing to infection.

- Skin color and age:
  - An increase in pigmentation of the skin will reduce the levels of vitamin D-3 production, which plays an important role in decreasing the incidence of scar formation
  - In younger patients, the increased amount of collagen production tends to result in hypertrophic scar formation
- Depth of burn:
  - Burn injuries that involve the reticular dermis are prone to hypertrophic scar formation
  - Burns involving the papillary dermis often heal without scarring
- Mechanical tension of the wound:
  - An increased wound tension will upregulate epidermis proliferation and angiogenesis, factors that lead to hypertrophic scarring
- Extended healing time owing to infection:
  - Deitch et al. reported that if the burn wound heals within 14 days, patients seldom had scar formation, with the exception of black patients.
  - When the burn wound healed between 14 and 21 days, 33% of the anatomic sites developed hypertrophic scarring
  - If the burn wound healed after 21 days, hypertrophic scars formed on 78% of the burn sites

Early active range of motion exercises and appropriate splinting can decrease the risk of hypertrophic burn scar formation. For severe hand burn patients, even with adequate initial treatment the normal healing process may lead to these deformities. Shortly after wound healing, it is recommended to apply almost 24 hours of constant pressure to the burn scar to minimize the occurrence of hypertrophic burn scars. A pressure garment is the recommended intervention for the prophylactic management of a hypertrophic burn scar. Steroid injections are considered helpful at the early phase of scar formation. Triamcinolone acetone can be administered as an intralesional injection at 10 mg/cm^2 of scar tissue.

Web space contracture

This is the most commonly reported deformity after web space burns. Surgical treatment is required for all web space contractures to increase abduction of the digits.

Z-plasty

A Z-plasty is recommended for the release of a simple web space contracture (**Figure 14.6**):

- Z-plasty transposition flaps are designed along the line of scar tension, and with an optimal rotation angle of 60°, web space length can improve by up to 75%
- These flaps are particularly useful to release linear web space contractures

Trapeze-flap plasty

Grishkevich reviewed over 500 web space contractures and identified three anatomical types of first web space contractures: edge, medial, and total.

- The study recommended the management with a trapeze-flap plasty (**Figure 14.7**) for a medial contracture. The flap is designed perpendicular to the contracted line and formed on the contracted surface and can result in 100% improvement in web space length. This flap is also suitable for thick and rough scars that are not easily rotated with a Z-plasty.

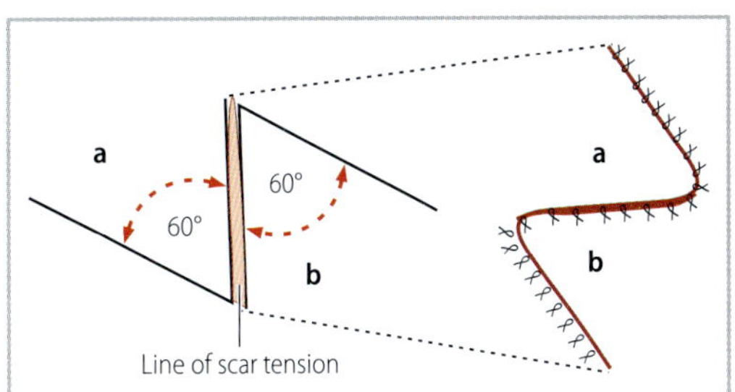

Figure 14.6 Z-plasty transposition flap for scar contracture revision.

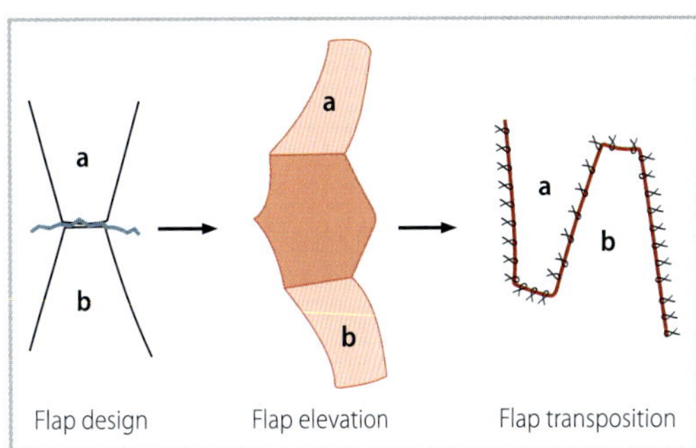

Figure 14.7 Trapeze-flap plasty for scar contracture revision.

Flaps

When the web space contracture is severe, local skin is often insufficient to fulfill the depths of the space. Free tissue transfers or regional flaps are recommended, including groin flaps, lateral arm flaps, and anterolateral thigh flaps.

OUTCOMES

- Zuijlen assessed the function of 143 burned hands by seven objective test criteria and found that 80% of the hands regained normal function with early excision and grafting treatment
- Ahmed Omar evaluated 40 patients with deep second- and third-degree burns, comparing the treatment of early excision and skin grafting versus delayed skin grafting
  - The study determined that 92% of patients managed in a timely fashion were able to return to normal function compared with only 65% of patients with delayed management
- Covey et al. treated deep hand burn injuries with early excision and grafting.
  - Seventy-five per cent of patients had normal TAM and 67% of patients obtained normal grip strength at one-year follow-up
- Holavanahalli reported that in 32 patients with fourth-degree burns, 50% had an amputation and 22% had a boutonnière deformity.

SUGGESTED READING

Chandrasegaram MD, Harvey J. Full-thickness vs split-skin grafting in pediatric hand burns – a 10-year review of 174 cases. Burn Care Res 2009; 30:867–871.

This study assessed the incidence of contractures following grafting of pediatric hand burns in 174 patients. The authors found that the incidence of contractures in the full thickness group was 2% versus 27% in the split-thickness graft group. In addition, when the grafted area was across the metacarpophalangeal (MCP) joints, the incidence of contractures in split-thickness group was documented as 43%. Where the skin grafting occurred on the palmar aspect of the hand, the incidence of contractures in the split-thickness group was 67%, with 50% requiring reoperative release. They concluded that full thickness skin grafts were preferred in the treatment of acute hand burns, particularly where the burn involved the surface of the palm and the MCP joints.

Deitch EA, Wheelahan TM, Rose MP. Hypertrophic burn scars: analysis of variables. J Trauma 1983; 23:895–898.

The authors evaluated the risks associated with the development of hypertrophic burn scars. They found that if the wound healed from 10 to 14 days, the risk of hypertrophic burn scar formation was lower than wounds that took longer than 14 days to heal. However, in patients that healed in 14–21 days, one third of the patients experienced wound problems, and for wounds that healed after 21 days, 78% of the burn sites became hypertrophic.

Grishkevich VM. First web space post-burn contracture types: contracture elimination methods. Burns 2011; 37:338–347. Epub 18 September 2010.

This study reported on the methods of contracture release in 500 cases with a first web space post-burn contracture. The authors preferred the trapeze-flap plasty technique for the three basic types of contractures, including edge, medial, and total adduction contractures. They concluded that a trapeze-flap plasty, providing a length gain of 100% to 200%, could be widely used in the treatment of hand border contractures.

Maslauskas K, Rimdeika R, Rapoliene J, Ramanauskas T. Analysis of burned hand function (early versus delayed treatment). Medicina (Kaunas) 2005; 41:846–851.

This study analyzed the hand functional outcomes in 79 patients with deep partial thickness hand burns treated by early and delayed surgery. Debridement and immediate split thickness skin grafting performing during the first 7 days after burn event were considered as the early treatment. At 12-month follow-up, the patients in the early treatment group obtained better outcomes than the delayed treatment group regarding key pinch and grasp pinch of the hand.

Mohammadi AA, Bakhshaeekia AR, Marzban S. Early excision and skin grafting versus delayed skin grafting in deep hand burns (a randomised clinical controlled trial). Burns 2011; 37:36–41.

The study compared early and delayed skin grafting by divided patients with hand burns into two groups, one group to be treated within 6.68 hours of burn injury, and the other group be treated at 32.4 hours after burn injury. They used the DASH questionnaire to evaluate the functional outcome after 6–8 months and found that the disability scores of five activities had no difference between the early excision group and delayed skin grafting group regarding function, sensation, scar formation, daily activity limitation, and overall satisfaction.

ELECTRICAL BURNS

EPIDEMIOLOGY

Electrical burns are the fourth leading cause of burn injury in the United States, accounting for 4% of total burn admissions from 2001 to 2011 in 91 burn centers. More than 500 deaths are also due to electrical injury per year. The majority of electrical injuries are work related (57%), with men at a higher risk of exposure to these burns. In the developing country of South Africa, low-voltage injuries are more common than high-voltage injury. Opara documented that the mortality rate for electrical burns was 12.5% in Nigeria. Luz found that the mortality rate was 11.5% for high-voltage injuries in Brazil, and that the majority of electrical burn patients were young men at the beginning of their professional lives. Vierhapper reported that the mortality rate was <5% in the developed country of Austria.

Electrical burns can be divided into two separate categories: (1) High-voltage electrical current burns (typically > 1000 volts) and (2) low-voltage electrical current burns (<1000 volts). In Brazil, Luz reported that among all electrical burn injury patients, low-voltage electrical burns accounted for 20%, 60% suffered high electrical burns, and 20% sustained a flash burn injury.

PATHOLOGY

An electrical injury is different from a thermal burn injury in two major aspects:

- The injury agent is electricity.
  - Tissue damage is caused by the conversion of electrical energy into heat
  - High-voltage injuries lead to extensive deep tissue damage, and the damage is far beyond what can be predicted by TBSA involvement
  - Experimental studies have shown that an electrical injury can cause skeletal muscle necrosis with only minimal thermal changes
- The mechanism of effect is the coagulation of tissue
  - The current passes through a point of contact (a small skin defect), and the generated heat destroys the deep tissue before exiting to an electrical sink
  - The exposure time and magnitude of current flow determine the extent of tissue damage

Voltage effects

- Current is converted into heat, which can be depicted by the formula $J = I^2 RT$
  - J indicates joules
  - I represents current
  - R is resistance
  - T designates time
  - According to Ohm's law, $I = V/R$, in which V signifies voltage
- Resistance is the tendency of tissue to resist the flow of electrical current
  - Each tissue has a specific resistance
  - The higher the resistance of the tissue, the greater heat will be generated by the electrical energy at any given current
- Resistance of tissue:
  - The highest resistance is found in bones, fat, and tendons
  - Skin has an intermediate resistance
  - The least resistance is found in nerves, blood, and muscles
    - Blood vessels with the least resistance can provide the most accessible path for a current
    - The generated heat may coagulate the blood vessels, and if both veins and arteries are destroyed in a high-voltage injury, the hand may have to be amputated
- In a low-voltage injury, the lesion is localized and limited to the contact area and subjacent tissue
- For a high-voltage injury, the generated thermal burn can destroy the skin and deep structures of the hand
  - The lesion involvement is larger and deeper than a low-voltage injury

INITIAL MANAGEMENT

The aim of management is to achieve maximum hand function outcomes and decrease amputation rates. According to the American Burn Association, all electrical burn victims should be admitted to the hospital for inpatient treatment.

History

- Determine the type of electrical source:
  - Low voltage or high voltage
  - Mechanism of injury:
    - Direct contact or indirect contact
- Medical history such as cardiac disease

Examination

A comprehensive evaluation of an electrical burn patient is crucial. Approximately 15% of patients with electrical burns also suffer from a traumatic injury. Often, the patient is thrown from their original position or falls from a high elevation upon exposure to electrical current. Physical examination should include:

- Cardiac injury: Cardiac involvement is not common, but it can be devastating. Electrocardiogram (ECG) and cardiac enzymes are helpful diagnostic tools
- Skin examination should be performed to assess the site of entry and the exit wound. A minimal entry or exit wound does not always indicate a minor electrical injury
- Hand and forearm examinations should test the function of muscles and nerves, capillary refill, and look for signs of compartment syndrome or possible fractures
  - Doppler ultrasonography is helpful to assess the perfusion of the palmar arch and distal digital capillary refill

It is important to monitor a patient's ECG for 24 hours after admission to the hospital. Patients require continued cardiac monitoring when these conditions are met:

- High-voltage injury regardless of the ECG result
- Low-voltage injury with an abnormal ECG at the emergency department
- A history of loss of consciousness regardless of voltage
- Abnormal ECG at the emergency department
- Past medical history of cardiac disease

Early treatment

- Fluid management is critical in patients with electrical burns. After an electrical injury, fluid extravasation into the third space compartment will lead to fluid loss. Muscle destruction may cause significant myoglobinuria, which can lead to renal failure
- Adequate fluid resuscitation with Ringer lactate or normal saline is essential
  - Initial fluid administration should produce a urine output at 70–100 mL/h until urine is cleared of pigment. Urine output should then be maintained at 30–50 mL/h or 0.5–1 mL/kg/h
  - Luce reported that the fluid resuscitation required when treating an electrical burn was approximately 1.7 times the calculated fluid requirement as that of a thermal burn of the same TBSA
- SSD cream and mafenide acetate (Sulfamylon) are to be used as indicated for thermal burns

SURGICAL PROCEDURES

Indications of surgical treatment

There are four main indications of surgical management of electrical burns:

1. Progressive neurologic dysfunction
2. Vascular compromise
3. Increased muscle compartment pressure (measurement >30 mmHg)
4. Systemic clinical deterioration from suspected ongoing myonecrosis

Timing of surgical procedure

Early exploration and surgical care is essential for high-voltage injuries. Observation is appropriate for low-voltage injuries, unless the patient shows signs of any of the four surgical indications described above. Early fasciotomy and nerve tunnel release help prevent extrinsic pressure on the nerves. Early exploration and decompression will prevent secondary tissue damage and associated complications resulting from tissue edema and necrosis. Delayed exploration and decompression of the compromised upper extremity may result in increased amputation rates and organ failure. Alexander reported escharotomy and fasciotomies were performed in 47% of the patients, all on the day of admission, with an amputation rate of 19.1%.

Surgical treatment options

- Exploration: The damaged tendons, muscles, nerves, and joint capsules need to be identified. Not only the superficial muscle, but also the deep layer muscle adjacent to the bone should be investigated
- Debridement: Any necrotic tissue should be removed, but the muscle with questionable viability should be preserved for re-exploration, and nerves should be left intact for potential functional recovery
- Fasciotomy: A forearm fasciotomy (**Figure 14.8a**) is used to decompress the carpal tunnel and the flexor compartment
  - The incision for a carpal tunnel release (**Figure 14.9**) should not be performed any further radial than the radial border of the ring finger. The extensor compartment incision is performed over the dorsal surface of the forearm (**Figure 14.8b**)
  - The intrinsic muscles of the hand should be decompressed to release the epimysium if it is causing constriction
  - Guyon canal and cubital tunnel release are considered when ulnar nerve dysfunction is present
- Repetitive debridement of necrotic tissue and subsequent closure: Muscle tissue may appear viable at first exploration and should be re-evaluated 2–3 days later until wound closure can be achieved. Before wound coverage, wound care is required similar to that for a thermal burn injury
  - Serial debridement is necessary to identify the extent of devitalized tissue. If bone, tendon, or joints are exposed after debridement, local or distal flap coverage is preferred, following the same guidelines as for thermal burns
  - Handschin et al. reported that a free flap is not recommended during the first 4 weeks after the inciting electrical injury event, for the following reasons:
    - Progressive endothelial damage to the arteries may lead to thrombosis during this period.
    - Local or distal pedicle-flap reconstruction can provide new blood supply and protect the wound from bacterial invasion.
- Amputation: When the electrical injury results in a septic hand or gangrene from deep tissue damage in association with destruction of vessels, amputation is necessary

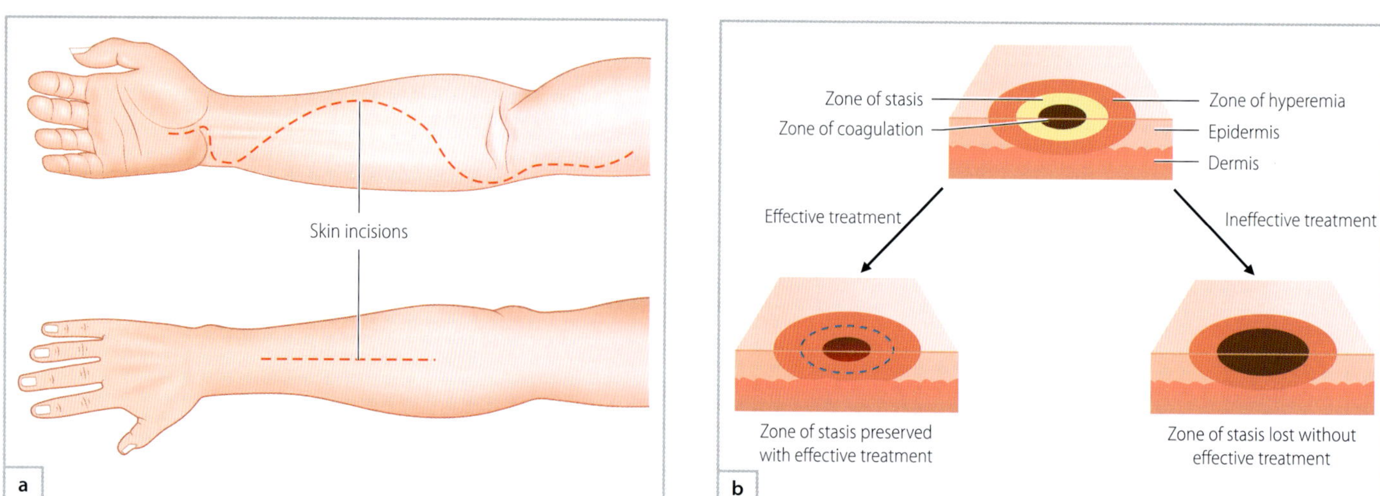

Figure 14.8 (a) Lazy S-shaped skin incision for volar fasciotomy. (b) Skin incision for extensor compartment.

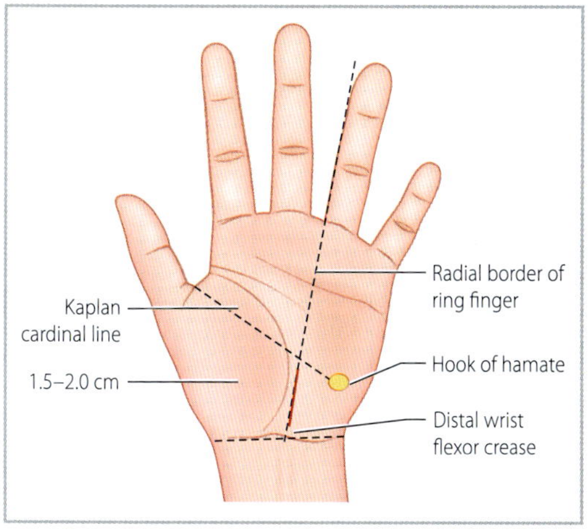

Figure 14.9 Skin incision for carpal tunnel release.

Hand therapy

Hand therapy should be initiated following the same guidelines as that of a thermal burn injury.

COMPLICATIONS

- Arnoldo documented complications in 700 electrical injury admissions:
  - Amputation rate was 37%
  - Muscle necrosis was 9.7%
  - Sepsis rate was approximately 1.6%
- Handschin reported an amputation rate of 19.1% in 68 patients with high-voltage electrical injuries
- Maghsoudi found the amputation rate to be 11% in 109 patients with high-voltage electrical injuries and 3.5% in 85 patients with low-voltage injuries
- Achauer et al. reported that 40% of patients required hand or digit amputation after severe electrical injuries

SUGGESTED READING

Achauer B, Applebaum R, Vander Kam VM. Electrical burn injury to the upper extremity. Br J Plast Surg 1994; 47:331–340.

This study presented experience on 22 patients with electrical injuries to the hand and described the guidelines in the formulated management of this injury. The authors preferred early extensive debridement of all damage tissues, including compartment release if indicated. The pedicled groin flap was the most commonly operative treatment used for salvaging hands severely injured by electrical burns. Guidelines for management of moderate to severe electrical hand injuries are also outlined.

Arnoldo BD, Purdue GF, Kowalske K, et al. Electrical injuries: a 20-year review. J Burn Care Rehabil 2004; 25:479–484.

This study reviewed 700 electrical injuries, finding that 95.4% of these injuries were men. Of all of the injuries, electrical arc injuries comprised the largest group (40%), with the lowest mortality rate (1.1%) and no amputation occurrence. The amputation rate was highest in high-voltage injuries (34%), with a mortality rate of 5.3%. Compared with high-voltage injuries, low-voltage injuries had a lower amputation rate (4%) and mortality rate (2.8%). Neurologic complications after all burn injuries were reported to be as high as 29%, more commonly in high-voltage group.

Chudasama S, Goverman J, Donaldson JH. Does voltage predict return to work and neuropsychiatric sequelae following electrical burn injury? Ann Plast Surg 2010; 64:522–525.

Reviewing the outcomes from 115 patients, this study looked at the differences between high- and low-voltage injuries, regarding the outcomes of neuropsychiatric sequelae and return to work. High-voltage injuries and low-voltage injuries experienced similar rates of neuropsychiatric sequelae and similar delays in returning to work. Final impairments rates for the high-voltage injuries (17.5%) were shown to be greater than that of low-voltage groups (5.3%).

Handschin AE, Vetter S, Jung FJ, et al. A case-matched controlled study on high-voltage electrical injuries vs thermal burns. J Burn Care Res 2009; 30:400–407.

This study provided and analyzed results on the surgical management of high-voltage electrical injuries compared with that of thermal burns using a case-controlled study design. Sixty-eight patients were placed in each group. The complication rate was 57.6% in the high-voltage electrical burn group versus 36.7% in the thermal burns group. The amputation rates (19.5% vs 1.5%), escharotomy/fasciotomy rates (47% vs 21%), and the total days of hospitalization (44 vs 32 days) were significantly (p <0.05) higher in the high-voltage electrical injury group compared with the thermal burn group. When performing flap coverage, a pedicled flap was preferred over a free flap for high-voltage electrical injuries treated within 4 weeks of trauma.

Mann R, Gibran N, Engrav L. Is immediate decompression of high voltage, electrical injuries to the upper extremity always necessary? J Trauma 1996; 40:584–587.

This study reviewed the treatment of 62 patients representing 100 upper extremities with electrical burns. In this study, 22% of the extremities were decompressed within 24 hours of injury. Immediate decompression was only required under the following conditions: numbness and tingling or neurologic deterioration, impending compartment syndrome include severe pain, and loss of arterial Doppler signal. The authors recommended selective decompression and early closure as the management protocol for high-voltage electrical injuries.

CHEMICAL BURNS

EPIDEMIOLOGY

Approximately 3% of all burn injuries are due to chemical exposure in the United States, with a higher frequency reported in males than in females. The majority of chemical injury was work related (51.8%) in the United States, according to a 2001–2011 report compiled by the American Burn Association. In China, chemical burn injuries account for 6.6–11.8% of all burn patients, and patients are mainly peasant workers. Maghsoudi reported that 58.7% of chemical burn injuries were sustained by peasant workers in the developing country of Iran. Hardwike found that >75% of chemical burns occurred in the domestic or industrial setting in the United Kingdom, with a male to female ratio of 6.4:1. Most chemical injuries occur while chemical substances are being handled, such as during transport or distribution, leaving the hands and upper extremity as the most frequent site of injury.

CLASSIFICATION

Chemical injuries can be classified into four groups:

- Acid burns
  - Sulfuric acid and hydrofluoric acid are the two most frequent chemical agents
  - Contact with very small amounts of acid can be fatal
  - Characterized by severe pain
- Alkali burns
  - Most common agent resulting in cutaneous burns
  - Characterized by a burning sensation
- Phosphorus burns
  - Common in military applications or fertilizers
- Chemical injection injury
  - Resulting from industrial accidents

Severity

The severity of chemical injuries typically depends on the:

- Composition of the agent
- Concentration of the agent
- Duration of contact with the agent
- Amount of substance contacting the skin

Chemical injuries have some important characteristics that distinguish them from to thermal burns:

- They occur through protein coagulation rather than a burning process
- There is a longer exposure to chemical substances, not just a momentary exposure
- The chemical agent will continue to cause progressive damage until entirely removed from the patient
- Chemical components may be absorbed, with a potential for systemic toxicity

INITIAL MANAGEMENT

According to the American Burn Association, all chemical burn victims should be admitted to the hospital for inpatient treatment.

History

- Obtain a detailed history of the injury that includes:
  - Type of chemical agent
    - Hydrofluoric/sulfuric acid
    - Strong alkali
    - Other substances
  - Medical history such as cardiac disease
    - For a hydrofluoric acid burn injury, calcium gluconate is administered for pain relief, which may cause cardiac arrhythmia

Physical examination

A comprehensive examination should be performed as a part of the initial evaluation to determine all of the affected areas and the presence of systemic toxicity. Chemical agents can penetrate and cause deeper necrosis, and it is difficult to determine burn depth during the initial patient evaluation. An area that is initially believed to be a partial thickness burn may turn out to be deep tissue burn, which would change the treatment protocol.

Initial treatment

- Remove the chemical agent:
  - The initial treatment involves removal of the chemical agent and any involved clothing that has been contaminated by the chemical
  - Powdered agents should be brushed from the skin without the use of water
    - Chemical powders such as dry lime react with water and need to be wiped off the skin
- Using neutralizing agents is controversial, with no clear consensus on an appropriate treatment regimen, and therefore, this type of treatment should be avoided
- Irrigate chemical fluids with copious amounts of water:
  - Skin areas in contact with a chemical fluid should be irrigated with copious amounts of water or isotonic saline
  - Irrigation must be continued until the tissue pH reaches a physiologic level
    - The length of time for irrigation varies greatly and can be up to 12 hours
    - Patients strong alkali should receive prolonged hydrotherapy
  - Avoid putting hands in a tub, because this may spread the chemical agent and damage other areas

Treatment

Conservative treatment

- Thorough debridement and cleaning of the wound
- Dressing changes should be performed every ≥ 2 days if necessary
- Topical agents, such as 1% silver sulphadiazine and mafenide acetate (Sulfamylon), are recommended as indicated for thermal burns

Surgical treatment

- Early excision and immediate split-thickness or full-thickness skin grafting and various skin flaps can be applied to cover the wounds, with the same principles as thermal burns

COMPLICATIONS

The complications resulting from chemical burns, including infections, hypertrophic scars, and contractures and the associated treatments are similar to that of thermal burn injury patients.

Compartment syndrome

Surgical release of the fascial compartment and carpal tunnel with delayed closure of the wound should be performed with the same guidelines as electrical injuries.

Systemic intoxication

Systemic toxicity occurs secondary to depletion of total body stores of calcium and magnesium, resulting in enzymatic and cellular dysfunction, and ultimately in cell death. It is uncommon, but patients with large TBSA exposed to chemical agents may have a high risk of systemic toxicity. Hemodialysis is an effective treatment for systemic intoxication.

SUGGESTED READING

Anderson WJ, Anderson JR. Hydrofluoric acid burns of the hand: mechanism of injury and treatment. J Hand Surg Am 1988; 13:52–57.
This study reported the outcomes of hydrofluoric acid burn injury of the hands in 14 adults, describing the mechanism as well as the treatment for these burns. The overall results were satisfying, and all patients returned to their previous job. The authors preferred prompt recognition and immediate skin cleaning management, using calcium gluconate for pain relief. Delayed treatment led to permanent impairment in two patients.

Cartotto RC, Peters WJ, Neligan PC. Chemical burns. Can J Surg 1996; 39:205–211.
This study discussed chemical burns and outlined the fundamental principles of chemical burn management. They found that chemical burns account for 2% to 4% of all burn admissions, and that immediate removal of the chemical agent was crucial for optimal results. After irrigation, local wound care and pain relief management were also recommended. The authors noted that it is important to be aware of any possible systemic absorption of the agent.

Palao R, Monge I, Ruiz M. Chemical burns: pathophysiology and treatment. Burns 2010; 36:295–304. Epub 28 Oct 2009.
The authors described the common agents of chemical injury, the basic management, and specific recommendations for proper treatment of these injuries. The key points in chemical burns treatment included removal of the chemical, dilution, examination of the burn, avoiding systemic toxicity, general support, and local care of the burn wound.

Young RC, Ho WS, Ying SY, Burd A. Chemical assaults in Hong Kong: a 10-year review. Burns 2002; 28:651–653.
This study assessed patients with chemical assault burn injuries in Hong Kong over a 10-year period. Chemical burn assault burn injuries were found to account for 0.8% of all burn patients, and 55% of these patients experienced upper limb burns. Alkaline chemicals were identified as the causal agent in 47% of all cases, whereas acid was responsible for 32% of these types of burns.

Chapter 15 High-pressure jet injection injuries

Keming Wang, Evan Kowalski, Kevin C. Chung

INTRODUCTION

Rees was the first to describe the high-pressure jet injection injury, documenting a diesel fuel injection injury in 1937. He determined that a pressure of only 700 kPa (100 psi) is sufficient to bleach the skin, but many different types of commercial and industrial equipment far exceed this pressure. A commercial spray paint gun may increase this pressure by as much as 30 times, and hydraulic machinery can reach pressures ranging from 14,000-20,000 kPa. Although the direct pressure from a high-pressure injection injury can cause substantial tissue damage, the injected material may lead to secondary events, including a damaging inflammatory response, compression ischemia, and progressive tissue necrosis.

EPIDEMIOLOGY

These injuries are more common in developing countries than in other parts of the world. Schoo et al. reported that high-pressure injection injuries of the hand were uncommon, with a rate of 0.1% among 3000 hand injuries emergency patients in Denver, Colorado, USA. Bekler reported that patients treated with high-pressure injection injuries of the hand accounted for 2% of all hand operations each year in the United Kingdom, most commonly to the index finger (35%) and nondominant hand (57%). Another study from Kentucky, USA, found that the majority (84%) of these injuries occurred in workers performing manual labor tasks, especially males between the ages of 19–64 years. Among 76 patients with high-pressure injection injuries of the hand, 65 patients sustained injuries to the digits, whereas 16 of the injuries occurred in other areas of the upper limb. Wong described the most commonly injured age group in China to be 35–40 years. The left hand and index finger were the most frequently involved sites, with injury rates of 89 and 64%, respectively.

Injectable materials

The composition of the injectable material has a direct influence on treatment outcomes. The most common agents involved in high-pressure jet injection injuries include grease, paint or paint thinner, water or air, and hydraulic fluid.

- Grease produces an inflammatory response that will lead to tissue necrosis if left untreated
- Paint and paint thinner have cytolytic properties that can lead to severe chemical injuries and a dangerous inflammatory response and often result in worse outcomes than grease or oil
- Water and air generally cause less toxicity and destruction to tissue than other substances, frequently resulting in good outcomes.
- Hydraulic fluid produces intense inflammation and extensive fibrosis formation

PATHOPHYSIOLOGY

- A high-pressure jet injury of the hand is characterized by
  - Small entry wound, one to several millimeters in diameter
  - Mild or absent pain
  - Severe internal damage with injected substances spreading along a superficial or deeper plane
  - Permanent functional loss or amputation
- Anatomic studies have shown that the distribution of the injected material was related to many factors including:
  - Angle of entry
  - Depth of penetration
  - Resistance of the object it contacts
- If the injection is over a fibrous tendon sheath, the substances diffuse to surrounding tissue, both distally and proximally. This may lead to extensive nerve and vessel damage, because the rigid and fibrous structure of the A-pulleys overlying the center of the phalanx may limit diffusion of the injected substances
- If the substance is injected into a fibrous tendon sheath, the material may travel a long distance. The hand, wrist, and even the elbow can be involved

Symptoms

- Immediate minor pain upon injection injury
- Discoloration or numbness of the hand or digits within 2 hours
- Intense throbbing pain at 4–6 hours
- Acute and chronic inflammatory reactions and associated subcutaneous emphysema will occur during the first 24 hours
  - The resulting pain will become intense
- The presence of pain that is disproportionate to the appearance of the hand may indicate compartment syndrome

Evaluation

- A detailed history should be obtained including:
  - The type of equipment involved
  - The force of the injection
  - The distance from the skin surface
  - The angle of the injection
  - The type of injected material
  - Time delay from injury to presentation
- General and local injury site examination should include:
  - The size of the entry wound and the extent of swelling
  - Temperature and general color of the skin
  - Subcutaneous emphysema, indicating the spread of the injection
  - Nerve and tendon function
  - Digits and wrist total range of motion (ROM)

- Compartments should be evaluated for signs of compartment syndrome, including the anterior forearm compartment, dorsal forearm compartment, and thenar and hypothenar compartments
- A careful neurovascular evaluation should be performed, assessing functions such as the capillary refill of the hands and digits
- An Allen test should be performed to determine the dual circulation of the hand and digits
- Radiographs may aid in revealing the quantity and distribution of the injected substance. Evaluation of the site of injury and adjacent regions is recommended

TREATMENT

Initial management

Appropriate treatment is reliant upon early recognition of the severity of the injury. It is also important to be aware of the deceptive nature of these injuries. Beneath a seemingly minor entry wound, deep extensive tissue destruction may be present. Prompt and effective treatment should be implemented to avoid subsequent complications.

Surgical intervention

Immediate surgical exploration, debridement, and lavage are critical to obtain adequate functional and postoperative results when treating high-pressure jet injection injuries. It is better to explore all injection injuries to be certain that most of the offending materials are removed, and the pressure over the hand and digits are decompressed, unless the injected substance was an innocuous material such as air or water. A high risk for amputation has been found in patients left untreated for over 10 hours.

- Stark treated 14 patients with paint-gun injuries, of which 7 patients were treated within 10 hours from the initial injection event
  - All seven patients treated within 10 hours regained adequate ROM following treatment
  - Among the seven patients who were seen over 10 hours after injury, three patients had fingers amputated and four patients experienced unsatisfactory outcomes after decompression
- Christodoulou assessed the functional outcome of 15 patients with high-pressure injection injuries of the hand, with an average delay in treatment of 11.7 hours
  - The amputation rate was 40%, and three patients changed their occupations after amputation
  - Pinto et al. found that the longer the interval between initial injury and surgery, the higher the risk of amputation

Treatment should proceed in the following order:

- Decompress the affected area
  - The incision should begin at the entry wound and reach the most proximal site of the injection
- Remove all of the injected material and devitalized tissue
  - This will help relieve the external pressure created by the injected material. If the fingers are involved, the A2 and A4 pulleys should be preserved when removing substances that have been injected into the tendon sheath. The neurovascular bundles should be carefully preserved during removal of the injected material.
- Obtain a culture to determine the appropriate antibiotic treatment
  - Prophylactic wide spectrum antibiotics can be used at the earliest stage and continued several days postoperatively
- Irrigate copiously with saline solution
- Wounds should then be loosely sutured with drainage tubes or left open for later closure
  - Pinto at the Mayo clinic reviewed 25 patients treated with open wound management that involved wide debridement, drainage, open packing, and delayed closure, and found that 84% of involved hands or fingers were salvaged, 64% returned to normal hand function, and 92% of patients were able to return to their previous jobs

Postoperative care

- Monitor the affected area for signs of compartment syndrome
- Re-exploration may be required for more extensive injuries or in the event of infection
- Steroid use is controversial and should not be a part of standard therapy until it has been proven to be effective through randomized controlled trials
- Hand exercises involving active and passive mobilization, and strength exercises are recommended for 6–12 months after surgical treatment. Splints are used initially to hold the fingers and hand in a functional position to avoid the development of a contracture or secondary deformity. Physiotherapy should begin as soon as possible, depending on the treatment method, to improve the likelihood of an optimal outcome

COMPLICATIONS

- Infection is usually not a primary concern; however, the risk of infection will increase over time because necrotic and injured tissue is vulnerable to secondary infection. Documented infection rates vary substantially, reported from 11.5 to 60%
- Amputation rates vary drastically, with reports showing rates from 19 to 80%
  - Patients who sustained injuries from a pressure <68.9 kPa who have immediate treatment had an amputation rate of 19%. For patients injured with a pressure of >68.9 kPa and delayed treatment over 10 hours after injury, the amputation rate reached 43%
  - Patients injured with paint solvents appear to have the highest amputation risk (60–80%)
  - Lewis conducted a 10-year review of 28 cases with high-pressure injection injury of the hand and reported an amputation rate of 21.4%

OUTCOMES

- Wieder reviewed 23 patients with 8.5 years follow-up and found that only 43% of patients returned to their previous jobs; metacarpophalangeal joint ROM was decreased on average by 8.1%. Proximal interphalangeal and distal interphalangeal joint ROM loss was found to be 23.9 and 29.7%, respectively. Two-point discrimination decreased by 49%
- Dailiana reported that patients who had proper treatment returned to their previous occupation at 8–16 weeks after injury

SUGGESTED READING

Bekler H, Gokce A, Beyzadeoglu T. The surgical treatment and outcomes of high-pressure injection injuries of the hand. J Hand Surg Eur Vol 2007; 32:394–399.

Hart RG, Smith GD, Haq A. Prevention of high-pressure injection injuries to the hand. Am J Emerg Med 2006; 24:73–76.
This study identified the particular population at risk in 76 patients with high-pressure injection injuries. They found that 84% patients were manual workers, and that within the whole cohort, 58% of patients injured the nondominant hand, whereas 33% of patients injured their nondominant index finger.

Lewis HG, Clarke P, Kneafsey B. A 10-year review of high-pressure injection injuries to the hand. J Hand Surg Br 1998; 23:479–481.
The study reported a review of 28 patients who underwent surgical treatment for high-pressure injection injury of the hand between 1986 and 1996. Six patients resulting in amputation had a mean surgical delay time of 11.8 hours. They concluded that amputation should be considered earlier in cases where initial tissue perfusion is poor.

Mizani MR, Weber BE. High-pressure injection injury of the hand. The potential for disastrous results. Postgrad Med 2000; 108:183–185, 189–190.
The authors reported on a patient who had the nondominant hand injected with air and presented with a benign initial appearance. Surgical exploration showed no sign of necrosis or foreign body and the patient returned to work within 3 weeks. In addition, they describe the management of high-pressure injection injuries, concluding that the surgeon should be aware of the potential damage of this type of injury and be careful not to miss the diagnosis in cases where the injury has a minor appearance.

Schoo MJ, Scott FA, Boswick JA Jr. High-pressure injection injuries of the hand. J Trauma 1980; 20:229–38.

Verhoeven N, Hierner R. High-pressure injection injury of the hand: an often underestimated trauma: case report with study of the literature. Strategies Trauma Limb Reconstr 2008; 3:27–33. Epub 2 February 2008.
This case study reported on a patient who injected oil-based paint into the nondominant index finger, and following surgical treatment, regained adequate outcomes. The authors then performed a literature review and described the mechanisms and symptoms of high-pressure injection injuries, as well as treatment options and key points in the treatment of this type of trauma. The immediate wide exploration and complete debridement of injected material and necrotic tissue were recommended.

Wieder A, Lapid O, Plakht Y. Long-term follow-up of high-pressure injection injuries to the hand. Plast Reconstr Surg 2006; 117(1):186–189.
This study evaluated the long-term functional outcomes of 23 patients after high-pressure injection injury and found that 78% of patients had cold intolerance, 22% had constant pain, and 22% had impairment of activities of daily living. In addition, 10 patients in this study returned to their previous form of employment. The reported delay from injury to treatment was an average 6.5 hours, with an amputation rate of 22%.

Chapter 16 Fundamental principles of microsurgery and replantation

Aaron WT. Gan, Yeong-Pin Peng

INTRODUCTION

Replantation is the surgical reattachment and restoration of circulation of a completely separated body part, whereas critical revascularization is the re-establishment of arterial perfusion and/or venous drainage to a body part, which is not completely separated. In critical revascularization, the circulatory-compromised extremity is still attached to the body by one or more tissue types.

FUNDAMENTAL PRINCIPLES OF MICROSURGERY

A high precision of clinical skill and deep understanding of the pathophysiology of vessels is required to perform microsurgery. As for microvascular anastomosis, the following principles should be applied:

- Precise clear-cutting of the vessels
- Preventing the adventitia from falling into the vessel lumen
- Ensuring the operative area always remains moist; otherwise, the vessels become less elastic
- Avoiding too much pull on the vessel stump
- Maintain the two vessel stumps in the appropriate position that will allow tension-free anastomosis
- Wash inside of the vessels using heparin saline solution prior to anastomosis
- Penetrating the needle perpendicular to the wall
  - It is preferable to do the back wall (posterior wall) first before the anterior wall is sutured
  - The suture can then be tied outside of the vessel
  - The anterior suture is then performed and tied without tension

For nerve repair, it is important to clear cut the nerve ends to avoid crushing the nerve and to provide clean stumps, and also to obtain a tension-free alignment of the two ends to perform epineural anastomosis.

INDICATIONS AND CONTRAINDICATIONS

The indications of replantation in the hand and upper limb include

- Major limb amputations (at or above the wrist level, within 6 hours of warm ischemia)
- Amputations through the hand
- Amputations in children
- Multiple digit amputations
- Thumb amputations

The contraindications include

- A severely crushed or mangled amputated upper extremity
- Multilevel injury to the amputated upper extremity
- Life-threatening conditions, which preclude replantation surgery
- Warm ischemia time of >4 hours in major limb amputations
- Amputations in mentally unstable patients

Single-digit amputations at the level of flexor zone II, in adult patients, it is a relative contraindication for replantation due to the likelihood of a resultant stiff digit. Digital amputations distal to the insertion of the flexor digitorum superficialis (FDS) (flexor zone I) should be attempted if the patient has a high requirement for hand performance, and the procedure can be carried out after having counseled the patient regarding:

- The requirement for hospital inpatient management and microsurgical monitoring of the replanted digit(s)
- The possibility of failure resulting in terminalization of the digit(s)
- The period of rehabilitation of the digit to restore motor and sensory function
- Possible need for further surgery - tenolysis for flexor and/or extensor adhesions, or removal of implants if necessary

CLASSIFICATION

Amputation injuries can be classified by level and type of injury.

Levels

- Major: Through wrist and proximal
- Hand: Transcarpus, transmetacarpal
- Digital:
  - Proximal to distal interphalangeal (DIP) joint
  - Distal to DIP joint

Digital amputations are classified based on the flexor tendon zones of injury classification. Different classifications have been proposed for distal amputations (distal to FDS insertion) (**Figure 16.1**).

Type of injury

- Clean-cut/guillotine-type
- Crush
- Avulsion

Clean-cut/guillotine-type amputations have the best chance of successful replantation compared with the other two injuries. Crush and avulsed amputated extremities have a large zone of injury, but successful replantation is still possible as long as adequate debridement of the injured zone and bone shortening is performed. This will allow tension-free arterial and venous anastomoses to be performed outside the zone of injury, with no risk of subsequent dieback of the skin and soft tissue. Often, the use of vein and nerve grafts is necessary due to the long segment of neurovascular injury in relation to the surrounding soft tissue.

Examples in the use of terms:

- One patient presented with a clean-cut amputation of the index finger at the level of the DIP joint

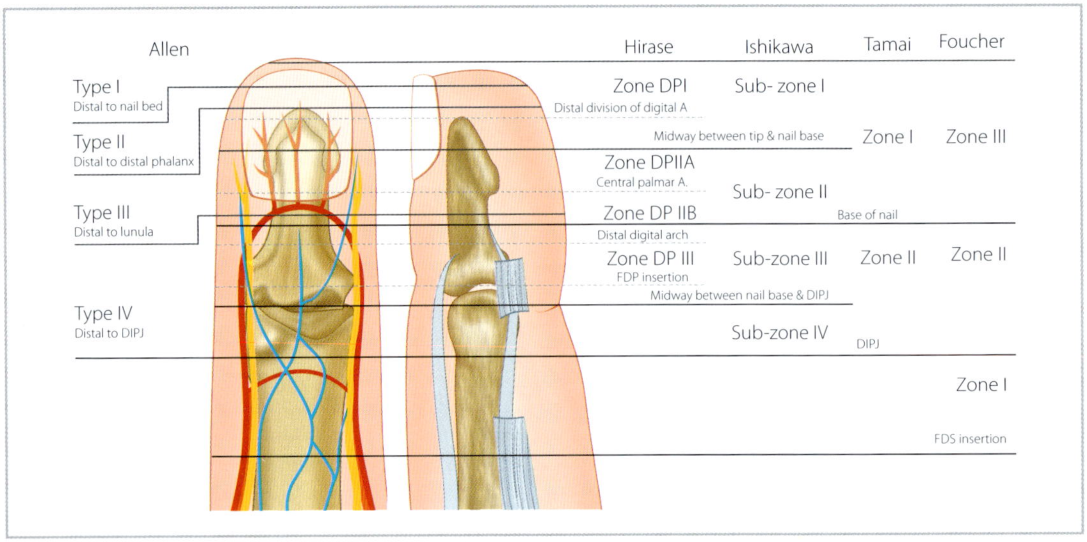

Figure 16.1 Classification of distal amputations (distal to flexor digitorum superficialis insertion).

- A patient has a crush amputation at the level of the junction between the proximal and middle thirds of the forearm, warm ischemia time is 4 hours

PREOPERATIVE MANAGEMENT

Resuscitate

It is crucial to prioritize injuries during the assessment of a patient with multiple traumas, giving the greatest threat to life the highest priority for treatment. The basic principles of advanced trauma life support should be applied during this evaluation.

Assess

Assess the patient's general condition, including pre-morbidities. Consider the following:

- Patient's age
- Handedness
- Occupation and hobbies
- Presence of premorbidities that may preclude replantation surgery or substantially increase the risk of replantation, such as a recent stroke, acute myocardial infarction, peripheral vascular disease, end-stage renal failure, diabetic vasculopathy, or neuropathy
- Assess the amputated extremity to ensure proper storage (kept cool and dry in water slightly above freezing) and suitability for replantation
- Assess the proximal stump to apply temporary hemostatic tamponade in the presence of active arterial bleeding, determine level of injury, and establish the amount of shortening and debridement to be performed and whether replantation of the amputated extremity will result in a functional hand or finger. Revision amputation is always an option.
- Investigations:
  - X-rays of the amputated extremity and proximal stump in orthogonal views
  - Group-and-cross matching of blood
  - Basic blood investigations including full blood count, urea, and electrolytes and coagulation profile
  - Electrocardiogram
  - Plain chest X-ray

Prepare for surgery

For major replantation

After determining that the injury is <4 hours from presentation and resuscitation is being carried out, immediate preparation involves

- Activation of another microsurgical team
- Alerting the anesthetic team regarding the high-priority case
- Placing the amputated extremity inside 1 bag and then another bag, and then cooling it in water slightly above freezing to avoid frostbite
- Starting intravenous (IV) antibiotics, such as 1 g of cefazolin, 8 hourly recommended.
- X-rays to be taken at the emergency department or in the operating room

In the operating room

- Perfuse the amputated extremity with cold saline or tissue preservation solution (at 4°C)
- Catheterize the patient
- Start transfusing packed cells
- Prepare one leg for harvesting of nerve, vein, and skin grafts if necessary

OPERATIVE TREATMENT

Sequence of replantation

Two-team approach

Team in charge of the amputated extremity:

- Step 1: Temporary perfusion of the amputated extremity

Connect a vascular shunt between the distal and proximal arterial stumps and allow the amputated extremity to perfuse for 15 minutes before clamping. There should be no venous connection, as any return of blood from the amputated extremity to the circulation at this time can cause a fatal reperfusion injury. Repeat perfusion every hour until arterial anastomosis is complete. Ensure that the anesthesiologist is actively transfusing blood to keep up with the intentional blood loss.

- Step 2: Preparation of stump and amputated extremity

Excisional debridement – Excision of all muscle tissue, leaving the tendons (**Figure 16.2a** and **b**):

  - Prophylactic fasciotomy to anticipate postoperative swelling from revascularization (refer to Chapter 9)

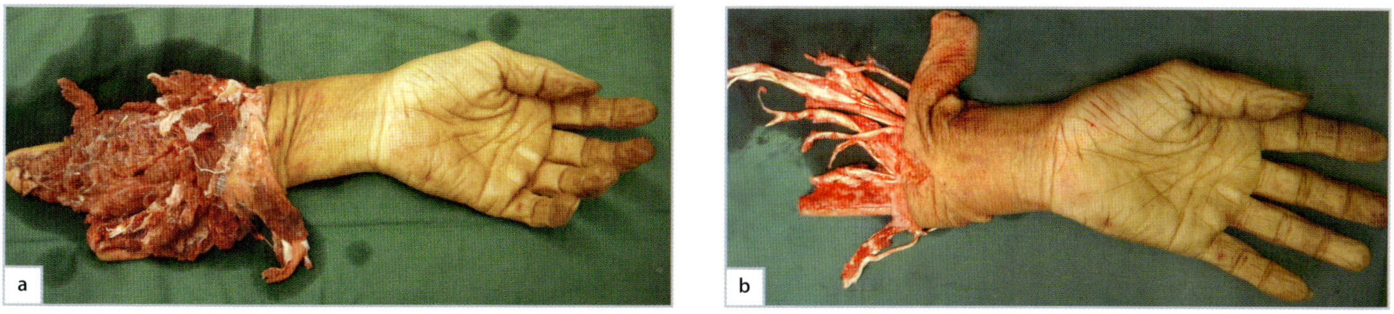

Figure 16.2 Major limb amputation through proximal forearm. (a) Before debridement. (b) After debridement.

  - Identify and mark nerves, arteries, and veins
  - Shorten the bone to allow primary anastomoses of vessels, neurorrhaphy of nerves, and closure of skin

Team in charge of the proximal stump:

- Excisional debridement of proximal stump
- Identify and mark nerves, arteries, and veins of the proximal stump
- Shorten the bone to allow primary anastomoses of vessels, neurorrhaphy of nerves, and closure of skin (**Figure 16.3**).

Sequence of operation thereafter:

- Step 3: Bone fixation (**Figure 16.4** and **16.5**)
- Step 4: Arterial anastomosis, allowing the limb to perfuse and veins to bleed out
- Step 5: Tendon repair
- Step 6: Venous anastomoses – Inform the anesthesiologist once venous connection is established to anticipate cardiac arrhythmias due to hyperkalemia from the ischemic amputated extremity
- Step 7: Nerve repair
- Step 8: Apposition of skin between the proximal and distal stumps, leaving the fasciotomy wounds open
- Ensure good hemostasis to prevent collection of hematomas. Consider placing subcutaneous drains

TREATMENT OF HAND/DIGITAL REPLANTATION

Preoperative management

The protocol is similar but less urgent as compared with major replantation:

- Alert the anesthetic team regarding the high priority case

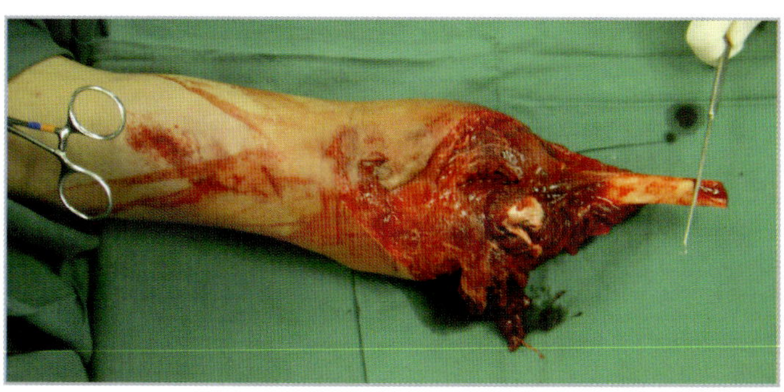

Figure 16.3 Preparation of proximal amputation stump.

- Cool the amputated hand or digit in water that is slightly above freezing as previously described.
- Start IV antibiotics – 1 g of cefazolin, 8 hourly preferred
- X-rays should be taken at the emergency department or in the operating room.

In the operating room:

- Catheterize the patient
- Prepare above the elbow level for harvesting of nerve, vein, and skin grafts from the forearm if necessary

Sequence of replantation

To save operative time, the amputated extremity can be taken to the operating room first for bench work while the patient is being prepped for surgery:

- Step 1: Excisional debridement
- Step 2: Prophylactic fasciotomies of the hand
- Step 3: Identification and marking of nerves and vessels under microscopic magnification. It is best to use a 10-0 or 9-0 nylon suture to mark these critical structures in the amputated digit
- Step 4: Bone shortening to allow primary anastomoses of vessels, neurorrhaphy of nerves, and closure of skin.

Sequence thereafter (when the patient has been put under anesthesia, cleaned, and draped). Under tourniquet control (try to complete these steps within 2 hours to minimize further tourniquet time):

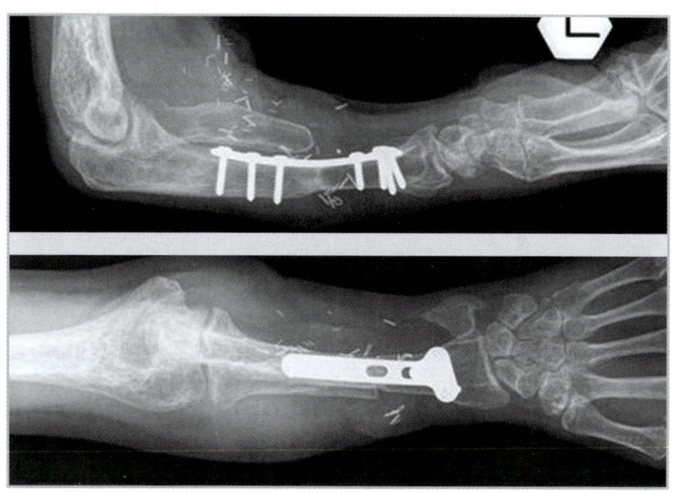

Figure 16.4 Late result of conversion to a one bone forearm and rigid fixation using plate and screws.

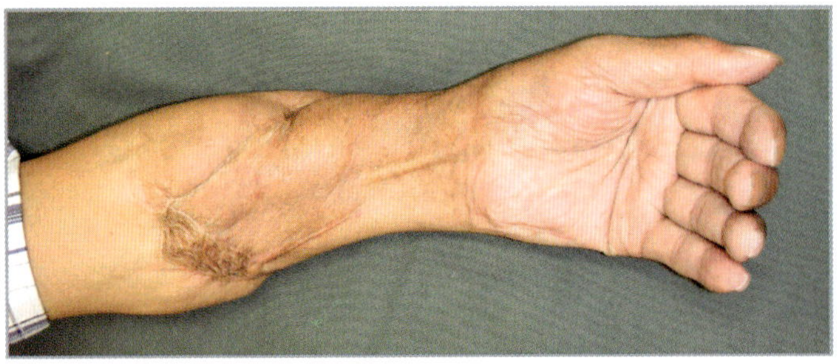

Figure 16.5 Result at 1 year after replantation of a major limb amputation.

- Step 5: Excisional debridement of the proximal stump and bone shortening
- Step 6: Bone fixation: straight transfixing Kirschner (K)-wires, crossed K-wires, Lister's technique of interosseous cerclage box wiring and an oblique K-wires through the fracture site, 90–90 cerclage wiring, plates, and screws (**Figure 16.6**)
- Step 7: Tendon repair
- Step 8: Nerve repair

With or without tourniquet control:

- Step 9: Arterial and venous anastomoses. Two veins for every artery preferred
- Step 10: Skin closure. Attempt to achieve good dermal apposition, as this will aid the early establishment of dermal connections for venous drainage

Strategies for managing the lack of veins for anastomosis

- Dermal pocketplasty: De-epithelialized index, middle, ring, and little finger tips anchored to the corresponding de-epithelialized area in the palm, ensuring good dermal contact. For the thumb, the dermal connection is made over the radial aspect of the proximal phalanx of the index finger
- Medical leeches
- Hourly bleeding of a de-epithelialized area over the replanted fingertip using heparinized saline

POSTOPERATIVE MANAGEMENT

- Use nonocclusive dressings
- Withhold food from patient in anticipation of urgent explorative surgery in the case of perfusion problems to the replanted part
- Hourly monitoring of vital signs and hourly microsurgical monitoring of replanted limb: color, temperature (charted and compared with a control), capillary refill, and turgor
- Keep limb elevated and warm
- Keep patient well perfused with IV fluids – monitor urine output
- IV morphine infusion: 1–2 mg hourly for pain relief and chemical sympathectomy to prevent vasospasm of the anastomosed artery
- IV cefazolin: 1 g every 8 hours

Optional anticoagulation/antiplatelet therapy:

- Aspirin: 100 mg daily after patient is allowed to take orally
- IV dextran: 500 mL every 24 hours
- Anticoagulation with subcutaneous heparin or low-molecular-weight heparin

For major replantation cases, in addition to the above:

- Admit patient to high-dependency unit or intensive care unit
- Commence oximeter monitoring of replanted limb (keep $\geq$95%)
- Blood investigations: Full blood count, urea and electrolytes, coagulation profile, urine for myoglobinuria
- Cardiology consultation, serial electrocardiograms, and acute coronary screening if hyperkalemic or cardiac arrhythmias present

Microsurgical monitoring and anticoagulation/antiplatelet therapy may be discontinued after 5 days if the replant is stable and healing well.

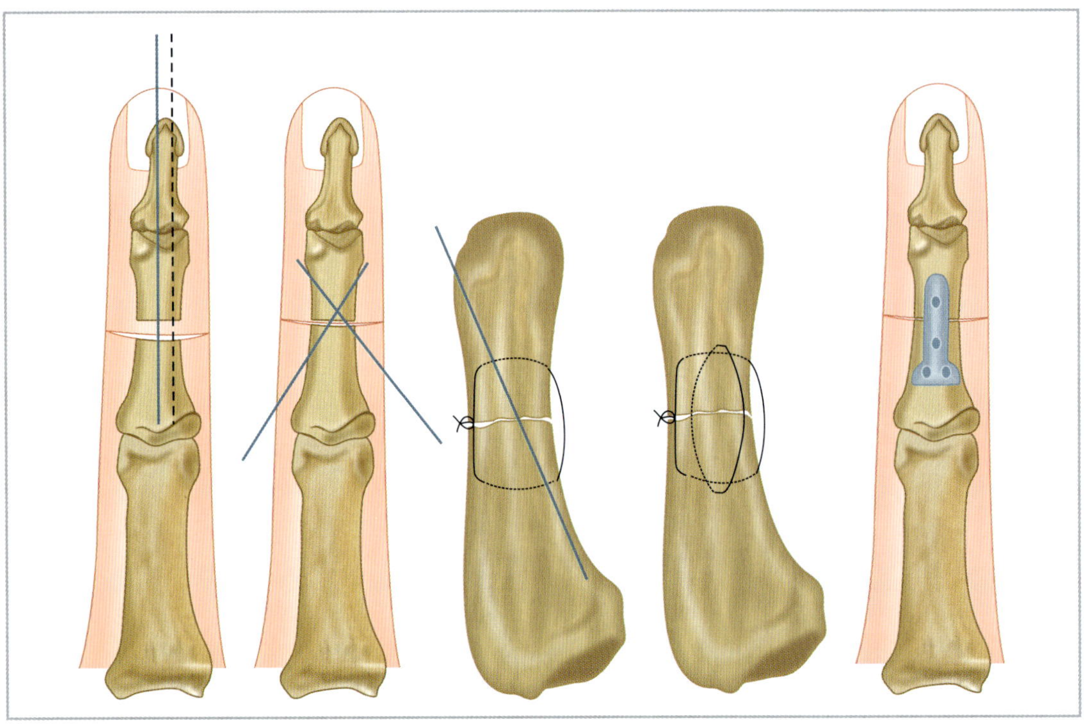

Figure 16.6 Different methods of bone fixation available for digital amputations.

IMMEDIATE AND EARLY COMPLICATIONS

Symptoms

- Arterial compromise: Replanted part looks pale, no capillary refill, poor turgor, feels cold (>2°C lower than the control)
- Venous congestion: Replanted part looks blue/purple, very brisk capillary refill, tense, feels cold (>2°C lower than the control)

Action

- Loosen dressings immediately, call senior for immediate evaluation at bedside and prepare for immediate exploration in operating room

Symptoms

- Persistent pain proximal to the replanted upper limb in major replantation. Suspect compartment syndrome/inadequate fasciotomy

Action

- Loosen dressings immediately, feel for tense and tender compartments and prepare for immediate fasciotomy in the operating room

SUGGESTED READING

Hattori Y, Doi K, Ikeda K, Estrella EP. A retrospective study of functional outcomes after successful replantation versus amputation closure for single fingertip amputations. J Hand Surg 2006; 31A:811–818.
A retrospective review supporting better functional outcome with fingertip replantation compared with revision amputation.

Komatsu S, Tamai S. Successful replantation of a completely cut-off thumb. Plast Recon Surg 1968; 42:374–377.
The first published case report on a successful thumb replantation. Scully RE, Hughes CW. The pathology of ischemia of skeletal muscle in man. A description of early changes in muscles of the extremities following damage to major peripheral arteries on the battlefield. Am J Pathol 1956; 32:805–829.
Morphological and histological study of muscle ischemia in humans.

Sebastin SJ, Chung KC. A systematic review of the outcomes of replantation of distal digital amputation. Plast Reconstr Surg 2011; 128:723–737.
An outcomes review article, which contains a summary of the classifications of fingertip amputations.

Chapter 17 Soft tissue coverage and thumb reconstruction

Keming Wang, Evan J. Kowalski, Kevin C. Chung

SOFT TISSUE

INTRODUCTION

Hand and forearm injuries constitute the largest patient group in emergency plastic surgery, with a frequency of 38–64%. Functional reconstruction of complex soft tissue defects in the hand can be challenging, especially with the involvement of exposed tendons, joints, nerves, and bone. Therefore, the surgeon needs to have a thoughtful approach when it comes to decision making for soft tissue reconstruction of defects in the hand and forearm. Multiple factors need to be considered before decision-making commences: patient factors, the genesis of the defect, the location, size, and depth of the defect, exposed structures, structures needing reconstruction, the degree of contamination, and the quality of surrounding tissues.

The reconstructive ladder theory can serve as a useful thought paradigm during the decision-making process, and it is based on the concept that reconstruction should always be attempted utilizing the most basic procedure that will successfully achieve closure for a given defect. The theory recommends that, when applicable, reconstruction should always be achieved by direct closure, followed by skin grafts, local flaps, and distant flaps. Mathes and Nahai later modified the reconstructive triangle for surgical decision making and included the principles of tissue expansion, local flaps, and microsurgery. They emphasized the necessity for selecting the treatment that will produce the best reconstructive result for each defect, instead of satisfying the minimum requirements for reconstruction by choosing the simplest treatment as in the old model. Janis et al. recently introduced two new techniques to the theory, negative-pressure wound therapy and dermal matrices, to create a more refined reconstructive ladder. Negative-pressure wound therapy can serve as a useful adjunct to various reconstructive methods, whereas dermal matrices can be used with skin grafts after the dermis substitute has revascularized.

Even with a simple defect, multiple factors should be considered while planning a reconstruction method. The choice of surgical treatment should be based on several variables, including the characteristics of the wound, the patient's medical condition, and the surgeon's experience. Key management includes defect analysis, assessment of surgical options, identification of surgical goals, execution of the operative procedure, postoperative care, and outcomes evaluation. The overall goal of a reconstructive procedure is to maximize the restoration of function and aesthetic appearance and minimize donor site complications.

PREOPERATIVE EVALUATION

During preoperative evaluation, a thorough history and physical examination should be obtained, which will influence selection of the reconstructive method. Soft tissue defects may result from trauma, infection, or tumor ablation. Traumatic injuries can be divided into two categories: (1) acute, caused by blunt or penetrating injury or (2) chronic, caused by infection. Acute traumatic defects with exposed nerves, vessels, and tendons require immediate flap coverage. On the other hand, chronic wounds with high bacterial load due to a prolonged exposure time should be treated with wound debridement and systematic antibiotic therapy until the infection clears. Penetrating injuries, such as electrical burns, may result in damage to underlying tissue, and the devitalized soft tissue may be the cause of a secondary infection. Any infection should be controlled before consideration of flap reconstruction.

History

A thorough history should include the cause of the defect, as well as the patient age, occupation, and motivation for correction:

- Use of tobacco products
  - Smoking or tobacco use adversely affects the survival rate of free flaps after reconstruction
- Patient age
  - Children are more tolerant to immobilization after hand reconstruction, but performing microsurgery in children is more challenging due to the small size of their blood vessels. Older patients are more likely to develop joint stiffness when immobilized for an extended period after reconstruction
- Patient occupation
  - A musician may wish to maintain maximum digit function and length and therefore may opt for a more complicated reconstruction, whereas a self-employed laborer may be treated with a relatively simple reconstructive procedure so that they can return to work as soon as possible
- Patient motivation and the desire for restoration of appearance also guide the choice of treatment
- Physical examination should include investigation of functional status, the location and geometry of the defect, exposed structures, bacterial contamination, and underlying vascular conditions
- Determining functional status involves examining tissue structures such as nerves and tendons, and these findings may indicate the need for nerve or tendon repair
- Conservative treatments such as nonadherent dressing for secondary healing by wound contracture are ideal for small defects (<1–1.5 cm^2) without exposed bone
- Skin grafting is appropriate for tissue loss without bone, tendon, or nerve exposure
- Flap coverage is indicated for defects with exposed tendons, bone, joints, or articular surfaces
- For a small defect in the fingertip, advancement flaps such as the bilateral V-Y flap, volar V-Y flap, and oblique triangle flap can be used to cover the defects

- For fingertip amputations involving loss of more than one third of the volar tissue, advancement flaps are not adequate to cover the defects. A cross-finger flap, reverse digital artery flap, or thenar flap can be considered for these circumstances
- For defects located on the radial or ulnar side of the dorsal metacarpal, or the dorsal surface of the finger, the dorsal metacarpal artery perforator flap is a good reconstructive option
- If soft tissue loss occurs at the first web space or dorsal surface of the hand, a reverse posterior interosseous flap, radial artery perforator flap, or radial artery flap can be considered for reconstruction
- When a patient presents with tissue loss over the dorsal aspect of the ring and little fingers as well as the palmar hand region, the ulnar perforator flap is preferred to cover the defects
- For soft tissue defects with damaged arm vessels, the forearm flap, local flap, and microsurgical flap are contraindicated. Instead, a distal pedicle flap is indicated for reconstruction, such as the intercostal flap or groin flap
- For major defects over the dorsum of the hand or those involving soft tissue loss at the forearm, a free anterolateral thigh (ALT) flap may be considered for reconstruction
- For chronic wounds that have poorly vascularized tissue at the base, multiple studies have shown that the use of negative-pressure wound therapy may increase the rate of granulation formation and control bacterial proliferation, enabling closure by second intervention or skin grafting
- When patients present with polytrauma, a long operation time is contraindicated

SURGICAL OPTIONS

After defects are evaluated to determine possible options for coverage, the proposed reconstruction should be performed at the earliest opportunity. As described previously, surgical options include primary closure, skin grafts, flaps, and free tissue transfers. These reconstructive procedures are generally preceded by the fixation of osseous structures and repair of tendons, vessels, and nerves.

Skin grafts

Skin grafts are harvested as either full-thickness or split-thickness grafts. A full-thickness skin graft contains the entire dermis, whereas a split-thickness skin graft contains only a portion of the dermis. The thickness of the grafted dermis determines the survival of the skin graft, because the nutrition is supplied to the graft via inosculation from the recipient bed. Therefore, full-thickness grafting requires a well-perfused vascular bed, whereas split-thickness skin grafts are able to tolerate a less vascular recipient site.

Skin grafts are usually the initial choice for covering open defects when primary closure is not possible, or wound closure may lead to undue tension of the skin. Contraindications for skin grafting include infection, a poor vascular recipient bed, or a defect with exposed bone or tendon. Full-thickness skin grafts are mainly used for relatively small defects, such as on the volar surface or pulp of the digit. The advantages of a full-thickness skin graft include a lower risk of contraction, better color match, and improved sensory recovery compared with a split-thickness graft. In children, when full-thickness grafts are used to reconstruct a defect, the graft maintains growth potential and can grow with the developing child. Split-thickness skin grafts are suitable for major defects in the dorsum of the hand, because they are able to tolerate decreased vascularity, but they often undergo a substantial amount of contracture.

It is important to understand the innate complexity of the hand before choosing a particular reconstructive method, as the anatomical configuration of the hand ultimately dictates which procedure is appropriate for a particular injury. The dorsal and palmar aspects of the hand are different with respect to their structure and function. Dorsal skin is thin and loose so as not to restrict finger flexion, whereas the palmar skin is thicker and tougher. Consequently, pinning the metacarpophalangeal (MCP) joints in 90° of flexion will maximize the amount of skin grafting on the dorsum of the hand, as it will provide the greatest surface area of skin and avoid secondary functional deformity (as described in Chapter 14). Full-thickness and glabrous skin grafts should be used to achieve coverage of the palmar skin, to match the toughness and durability of this skin surface. Fluffed gauze and circumferential wrap should be applied to all skin grafts to assure contact of the graft with the host bed.

Postoperative care and complications

- Initial dressing change should occur 14 days after skin grafting
- Hands should be immobilized with a splint for 7–9 days
- Complications: Skin graft failure can be caused by a poor wound bed, sheer of the skin graft, hematoma under the skin graft, and infection

Local flaps

Bilateral V–Y advancement flap

The bilateral V-Y advancement flap was first described by Kutler in 1944, and is indicated in cases of transverse or volar oblique distal fingertip amputations (**Figure 17.1**).

Surgical technique

- Two triangular flaps are developed from the midlateral aspect of each side of the digit
- The soft tissue is then mobilized as a V-Y advancement flap (**Figure 17.2**)
- The flaps are then advanced distally to the midline to cover the exposed distal phalanx
- Typically, the advancement is no greater than 3–4 mm
- Complications include superficial necrotic skin and incomplete skin coverage

Volar V–Y advancement flap

The volar V-Y advancement flap was first reported by Atasoy in 1970, and it remains applicable for the reconstruction of transverse or dorsal amputations at the distal fingertip, with or without bone exposure. However, this flap is contraindicated in cases involving greater palmar pulp loss than dorsal skin loss, because this will leave insufficient skin tissue to design the flap.

Surgical technique

- The triangular flap is designed from the distal interphalangeal (DIP) joint crease to the distal edge of the amputation (**Figure 17.3**)
  - The blood supply of this flap originates from the fibrous septa, which connects the skin and the deep tissue structures
- To mobilize the flap, the fibrous septa must be gently divided by spreading of the scissors to divide variable amounts of the septa
- The flap can then be advanced up to approximately 1 cm

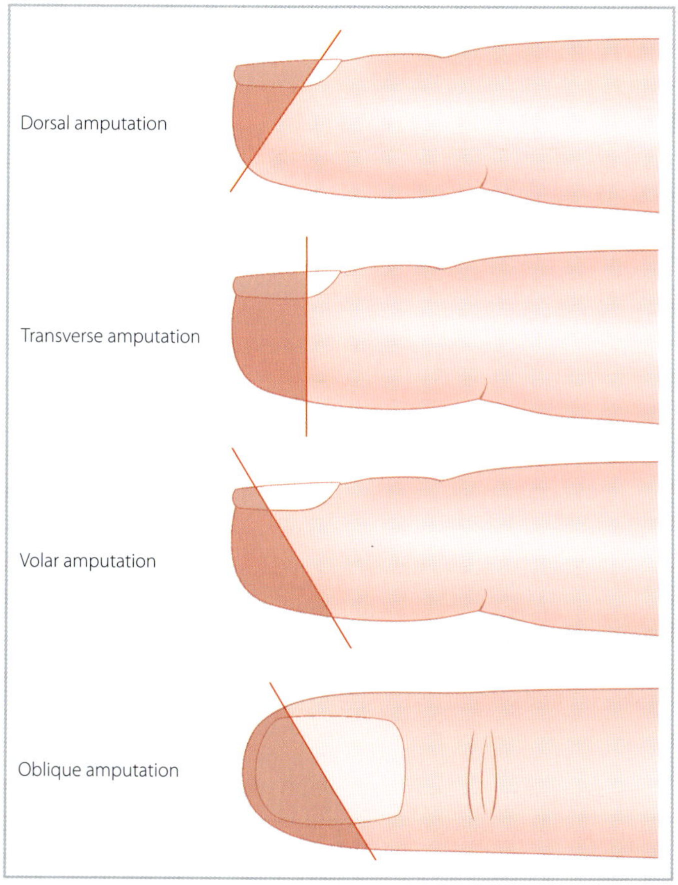

Figure 17.1 Planes of injury in fingertip amputations.

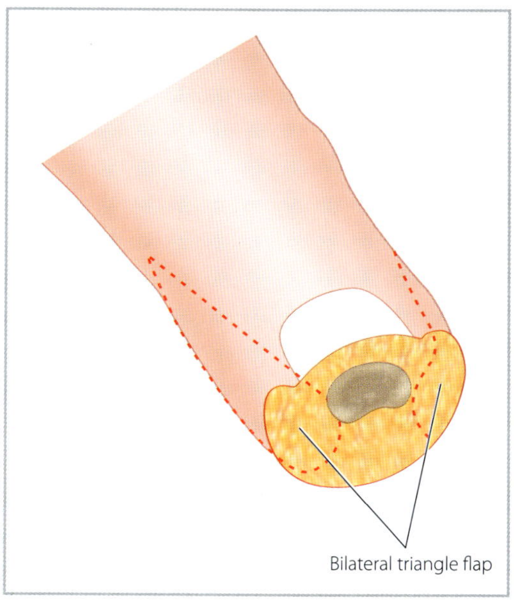

Figure 17.2 Illustration of the bilateral V–Y advancement technique.

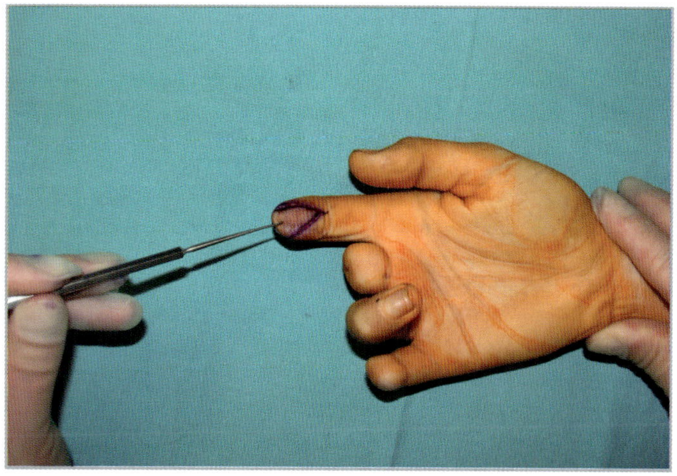

Figure 17.3 The design for a V–Y advancement flap.

Postoperative care

Complications include partial or full necrosis due to tension at closure.

Oblique triangular flap

Venkataswami first described the oblique triangular flap for reconstruction of oblique amputations of the fingertip and thumb.

Surgical technique

- The flap is designed in the radial side or ulnar side of the finger (**Figure 17.4**), with a length of approximately 2–2.5 times the base of the triangular flap
- Typically, this flap is advanced no greater than 7 mm, but if the defect requires > 1 cm of flap advancement (up to 2 cm), the flap can be elevated above the pedicle, similar to a neurovascular island flap, and the vascular bundle traced proximally as far as the MCP joint to enable extended coverage
- During flap elevation, on the straight side of the triangle, the skin incision should be dorsal to the neurovascular bundle to allow for incorporation of the neurovascular bundle within the flap. Near the apex of the flap, the neurovascular bundle enters from the oblique side, and the fibrous septa should be gently divided under magnification, providing mobility to the flap
- As the flap is advanced it is rotated toward the volar aspect of the thumb
- For palmar oblique amputations that mainly involve the lateral side of the finger, Lanzetta et al. recommends designing the flap on the injured side to preserve the length of the finger and digital nerve peripheral branches

Complications

A common complication is a proximal interphalangeal (PIP) joint flexion contracture, which can be avoided by using a night extension splint for the PIP joint from 7 days postoperatively.

Cross-finger pedicle flap

When a fingertip amputation results in the loss of more than one third of the volar tissue and leaves exposed tendons, joints, or bone, an advancement flap is not sufficient to cover the defect. First described by Gurdin and Pangman in 1950, the cross-finger pedicle flap is well suited for such circumstances due to the proximity of this flap to the defect itself. The cross-finger flap can be a very useful treatment for partial fingertip amputations, but this technique does have limitations. Contraindications include patients with an impaired adjacent digit and those experiencing limited joint motion from diseases such as arthritis and Dupuytren disease. The main disadvantage of this flap is the required 2–3 weeks' immobilization period before separation from the donor site, which has the potential to cause joint stiffness, especially in elderly patients. As a result, avoiding this procedure in elderly patients is recommended to reduce the occurrence of joint stiffness. Other disadvantages of this flap include limited width, poor sensation of the fingertip, and contour deformity of the donor site.

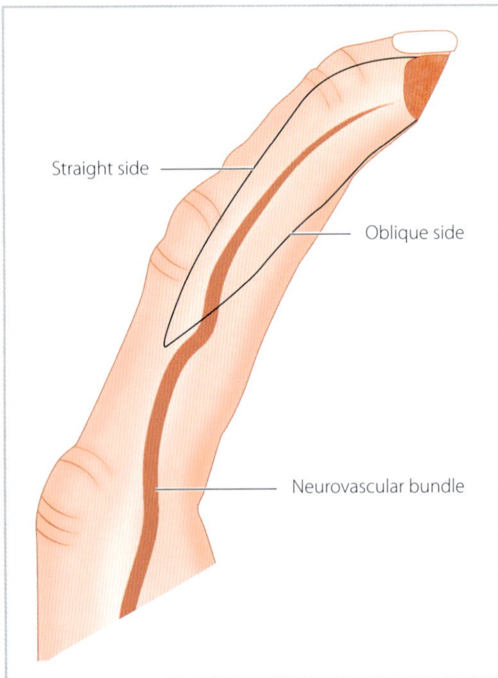

Figure 17.4 Schematic drawing demonstrating avulsion amputation of the fingertip covered by the oblique triangle flap. Note that the straight side of the triangle flap should be dorsal to the neurovascular bundle to allow incorporation of the bundle within the flap.

Surgical technique

- This rectangular flap is designed over the dorsal surface of the middle phalanx of the adjacent digit (**Figure 17.5a**). The flap area should be increased to make it approximately 25% larger than the defect so as to prevent tension on the pedicle
- The flap is then elevated superficial to the extensor paratenon and folded over, similar to turning the page of a book (**Figure 17.5b**)
- This technique can maintain the remaining length of the injured fingertip, but the donor site requires a full-thickness skin graft for adequate coverage
- The cross-finger flap can also be designed as an axial flap based on the dorsal branches of the digital vessels, often referred to as a flag flap, and is useful in smaller areas of tissue loss

Postoperative care

Immobilization of both fingers is required until the pedicle is divided.

Thenar flap

In 1926, Gatewood described the thenar flap for coverage of fingertip defects involving the index and middle fingers. Compared with the V-Y advancement flap and cross-finger flap, this flap can provide a good color and texture match for pulp and sufficient subcutaneous soft tissue for preservation of length of the injured finger. The indications for this flap include acute traumatic oblique and volar amputations of the index and long finger. Contraindications are any connective diseases that may lead to finger stiffness after 2–3 weeks of immobilization. It is recommended that this technique is avoided in elderly patients due to the potential this procedure has for causing joint stiffness.

Surgical technique

- The thenar flap is designed on the thenar eminence, the distal border lying in the MCP flexion crease of the thumb. A rectangular flap is marked on the skin of the thenar eminence (**Figure 17.6**)
- The flap is raised just superficial to the muscle fascia in a proximal to distal direction, carrying the subcutaneous tissue (**Figure 17.7**)

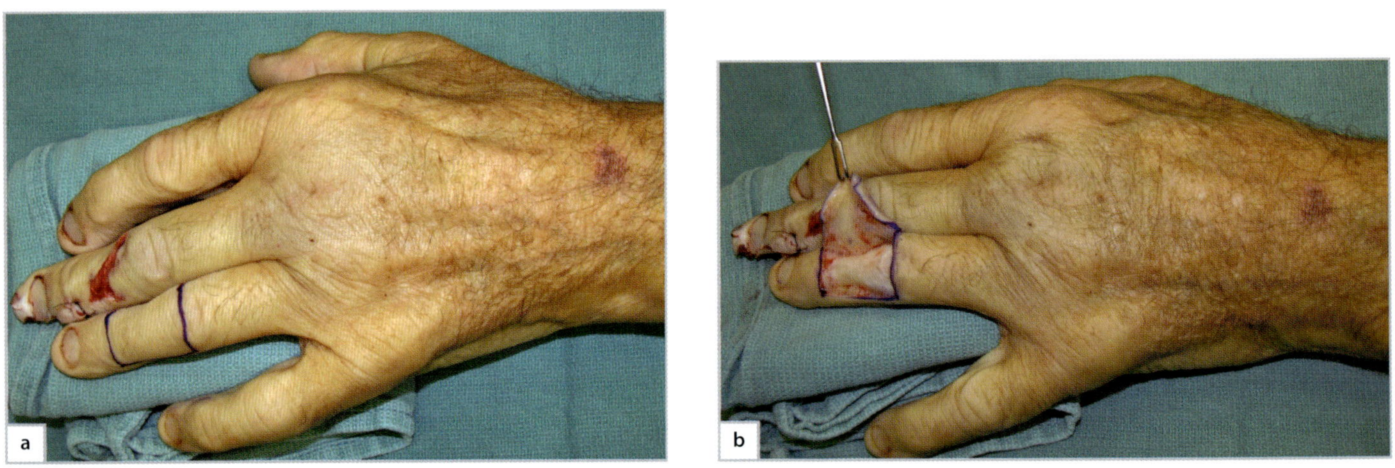

Figure 17.5 Intraoperative view of a cross-finger flap. (a) The flap is designed over the middle phalanx of the adjacent finger. (b) The pedicle is adjacent to the injured finger and the paratenon of the extensor tendon is left intact.

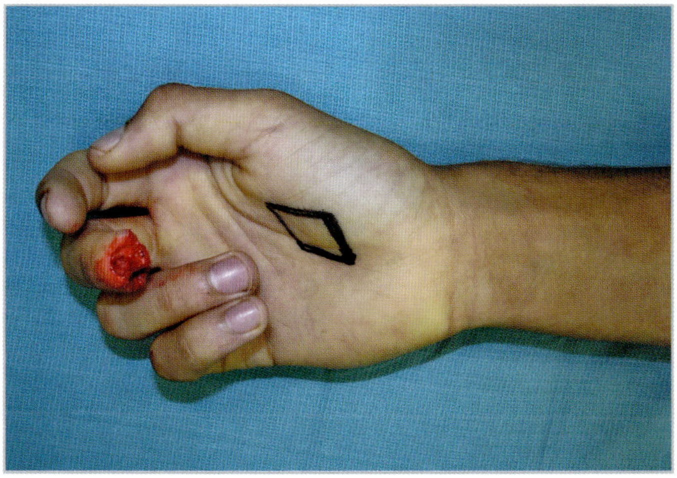

Finger 17.6 A thenar flap is planned on the thenar eminence.

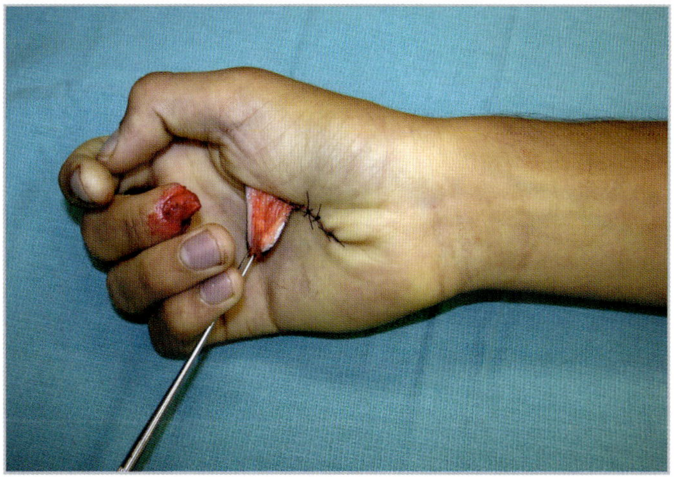

Figure 17.7 The flap is designed to rotate and close the donor site.

- The flap's distal hinge is limited to the line demarcating the radial digital nerve of the thumb, which should be preserved
- The flap is then sutured to the defect, with the MCP joint of the injured finger held in maximum flexion (**Figure 17.8**)
- The donor site of the thenar area can then be closed primarily without skin grafting

Postoperative care

Two to three weeks after flap division, active range of motion exercises can be initiated.

Regional flaps

Reverse digital artery flap

The reverse digital artery flap, first reported by Lai, uses a distally based vascular pedicle and can be used to cover any defect from the proximal phalanx to the fingertip. This flap is designed on the ulnar or radial side of the proximal phalanx of the finger according to the size and shape of the defect (**Figure 17.9**). The advantage of this flap is that it can be completed as a one-stage operation, with no splint immobilization of the hand and only a short period of disability of the hand. The disadvantage is the potential risk of venous insufficiency, which may cause problems in an already traumatized finger. To avoid such problems, the hand should be elevated postoperatively to minimize any venous congestion.

Surgical technique

- The flap is raised from the lateral aspect of the proximal phalanx, containing a digital artery and a generous cuff of subcutaneous tissue around the perivascular pedicle, which allows for a wide arc of transposition
- The pedicle can be dissected approximately 5-mm proximal to the DIP joint (**Figure 17.9**)
- The digital nerve can be left intact or included in the flap
  - If the digital nerve is included, it may improve sensation of the flap
- Once the flap is transferred and sutured to the defect, the donor site can be covered with a full-thickness skin graft

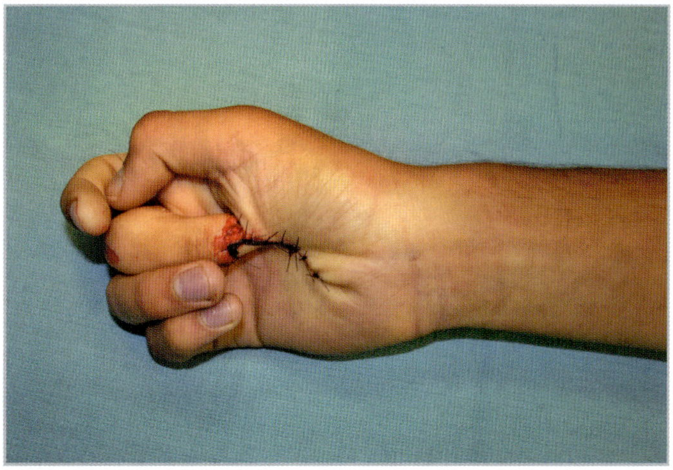

Figure 17.8 The middle finger is inserted into the flap.

Dorsal metacarpal artery perforator flap

The dorsal metacarpal artery perforator flap was first described by Quaba and Davison in 1990. The blood supply of this flap is based on a direct cutaneous branch of the dorsal metacarpal artery. The cutaneous branch occurs primarily distal to the juncture tendinea in the distal one third of the dorsum of the hand and supplies blood to skin tissue over the proximal half of the intermetacarpal space (**Figure 17.10**). This flap is applicable for resurfacing web spaces as well as skin defects of the dorsal metacarpal, proximal phalanx, and middle phalanx regions. It is indicated when a defect is too large for coverage by homodigital or heterodigital flaps or when there is a need for early mobilization of the hand. Sebastin suggests that this flap is indicated for defects of the web space, lateral side of the finger, and dorsal soft-tissue defects on the finger. The main drawback of this flap is the potential for venous congestion due to rotation and compression of the pedicle bridge. In addition, the scar appears conspicuous at the dorsum of the hand.

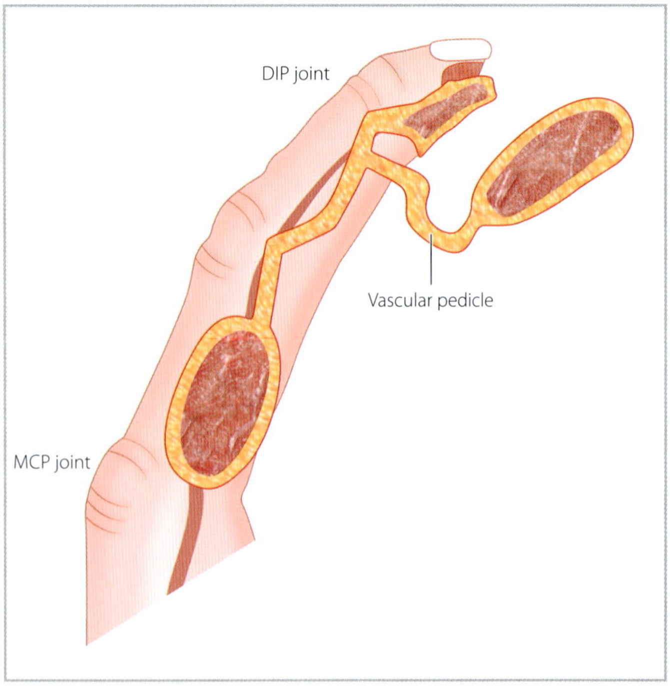

Figure 17.9 The reverse digital artery flap is designed on the ulnar or radial side of the injured finger, requiring the sacrifice of one digital artery.

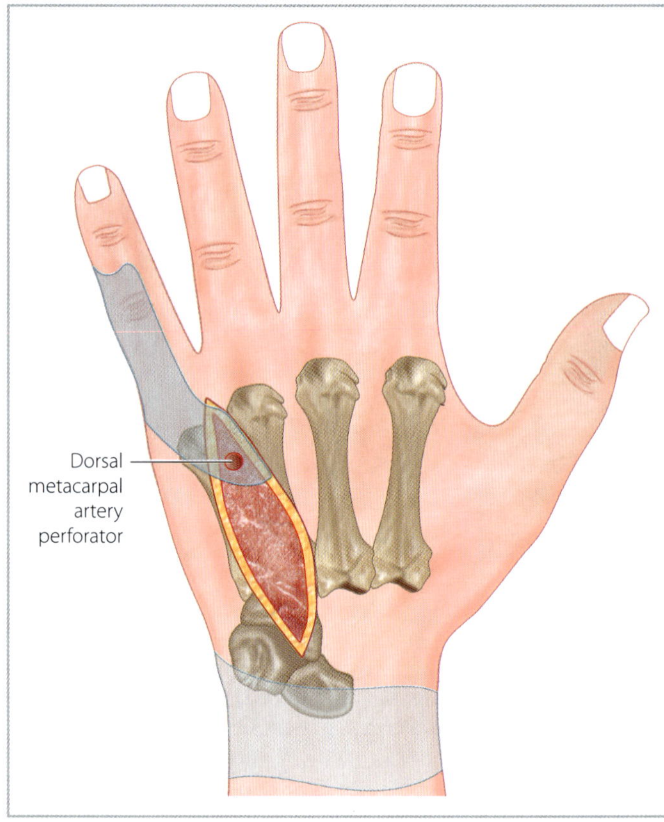

Figure 17.10 The design of the dorsal metacarpal artery perforator flap.

Surgical technique

- The flap can be designed on the second, third, or fourth intermetacarpal spaces (**Figure 17.11a**)
- The width varies from 1 to 3.5 cm and 0.5–1 cm proximal to the adjacent metacarpal joint
- The flap is elevated from proximal to distal in the loose connective tissue plane superficial to the extensor tendon
  - The perforators can be visualized immediately distal to the juncturae tendinum (**Figure 17.11b**)
- Following flap rotation into the defect (**Figure 17.11c**), compression of the perforators should be avoided, keeping the PIP joint and MCP joint in extension or putting gauze between the fingers to keep the web space open

Postoperative care

A volar splint should be applied to keep the fingers and wrist in extension for 1 week after the procedure, after which time the patient can initiate range of motion exercises once the splint has been removed.

Radial forearm flap

The radial forearm flap was first described as a free flap for oral and facial reconstruction by Yang in 1981, and later modified by Lu into the reverse pedicled radial forearm flap for hand reconstruction in 1982. This flap can be used for coverage of defects in both the palmar and dorsal surfaces of the hand or thumb in a single-stage procedure. Because the flap pedicle is based on the radial artery in the hand, a normal Allen test is required preoperatively to confirm adequate perfusion of the hand by the ulnar artery alone. The blood supply of the radial forearm flap is based on the retrograde flow that courses through the deep palmar arch and associated venae comitantes. In the hand, the radial artery has an average diameter of 1.9 mm and lies just beneath the margin of the brachioradialis on the pronator teres and the flexor carpi radialis (FCR), where it is accompanied by two or more venae comitantes. Regarding flap size, more distal flaps will require longer vascular pedicles, and therefore, a more distal defect will need a more proximal skin paddle.

Surgical technique

- The flap and the pedicle are marked out on the forearm (**Figure 17.12**) over the course of the radial artery, which lies between the FCR and brachioradialis tendons (**Figure 17.13a**)
- The radial artery and venae comitantes are dissected from the adjacent tissues to the pivot point, which is close to the radial styloid (**Figure 17.13b**)
- Care should be taken to identify and ligate any small side branches, preserve a perivascular cuff of adventitial tissue, and identify and preserve the superficial radial nerve
  - The cephalic vein is most frequently left intact
- After flap insertion, the donor site is closed directly (**Figure 17.13b**) or with a skin graft

  There are two main disadvantages to this flap:
  - The poor appearance of the donor site, particularly in the younger patient
  - The required sacrifice of the radial artery potentially compromising the vascular supply of the hand, which is the dominant vessel of the hand in 12% of the population. To avoid this problem, a cephalic vein graft can be harvested and interposed to reconstruct the radial artery segment taken with the flap after the flap is elevated

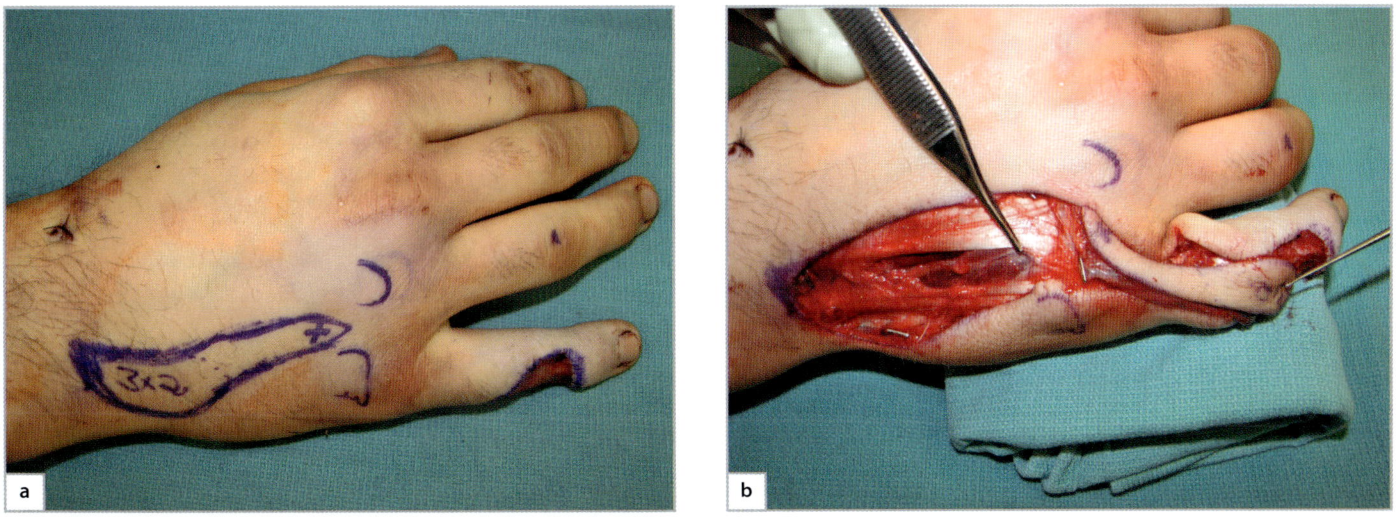

a

b

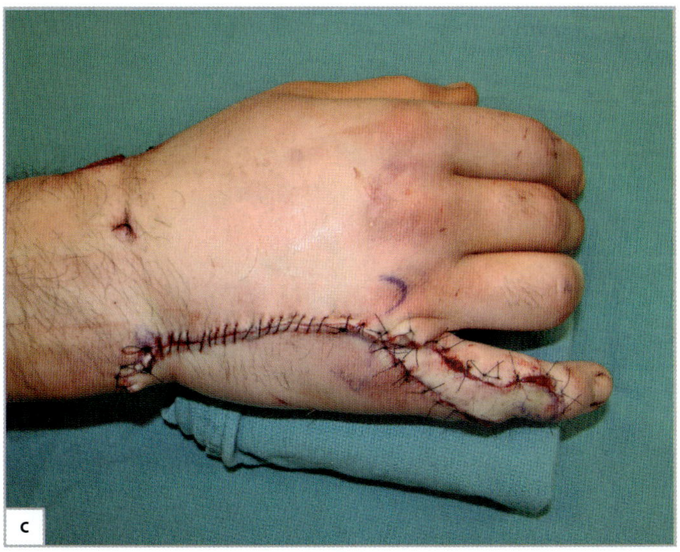

c

Figure 17.11 (a) Intraoperative view of the dorsal metacarpal artery perforator flap. (b) That flap is elevated, and the pivot point is located at the juncturae tendinum. (c) The flap is transferred into the defect and the donor site closed primarily.

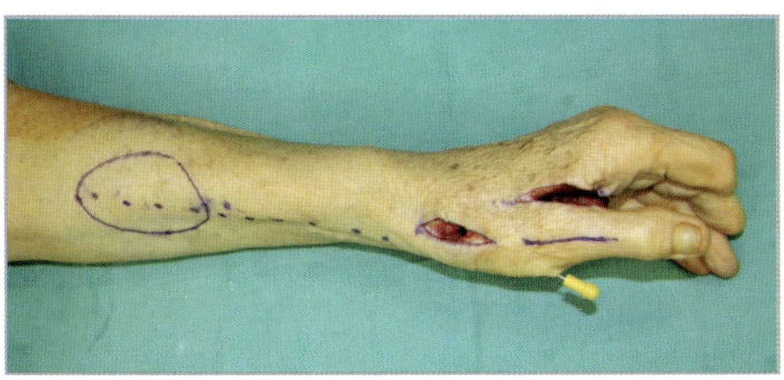

Figure 17.12 First web space contracture. A template is used to mark out the pedicled radial artery perforator flap on the volar forearm.

Radial artery perforator flap

To overcome the drawbacks of the radial forearm flap, Zhang described the radial artery perforator flap in 1988, based on the septocutaneous perforators originating from the distal radial artery. The main advantage of the perforator flap over the reverse radial forearm flap is the preservation of the radial artery. This flap is indicated for coverage of defects over the volar or dorsal aspects of the hand, as well as the first web space. Defects distal to the MCP joints of the hand are contraindicated due to size constraints of the flap. There are approximately 10 small perforating vessels that originate from the radial artery at the distal forearm, which is located 2–4 cm proximal to the radial styloid process (**Figure 17.14**). These septocutaneous perforators form a longitudinal vascular plexus along the course of the artery that can be developed as an adipofascial pedicle flap or adipofasciocutaneous flap.

Surgical technique

- This flap is designed over the proximal volar forearm, and the pivot point marked 2–4 cm proximal to the radial styloid process
- The island flap is marked in accordance with the size of the defect, along the axis of the pedicle
- Flap elevation should begin from the lateral margin toward the distal septocutaneous perforators
  - The perforators should not be isolated or skeletonized to preserve the blood supply for the flap

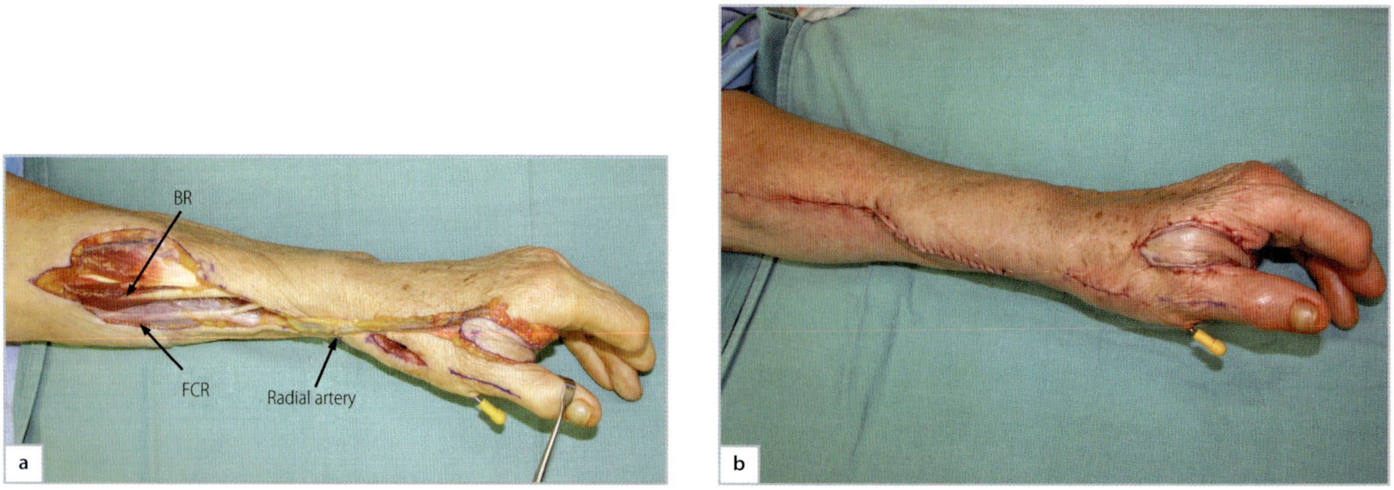

Figure 17.13 (a) A pedicled radial forearm flap based on radial artery was raised up in a fascia level. Note that the radial artery is located between the flexor carpi radialis and brachioradialis. (b) The flap is inset into the first web space and the donor site closed primarily.

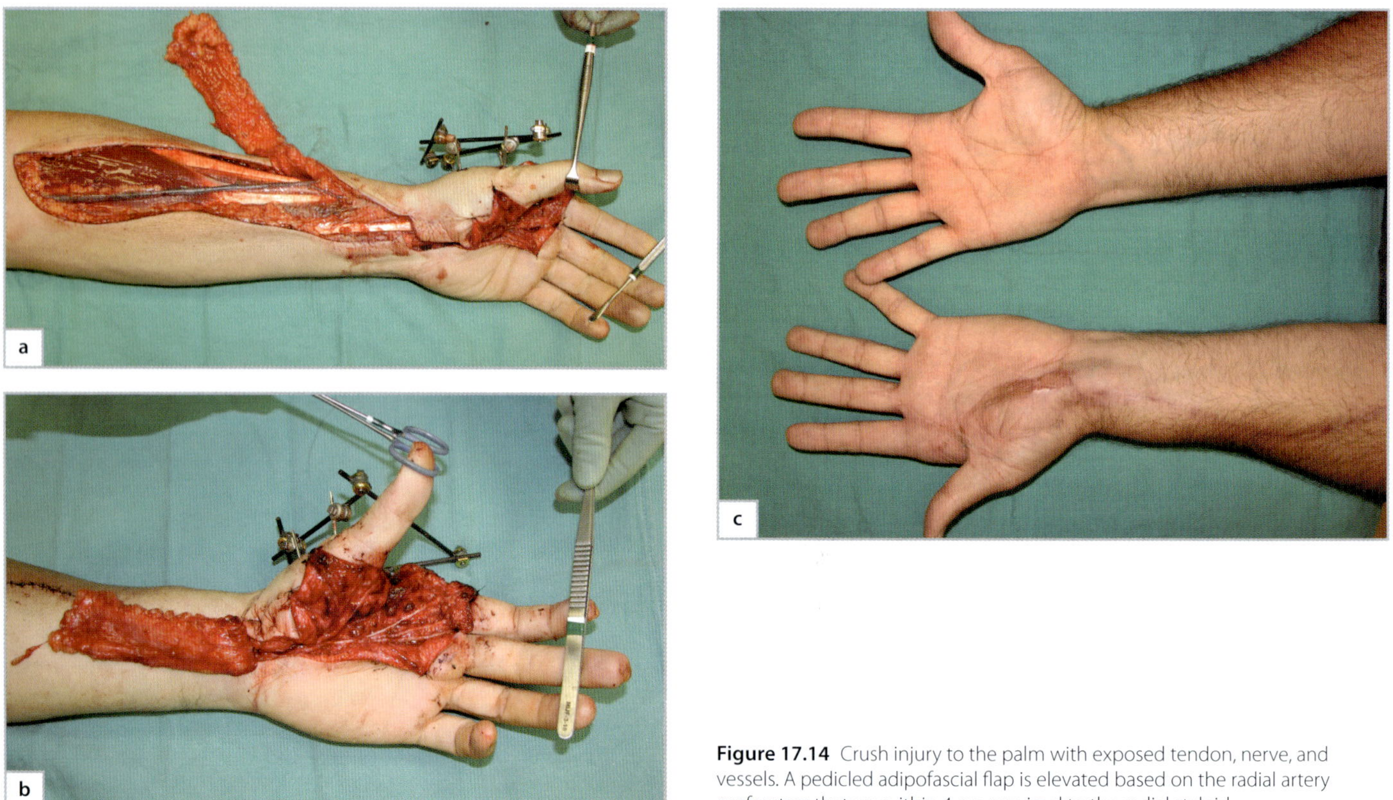

Figure 17.14 Crush injury to the palm with exposed tendon, nerve, and vessels. A pedicled adipofascial flap is elevated based on the radial artery perforators that are within 4 cm proximal to the radial styloid.

  - During flap elevation, care should be taken to preserve the integrity of the superficial branch of the radial nerve
- After visualization of the septocutaneous perforators, the medial border of the flap is incised
- The flap pivot point is located at least 2 cm proximal to the radial styloid process
- The flap is then rotated and applied to the recipient site
- The donor site can be closed primarily or covered with skin grafts, depending on the degree of skin laxity

Postoperative care and results

The poor appearance of the scar after harvest of a fasciocutaneous flap remains an issue. An adipofascial flap used in combination with a skin graft for coverage of a soft tissue defect will obviate the necessity of a skin graft to the donor sites.

Reverse posterior interosseous flap

Lu first described the reverse posterior interosseous flap in 1986 to reconstruct a wide variety of soft tissue defects of the hand, including defects of the first web space as well as on the dorsal and palmar aspects of the hand. As the posterior interosseous artery is ligated during flap harvest, the pedicle for this flap is ultimately supplied by the anterior interosseous artery via anastomosis between the two arteries. Previous studies have found the posterior interosseous artery to be absent in 2.5–5.7% of patients, but when present the artery lies in the septum between the extensor carpi ulnaris and the extensor digiti minimi. Due to the absence of the posterior interosseous artery in certain patients, a preoperative Doppler test is essential to confirm the presence of anastomosis between the posterior and anterior artery.

There are two main advantages to this flap:

1. It allows for reconstruction of large hand defects without sacrificing any major arteries and disrupting the vascular supply of the hand
2. It can be used even in the presence of extensive vascular damage to the hand

Surgical technique

- The flap is marked out along the line between the lateral epicondyle of the humerus and the distal radioulnar joint (DRUJ) while the forearm is held in full supination
- The flap is dissected from proximal to distal along its course until the pivot point is reached, which is approximately 2 cm proximal to the DRUJ (**Figure 17.15**)
- During flap elevation, the posterior interosseous nerve travels along the radial side of the posterior interosseous artery and needs to be separated from the vascular pedicle
- The flap is then transferred and inserted onto the defect through an open or closed subcutaneous tunnel
- It is advisable to keep the proximal artery longer when dividing the pedicle in case the flap needs to be converted into a free flap because of potential vascular insufficiency from the anastomotic vessels

Postoperative care and complications

Similar to other flaps, the hand must be elevated to minimize the potential for postoperative venous congestion after surgery. The limb should then be splinted for 7 days, after which time the patient should begin active and passive mobilization exercises. Complications after posterior interosseous flap elevation include injury to the posterior interosseous nerve, delayed healing of the donor site, and partial necrosis of the flap.

Distal ulnar artery flap

The distal ulnar artery flap can be used to cover defects located on the dorsal wrist, volar or dorsal aspects of the hand, the first web space, and the thumb. The flap is based on the distal dorsal branch of the ulnar artery, arising from the ulnar artery approximately 3–5 cm proximal to the pisiform bone. The branch runs from the palmar to dorsal region, passing between the ulnar bone and the flexor carpi ulnaris (FCU), and the flap is typically designed over the medial aspect of the distal forearm and hand (**Figure 17.16**). It can be raised as a pedicle, island, or free flap and harvested as a fascial flap or fasciocutaneous flap.

There are several advantages to this flap, including

- Ease of harvesting
- No exposure of the flexor tendons
- No sacrifice of a major artery
- The donor site scar is in a concealed area on the medial side of the forearm

The disadvantage of the flap is the short length of its pedicle (3 cm), which does not reach the distal surface of the palmar hand.

The dorsal branch of the ulnar artery diverges from the main vessel 3–5 cm proximal to the pisiform, with a diameter of approximately 1.17 mm at its origin. After traveling below the FCU and above the ulnar nerve, the main trunk of the perforator divides into three branches:

1. The proximal branch supplies the FCU
2. The middle branch is a cutaneous branch, which is the perforator of the ulnar artery perforator flap and travels between the ulna and the FCU, supplying the skin on the medial aspect of the distal forearm
3. The distal branch leads to the pisiform

Surgical technique

- The flap is designed on the line between the pisiform and the medial epicondyle of the humerus
  - The pivot point is 3–5 cm proximal to the pisiform
- The length of the pedicle depends on the distance from the pivot point to the proximal edge of the recipient site
- The flap can be elevated through the deep fascia from the radial side toward the FCU muscle (**Figure 17.17**)
- Gentle dissection must be carried out below the FCU tendon to expose the distal cutaneous branch of the ulnar artery
- After visualizing the pedicle in the distal third of the flap, the ulnar side of the flap is elevated
- The flap can then be rotated and inset to cover the defect (**Figure 17.18**)

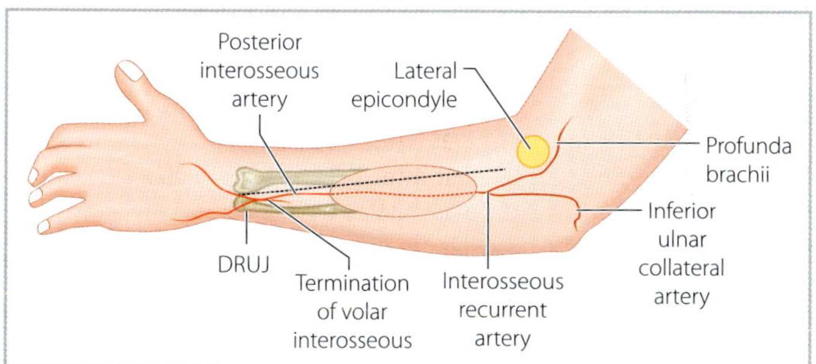

Figure 17.15 Anatomy of the posterior interosseous artery flap. The axis of the flap runs from the lateral epicondyle to the distal radioulnar joint.

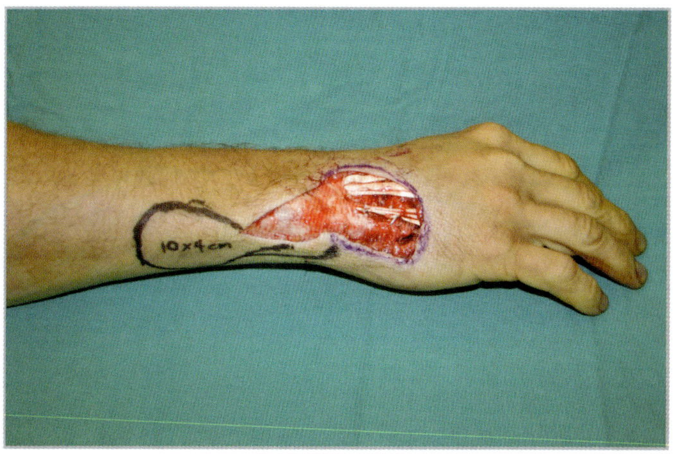

Figure 17.16 Intraoperative design of the ulnar perforator flap.

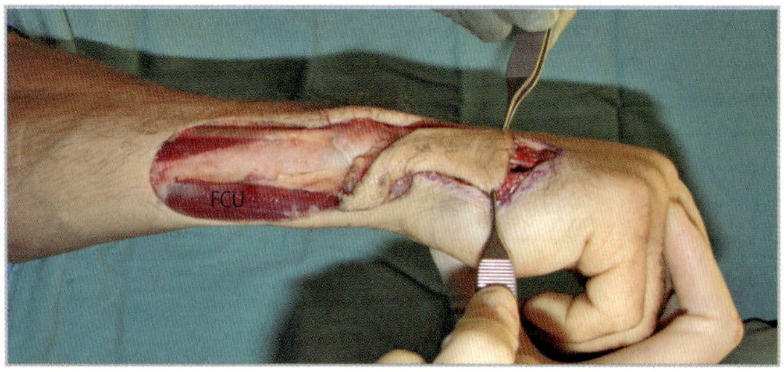

Figure 17.17 The flap is raised up through the deep fascia.

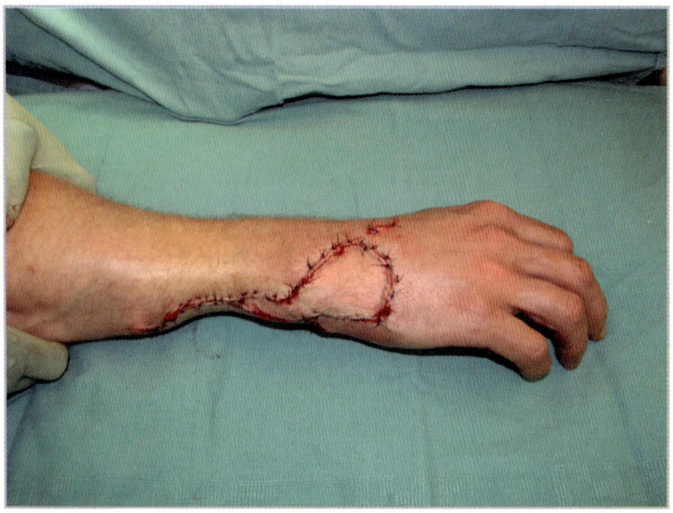

Figure 17.18 The flap is then transferred to the recipient site, and the donor site closed primarily.

- The donor site is closed primarily or covered with a full-thickness skin graft

Postoperative care and complications

After surgery, the hand and wrist should be immobilized for 2 weeks in a plaster splint. One functional drawback to this flap is the potential for scar contracture on the ulnar side of the forearm because this area is frequently bearing the weight of the arm when resting/placing the arm on a surface. The risk of this complication can be reduced by using a full-thickness skin graft to cover the donor site.

DISTANT FLAPS

Lateral arm flap

Song et al. first described the lateral arm flap in 1982, and it is based on the posterior radial collateral artery, which travels in the lateral intermuscular septum between the triceps posteriorly and brachialis and brachioradialis anteriorly. This flap is extremely versatile and can be applied to many different reconstructive scenarios:

- A reverse lateral arm flap based on the distal pedicle vascular communication can be used to cover elbow defects
- A free lateral arm flap can be used in severe hand reconstruction
- A contralateral pedicled arm flap is another good choice for hand reconstruction, especially for coverage of multiple large defects in the distal digits or when the preservation of potential recipient vessels for secondary reconstructive procedures of the hand is required

The main disadvantage of this flap is the potential for unintentional damage of the posterior cutaneous nerve of the forearm during flap harvesting.

Surgical technique

- The flap is designed along the line extending from the deltoid insertion to the lateral humeral epicondyle
  - It can be extended onto the proximal forearm area passing the lateral epicondyle 1–2 cm distally (**Figure 17.19**)
- The flap is elevated between the epimysium of the muscles and the deep fascia
  - Care must be taken to identify the radial nerve and the posterior cutaneous nerve of the forearm
- The flap is then isolated from the intermuscular septum attached to the humerus (**Figure 17.20**)
- If a free flap is required, the pedicled septum can be traced and elevated cephalad by sharply dissecting off the humerus (**Figure 17.21**)
  - The posterior radial collateral artery and venae comitantes can be divided and used as the pedicle of the free lateral arm flap

This flap is advantageous because it has a predictable vascular anatomy compared with other flaps, and the donor site can be closed primarily, even when a flap up to 8 cm in width is taken.

Postoperative care

Patients should initiate intensive therapy three times a day in the immediate postoperative period to prevent stiffness of the shoulder, elbow, and wrist, with care to protect the pedicle.

Groin flap

The groin flap was first described by Mcgregor and Jackson in 1972, and it is based on the superficial circumflex iliac artery (SCIA) and

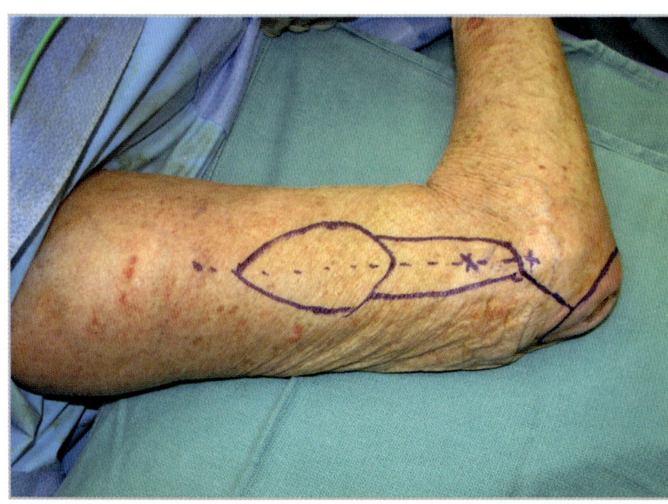

Figure 17.19 Design of the lateral arm flap. The humeral insertion of the deltoid and the lateral epicondyle are both identified.

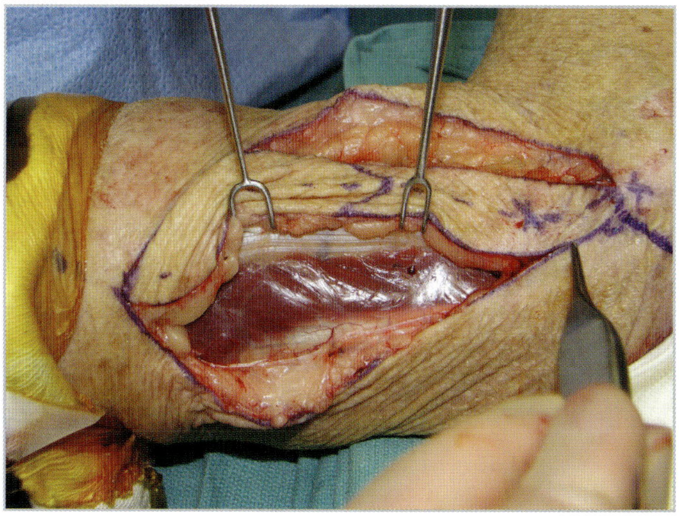

Figure 17.20 The flap is raised up from the epimysium of the muscles.

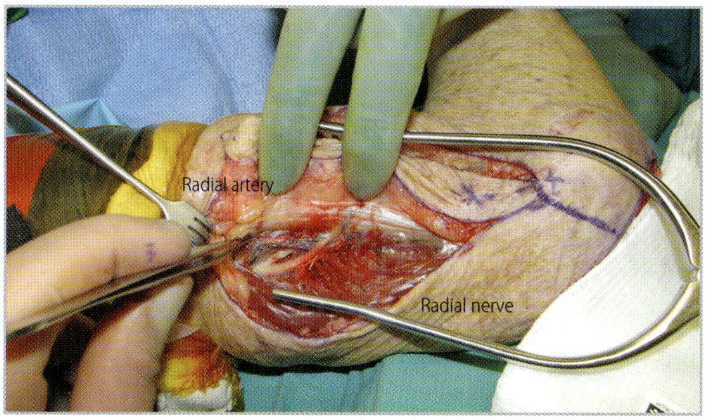

Figure 17.21 The pedicle can be found coursing alongside the radial nerve. Care should be taken to protect the radial nerve.

concomitant vein arising from the femoral artery and venae 2.5–3 cm inferior and parallel to the inguinal ligament. The point of origin of the SCIA is within the femoral triangle, which is formed by the inguinal ligament superiorly, the medial border of the sartorius laterally, and the lateral border of the adductor longus medially. The SCIA is located proximally over the deep fascia of the sartorius muscle and then penetrates the deep fascia at the lateral border of the sartorius muscle, entering distally into the fatty tissue. This flap is considered an axial-based flap extending between the femoral vessels and the posterior iliac spine (**Figure 17.22**). Indications for this flap include soft tissue defects in the finger, thumb, and dorsal hand, and it can be used as a pedicled groin flap, free groin flap, or SCIA perforator flap.

Surgical technique

- Flap dissection begins at the anterior superior iliac spine, in a lateral-to-medial direction (**Figure 17.23**), in a plane directly superficial to the fascia lata
- Once the sartorius muscle is visualized, flap dissection is initiated deep to the fascia plane, from the superficial plane to the muscle belly (**Figure 17.24**)
  - Excess fat tissue can be removed from the deep surface of the flap lateral to the lateral edge of the sartorius muscle

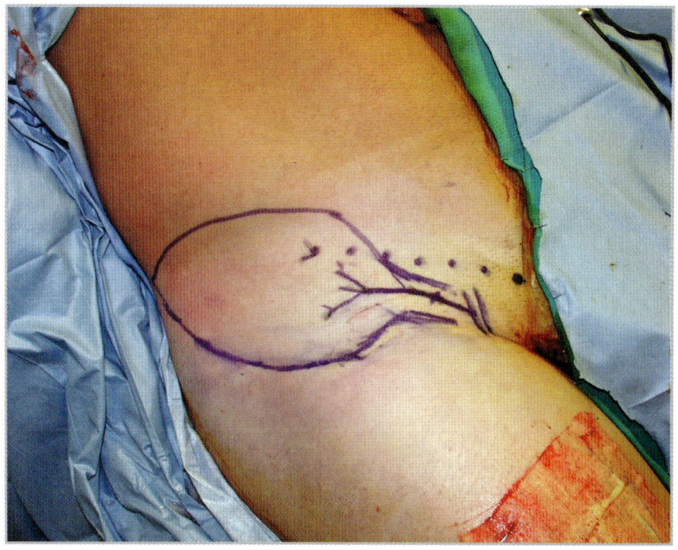

Figure 17.22 Preoperative marking of a groin flap showing the inguinal ligament and superficial circumflex iliac artery.

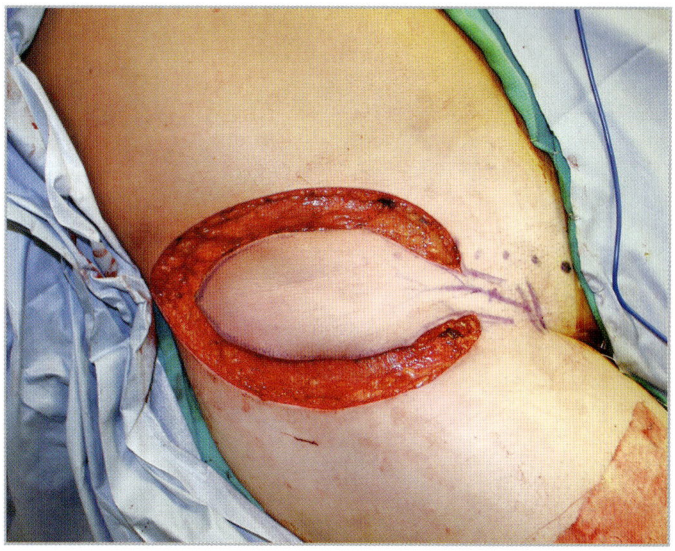

Figure 17.23 The flap is raised from lateral to medial.

- If required, the proximal portion of the flap can be tubed
- Skin edges should then be sutured to the defects of the hand
- The donor site can be closed primarily as long as the flap width does not exceed 10 cm. The donor site should be closed first before insetting the flap to facilitate ease of donor site closure

Postoperative care

Cheng et al. reported on an ischemic preconditioning concept, which allows the flap to be divided early, at approximately 8.4 days postoperatively, with no degree of flap loss. To condition the flap, the investigators recommend clamping the pedicle of the flap for a set time to induce ischemia and encourage the flap to create microvascular connections with the recipient site, followed by several hours of reperfusion. The pedicle is initially clamped for 30 minutes, followed by 7 hours of reperfusion, and the duration of induced ischemia is increased while the reperfusion time is decreased over the course of several days. From postoperative day 3 to the day of flap division, the induced ischemia time can be progressively increased to 2 hours and reperfusion time progressively decreased to 6 hours.

Pedicled intercostal perforator flap

Dibbell first described the intercostal flap in 1974, and it is based on the intercostal neurovascular bundle in the 7th–11th intercostal spaces. In 1994, Gao et al. described the pedicled intercostal perforator flap, which they based on the intercostal cutaneous perforators of the fourth–seventh intercostal spaces. This flap is indicated for covering defects of the fingers, hands, forearm, and elbow. The advantage of this flap is the ability to achieve a color match and hairless texture. Compared with the groin flap, the disadvantages include abdominal scarring on the upper abdomen and the bulkiness of the flap in the recipient cite. A recent anatomical study conducted by Oki et al. demonstrated that the cutaneous perforators were dense along the rib cages in the fifth–eighth intercostal spaces, penetrating the interdigitations of the serratus anterior muscle and the external oblique muscle.

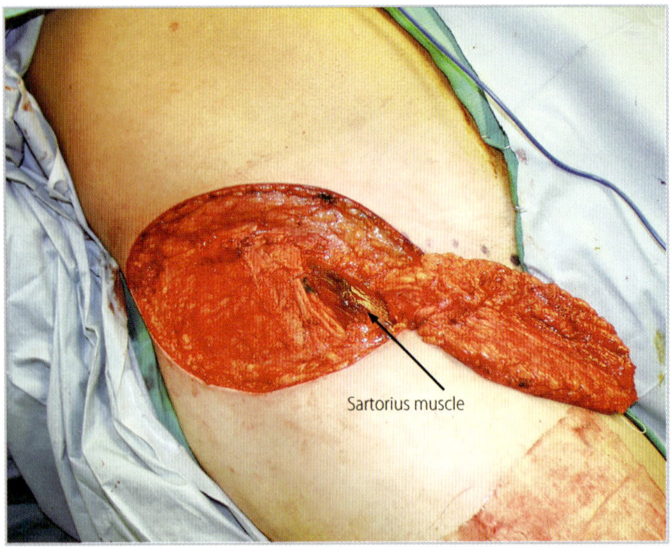

Figure 17.24 The dissection progresses deep to the fascia, and a piece of the sartorius fascia is removed.

Surgical technique

- Preoperatively, a handheld Doppler can be helpful to detect the perforators in the fifth–eighth intercostal spaces
- Once the correct perforators are identified, the flap can be marked in a vertical or oblique course (**Figure 17.25a and b**), from the upper abdominal area toward the umbilicus
- The pedicle of the flap should measure 3–5 cm in width by 3–5 cm in length, which includes the intercostal perforators of the fifth–eighth intercostal spaces
- The wide distal aspect of the flap should be marked 2 cm wider than the defects, and the medial border at least 2 cm off the midabdominal line
- The flap is then elevated at the superficial layer from the distal end toward the pedicle
- Flap dissection should be stopped before the point where the perforator vessels arise from the fascia
- To preserve vessels, the perforators should not be exposed, so the pedicle is rolled into a tube shape (**Figure 17.26a**)
- Finally, the flap is transposed to the defects (**Figure 17.26b**), and 10–14 days postoperatively the flap can be divided

Postoperative care

The flap can be divided on average at 13.8 days postoperatively.

Anterolateral thigh flap

The ALT flap was first described by Song in 1984, based on either the musculocutaneous perforators (87%) or septocutaneous vessels (13%) derived from the lateral circumflex femoral artery. This flap can be used as a free flap to cover soft tissue defects on the dorsal and palmar aspects of the hand, thenar web space, and forearm that are too large to be covered with local flaps. In addition, some investigators

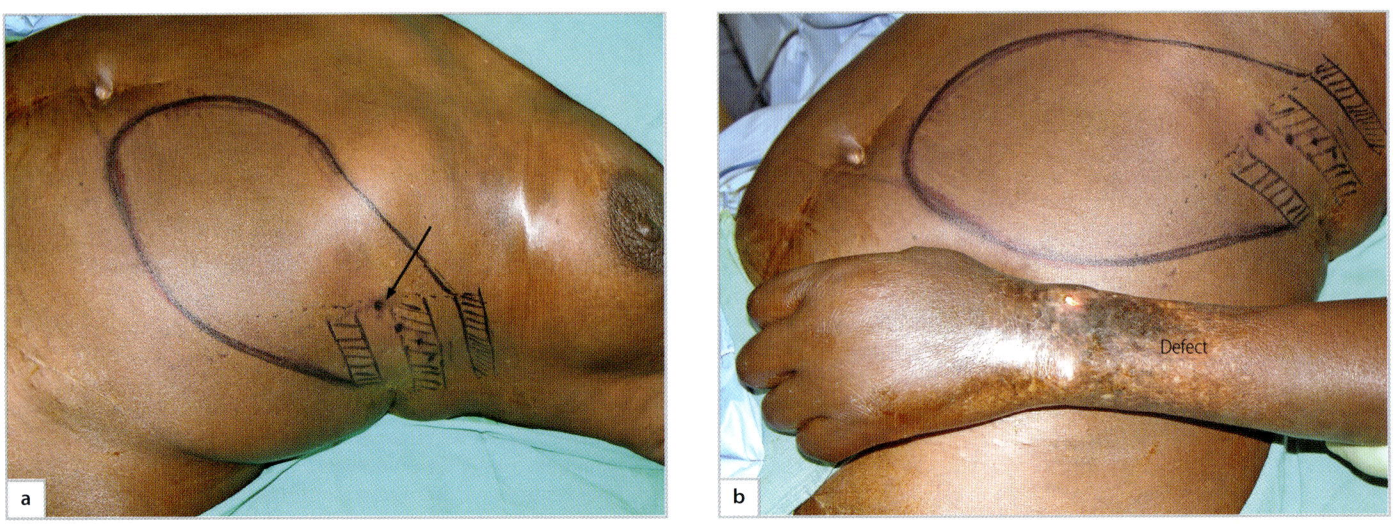

Figure 17.25a and b The design of the pedicled intercostal flap and the location of the intercostal cutaneous perforators.

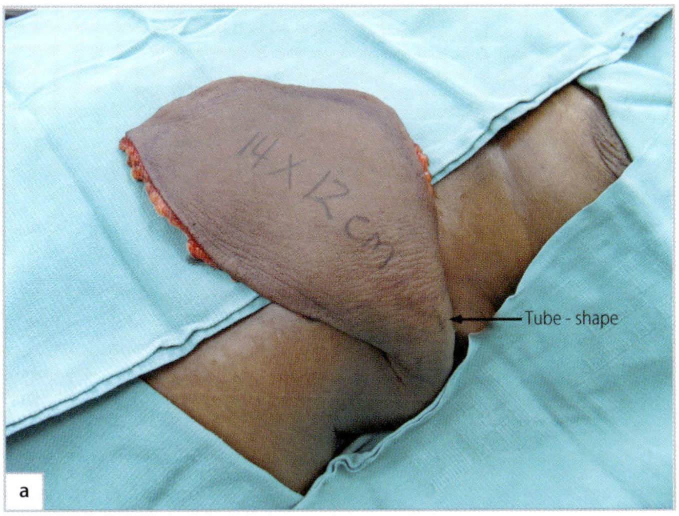

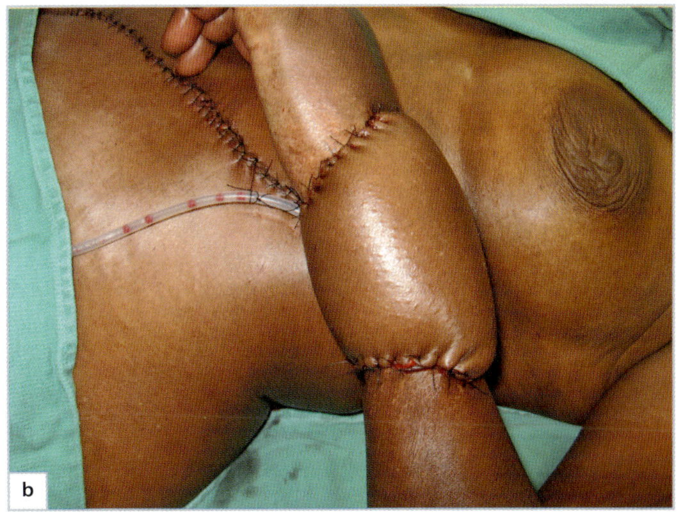

Figure 17.26 (a) The flap is elevated, and the pedicle is formed into a tube shape. (b) The flap is transposed to the wrist.

have concluded that the ALT flap can provide a large volume of soft tissue coverage with improved aesthetics and function compared with other flaps.

The ALT flap is harvested from the middle third of the lateral thigh, where the medial border is the medial border of the rectus femoris, and the lateral border is the lateral intermuscular septum between the lateral edge of the tensor fascia lata, vastus lateralis, and biceps femoris muscles. The pedicle is based on the descending branch of the lateral circumflex femoral artery (**Figure 17.27**), which originates from the profunda femoris, and then immediately divides into ascending, descending, and transverse branches. Among the three branches, the descending branch is the largest, traveling downward in the intermuscular septum between the rectus femoris and vastus lateralis muscles for a variable distance before entering the vastus lateralis muscle. Proximally, near its origin from the lateral circumflex femoral artery, a dominant branch splits off to the rectus femoris muscle, and should be preserved during flap elevation.

Surgical technique

- Preoperative Doppler examination will aid in identifying the location of cutaneous perforators, but it is not always accurate due to the thick subcutaneous tissue in this region
- The flap is marked around a line between the anterior superior iliac spine and the superolateral corner of the patella (AP line) (**Figure 17.28**)
- The main cutaneous perforators are located around the midpoint of this line, on average 1.0–1.5 cm lateral to the line
  - Yu described the ABC system to identify the location of the cutaneous perforators for the ALT flap (**Figure 17.28**)
  - Perforator B is commonly located in the vicinity of the midpoint of the AP line
  - Perforator A and C, if present, would be found approximately 5 cm proximal and distal to perforator B

The flap can be elevated from the subfascial plane either from medial to lateral or from lateral to medial.

Medial to lateral incision:

- If a medial incision is made first, the flap can be elevated off the rectus femoris muscle; the vastus lateralis is then identified to gain an approach (expose) to the intermuscular septum

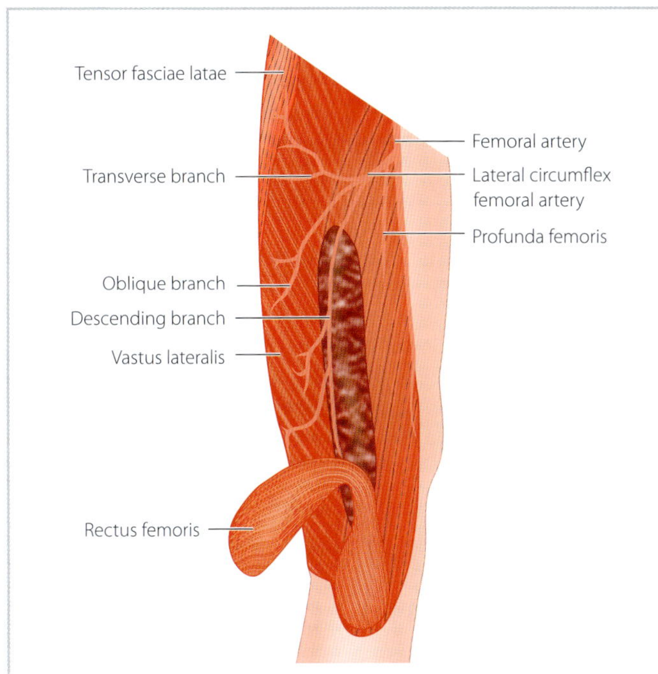

Figure 17.27 Schematic drawing illustrates the location of the oblique branch and the descending branch of the lateral circumflex femoral artery in the lateral thigh.

- Once the intermuscular septum between the rectus femoris and vastus lateralis is exposed, the descending branch of the lateral circumflex femoral artery will be visualized
- If the perforator supplying the flap is septocutaneous that means the perforator lies in the intermuscular septum between the rectus femoris and vastus lateralis, and the dissection will be easy
- For musculocutaneous perforators, the perforators take an intramuscular course, and intramuscular dissection is required for mobilization (**Figure 17.29a and b**)
- Wei et al. described the modified technique to separate the perforators from the muscles, unroofing the muscle over the musculocutaneous

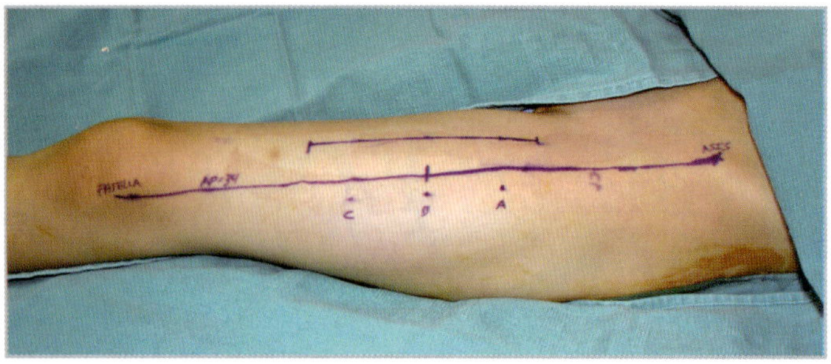

Figure 17.28 Perforator location and flap marking. The cutaneous perforators (A, B, C) may be found in the anterolateral thigh flap, with perforator B located near the midpoint between the anterior superior iliac spine and superolateral patella.

perforators. They stated, 'Unroofing of musculocutaneous perforators is safe, minimally devascularizes the muscle, and can be done quickly with minimal bleeding.' The perforators can be traced from distal to the origin of the main pedicle. The branch deriving from the lateral circumflex femoral artery supplying the rectus femoris muscle should be preserved to avoid the risk of muscle necrosis. After elevation of the flap, thinning of the flap may be required for removal of the fatty tissue, with caution taken to preserve the perforators. The flap can be transferred to the defects and the vessels anastomosed to the radial or ulnar artery in an end-to-end manner or end-to-side manner. The donor site can then be closed primarily

Lateral to medial incision:

- If the flap is elevated lateral to medial, the perforators should be identified first
- The proximal and distal margins of the flap are then elevated to allow exposure of the intermuscular septum between the vastus lateralis and the rectus femoris
- The descending branch of the lateral circumflex femoris and the original location of the perforators can be visualized
- Further dissection to the proximal end of the lateral circumflex femoral vessels will expose the long vascular pedicles
- After the incision at the medial side, flap elevation can be safely completed

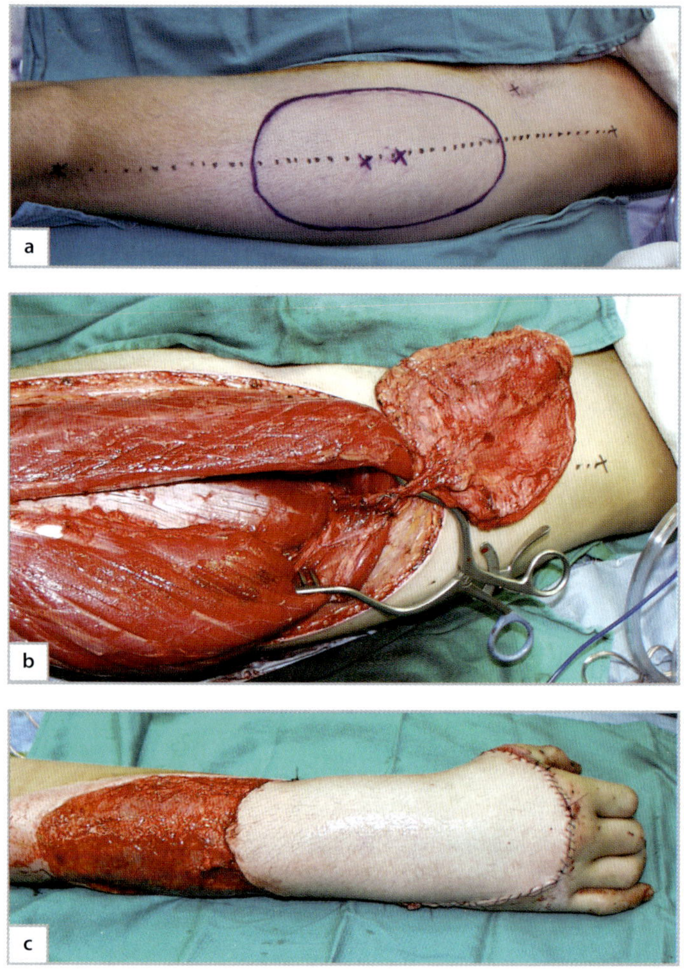

Figure 17.29 (a) Intraoperative pictures demonstrate the anterolateral thigh (ALT) flap design. (b) The flap is raised up and the pedicle is traced as long as possible. (c) The free ALT flap is transferred to the dorsum of the hand with a crush injury.

SUGGESTED READING

Dibbell DG. Use of a long island flap to bring sensation to the sacral area in oung paraplegics. Plast Reconstr Surg 1974; 54:220–223.

Gao JH, Hyakusoku H, Inoue S et al. Usefulness of narrow pedicled intercostal cutaneous perforator flap for coverage of the burned hand. Burns 1994; 20:65–70.

Goertz O, Kapalschinski N. The effectiveness of pedicled groin flaps in the treatment of hand defects: results of 49 patients. J Hand Surg Am 2012; 37:2088–2094.
The study reported on 49 cases of soft tissue defects in which groin flaps were used for reconstruction. On average, the authors performed 4.6 operations on each patient in total, and most patients were satisfied with the results.

Gurdin M, Pangman WJ. The repair of surface defects of fingers by trans-digital flaps. Plast Reconstr Surg 1950; 5:368–71.

Ho AM, Chang J. Radial artery perforator flap. J Hand Surg Am 2010; 35:308–311.
This study reported the anatomy, indications, and operating technique of the radial artery perforator flap for upper limb reconstruction.

Innocenti M, Baldrighi C, Delcroix L, Adani, R. Local perforator flaps in soft tissue reconstruction of the upper limb. Handchir Mikrochir Plast Chir 2009; 41:315–321. doi: 10.1055/s-0029-1237357. Epub 2009 Dec 18.
In this study, the authors described their experiences using local perforator flaps for upper extremity reconstruction and recommended preoperative Doppler to identify the perforators. Local perforator flaps are usually based on the two main arteries of the forearm and can cover the defect while sparing the main vessels.

Lanzetta M, Mastropasqua B, Chollet A et al. Versatility of the homodigital triangular neurovascular island flap in fingertip reconstruction. J Hand Surg Br 1995; 20:824–829.

Mathes SJ, Nahai F (eds). Reconstructive surgery: principles, anatomy and techniques. New York; Churchill Livingstone, 1997:11–12.

McGregor IA, Jackson IT. The groin flap. Br J Plast Surg 1972; 25:3–16.

Ng SW, Teoh LC, Lee YL. Contralateral pedicled lateral arm flap for hand reconstruction. Ann Plas Surg 2010; 64:159–163.

This retrospective study reported on 22 patients with hand defects that were treated with a contralateral pedicled lateral arm flap. The authors reviewed the indications for this technique and the outcomes, as well as complications. The size of the flaps ranged from 18 cm^2 to 127.5 cm^2, and the flaps were divided 3 weeks after 1 week of ischemia preconditioning.

Quaba AA, Davison PM. The distally-based dorsal hand flap. Br J Plast Surg 1990; 43:28–39.

Sebastin SJ, Mendoza RT, Chong AK, et al. Application of the Dorsal metacarpal artery perforator flap for resurfacing soft-tissue defects proximal to the fingertip. Plast Reconstr Surg 2011; 128:166e–78e.

This paper discusses the application of 58 dorsal metacarpal artery perforator flaps in 56 patients from surgery to 5-year follow-up. The average flap size was 4.6 × 2.3 cm, and the patient satisfaction rate was very high, with a low rate of complications including venous congestion in six flaps and arterial insufficiency in three flaps.

Venkataswami R, Subramanian N. Oblique triangular flap: a new method of repair for oblique amputations of the fingertip and thumb. Plast Reconstr Surg 1980; 66:296–300.

Yu P. Characteristics of the anterolateral thigh flap in a Western population and its application in head and neck reconstruction. Head Neck 2004; 26:759–769.

The author introduced a simple classification system of vascular anatomy to assist anterolateral thigh (ALT) flap dissection. The cutaneous perforator can be found in the territory of the ALT flap in a predictable pattern, which they labeled as A, B, and C.

TRAUMATIC THUMB RECONSTRUCTION

INTRODUCTION

The thumb is responsible for 40% of total hand function, enabling maneuvers such as pinching, grasping, and fine manipulation that are essential in daily life. The loss of the thumb not only causes a functional disability of the hand, but it also contributes to lower self-esteem and poor body image. Therefore, replacing a lost thumb optimizes both hand function and aesthetics. When replantation is not feasible, thumb reconstruction is necessary, with all efforts made to restore skeletal stability, length, position, delicate sensation, appearance, and durability of the thumb. Many factors, such as patient occupation and motivation for reconstruction, as well as the cause of defects, should be carefully considered in the preoperative evaluation. The use of reconstruction methods primarily depends upon the level of the amputation, depth of tissue loss, and the size of the defect. The treatments include homodigital and heterodigital flaps, partial-toe transfer, great-toe wrap-around flap, great-toe transfer, and second-toe transfer.

VASCULAR ANATOMY OF THE THUMB

An appreciation for the vascular anatomy of the thumb is essential in understanding the steps required to successfully perform a thumb reconstruction procedure. Blood flow to the thumb has some variations, but it is mainly provided by three fundamental artery systems: the radial artery, the princeps pollicis artery, and the terminal branches of the superficial palmar arch (**Figure 17.30**). The princeps pollicis artery arises from the radial artery at the base of the first metacarpal bone and then divides into the dorsal ulnar artery at the MCP joint of the thumb. At the trapeziometacarpal joint of the thumb, the dorsal radial artery originates from the radial artery, and travels to the distal phalanx of the thumb. The first palmar metacarpal artery originates from the superficial palmar arch and later splits into the ulnar and radial palmar digital arteries at the base of the thumb metacarpal bone. The first dorsal metacarpal artery (FDMA) arises from the radial artery in the anatomical snuffbox, proximal to the trapeziometacarpal joint. It runs along the dorsal aspect of the thumb metacarpal, passing distal to the insertion of the adductor pollicis longus tendon and deep to the extensor pollicis brevis tendon. The artery divides into the radial collateral dorsal artery of the thumb, with the intermediate branches supplying the first web space, and the ulnar branch providing blood to the index finger.

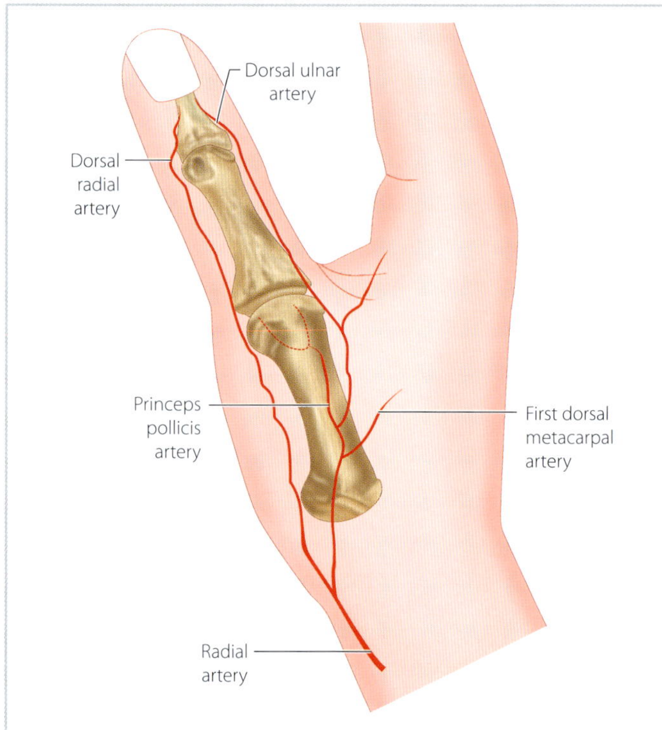

Figure 17.30 The fundamental artery system of the thumb.

RECONSTRUCTION CONCEPTS

The main principles of thumb reconstruction are to restore the maximum amount of stability, position, length, and sensation. Additional pertinent considerations include strength, mobility, and aesthetic appearance.

- Sensation: Every attempt should be made to provide the most durable and painless, sensate skin coverage
- Mobility: The mobility of the thumb is essential for positioning, to permit opposition of the thumb to one or more fingers
- Stability: The stability is a more critical aspect than mobility because the fingers can compensate for an immobile thumb but not for an unstable thumb
- Length: Maintaining the appropriate length is paramount for patients who need fine motor or precise pinch. However, patients without this requirement may do well with a shorter thumb
- Strength: The strength of the thumb is dependent upon adequate length and stability. Power grip and key pinch are made possible by adequate strength and mobility.

When assessing candidates for thumb reconstruction, a surgeon should tailor an individual treatment plan for each patient. The concepts of adequate function and optimal function of the thumb must be discussed with the patient to appropriately customize treatment. For patients who only expect adequate function of the thumb, retaining some length of the proximal phalanx of the thumb may achieve the required function. However, for patients who have higher requirements and a desire for optimal functional outcomes over adequate function, the full length of the thumb needs to be reconstructed. Under such circumstances, a toe transfer or pollicization should be considered. Finally, it cannot be overemphasized that, whenever possible, an amputated thumb must be replanted or reconstructed by one of the many available options for post-traumatic thumb reconstruction.

Soft tissue injuries of the thumb are treated similar to wounds found elsewhere in the hand. When there is a defect on the thumb, whether immediate reconstruction is feasible or a simple primary repair is undertaken, a plan for subsequent management should be visualized. The selection of an ideal reconstruction method should be based on the level and type of thumb injury, the degree of tissue loss, patient preferences, and decision-making skills of the surgeon. It will be helpful to classify the defects according to the level of amputation so as to organize the various surgical options, i.e. distal third, middle third, and proximal third.

- The distal third of the thumb is defined as distal to the interphalangeal (IP) joint
- The middle third refers to the location from the IP joint to just proximal to the MCP joint
- The proximal third extends to the carpometacarpal (CMC) joint level

Distal third

Most of the unique features of the thumb's function, such as pulp pinch, pulp stability, and sensation, lie in the distal third of the thumb. The distal third of the thumb provides powerful and precise opposition to one or more fingers, and the volar pulp of the thumb is critical in lateral or key pinch movements. Therefore, when the distal third of the thumb needs to be reconstructed, the treatment should provide a sensate, durable, and padded distal thumb.

For a minimal thumb pulp loss injury, allowing the wound to heal spontaneously by secondary intention is a good option. A full-thickness skin graft can be used to cover defects that do not have bone or tendon exposure. If more extensive pulp loss occurs through the terminal phalanx, a V-Y advancement flap can be designed appropriately for defects <1-cm long. A Moberg flap can be used to cover a relatively large defect ≤2 cm in longitudinal diameter at the palmar tip of the thumb and will also provide the donor site with the durable pulp of the distal thumb. For defects >2 cm, a full-thickness skin graft may adequately cover the defect. However, a cross-finger flap or first metacarpal artery flap will provide a better sensory return, aesthetic appearance, and functional outcome compared with a skin graft. Each of these techniques can maintain the normal length of the thumb, so the surgeon should avoid shortening the bone to facilitate the closure.

Tissue or bone loss distal to the IP joint is unlikely to cause substantial functional impairment, and flap coverage is adequate to preserve the functional requirement of the thumb. However, for patients who demand better aesthetic outcomes, a wrap-around great-toe transfer is preferred due to the improved cosmetic result it provides.

Middle third

When amputation occurs distal to the MCP joint, only two tendons are destroyed, the flexor pollicis longus (FPL) and the extensor pollicis longus (EPL). In this situation, the CMC joint and thenar muscles are intact, which provide mobility and stability to the remaining thumb. Therefore, when tissue loss of the thumb occurs through the middle third level, acceptable function is still possible. In general, for amputation at this level, the functional capability depends on the remaining skin and length of the thumb. To provide adequate functionality, the thumb should be long enough to contact the other digits. If the remaining thumb does not have adequate length, additional length and sensibility should be considered when performing reconstruction. If healthy, sensate skin exists in the remaining soft tissue covering the site of amputation, the thumb can maintain the ability to discriminate between objects.

- Z-plasty: Z-plasty and deepening of the web space can improve the grasping ability of the thumb. Simple Z-plasty, four-flap Z-plasty (**Figure 17.31**), and five-flap Z-plasty (**Figure 17.31**) can increase the hand span and deepen the first web space. Indications for Z-plasty include minimal scarring at the web space, no muscle contracture, and amputation of the thumb metacarpal bone distal to the middle portion of the proximal phalanx

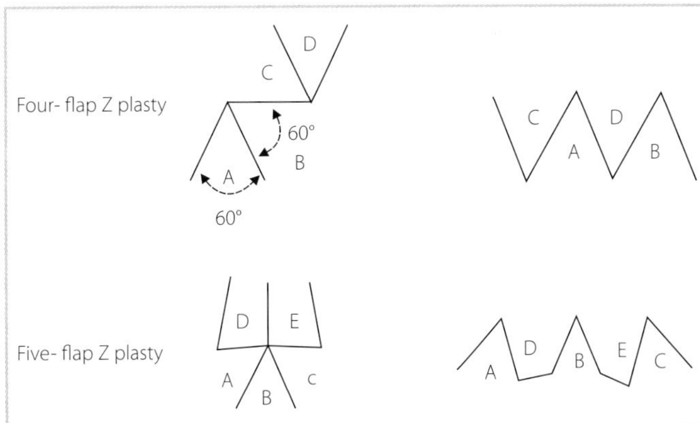

Figure 17.31 Four-flap and five-flap Z-plasty techniques.

- Distant flap: For patients with extensive scarring of the web space or an adduction muscle contracture, a Z-plasty may be inadequate for thumb phalangization. In this setting, a pedicled flap such as a radial forearm flap, radial artery perforator flap, reverse posterior interosseous flap, or lateral arm flap from the uninjured opposite arm can be sought to provide sufficient coverage of the web space. These procedures provide excellent skin and subcutaneous tissue both palmarly and dorsally. Following web space deepening and expansion, the hand will have improved function
- Bone lengthening procedures can stretch the bone and soft tissue to an appropriate length for functional restoration. The distraction apparatus is applied to the proximal and distal bone segments to enable gradual lengthening of the bone. Once adequate length is achieved, a bone graft is fixed to the distracted gap for rapid healing
- A composite radial forearm island flap can be used for patients who demand improvements in the length and function of the thumb, but not for good motion. This procedure can achieve bone lengthening in one stage and avoid staging osteoplastic procedures. A bone flap ranging from 2 to 4 cm is harvested on the lateral side of radius, which includes the perforating branches from the radial artery
- Microsurgical toe-to-thumb transfer provides better sensory recovery, functional results, and aesthetic outcomes compared with the previously described techniques. The toe-to-thumb transfer may best treat the proximal middle third amputation in a patient with a high functional demand. This technique can also carry the extensor and flexor tendons from the toe to the thumb, which are destroyed during a middle third amputation. The disadvantages of the toe-to-thumb transfer are that it is time consuming and may not be successful. To achieve optimal outcomes, collaboration between the patient and a skilled surgeon is required

Toe-to-thumb transfer

There are four established toe transfer methods: (1) Great-toe transfer, (2) Wrap-around great-toe transfer, (3) trimmed great-toe transfer, and (4) Second-toe transfer. A recent systematic review of toe-to-thumb transfer revealed that there were no differences in any objective functional parameters among the four transfer techniques.

- The great-toe transfer is indicated for patients who demand the best function and appearance. Generally, for a patient with a thumb amputation at the MCP joint, the size of the great toe is similar compared with the uninjured thumb, making it suitable for replacement of the missing MCP and IP joints of the thumb.

When a great-toe transfer is considered for thumb reconstruction, the metatarsophalangeal joint of the toe should be preserved for important function such as push-off
- A trimmed great-toe transfer may be indicated when the great toe is much larger than the normal thumb
- A second-toe transfer is preferred for those patients who do not want to lose the function of the great toe, which is important for push-off during walking
- A great-toe wrap-around transfer is not suitable for a middle third amputation of the thumb, but it is indicated for a thumb with an avulsion injury at the distal third
- Total great-toe, great-toe wrap-around, and trimmed great-toe techniques provide a broader, stronger thumb tip for pinching and grasping compared with a second-toe transfer. However, for patients who require a more precise pinch, trimmed great-toe and second-toe transfer techniques may be more suitable than a total great-toe transfer

Proximal third

The intrinsic thenar muscles responsible for stability and mobility of the basal joint are usually injured during amputations proximal to the MCP joint. In this situation, a toe-to-thumb transfer will not provide the reconstructed thumb with sufficient stability because a toe-to-thumb transfer can only provide the extensor and flexor tendons of the thumb. Index pollicization can provide acceptable stability and mobility for reconstruction of amputations proximal to the MCP joint. Index pollicization is also indicated for severe congenital thumb hypoplasia, and the transferred digit will retain growth potential. The presence of the thenar muscle is the key to the intrinsic muscle reconstruction of the thumb. If the thenar muscle is destroyed after severe traumatic total thumb loss, pollicization using the index finger will not be able to achieve control of thumb movement due to a lack of the intrinsic muscle. Instead, the procedure will only arrange the index finger into a posture that will allow the rest of the fingers to flex toward it, with no control over the index finger. Pollicization or a tube-pedicled skin flap with bone graft is recommended for traumatic thumb loss at the proximal third. The second toe to thumb transfer is suitable for the patient who does not want to sacrifice a normal finger, but the functional outcomes of pollicization are better than that of a second toe-to-thumb transfer.

The disadvantage of pollicization is that a normal finger must be sacrificed to create a thumb in which function may not be normal. In addition, removing one ray narrows the hand, reducing grip strength by 20%, possibly causing difficulty for manual laborers. For patients with associated digital injuries in addition to thumb loss, pollicization of the injured digit is an ideal choice for thumb reconstruction.

SURGICAL TECHNIQUE

Distal third loss of the thumb

When the pulp of the thumb needs to be reconstructed, the original pulp thickness and color should be considered, and the result of reconstruction should be stable and durable. In addition, adequate thickness and good two-point discrimination is preferred in the pulp. There are various reconstructive options based on the shape and size of the defect. The V-Y advancement flap is suitable for defects no > 1 cm, and the Moberg flap is indicated for pulp defects < 2 cm. If a defect is > 50% of the thumb pulp pad and has exposed tendon or bone, the function and length of the thumb should be carefully considered during the decision-making process. Under such circumstances, a cross-finger flap or conventional kite flap should be used for reconstruction.

Moberg flap

The volar advancement flap was first described by Moberg in 1964. The blood supply of this flap is based on the two digital arteries of the thumb, which are branches of the princeps pollicis artery. This flap is particularly suited for the thumb because of the dual volar and dorsal blood supply to the thumb. In the fingers, however, the use of this flap is limited due to the increased risk of flexion contracture that will affect finger function and the potential for dorsal skin necrosis. This flap is contraindicated when the injury involves the dorsal arteries, because this increases the risk of dorsal skin and nail bed necrosis.

Surgical technique

- The flap can be designed from the defect to the proximal thumb crease (**Figure 17.32**)
- Mid-lateral incisions are made on the radial and ulnar sides of the thumb, dorsal to the digital arteries
- The flap is then elevated in a distal to proximal manner, exposing the flexor tendon sheath (**Figure 17.33**)
- To preserve the blood supply for the flap, the flap should include the subcutaneous tissue and neurovascular bundles
- The mobility of the flap can be tested by distal traction to determine if any more tissue release is required to cover the defect
- Once the flap's dorsal attachment is detached distal to the MCP joint, the tourniquet should be released to confirm adequate perfusion
- It is recommended to hold the IP and MCP joints of the thumb in 30°–45° of flexion during flap advancement. Then the flap can be advanced toward the defect and sutured to the nail bed or remnant skin edge (**Figure 17.34**)

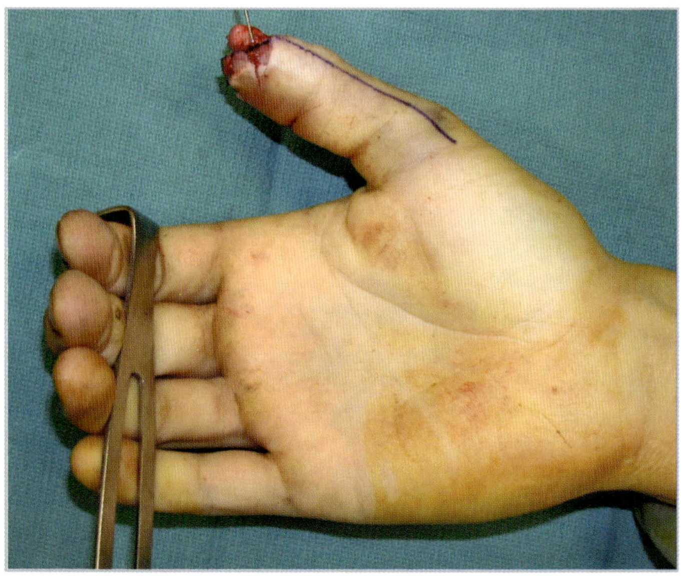

Figure 17.32 The skin markings for a Moberg flap.

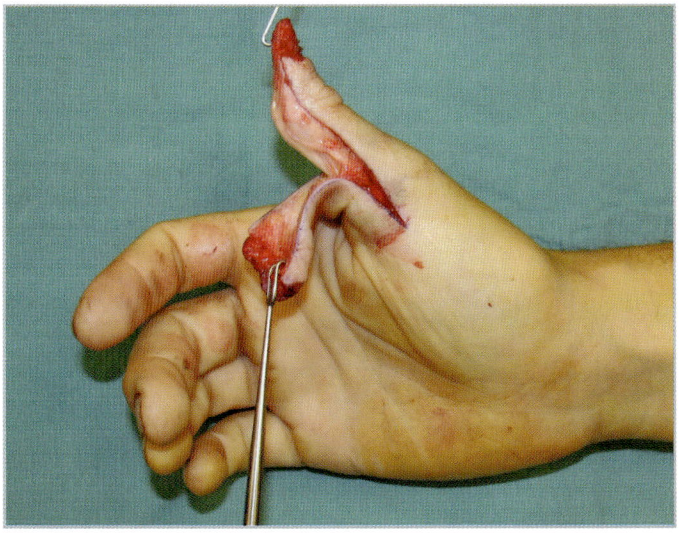

Figure 17.33 After the flap is elevated from distal to proximal, the flexor tendon sheath is exposed.

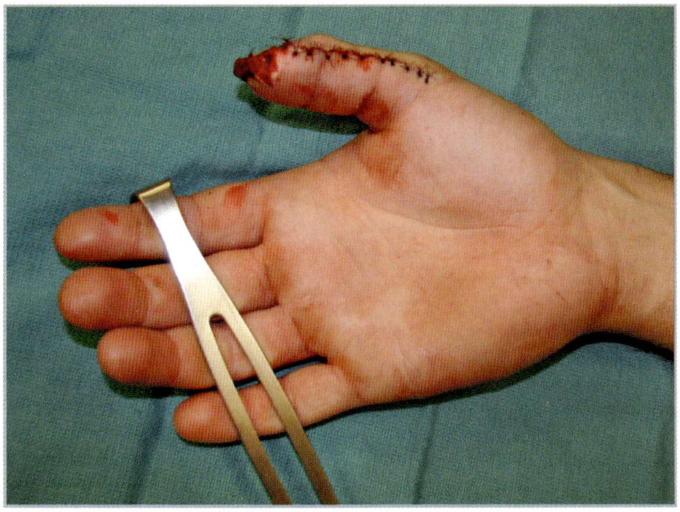

Figure 17.34 The flap is advanced to the defect and sutured in place.

Postoperative care and complications

Postoperatively, active range of motion exercises can be started at 3 weeks (**Figure 17.35**). The main drawback of this technique is the potential risk for a flexion contracture.

Kite flap (the FDMA flap)

The kite flap is indicated when there is a loss of thumb pulp coupled with exposed tendon or bone or a dorsal thumb defect that is too large to be covered by a Moberg flap. Based on the FDMA, and innervated by the superficial radial nerve sensory branches, this flap is particularly useful in resurfacing volar or dorsal distal thumb defects. The FDMA arises dorsally from the radial artery at the CMC joint, superficial to the first dorsal interosseous muscle. The kite flap is contraindicated when the first dorsal web space is not intact, because the FDMA may have been damaged and the flap may not provide adequate coverage of the defect.

Surgical technique

- Using Doppler ultrasound, mark the radial artery and the FDMA, from the radial aspect of the index finger to the proximal pivot point at the juncture of the thumb and index metacarpals
- After identifying the FDMA, the flap can be designed on the dorsal aspect of the index finger over the metacarpal head and MCP joint (**Figure 17.36**)
- An incision is then made over the line of the FDMA, and the flap can be dissected down to the first dorsal interosseous muscle, elevating muscle and all superficial tissue within the flap from distal to proximal, up to the branching point of the FDMA
  - Care should be taken at the radial border of the MCP joint where the FDMA travels subcutaneously from the muscle to the superficial tissue
- Do not isolate the artery, but instead harvest the pedicle with a width of approximately 1.5 cm of surrounding tissue (**Figure 17.37**)
- After creating a tunnel under the intact skin of the first web space, the FDMA flap, including the first interosseous muscle, FDMA, superficial veins, and the surrounding fat, can be transferred to a defect of the thumb

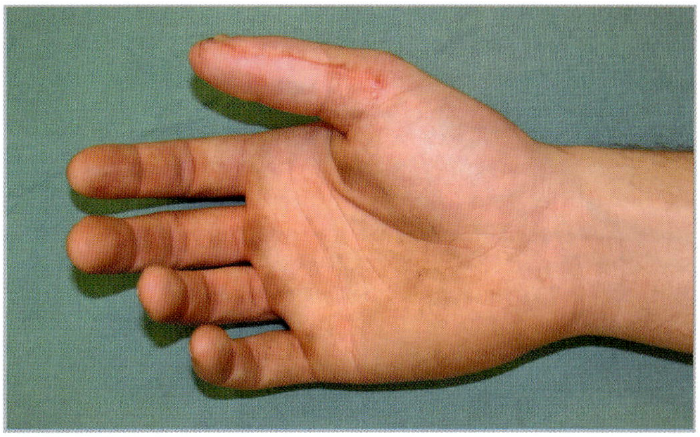

Figure 17.35 Patient treated with Moberg flap at 3-week postoperative follow-up.

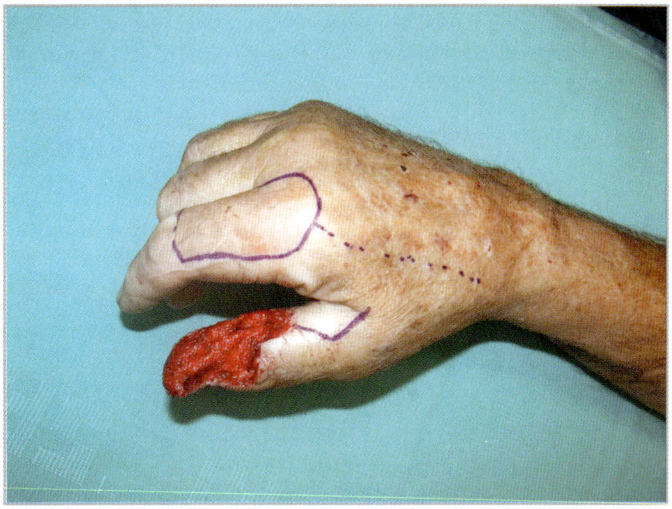

Figure 17.36 The design of the kite flap.

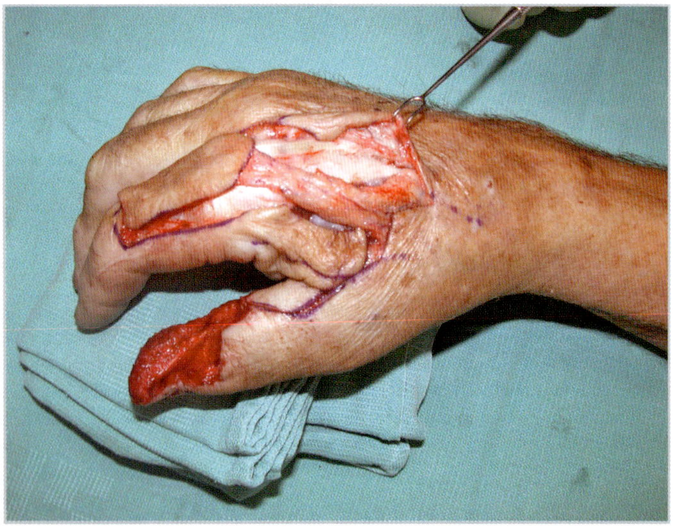

Figure 17.37 The pedicle should be harvested with approximately 1.5 cm of surrounding tissue.

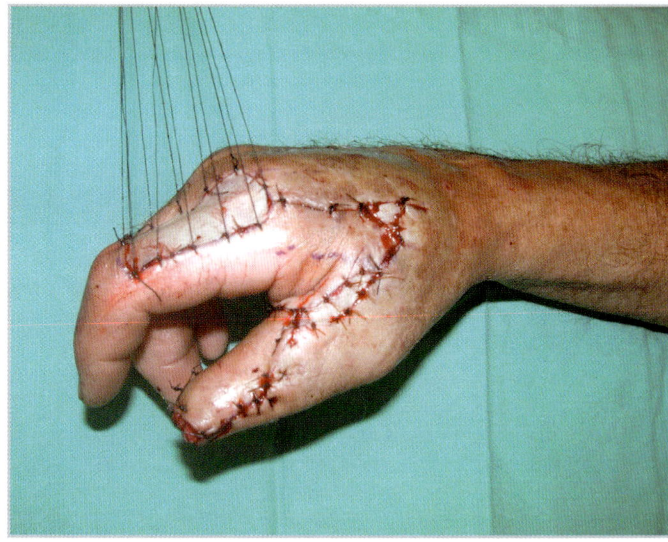

Figure 17.38 The flap is transferred and sutured to the defect, and the donor site is covered with a full-thickness skin graft.

- This flap has a wide arch of rotation and can reach the palmar or radial aspects and the pulp of the thumb (**Figure 17.38**)
- The donor site of the index finger can be closed with a full-thickness skin graft

Postoperative care and complications

The thumb should be immobilized with a padded spica splint and kept elevated. Complications include vascular compromise to the flap and donor site morbidity, such as stiffness and hypertrophic scarring.

Middle third loss of the thumb

Second-toe transfer

The authors prefer the second-toe transfer for thumb reconstruction at the middle third level due to the low donor-site morbidity associated with this technique. There are several anatomic variations in the first interosseous space, and therefore, it is necessary to identify the dominant vascular pattern (**Table 17.1**) before attempting to harvest the second toe, because different anatomic variations require different harvesting techniques. The free second-toe transfer is based on the dorsalis pedis artery and the first dorsal metatarsal artery system. The first dorsal metatarsal artery originates from the dorsalis pedis artery, which is a continuation of the anterior tibial artery from the leg (**Figure 17.39**). The anterior tibial artery becomes the dorsalis pedis artery under the extensor retinaculum, running laterally to the extensor hallucis longus. The dorsalis pedis artery divides into the first dorsal metatarsal artery and the deep plantar metatarsal artery at the level of the first metatarsal. Over the first dorsal interosseous muscles, the first dorsal metatarsal artery branches to the lateral digital artery

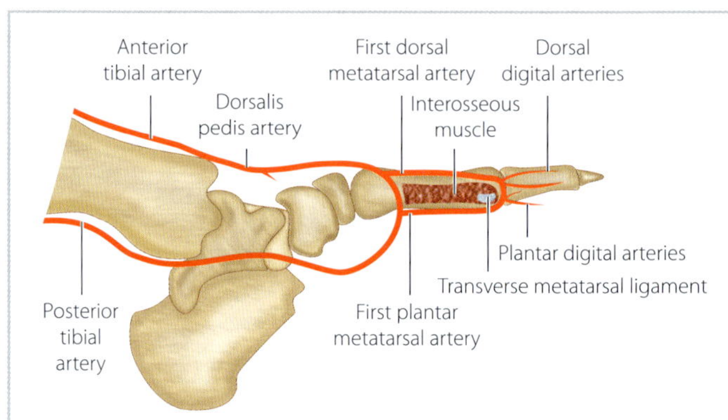

Figure 17.39 The anatomy and origins of the first dorsal metatarsal artery.

Table 17.1 Gilbert classification of anatomic variations of first dorsal metacarpal artery

Type	FDMA location
Ia	Superficial to the first dorsal interosseous muscle
Ib	Within the superficial part of first dorsal interosseous muscle
IIa	Deep to the interosseous muscle but becoming superficial to the deep intermetatarsal ligament distally, small branch of dorsalis pedis artery (DPA) present within the first dorsal interosseous muscle
IIb	Same to IIa, but no DPA present
III	Insufficient or absent of FDMA. The first plantar metatarsal artery is larger and splits from DPA at the base of the second metatarsal and passes deep to the deep intermetatarsal ligament

FDMA, first dorsal metacarpal artery.

of the great toe and the medial digital artery of the second toe, as well as the communicating branch to the first plantar metatarsal artery.

Surgical technique

Donor site

- Doppler ultrasound is recommended to mark the course of the dorsalis pedis artery and first dorsal metatarsal artery, as well as the course of the dorsal veins to the greater saphenous vein
- A curvilinear incision can then be designed on the dorsal and plantar surfaces, from the ankle joint extending to the first web space (**Figure 17.40**)
- Dissection can be carried out from the first web space to identify the arterial anatomy
  - If the artery present is type I or type II (Gilbert classification), a dorsal dissection should be relatively easy to perform by isolating the first dorsal metatarsal artery proximally until an adequate length is obtained. The communicating branches of the first dorsal metatarsal artery should be ligated; however, the major draining vein and toe extensor tendon are usually harvested with the flap
  - If the artery present is type III, the dissection of the first dorsal metatarsal artery can be difficult, making a combination dorsal and plantar approach preferable. The dorsal dissection isolates the extensor tendon and a dorsal vein, and the plantar dissection is carried out to expose the first dorsal metatarsal artery, the flexor tendons, and nerves, as well as the detachment of the deep intermetatarsal ligament
- Once the plantar digital nerves, flexor digitorum superficialis, and profundus tendons are isolated (**Figure 17.41**), the osteotomy can be performed with an oscillating saw, with care taken to keep the pedicle and draining vein intact
  - The proximal osteotomy is determined by the level of amputation, and the length is dependent on the measurement of the recipient site
- After the osteotomy, the nerves and tendons can be detached
- Release the tourniquet and perfuse the toe for 5 minutes to check the vascular status of the toe graft
  - If the dorsalis pedis artery and vein are well perfused, they can be detached with scissors

Thumb recipient site

- The middorsal (**Figure 17.42a**) and midvolar (**Figure 17.42b**) incisions are made over the stump of the thumb
- Several important anatomies should be exposed for thumb reconstruction, including the radial artery at the snuffbox, cephalic vein, branch of the superficial radial nerve, flexor and EPL, and both volar digital nerves (**Figure 17.43**).
  - Any scar tissue surrounding the bony stump should also be removed
- The EPL and FPL should be checked to ensure the tendons are free of adhesions
- If the EPL is not available, the extensor indicis tendon can be transferred for restoration of the EPL function
- It is important to preserve the attachment of the thenar muscle at the level of the metacarpal
- Care should be taken to dissect both thumb digital nerves to a level of healthy fascicles

Skeletal stabilization

- The sequence of repair include
  - Bone
  - Flexor tendons
  - Volar digital nerves
  - Arteries
  - Veins
  - Dorsal digital nerves
  - Remove clamps to perfuse thumb

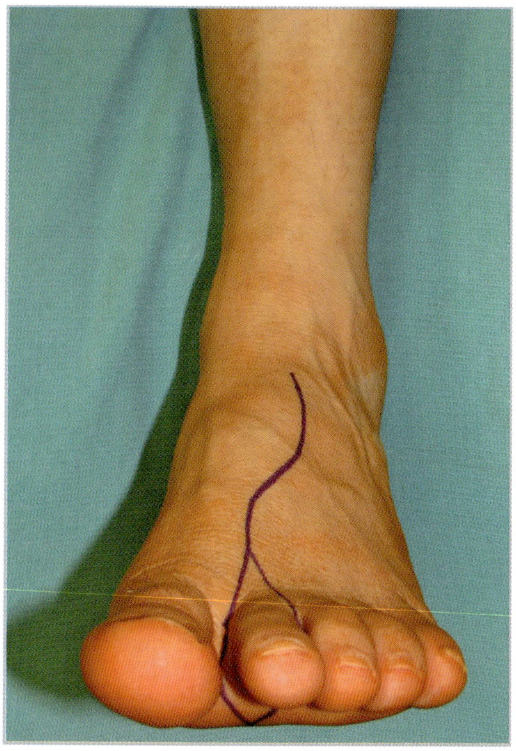

Figure 17.40 A curvilinear incision is designed over the second toe.

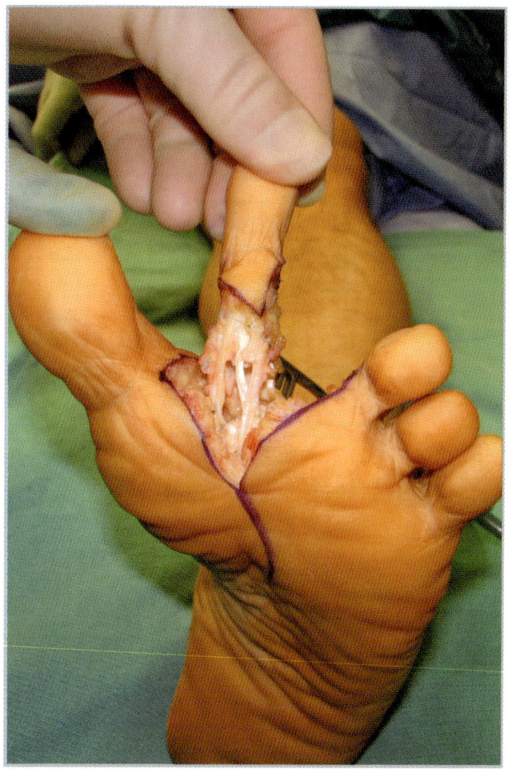

Figure 17.41 Exposure of the plantar digital nerves, flexor digitorum superficialis, and profundus tendons.

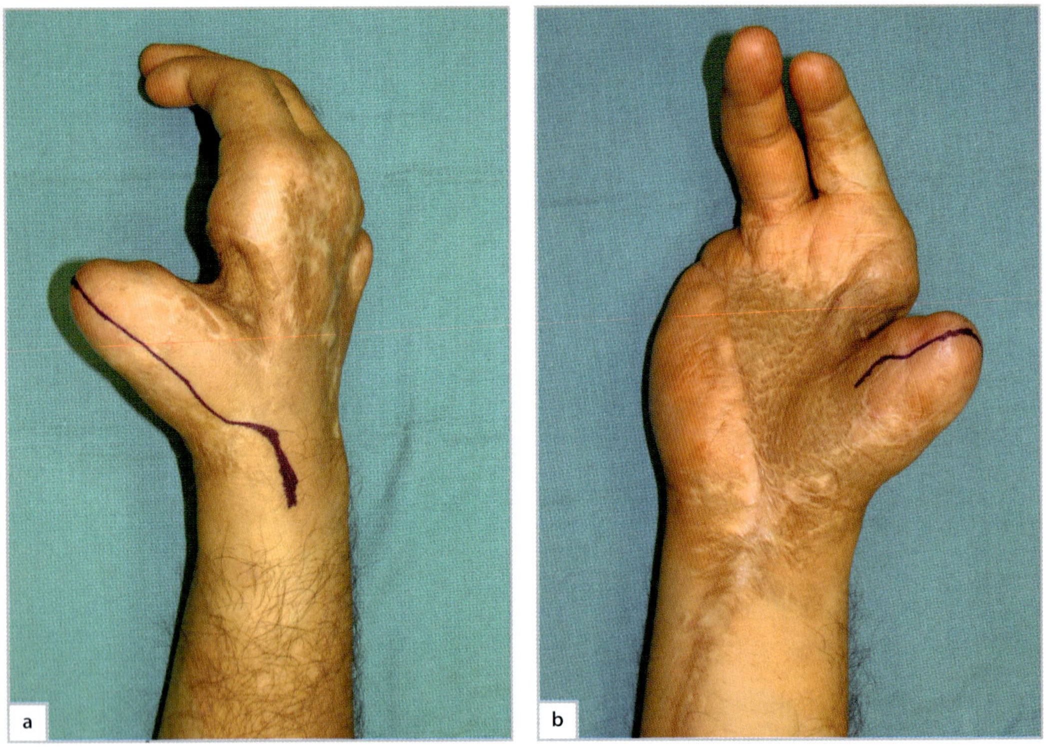

Figure 17.42 (a) Middorsal incision over the stump of the thumb. (b) Midvolar incision over the stump of the thumb.

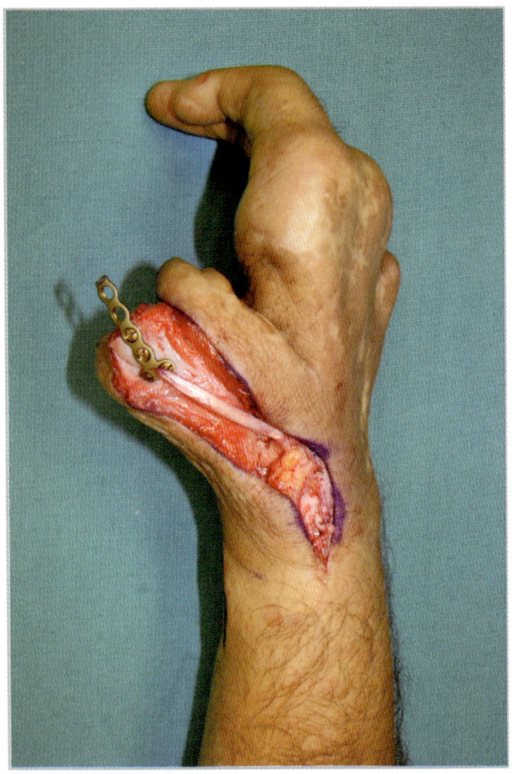

Figure 17.43 Exposure of the radial artery in the snuffbox and the extensor pollicis longus. A plate is used to secure the second toe skeleton to the thumb.

- Extensor tendons
- Skin

- The critical step of this operation is the stabilization of the skeleton between the second toe and the carpal bones. Kirschner wires (K-wires) or a miniplate is recommended for bony fixation
- The thumb should be stabilized in a position of abduction so that the pulp of the transferred thumb can point to the other fingers (**Figure 17.44**)

Tendon and nerve repair

- The extensor and flexor digitorum tendons of the second toe are attached to the EPL and FPL of the thumb, respectively
- The superficial peroneal nerves are coapted to the superficial radial nerve branches, which are helpful to promote sensory recovery. The digital nerves of the thumb are then coapted to the toe digital nerves
- The dorsalis pedis artery can be anastomosed to the radial artery at the snuffbox in an end-to-end fashion
- Finally, the soft tissue can be closed around the thumb
- Before closing the foot wound, the intermetacarpal ligament over the head of the metatarsal bone should be reconnected
- After surgery, the thumb joint should be maintained in full extension for 4 weeks

Proximal third loss of the thumb

Pollicization of index or injured finger stump

Indications include

- Thumb amputation at the CMC joint or proximal to the MCP joint
- Thumb amputation at the MCP joint or more proximally, with a complete or partial amputation of the index finger at or distal to the PIP joint
  - In this instance, the salvageable portion of the index finger can be transferred to the remaining stump of the thumb

Surgical technique

- A 'V' incision is designed around the base of the MCP joint of the index finger, and the skin flaps raised up

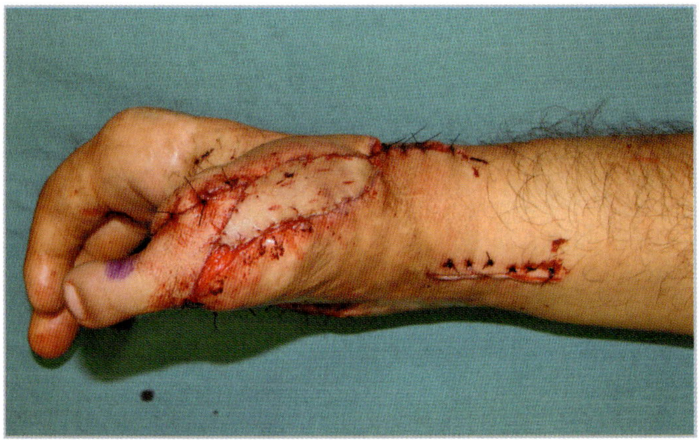

Figure 17.44 The thumb is stabilized in 45° of abduction and 100°–120° of pronation to oppose the fingers.

- The radial side neurovascular bundle of the index finger is identified and isolated with care
- Dissection is carried out in the second web space to identify the common digital artery, as well as the proper digital artery to the ulnar side of the index finger and radial side of the middle finger. Then, the proper digital artery to the middle finger is ligated just distal to the bifurcation to allow tension free index finger pollicization
- Identify and preserve the digital nerve by splitting the common digital nerve between the index and middle finger
- Dissection is alternated from the palm to the dorsum and the transverse intermetacarpal ligament is divided
- Any juncturae tendinum connected to the index extensor tendons should be divided
- Elevate the first dorsal and palmar muscles from the index metacarpal and MCP joint
- The interossei are separated down to the proximal aspect of the intermetacarpal interval through blunt dissection. This muscle will be transferred as the thenar muscle
- The index metacarpal is exposed, using a reciprocating saw to divide it at the base. The amount of additional metacarpal to be removed depends on the extent of thumb loss, but typically the bone is divided just proximal to the metacarpal neck
- Crossed K-wires are applied to stabilize the transferred digit. The index finger should be positioned into 45° of abduction and 100°–120° of pronation to be able to oppose with the middle, ring, and small fingers.
- The extensor tendons of the extensor indicis proprius and extensor digiti communis are either transferred intact or repaired to the EPL
- The first dorsal interosseous and thenar muscles are reattached to the radial lateral band, and the first palmar interosseous is reattached to the ulnar lateral band
- The skin can then be closed

Postoperative care

Postoperatively the arm is elevated, and the dressings are removed 3–4 weeks after surgery, at which point therapy can be initiated.

SUMMARY

As many options are available for thumb reconstruction, treatment for each patient should be determined based on the level of the tissue loss. The treatment plan should be derived from a careful assessment of each patient's functional status and specific reconstructive requirements, to achieve the best aesthetic and functional results.

SUGGESTED READING

Ramirez AR, Gonzalez SM. Arteries of the thumb: description of anatomical variations and review of the literature. Plast Reconstr Surg 2012; 129:468e–476e.

In this paper, the authors described the variations in the vascular anatomy of the thumb. It is important to be aware that the hand vasculature may course in a different fashion than expected because these variations may require the steps of a thumb reconstruction procedure to be modified.

Ray EC, Sherman R, Stevanovic M. Immediate reconstruction of a nonreplantable thumb amputation by great toe transfer. Plast Reconstr Surg 2009; 123:259–267.

The authors highlight the advantages of immediate reconstruction compared to delayed reconstruction of the thumb with a great toe transfer. The authors suggest immediate reconstruction decreases hospitalization, operative, and recovery time, and that increased time waiting for reconstruction may amplify the economic hardship of the patient. The study determined that immediate reconstruction with a great toe transfer can be performed safely and effectively in select patients upon their initial presentation to the hospital.

Stern PJ, Lister GD. Pollicization after traumatic amputaiton of the thumb. Clin Orthop Relat Res 1981; 155:85–94.

This paper describes the indications and surgical technique for pollicization of a hand after traumatic amputation of the thumb. The advantages of pollicization include lower morbidity, greater success rate, and completion in a one-stage operation. This procedure is particularly useful when part or all of the metacarpal bone has been lost. In addition, this technique can be performed without extensive microsurgical training.

Wei FC, Chen HC, Chuang CC, Chen SH. Microsurgical thumb reconstruction with toe transfer: selection of various techniques. Plast Reconstr Surg 1994; 93:345–351; discussion 52–57.

This paper provides a set of guidelines that help determine the type of toe-to-hand transfer that will provide the most benefit to the patient. They highlight the indications of the second toe transfer, total great toe transfer, great toe wrap-around transfer, and the trimmed great toe transfer. There is no consensus on the best overall toe-to-hand transfer technique, mainly because each technique has advantages and disadvantages. Therefore, patients should be evaluated on an individual basis to determine the most appropriate technique.

Zhang X, Shao X, Ren C, et al. Reconstruction of thumb pulp defects using a modified kite flap. J Hand Surg 2011; 36:1597–1603.

The authors describe a modified kite flap to treat thumb pulp defects that will help increase pulp sensation. By harvesting the radial branch of the first and second dorsal digital nerve with the flap and coaptating the nerves with the radial or ulnar proper digital nerves of the thumb, flap sensation was improved.

Chapter 18 Approach to complex hand trauma

Amitabha Lahiri

INTRODUCTION

There is no precise definition for complex hand trauma, but the term may be described as an injury to the hand, involving multiple structural elements, with tissue loss and/or devascularization. Although many classification systems have been devised, none of these systems is comprehensive enough to accurately include all possible patterns of injury into strict categories. Injury patterns are unique for each patient, and each patient has unique functional needs; therefore, the problem in management arises from the complexity of the injury itself. The surgeon has to make decisions on the operating table and must quickly create a roadmap for the entire course of management. There are no cookbook solutions to these injuries; however, principles and guidelines of managing complex hand trauma have evolved over the last 30 years with a deeper understanding of wound healing, infection, development of implants, and the evolution of microsurgery and free flaps.

The restoration of maximal possible hand function in the shortest period of time should be the guiding principle for hand reconstruction in complex trauma. One should avoid falling into the trap of endless cycles of revisions and reconstructive procedures, because these become frustrating for the patient and the surgeon alike. The ideal reconstructive outcome is a fully functioning and sensate hand, which, in general, is rarely achieved in a complex trauma situation. Nevertheless, good surgical outcomes equally depend on the collaborative efforts of the surgeon, hand therapist, and patient. This chapter is not intended to be a set of strict instructions or guidelines, but rather a conceptual guide in aiding the emergency management of severe and complex hand trauma. Junior doctors and inexperienced surgeons are advised to seek advice from their senior colleagues in the setting of these complex trauma situations. The surgeons or teams undertaking reconstruction of complex hand trauma should be proficient in skeletal fixation,microsurgery, and tissue transfer procedures.

PATIENT ASSESSMENT

The first step in the management of complex trauma is to stabilize a patient's vital signs (e.g. blood pressure, pulse, and respiration) and to exclude associated life-threatening injuries (e.g. severe hemorrhage or tension pneumothorax). Hand reconstruction is then prioritized in the perspective of the overall patient assessment.

History

A careful medical and surgical history should be obtained. The following three questions are essential in the understanding of the type and nature of the injury and will further guide a surgeon's approach in the preoperative planning and the decision-making process:

- When: Time of Injury
- How: Mechanism of injury
- Where: Environment in which the injury took place

ANTIBIOTIC AND TETANUS PROPHYLAXIS

Antibiotics should be started immediately and continued postoperatively. Commonly used antibiotics are crystalline penicillin, amoxicillin with clavulanic acid, or clindamycin. Before administering antibiotics, it is imperative to check a patient's allergy status to avoid the development of drug anaphylaxis. The choice of antibiotic therapy should be tailored based on the environment in which the injury has occurred as well as the results of postoperative cultures. Advice from a hospital microbiologist is always helpful to further guide the optimal antibiotic therapy.

In dirty and heavily contaminated wounds, a tetanus booster may prove to be life saving. Check a patient's immunity status and administer a dose of tetanus immunoglobulin followed by a shot of tetanus vaccine, especially in unimmunized patients. Further information and guidelines regarding tetanus immunization and prophylaxis are usually widely available through the national and local health authorities.

ASSESSMENT OF THE INJURED HAND

It is usually impossible to perform a formal examination of sensory and motor functions of the hand in the setting of severe trauma, due to a patient's poor general condition and the nature of trauma or pain, which often precludes full examination of the hand. However, a careful visual assessment combined with the knowledge of anatomy can provide a wealth of information without the need for a physical examination and can be used for preoperative planning a comprehensive assessment of structures involved or damaged by the injury can be performed under general anesthesia after an initial assessment.

Visual assessment of the hand (Figure 18.1)

- Tissue loss and viability: Inspection of wounds allows the surgeon to assess the vascularity/viability of the injured structures (e.g. digits and soft tissue). Viable healthy tissues appear pink, whereas traumatized devitalized tissue or ischemic digits appear pale white or black. Wound inspection also provides important details regarding the extent of the injury (i.e. size of soft tissue defect, exposure of underlying structures such as bone and tendons)

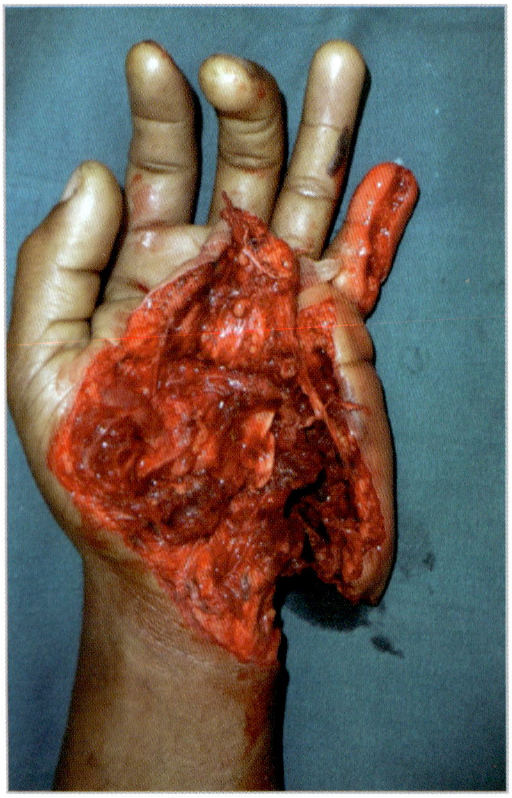

Figure 18.1 Visual assessment A roller injury to the hand. Visual assessment can confirm degloving and likely devascularization of the palmar skin, as well as loss of flexor tendons to the ring and middle fingers, with crush injury to both thenar and hypothenar muscle groups. The extent and the depth of the injury indicates the ulnar and median nerves are likely to be injured along with the tendons (although not visualized). The thumb, index, middle, and ring fingers have intact vascularity. The little finger is the most severely injured out of all the rays.

- Degree of wound contamination: Wound debris and foreign bodies may be obvious by initial inspection of the wounds, and the wound should be cleansed and all debris and foreign bodies removed
- Posture and deformities: Abnormal posture indicates injuries to the tendons in the hand, deformities of digits indicate underlying skeletal injuries
- Surface anatomy: The anatomical location of wounds may give the surgeon an idea to the extent of underlying tissue or structural damage. For example, a deep wound over the volar surface of wrist may be suggestive of underlying damage to vital structures such as nerves (e.g. median or ulnar nerves), tendons, or vessels (e.g. radial or ulnar arteries)
- Documenting severity of injury: After inspection of the wound, it is essential to carefully document the extent of injury and take clear photographs of the entire wound. Obtaining medical photographs has many benefits in the setting of complex trauma. First, it allows other doctors involved in the patient's care to have a good idea regarding the nature and extent of injury without repeatedly exposing a patient's wounds. Second, in severely crushed or badly traumatized extremities, limb-salvage procedures may not be feasible. Thus, medical photographs are useful for medicolegal purposes and also for explaining the magnitude of injury to patients and their families

Radiographic examination

Standard X-ray views (anteroposterior and lateral) should be obtained in the emergency department to assess bony injuries. However, the quality of these X-ray films is usually unsatisfactory due to the poor positioning of patients in the X-ray machines as well as the decreased penetrance of X-ray through a patient's bandage and bulky dressings. Therefore, X-rays should be repeated in the operating room when the patient is anesthetized.

Wound evaluation

A clear and organized assessment of tissue injury or loss makes reconstruction planning easier. One method is to classify the injury according to the type of tissue loss (e.g. soft tissue, bone, nerves, or a combination of all). Another style of assessment involves the evaluation of the structures affected by trauma from superficial to deep. Here, we present one method of wound assessment as follows:

- Dorsal skin
- Extensor tendons
- Bones and Joints
- Flexor tendons
- Vessels
- Nerves
- Palmar skin

SURGICAL MANAGEMENT OF COMPLEX HAND INJURIES (FIGURE 18.2)

Emergency surgery

A diagnosis of compartment syndrome or a vascular compromise that threatens the viability of the hand or upper-limb should be taken to the operating room as urgently as possible to decompress the affected compartments or to revascularize ischemic limbs. Such cases are easily missed! Recognition of compartment syndrome and ischemic situation is paramount to a successful limb salvage.

Surgical planning

After an initial assessment of wounds in the emergency department and/or operating room, a plan should be formulated to determine the structures that need to be repaired or reconstructed and the source of tissues required for reconstruction.

Timing of surgery

Complex hand injuries should receive immediate surgical treatment. Delaying treatment may result in critical ischemia of damaged tissues and skeletal muscles and increase the risk of infection, or may result in desiccation of exposed tissues, thus making subsequent surgery difficult or even impossible to perform.

Goals of reconstruction

The final goal of any reconstruction is a basic prehensile hand, i.e. a stable thumb post with two or more mobile digits that can perform pulp-to-pulp contact with the thumb. The digits and the thumb should be sensate and pain free. There is a debate in the literature regarding dichotomization of one-stage and multiple stage reconstruction of the hand, but the concept illustrated in this chapter follows the logical process of staging the reconstruction based on the priority in which different tissues should be addressed. The process described is illustrated though the single stage reconstruction of an injured hand in **Figures 18.1–18.6**.

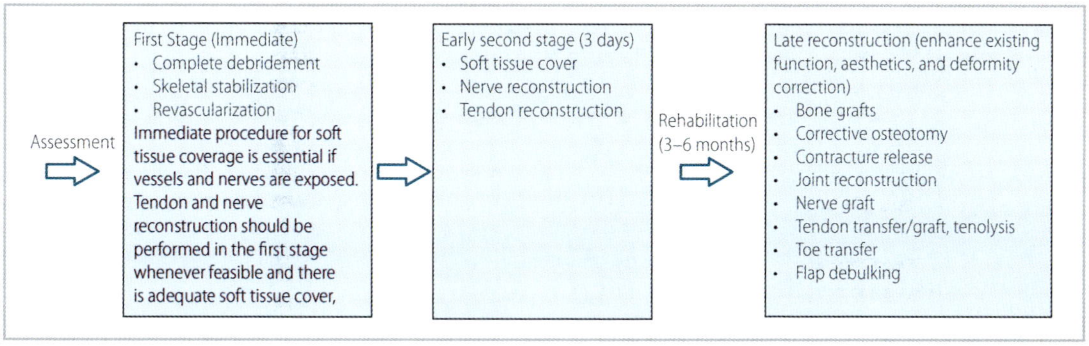

Figure 18.2 Outline of the reconstructive approach in complex hand trauma.

Surgical preparation and sources of tissues

- Prep the lower limb if anticipating the need for vein graft, skin graft, sural nerve graft
- Prep the Iliac crest if anticipating bone graft
- Prep the groin or the abdomen if anticipating a groin flap or an abdominal flap
- Spare parts can be obtained from nonsalvageable digits, e.g. nerves, tendons, and bone and skin grafts

THE FIRST STAGE OF RECONSTRUCTION (EMERGENCY SURGERY)

Primary surgery should aim to achieve complete reconstruction whenever possible. The essential components of the emergency surgery are:

1. Adequate debridement
2. Skeletal stabilization
3. Vascular reconstruction
4. Nerve and tendon reconstruction. Should be performed in the first stage itself if feasible, but can be performed in the early second stage or as late reconstruction
5. Definitive soft tissue coverage is essential in the first stage if the reconstructed vessels are exposed

Adequate debridement (Figure 18.3)

- Debridement in layer by layer fashion is carried out with the preservation of neurovascular structures. All devitalized tissue layers should be excised to create a new surgical margin
- Precise and adequate debridement facilitates accurate assessment of tissue loss and reconstruction planning. Inadequate debridement leaving behind contused or necrotic tissue that promotes secondary infection and may jeopardize future reconstruction

Skeletal stabilization

- This is the first and immediate step to stabilize bone fractures and forms the foundation for the rest of the reconstruction as well as for the rehabilitation. External as well as internal fixators can be used, depending on the type of fracture and the nature of trauma. For example, a multifragment comminuted fracture can be initially stabilized using an external fixator, which can be revised later after the soft tissue reconstruction
- The basic principles include the restoration of articular congruity, bone alignment, and the preservation of skeletal length. In cases of bone loss, skeletal length can be maintained using an external fixator, bridge plate, and a primary bone graft. In severely affected joints with loss of supporting ligaments and articular surfaces, primary joint fusion should be considered

Vascular reconstruction

This is an essential aspect of primary surgery and should be carried out immediately after the skeletal and tendon reconstruction. Occasionally, vascular reconstruction may precede tendon reconstruction if the ischemia time of the tissues has been long.

Nerve, tendon, and soft tissue reconstruction

The following procedures should also be included in the first stage of reconstruction, but they may be considered for the early second stage:

- Nerve reconstruction
  - Primary nerve repair or nerve graft should be carried out in the first stage but if necessary can be postponed to the early second stage or late reconstruction stage
- Tendon reconstruction (**Figure 18.4**)
  - Tendon repair and grafts are carried out immediately but can be carried out in the early second stage with definitive soft tissue coverage
- Definitive soft tissue coverage (**Figure 18.5**)
  - Preferably immediate or early second stage (within 72 hours). Commonly available options include skin grafts, a groin flap, abdominal flaps, a lateral arm free flap, or flow-through flaps when soft tissue reconstruction is combined with vascular reconstruction. Definitive soft tissue coverage can be postponed to the early second stage if there is a significant risk of infection such as in cases of farmyard injuries or technical expertise for free tissue transfer is not available immediately. During this time, the exposed tissues should be adequately protected from desiccation and secondary infection

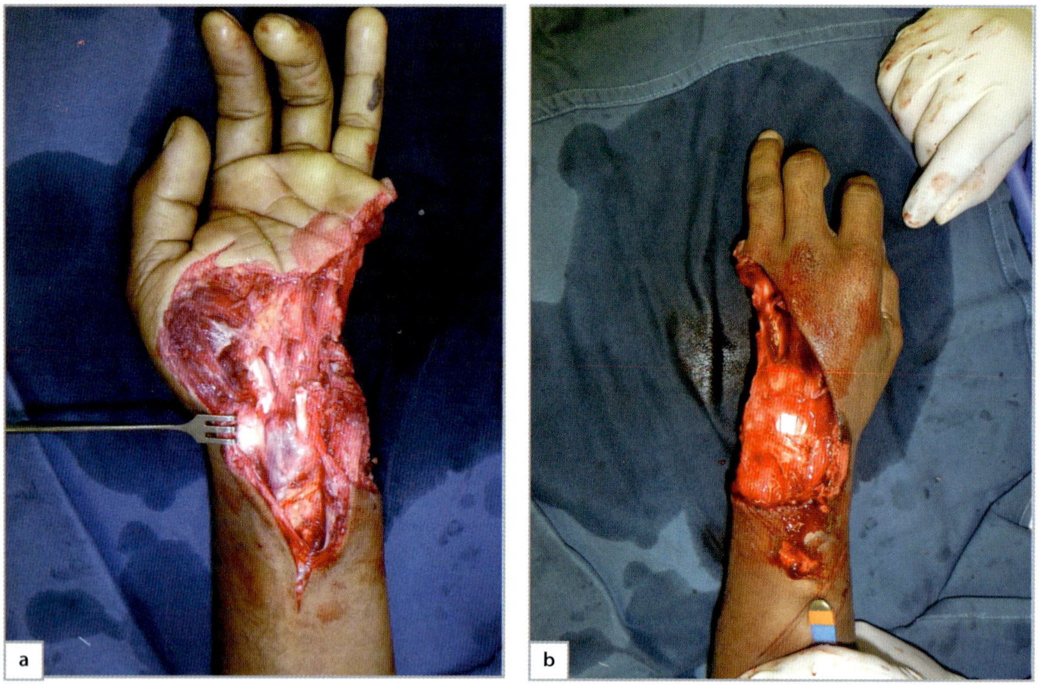

Figure 18.3 (a and b) The same hand as Figure 18.1 following complete debridement with healthy skin edges. The little finger is sacrificed due to crush injury to all component tissues.

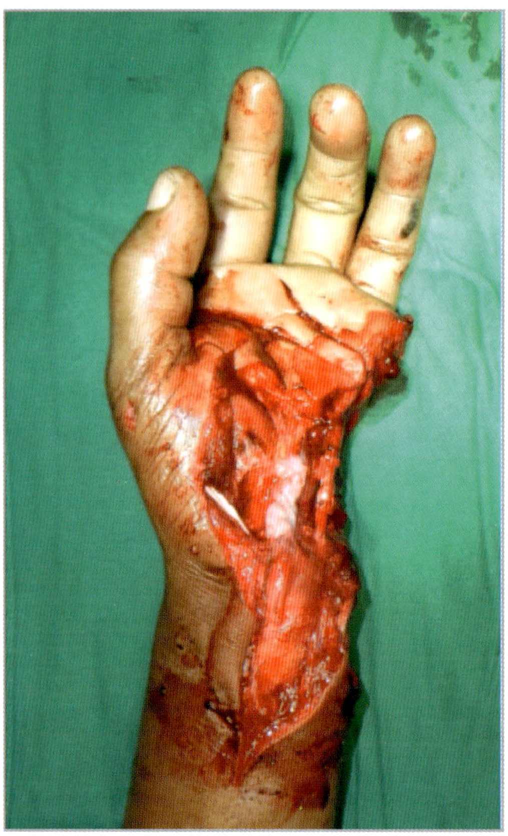

Figure 18.4 Immediate recontruction. Camitz transfer using tendon graft from the little finger and tendon graft to reconstruct the flexor digitorum profundus to the ring finger. Median nerve reconstructed using nerve grafts from the little finger (not seen in the picture).

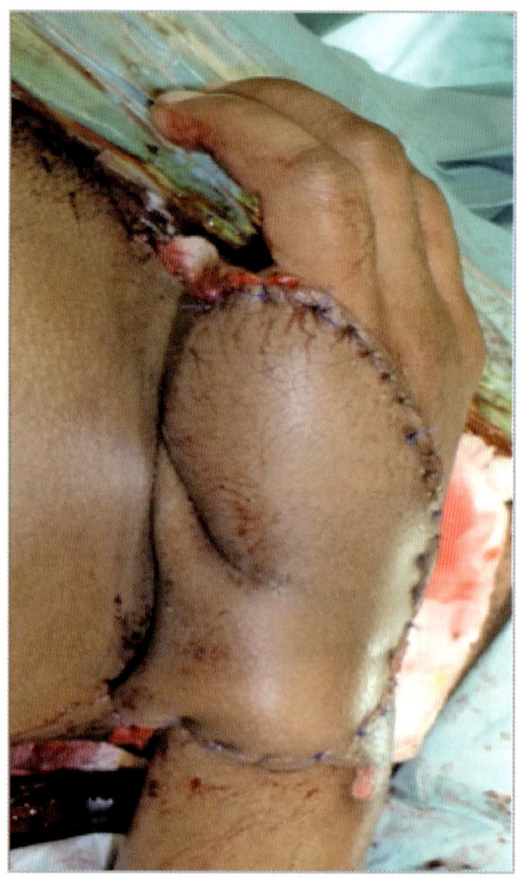

Figure 18.5 Immediate soft tissue cover. Bilobed groin and superficial epigastric flap with skin graft to the flap donor site. The surgical preparation was planned to include the abdomen and the left lower limb for skin grafting and possibly sural nerve grafting.

Prioritizing salvage during surgery (intraoperative 'triage')

In complex trauma, the injury is typically nonuniform, leading some areas to have greater structural damage than others. Nevertheless, all attempts must be made to preserve the thumb. Digits/rays that can be reconstructed with a good functional outcome should be distinguished from digits that should be sacrificed for use as spare parts. The least injured digits with the maximum functional potential should be reconstructed as priority.

A general guideline for severity of injury in the digit is the number of tissues that are injured that require reconstruction. Poor outcomes are expected if there is extensive tissue loss. This assessment is relative and the decision should be made in the perspective of the entire hand.

- Significant soft tissue loss
- Substantial bone loss
- Joint injury involving ligaments or the cartilage
- Tendon injury or loss
- Vascular injury
- Nerve injuries or loss

Spare-parts concept

- The concept of spare-parts surgery should always be kept in mind. Nonsalvageable rays or digits can be a source of skin grafts, nerve grafts, tendon grafts, bone grafts, and articular grafts. Structures that are sacrificed should not be discarded until the end of the surgical procedure.

All efforts should be made to prevent repeated trips to the operating theatre for piecemeal debridement. The first surgery should set a clear stage for the execution of the early second stage. The only exception being wounds with biological activities where there is ongoing infection that may jeopardise soft tissue reconstruction.

THE EARLY SECOND STAGE OF RECONSTRUCTION

This stage essentially consists of definitive soft tissue coverage of the defect using either pedicled flaps or free tissue transfer, but it may also include the following:

- Skeletal reconstruction or revision of fixation
- Nerve reconstruction
- Tendon reconstruction

The early second stage of reconstruction should be planned within 72 hours of the primary surgery before the wound is contaminated in the form of granulation tissue. At this stage, it is essential to provide definitive soft tissue coverage upon completion of nerve and tendon reconstruction if possible. The provision of a definitive soft tissue coverage also sets the stage for future reconstruction such as tendon grafting, nerve grafting, or procedures such as toe transfer.

REHABILITATION: ACTIVE AND PASSIVE MOBILIZATION (FIGURE 18.6)

Rehabilitation should commence as soon as feasible after soft tissue coverage, as it remains an integral part of management and is essential for functional recovery. The therapy is aimed to maintain joint mobility and prevent adhesions. A stable skeletal fixation and strong tendon repair in the previous stages allows for early mobilization.

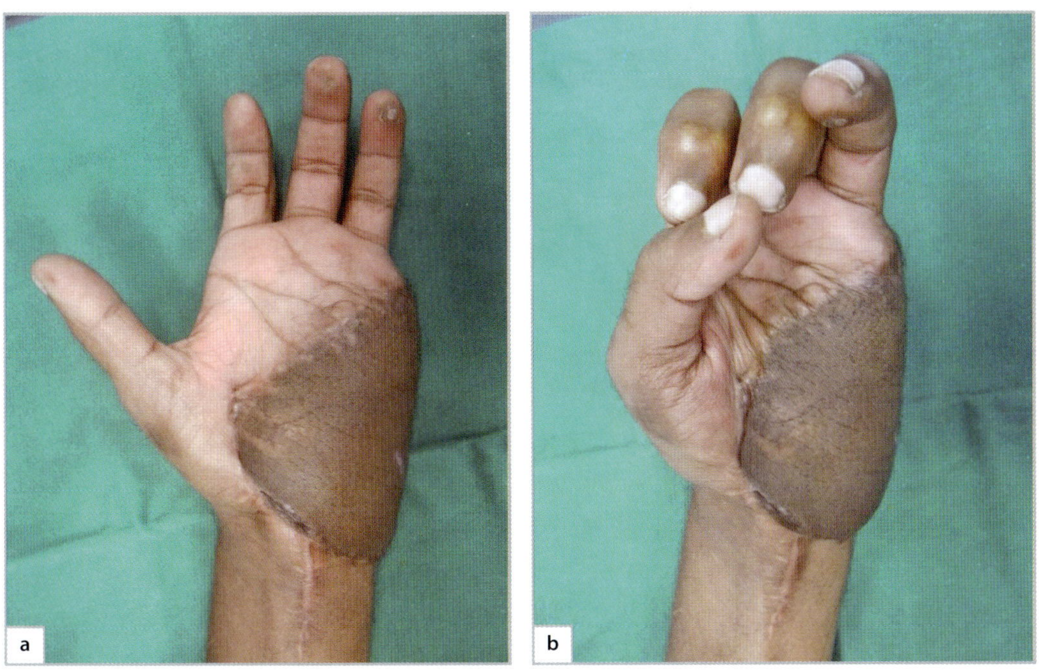

Figure 18.6 (a and b) Restoration of a functional hand with basic grip and pinch function at 8 weeks postsurgery with fingers showing purely extrinsic function. A delayed procedure may be advised to include flexor tenolysis for the ring finger to improve the range of motion.

THE LATE STAGE OF RECONSTRUCTION (PERFORMED 3–6 MONTHS AFTER THE RECONSTRUCTION)

At this stage, all the tissues have healed and the hand function has reached its maximum potential. Surgery should be aimed to enhance existing function, correct deformities, or improve the aesthetics of the hand. This includes flap debulking, tendon or nerve grafting, or correction of deformities.

A strict timeline sharpens the focus on reconstruction and enforces clear decision making, thus decreasing the potential for half-hearted and unrealistic decisions. The procedures performed at this stage usually include:

- Tendon graft/tendon transfer/tenolysis
- Nerve graft/neurolysis
- Bone graft/bone lengthening/corrective osteotomy
- Joint fusion
- Contracture release
- Toe transfer
- Debulking the flap

SUGGESTED READING

Brown PW. Less than ten – surgeons with amputated fingers. J hand Surg 1982; 7A:31–37.
An interesting paper that provides an insight into the functional aspects of digit amputation on surgeons and reemphasizes the adaptability of the hand. It provides a perspective on situations when some digits may need to be sacrificed for the overall benefit of hand function.
Entin MA. Salvaging the basic hand. Surg Clin North Am 1968; 48:1063–1081.
The paper rationalizes the basic principles of hand reconstruction and lays down the basic characteristics of a functional hand.
Vilkki SK. Free toe transfer to the forearm stump following wrist amputation – a current alternative to the Krukenberg operation. Handchir Mikrochir Plast chir 1985; 17:92–97.
The paper is a superb example of out-of-the box thinking in hand reconstruction and the need to fall back to the basic nature of hand function. Professor Vilkki created a pincer function in individuals who did not have a hand at all.
Chase RA. Functional levels of amputation in the hand. Surg Clin North Am 1967; 40:415–423.
This article attempts to correlate the functionality of the hand with the progressive loss of functional elements of the hand.
Wei FC, El-Gammal TA, Lin CH, Chuang CC. Metacarpal hand: classification and guidelines for microsurgical reconstruction with toe transfers. Plast Reconst Surg 1997; 99:122–128.
Professor Wei compiles his experience of toe-to-hand transfer into a rational approach for hand function restoration when all of the fingers are lost.

Section 3

Elective hand surgery

Chapter 19 System-specific examination of the hand

Shady A. Rehim, Kevin C. Chung

INTRODUCTION

The first clinical appointment between the patient and the hand surgeon is a good introduction for the surgeon to get to know the patient and understand his/her problem. More than one clinic appointment may be required for the surgeon to make the correct diagnosis and determine the best treatment option according to patient's individual needs. To achieve this goal, the surgeon must have a good knowledge of the basic anatomy and biomechanics of the hand. In addition, the surgeon must obtain a careful medical and surgical history and perform a meticulous physical examination of the patient's hands. In this chapter, we will review the key elements of a hand physical examination performed in the outpatient clinic setting.

HAND EXAMINATION

After the initial introduction and procurement of the relevant patient history, the examiner should sit opposite to the patient with the patient's hands lying straight across a table between the patient and the examiner. The hand should be fully exposed from the fingers to the elbow (**Figure 19.1**). The physical examination usually consists of two parts; a basic general examination followed by a focused system-specific examination of the hand. This examination sequence is occasionally referred to as 'primary and secondary surveys.' In the following sections, we will demonstrate different hand examination techniques that will help the surgeon reach the correct diagnosis of the most common conditions affecting the hand and wrist.

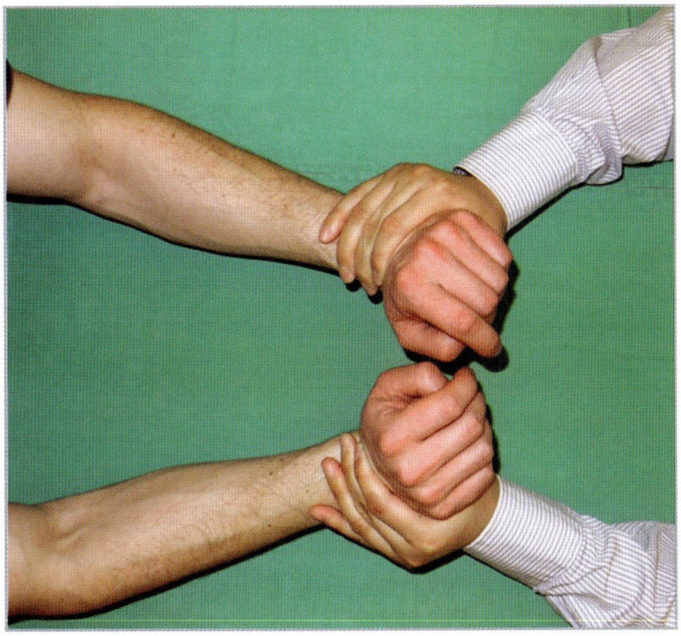

Figure 19.1 Correct clinical examination posture. The patient should sit opposite to the examiner with the patient's hands exposed all the way up to the elbow.

HAND INSPECTION

The physical examination begins with a general inspection of the palmar and dorsal surfaces of a patient's hands to assess the following:

- Gross morphologic appearance of the hand: Assess hand posture at rest; look for obvious deformities resulting from neurological disorders (e.g. claw hand and fingers drop) or characteristic features of skeletal deformities resulting from previous fractures or systemic conditions (e.g. ulnar drift of fingers in advanced rheumatoid arthritis)
- Skin and soft tissue: Look for old scars, soft tissue swelling, bruising, signs of infection, etc. Systemic conditions may be associated with skin and soft tissue changes, such as connective tissue diseases (scleroderma) that may result in a tight, glistening appearance of the skin. In addition, conditions resulting in contractures of the skin and fascia, such as Dupuytren disease, usually lead to a characteristic flexion deformity of the fingers. Moreover, in denervated areas of the hand and fingers, the skin may appear coarse and dry due to failure to secrete sweat that is mediated by sympathetic nerves
- Nail changes: Assess nails for discoloration or deformities. Several conditions may lead to nail deformation. Examples include dermatologic conditions (e.g. psoriasis), fungal infections (e.g. onychomycosis), trauma (e.g. subungual hematoma), or malignancy (e.g. subungual melanoma)
- Muscle atrophy/wasting: Muscular atrophy is commonly associated with conditions of hand denervation. Examples include:
  - Ulnar nerve palsy: Associated with atrophy of the muscles of the hypothenar eminence and interosseous muscles, often resulting in wasting of the dorsum of the first web space as well as guttering of the dorsal intermetacarpal spaces
  - Median nerve palsy: Associated with atrophy and flattening of the muscles of the thenar eminence
  - Radial nerve palsy: Associated with finger drop deformity ± wrist drop deformity

SYSTEM-SPECIFIC EXAMINATION

In this part of the hand examination, we will concentrate on the clinical evaluation of the following four categories:

1. Muscle and tendon function
2. Motor and sensory function
3. Hand vascularity
4. Bone and joint stability

Within each group, we will give a brief account of a patient's symptoms and will demonstrate the relevant examination techniques of common conditions affecting the hand and wrist.

Assessment of muscle and tendon function

Tendon disorders are among the most common complaints evaluated by hand surgeons. Tendinopathy is a general term used to describe painful conditions affecting tendons of the hand. Nonetheless, several nomenclatures exist, such as tenosynovitis, tendinitis, or tendovaginosis, which are used to describe the different etiologies of tendon disorders that can be infectious, inflammatory, or degenerative in nature.

- Proliferative tenosynovitis: An inflammatory condition affecting the synovial lining of a tendon sheath. Causes include inflammatory tenosynovitis (rheumatoid arthritis), septic tenosynovitis (bacterial, viral, or fungal), crystalline tenosynovitis (gout, pseudogout), and deposition diseases (amylodosis, sarcoidosis). The clinical presentation can be either acute or chronic. In acute septic tenosynovitis (**Figure 19.2**), look for the presence of Kanavel's four cardinal signs: (1) fingers fusiform swelling, (2) fingers flexed position at rest, (3) intense pain on passive extension of the fingers, (4) localized tenderness along the flexor tendon sheath. In a chronic disease, the clinical presentation is usually less severe, and clinical signs include swelling of the palm and fingers, decreased range of movement, and localized crepitus over the affected tendon sheath
- Trigger finger: A pathological disproportion between the volume of the flexor tendon sheath and its contents. The term tendovaginosis appropriately describes trigger finger, which has been shown to occur due to mechanical entrapment of the tendon within a fibrosed tendon sheath rather than an inflammatory condition. Although pain can be present, the most common patient complaint is 'catching and locking' of the affected fingers. The physical examination involves feeling for a nodular thickening over the A1 pulley and localized tenderness. In addition, flexion deformity of the proximal interphalangeal joint and the inability of a patient to fully flex the fingers into the palm may also be seen
- de Quervain disease: This is another example of a tendon entrapment disorder, occurring in the first extensor dorsal retinacular compartment of the wrist, which contains the abductor pollicis longus (APL) and extensor pollicis brevis (EPB). Patients often complain of pain over the radial styloid process that can be reproducible by performing the Finkelstein test. The Finkelstein test is performed by holding the patient thumb in adduction while ulnary deviating the wrist (**Figure 19.3**). Development of pain at the first extensor compartment is considered a positive Finkelstein test. Another way of evaluating the presence of de Quervain disease is by simply pressing over tendons of the first dorsal compartment, which will result in a consistent localized tenderness over that area. A distinct but similar condition, known as intersection syndrome, occurs more proximal in the forearm. Symptoms usually include swelling, pain, and tenderness over the muscle bellies of the APL and EPB, as they cross over the wrist extensors. Intersection syndrome can be examined by eliciting a localized tenderness in the same manner as described earlier for de Quervain disease by performing the Finkelstein test
- Extensor carpi ulnaris (ECU) tendinitis: A broad spectrum of pathology involving the ECU, which may occur due to tenosynovitis, tendinosis, tendon subluxation, or tendon rupture. Concomitant injuries of the ulnar-sided structures of the wrist or distal radioulnar joint (DRUJ) may make the diagnosis difficult. Therefore, the ECU synergy test was described to distinguish between tendon and joint pathology. This test is performed by asking patients to flex their elbow to 90° and fully supinate the forearm. The examiner then resists the radial abduction of a patient's thumb while applying counter pressure on the long finger. The development of pain on the dorsoulnar aspect of the wrist is considered a positive test. In the case of ECU tendon subluxation, the examiner may hear a tendon snap or palpate a volar displacement of the ECU tendon upon pronation and ulnar deviation of the wrist joint
- Flexor carpi radialis (FCR) tendinitis: The tendon of the FCR muscle passes through a narrow lumen of a fibrous sheath lined by synovial tissue and surrounded by the tubercle of the trapezium, making the FCR prone to stenotic tendovaginitis and attrition rupture as the tendon rubs against the tubercle of the trapezium. Patients suffering from FCR tendinitis often complain of pain

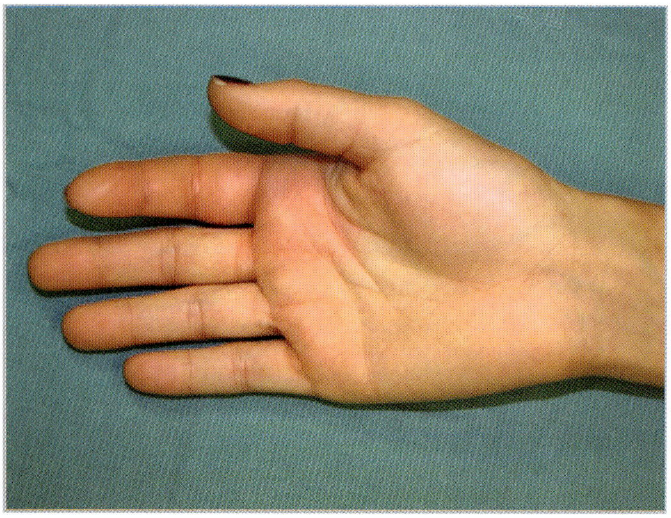

Figure 19.2 Septic tenosynovitis. Look for the four Kanaval signs.

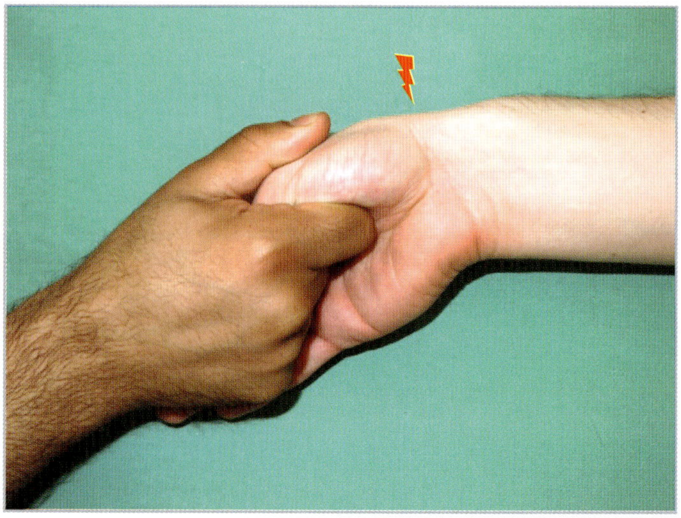

Figure 19.3 Finkelstein test. This maneuver elicits tenderness at the site of the first dorsal compartment (arrow).

and tenderness near the scaphoid tubercle. Physical examination usually demonstrates increased pain and occasional crepitus over the tendon of the FCR with flexion and radial deviation of the wrist

Assessment of motor and sensory function

The upper extremity is supplied by motor and sensory branches arising from the brachial plexus (C4/5-T1/2), including the median, ulnar, and radial nerves. The dermatome distribution of cutaneous nerves of the upper limb is shown in **Figure 8.7**. The nerves of the upper extremity are subject to mechanical compression and other pathological conditions throughout their course at different anatomic locations. Therefore, it is essential for the examiner to perform the correct examination to differentiate between the various conditions arising from nerve injury at different sites. The general examination of the nerve function, including light touch, pinprick, and two-point discrimination tests, is explained in detail in Chapter 8. The specific-examination techniques of nerves dysfunction associated with common pathological conditions of the hand are described below.

Median nerve

- Carpal tunnel syndrome (CTS): A compressive neuropathy of the median nerve at the wrist joint, resulting in various sensory (numbness, paresthesia, and pain) and motor (muscle weakness) symptoms. Hand inspection may show flattening of the thenar muscles. The motor recurrent branch of the median nerve can be reliably tested by evaluating the action of the abductor pollicis brevis muscle. This is performed by laying the dorsum of the patient's hand on a flat surface and then asking the patient to abduct the thumb palmarly against resistance. Weakness or inability to abduct the thumb indicates median nerve injury/palsy (**Figure 19.4**). Provocative tests: In general a positive finding with provocative tests indicates the presence of an ongoing nerve regeneration process, and hence, a nerve insult. Provocative tests that assist in diagnosis of CTS include:
  - Durkan test (**Figure 19.5**): It is the most sensitive clinical test to diagnose CTS. This test is performed through pressing over the carpal tunnel by the examiner's thumb for approximately 30 seconds. Development of numbness or paresthesia over the cutaneous distribution of the median nerve (radial two and half fingers) is suggestive of CTS
  - Tinel sign (**Figure 19.6**): It is performed by repeatedly tapping/percussing over the carpal tunnel. Development of numbness or paresthesia over the cutaneous distribution of the median nerve is suggestive of CTS
  - Phalen test (**Figure 19.7**): It is performed by asking patients to maximally flex and oppose their wrists for approximately 60 seconds. Again, the development of sensory symptoms indicates CTS
- Pronator syndrome: A compressive neuropathy of the median nerve at the elbow joint. Common sites of median nerve entrapment occur between the two heads of the pronator teres, bicipital aponuerosis, or flexor digitorum superficialis (FDS) aponeurotic

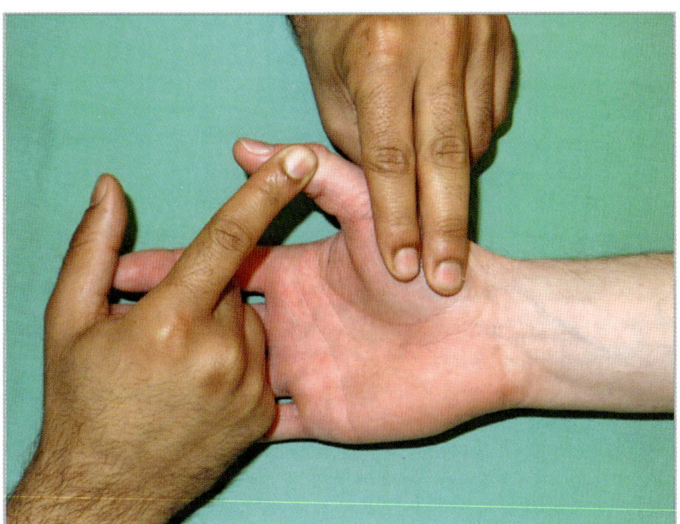

Figure 19.4 Assessment of action of the abductor pollicis brevis reliably tests the motor function of the median nerve in the hand.

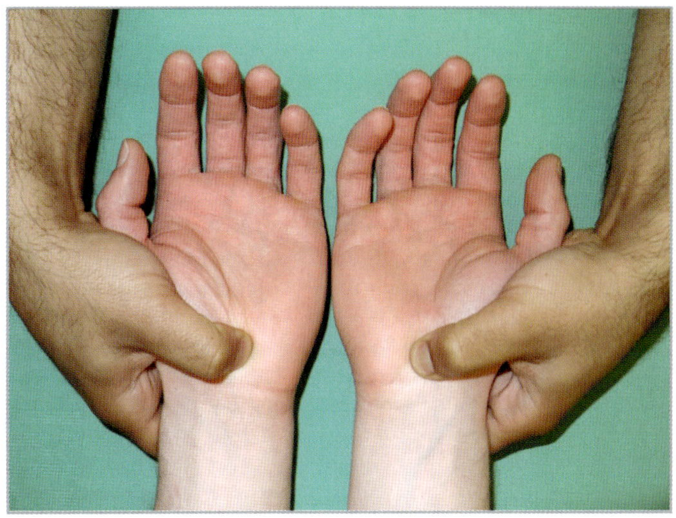

Figure 19.5 Durkan test.

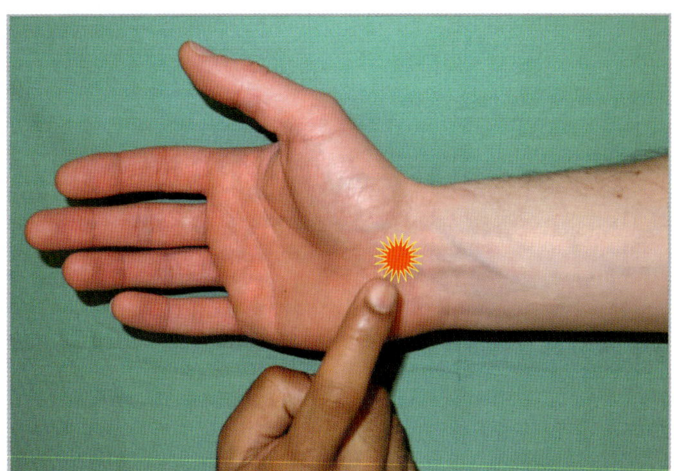

Figure 19.6 Tinel sign is performed by tapping over the site of nerve compression (circle), numbness and paresthesia indicate nerve injury and regeneration.

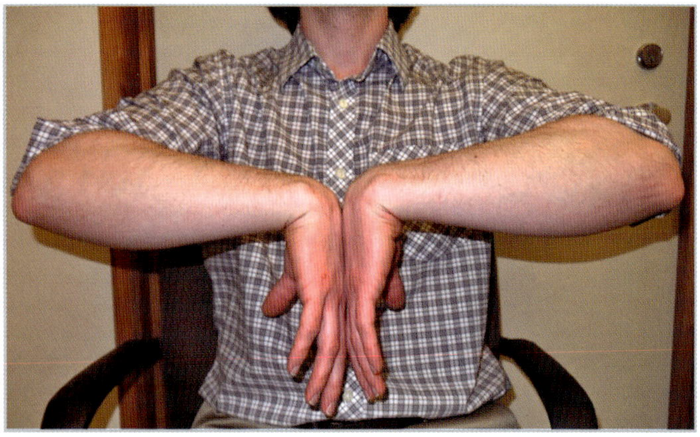

Figure 19.7 Phalen test. Forced flexion increases intracarpal tunnel pressure and elicits symptoms of median nerve compression.

arch. Symptoms include numbness, pain, and paresthesia over the cutaneous distribution of the median nerve. Pronator syndrome can be distinguished from CTS by the presence of numbness and paresthesia over the palm, which is an area supplied by the palmar cutaneous branch of the median nerve (spared in CTS). Other distinguishing features include the presence of aching pain over the volar side of the forearm and lack of night symptoms (patients with CTS often complain of interrupted night sleep due to pain and paresthesia developing in the affected hand at night time). Provocative tests include:

- Positive Tinel sign over the volar forearm
- Resisted forearm pronation and supination with elbow flexion and extension produces sensory symptoms due to nerve entrapment between the two heads of pronator teres and bicipital aponeurosis, respectively. Similarly, numbness and paresthesia can be reproduced with flexion of the long finger (FDS) due to nerve compression at the FDS aponeurotic arch (**Figure 19.8a–c**).

- Anterior interosseous nerve (AIN) syndrome: A compressive neuropathy of the AIN, which manifests as a purely motor disorder with no sensory loss. The motor function of four muscles is affected, namely, the flexor pollicis longus (FPL), flexor digitorum profundus (FDP) of the index and long fingers, and pronator quadratus muscle. Motor function examination shows weakness of handgrip, pinch strength, and forearm pronation. Patients will also demonstrate an inability to do the OK sign (opposition of pulp of thumb and index fingers, **Figure 19.9**)

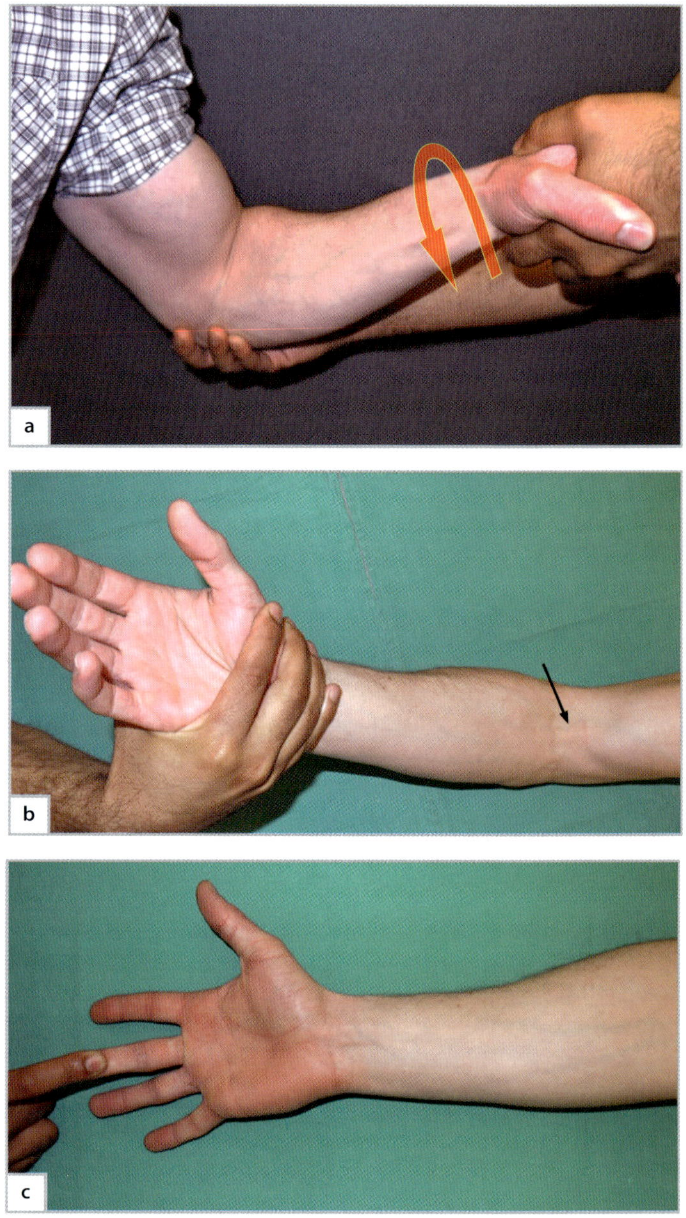

Figure 19.8 (a) Resisted forearm pronation and supination produces pain and paresthesia due to median nerve compression between the two heads of pronator teres. (b) Resisted elbow flexion produces pain and paresthesia due to median nerve compression underneath the bicipital aponeurosis (arrow). (c) Resisted long finger flexion produces pain and paresthesia due to median nerve compression at the flexor digitorum superficialis aponeurotic arch.

Ulnar nerve

- Compression of ulnar nerve in Guyon canal: A compressive neuropathy of the ulnar nerve in Guyon canal. A patient's symptoms can be sensory (pain and paresthesia) along the cutaneous distribution of the ulnar nerve (ulnar one and a half fingers), motor, or mixed. Hand inspection may show finger clawing of the ring and little fingers. The ulnar nerve innervates intrinsic muscles of the hand (palmar and dorsal interossei and the two ulnar lumbricals), which flex the metacarpophalangeal (MCP) joint and extend the interphalangeal (IP) joints. Therefore, in the presence of intrinsic muscle paralysis resulting from ulnar nerve palsy, claw fingers deformity is seen due to the unopposed MCP joint hyperextension by the long extensors and IP joint flexion by the long flexors. The motor function of the ulnar nerve can be evaluated by the following:
  - Weakness of pinch strength due to the weakness of adductor pollicis muscle (supplied by ulnar nerve) as well as an overall weakness of handgrip
  - Cross-finger test (**Figure 19.10**): Abduction and adduction movement of the fingers is executed by the dorsal and palmar interossei, respectively. Thus, the cross-finger test is utilized to assess the function of interosseous muscle by asking a patient to cross the index finger over the long finger or move the long finger from side-to-side. A patient inability to cross the fingers or move the long finger from side-to-side indicates ulnar nerve palsy and weakness of interosseous muscles

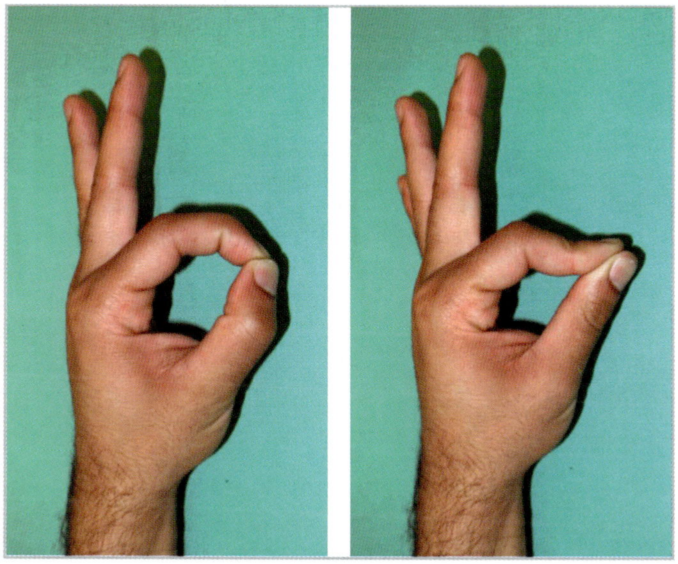

Figure 19.9 In anterior interosseous nerve syndrome, patients are unable to do the OK sign due to weakness of the flexor pollicis longus and flexor digitorum profundus of the thumb and index fingers, respectively.

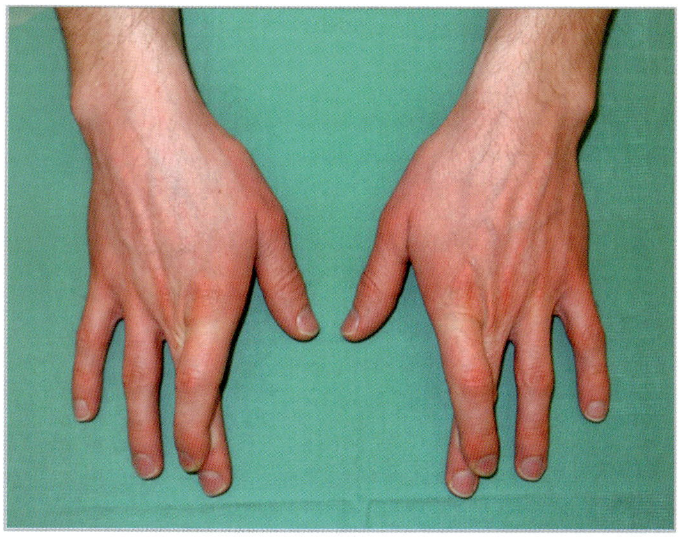

Figure 19.10 Cross-finger test. Crossing fingers indicates an intact function of the interosseous muscles, which indicates an intact ulnar nerve function.

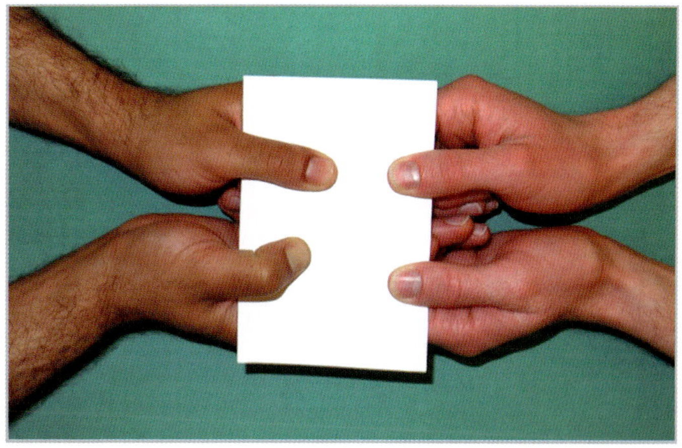

Figure 19.11 Froment sign. Note how the patient flexes the distal phalanx of the thumb to keep the paper between the thumb and index instead of adducting the thumb.

- Froment sign (**Figure 19.11**): The presence of a Froment sign indicates an ulnar nerve injury/palsy. This sign is demonstrated by asking the patient to hold a piece of paper between the thumb and the index finger and having the examiner pull the paper out of the patient's hand. With ulnar nerve palsy, the patient tries to keep the paper by flexing the distal phalanx of the thumb through the action of the FPL (supplied by the median nerve) instead of adducting the thumb by the adductor pollicis muscle (supplied by the ulnar nerve)

- Cubital tunnel syndrome: A compressive neuropathy of the ulnar nerve at the elbow joint most commonly occurring between the two heads of the flexor carpi ulnaris (FCU) muscle. Symptoms include numbness, pain, and paresthesia over the cutaneous nerve distribution of the ulnar nerve, including the ulnar one and a half fingers as well as the ulnar half of the dorsum of the hand, which is supplied by the dorsal cutaneous branch (usually spared in distal ulnar nerve compression) of the ulnar nerve. Hand inspection may reveal wasting of the first dorsal web space and clawing of the ring and little fingers. However, the degree of finger clawing is usually less severe than with the distal/low ulnar nerve palsy due to the paralysis of the long flexors (two ulnar FDP tendons) resulting in less amount of finger flexion. Less clawing of the fingers with high ulnar nerve palsy (e.g. cubital tunnel syndrome) compared with low ulnar nerve palsy is often called 'ulnar nerve paradox.' Assessment of ulnar nerve motor function in cubital tunnel syndrome is performed using the same examination techniques described earlier for the distal compression of the ulnar nerve, which include a positive Froment sign, weakness of handgrip, and the inability to cross fingers. Provocative tests include:
  - Tinel sign over cubital tunnel
  - Elbow flexion test: It is performed by asking the patient to maintain elbow flexion for 60 seconds. Sensory symptoms (pain, paresthesia) over the cutaneous nerve distribution of ulnar nerve develop due to nerve compression

Radial nerve

- Posterior interosseous nerve (PIN) compression syndrome (**Figure 19.12a and b**): A compressive neuropathy of the PIN (predominantly a motor branch of the radial nerve) in the forearm. The PIN supplies most of the extensor compartment of the forearm, with the exception of two muscles, the extensor carpi radialis longus (ECRL) and the brachioradialis muscle. Therefore, PIN palsy leads to finger drop deformity due to loss of extensor muscle function. On physical examination, wrist extension can still be achieved utilizing the intact ECRL tendon (supplied by the radial nerve above the elbow). Regarding finger extension, patients are unable to extend the MCP joints due to the complete paralysis of the long extensors; however, some degree of IP joint extension is preserved by the intact function of the interosseous muscles, which are supplied by the ulnar nerve
- Radial tunnel syndrome: A compressive neuropathy of PIN that can be distinguished from PIN compression syndrome by the lack of muscle weakness. Patients primarily complain of pain due to nerve compression between the supinator muscle and

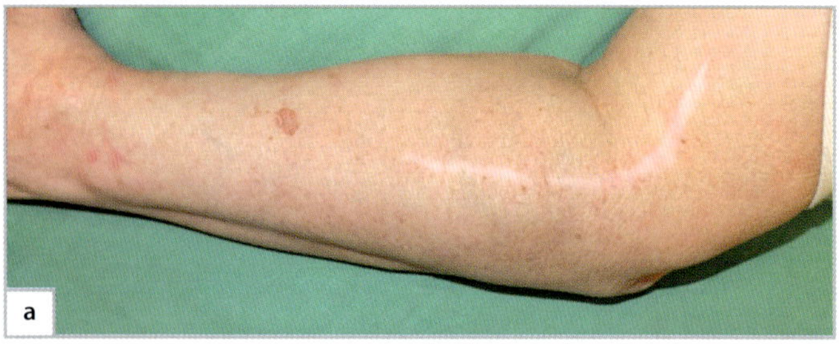

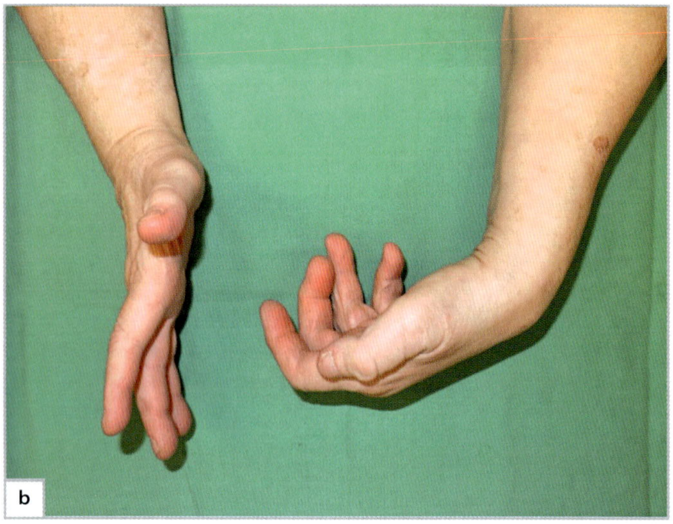

Figure 19.12 A case of iatrogenic injury of the posterior interosseous nerve. The patient is unable to extend the fingers (finger drop deformity).

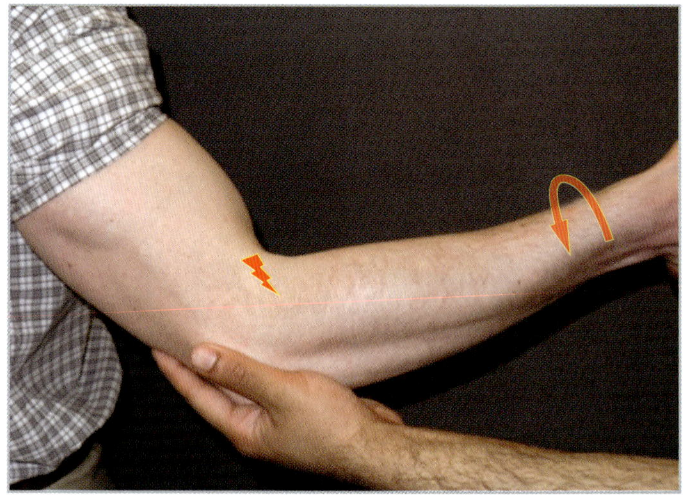

Figure 19.13 Supinator compression test. Resisted supination produces pain in the proximal forearm due to radial nerve compression in the radial tunnel (arrow).

lateral intermuscular septum at the proximal forearm, with no other sensory or motor loss. Provocative tests that compress the PIN in the proximal forearm (radial tunnel) may reproduce a patient's symptoms. This includes supinator compression test (**Figure 19.13**), where resisted forearm supination with the wrist and elbow in extension reproduces the pain

- Wartenberg syndrome: A compressive neuropathy of the superficial sensory branch of the radial nerve in the distal forearm. Symptoms include pain and paresthesia over the dorsum of the first web space supplied by the radial nerve. Patients often refrain from wearing a watch on the affected hand. Performing the Finkelstein test as described previously can reproduce a patient's symptoms

Assessment of hand vascularity

Disruption of the blood supply to the hand may be due to an acute traumatic injury or chronic systemic or local disease. At the outpatient clinic, the surgeon is often presented with chronic conditions that may have primary or secondary vascular involvement. A patient's history, including relevant risk factors such as smoking or systemic diseases such as atherosclerosis or diabetes, as well as the history of drugs affecting the tonicity of blood vessel, should be obtained.

Chronic conditions affecting the blood supply of the hand are usually due to vascular insufficiency that may result from a single or multiple disorders, e.g. vasospastic (Reynaud disease), vaso-occlusive (thrombus or emboli), vasculitis (thromboangiitis obliterans/Buerger disease), aneurysm, or arteriovenous fistula. Regardless of the etiology or predisposing factors, in the presence of inadequate blood supply and collateral circulation, the final outcome is tissue ischemia, which is defined as a lack of adequate blood supply that is required to meet the cellular metabolic requirements to keep the tissues alive. The physical examination usually reveals symptoms and signs of vascular insufficiency that include pain and tenderness, trophic changes, cold intolerance, numbness, ulceration, tissue necrosis, and gangrene of the hand and digits.

Evaluation of upper-limb tissue perfusion involves the assessment of skin turgor, capillary refill time, and arterial pulsation, as well as the presence of any abnormal pulses or thrills (e.g. arterial aneurysm). The Allen test (as described in Chapter 8) and its modification, the digital Allen test, should be performed to assess the blood flow and patency of the radial and ulnar arteries and radial and ulnar digital branches of the common digital arteries (**Figure 19.14**). A hand-held Doppler may also be a useful tool to assess the presence of blood flow in the major arteries of the upper limb. Examples of vascular disorders and their examination techniques are described below.

Raynaud phenomenon and disease: Raynaud disease occurs without an associated or underlying disease; therefore, it is an idiopathic (primary) disease. In contrast, Raynaud phenomenon commonly occurs secondary to an underlying disease and, therefore, is considered a secondary disease. To avoid confusion, the condition is called Raynaud phenomenon whenever there is an identifiable cause of patient's symptoms. There are a number of medical disorders that may cause Raynaud phenomenon including connective tissue diseases, such as scleroderma, arterial disease (e.g. vasculitis), trauma, endocrine, and hematological disorders are among others. On clinical examination, one can look for signs of coexisting disease, if present. However, in both conditions there is a characteristic color change of the fingers resulting from alterations of the blood flow to the hand as described by Maurice Raynaud in 1862, which includes three phases: a phase of ischemia resulting in pallor, followed by a phase of stasis and cyanosis resulting in bluish discoloration of the fingers, and finally a phase of hyperemia resulting in redness of fingers.

Apart from the presence or absence of a coexisting disease, there are other features that can differentiate Raynaud disease from Raynaud phenomenon. For example, digital ischemia may occur in both conditions; however, the presence of trophic changes, ulceration, and digital gangrene are more common in the Raynaud phenomenon. In addition, Raynaud phenomenon results from a structural damage

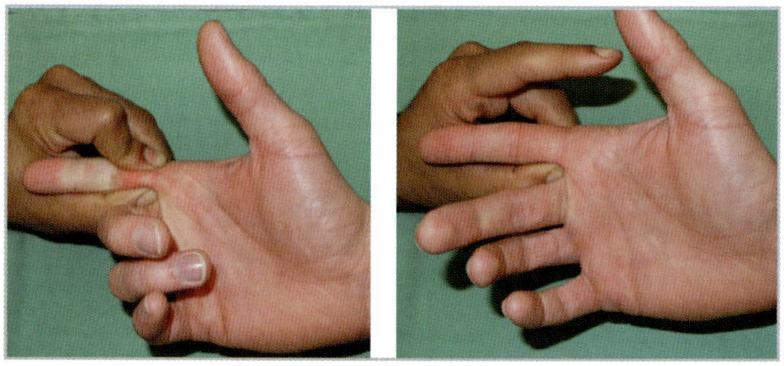

Figure 19.14 Digital Allen test is performed by compression and alternate release of the radial and ulnar digital arteries to assess blood flow to the fingers by evaluating patency of the digital arteries.

to the blood vessels; therefore, the condition tends to be unilateral and asymmetric occurring at a distal site to the vascular injury, whereas Raynaud disease is a functional problem resulting from vasospasm of the blood vessels and is usually bilateral and symmetric. When the Allen test is performed, the test is usually negative in Raynaud disease (i.e. normal blood flow within digital arteries) due to the absence of peripheral vascular occlusion, whereas the test is usually positive in Raynaud phenomenon due to the presence of vascular damage and occlusion of the digital arteries.

Hypothenar hammer syndrome: A post-traumatic vaso-occlusive disease that results from damage of blood vessels elastic lamina, which leads to thrombosis, and occlusion of the ulnar artery (within the Guyon canal) and the superficial palmar arch. The predisposing injury is a repetitive movement/trauma; hence, the condition is commonly seen in manual laborers and in certain sports such as golf and baseball catchers. Symptoms include distal pain, cold intolerance, numbness, and weakness of handgrip. Assessment of blood flow by the Allen test may demonstrate lack of blood flow in the ulnar artery. Other signs may include decreased sensation of the ulnar aspect of the hand, nail changes, skin ulceration, and chronic gangrene. More details on the diagnosis and treatment of vascular insufficiency can be found in Chapter 24.

Assessment of bone and joint stability

Obvious fractures and joint dislocations of the hand are usually diagnosed in the emergency department; however, subtle bony injuries and ligamentous disruption are often missed and are difficult to treat. Moreover, patients suffering with these types of injuries often present late to the hand clinic. Therefore, a general assessment of the hand including measurements of the active and passive range of motion of individual joints using a goniometer (**Tables 19.1** and **19.2**) may reveal the presence of joint stiffness, laxity, or flexion/extension deformities that warrant more specific examination. This may include the following injuries:

Bone injuries

- Scaphoid fracture: This is the most commonly fractured carpal bone, with the typical mechanism of injury involving a fall on an outstretched hand. Scaphoid bone fractures may not be evident on plain radiographs within the first 2 weeks after the initial injury. On inspection, swelling and bruising may be seen on the palmar surface of the hand. Eliciting pain over the scaphoid region by palpation is suggestive of a scaphoid fracture. Physical examination includes:
  - Tenderness over anatomical snuffbox: Local tenderness elicited by pressing over the anatomical snuffbox (proximal pole of the scaphoid) or by palpating the scaphoid tubercle on the palmar surface of the hand is indicative of a scaphoid fracture (**Figure 19.15**)
- Hook of hamate fracture: May be associated with racquet sports injuries such as golf or tennis, commonly occurring when patients miss the ball and hit the ground. Physical symptoms include sensory and motor dysfunction of the ulnar nerve due to nerve compression inside Guyon canal. Evaluation of hook of the hamate fractures can be performed by:
  - Ring and small finger flexion test: Resisted flexion of the ring and little fingers induces pain due to irritation of the flexor tendons caused by the fractured hook of the hamate
- Pisiform bone fracture: Associated with a fall on an outstretched hand. Pisiform fractures are not associated with motor or sensory

Table 19.1 Normal range of motion of the finger joints

Digit	Distal interphalangeal joint	Proximal interphalangeal joint	Metacarpophalangeal joint		Carpometacarpal joint	
	Extension–flexion	Extension–flexion	Extension–flexion	Adduction–abduction	Extension–flexion	Adduction–abduction
Thumb	-	0°–90°	-10°–70°	-10°–10°	-10°–30°	0°–50°
Index finger	0°–80°	0°–100°	-20°–90°	-20°–20°	0°	Nil
Long finger	0°–80°	0°–100°	-20°–90°	-20°–20°	0°–10°	Nil
Ring finger	0°–80°	0°–100°	-20°–90°	-20°–20°	0°–20°	Nil
Small finger	0°–80°	0°–100°	-20°–90°	-20°–20°	-10°–30°	Nil

Table 19.2 Normal range of motion of the wrist joint

	Flexion	Extension	Radial deviation	Ulnar deviation	Pronation	Supination
Wrist joint	0°–80°	0°–70°	0°–20°	0°–30°	-	-
Midcarpal joint	54°	42°	12°	18°	-	-
Radiocarpal joint	26°	28°	8°	12°	-	-
Distal radioulnar joint	-	-	-	-	0°–80°	0°–70°

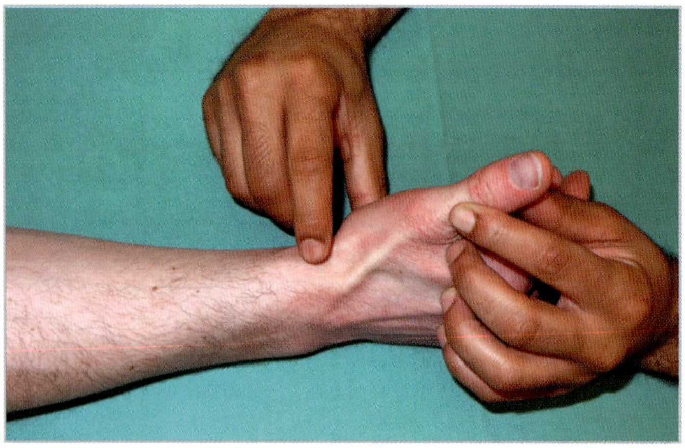

Figure 19.15 Tenderness over the anatomical snuffbox is suggestive of a scaphoid fracture after a fall on an outstretched hand.

loss, and the clinical presentation is often delayed. Patients may complain of ulnar-sided wrist pain over the hypothenar eminence. Physical examination may show soft tissue swelling or bruising by hand inspection, as well as localized tenderness by palpation over the pisiform bone

Specific joint injuries

- Thumb collateral ligament injury: The soft tissue support of the thumb MCP joint includes the radial (RCL) and ulnar (UCL) collateral ligaments. The UCL is more commonly injured than the RCL, and the mechanism of injury involves hyperabduction of the thumb, which is often referred to as a Gamekeeper or Skier thumb injury. Patients often complain of pain and swelling on the ulnar aspect of the thumb as well as thumb instability, especially with key pinch grip. By inspection, swelling and bruising may be seen on the ulnar side of the thumb. Joint laxity due to UCL injury can be assessed by the following test:
  - Varus stress test (**Figure 19.16**): The examiner holds the thumb in a semiflexed position and stresses the UCL by pushing on the radial aspect of the thumb MCP joint. Laxity greater than 35° compared with the uninjured side indicates a rupture of the proper collateral ulnar ligament. The same test is repeated with the thumb in extension, and when positive, it indicates a rupture of the accessory UCL. When comparing the injured to noninjured thumb, the affected MCP joint demonstrates a high degree of laxity with the stress test, often referred to as an 'open book.' The UCL injuries can also be diagnosed by ultrasonography; however, the diagnosis is mainly clinical
- Scapholunate (SL) dissociation: This consists of three parts, dorsal, proximal, and palmar, with the dorsal aspect being the strongest ligament. A fall on an outstretched hand with the wrist extended and ulnarly deviated disrupts the SL ligament, leading to SL dissociation and carpal instability (DISI-dorsal intercalated segmental instability). DISI deformity occurs when the lunate bone is regarded as an intercalated segment and appears abnormally extended relative to the radius and capitate. The following tests have been described to help in the clinical diagnosis of SL dissociation
  - Scaphoid shift test (Watson test, **Figure 19.17**): First, the examiner holds the patient's hand by wrapping his/her fingers around the dorsum of the patient's wrist and firmly pressing the thumb over the distal pole of the scaphoid. With the other hand, the examiner moves the patient's wrist back and forth from extension

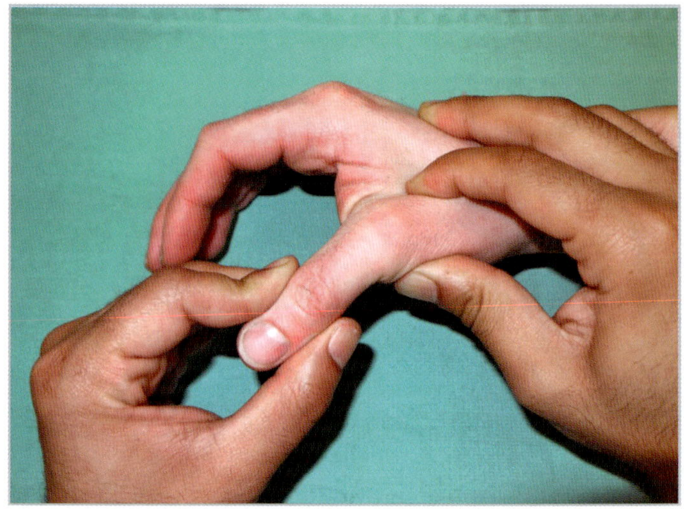

Figure 19.16 Varus stress test to assess the integrity of the ulnar collateral ligament of the thumb metacarpophalangeal joint.

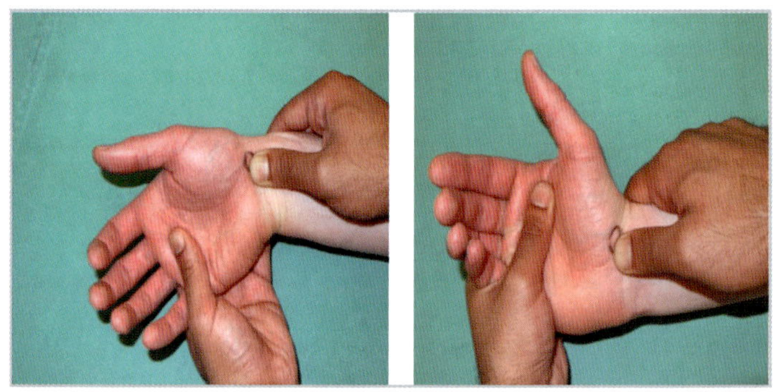

Figure 19.17 Scaphoid shift test (Watson test).

and ulnar deviation to flexion and radial deviation. Normally, in wrist extension, the scaphoid assumes an extended position in line with the forearm, and when the wrist is flexed the scaphoid flexes. However, in this test, scaphoid flexion is prevented by the pressure applied by the examiner's thumb. If the SL ligament is incompetent, the proximal pole of the scaphoid would dorsally sublux on the distal radius, and when the examiner removes his/her thumb and relieves the pressure over the patient's scaphoid, a typical 'snap/clunk' is heard as the scaphoid moves back into its normal position at the scaphoid fossa

- Lunotriquetral (LT) dissociation: A relatively subtle type of injury that ranges from mild instability of the LT joint to global carpal collapse. The mechanism of injury often involves a fall on an outstretched hand with the wrist extended and radially deviated. Depending on the magnitude and extent of injury, different patterns of LT dissociation may exist. Injury resulting in the LT dissociation is frequently associated with other injuries, such as an injury of the triangular fibrocartilage complex (TFCC), and often presents with ulnar-sided wrist pain. Several provocative/stress tests and their modifications have been described to assess carpal stability of the LT joint, and these tests include the following:
  - Reagan test/LT ballottement test (**Figure 19.18**): This test evaluates LT joint instability. The examiner stabilizes the lunate between the thumb and index finger with one hand and

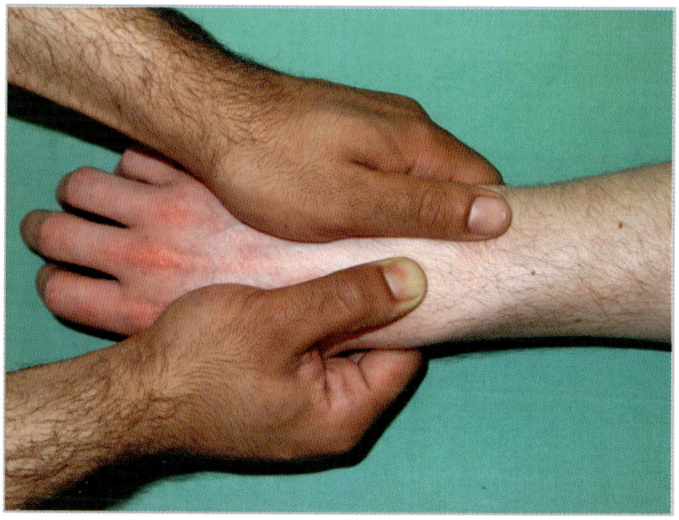

Figure 19.18 Reagan test/LT ballottement test.

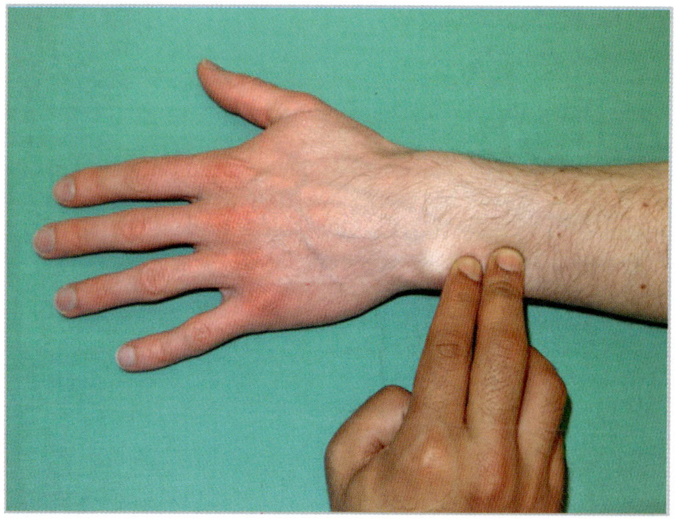

Figure 19.19 Piano key sign to test for distal radioulnar joint instability.

manipulates the triquetrum and pisiform dorsally and volarly using the other hand. The presence of pain, crepitus, and laxity of the LT joint is considered a positive test
  - Kleinman test/LT shear test: This is a modification of the LT ballottement test, where the examiner stabilizes the dorsal surface of the lunate and applies volar pressure on the pisiform to create a shearing force on the LT joint, which elicits pain and instability of LT joint
- DRUJ instability: This may result from arthritis or traumatic injuries. The clinical assessment of DRUJ instability must also take into account pathology of other anatomically and functionally related joints, such as the LT, ulnocarpal, and proximal radioulnar joint. Several provocative or stress tests have been described to assess DRUJ instability, which include the following:
  - Piano key sign (**Figure 19.19**): This test is performed by asking the patient to lay the hand and forearm in a pronated position. The examiner then presses or 'ballots' the distal ulna head. Little resistance in addition to movement of the ulna head back and forth resembling the movement of a piano key indicates laxity of the DRUJ
  - Radioulnar shuck test: With the patient's forearm in supination, the examiner holds the distal part of the ulna between the thumb and index fingers and assesses the dorsal and volar displacement of the distal part of the ulna. Increased laxity as compared with the contralateral side indicates DRUJ instability or a peripheral TFCC tear
  - Ulnar foveal sign (**Figure 19.20**): With the forearm in a neutral position, the examiner palpates the area proximal to the pisiform between the FCU and ulnar styloid. Presence of pain and tenderness indicates a TFCC injury, which is frequently associated with DRUJ instability.
- Ulnocarpal instability: This is part of the differential diagnosis of conditions resulting in ulnar-sided wrist pain. Ulnocarpal instability can be evaluated by:
  - Pisiform boost maneuver: With the forearm in a neutral position and the wrist in passive ulnar deviation, the examiner simultaneously pushes the ulnar head with his fingers from a dorsal to volar direction while pushing the pisiform using his thumb in the opposite direction (volar to dorsal). In a positive test, this maneuver demonstrates joint laxity and induces pain.

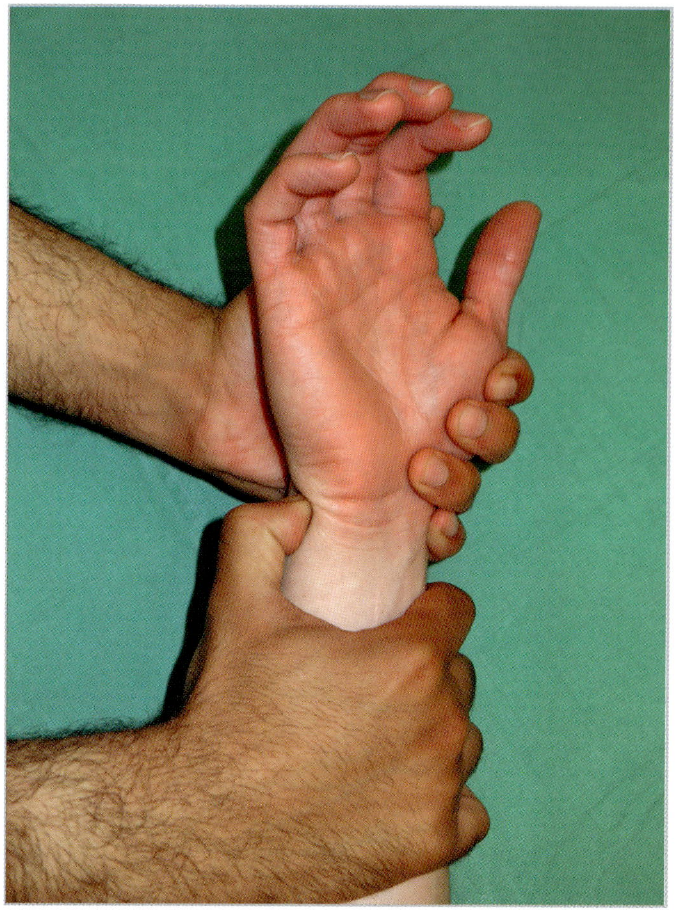

Figure 19.20 Ulnar foveal sign; eliciting pain and tenderness at the area proximal to the pisiform between the flexor carpi ulnaris and ulnar styloid indicates injury of the triangular fibrocartilage complex.

- Midcarpal instability: This condition is considered a type of non-dissociative carpal instability. Non-dissociative carpal instability is a type of carpal dysfunction where there is no disruption between the carpal bones, but rather a malalignment of the carpal rows resulting in a volar displacement or sag of the wrist joint. This is in contrast to dissociative carpal instability, where there is disruption between carpal bones such as S-L dissociation and L-T dissociation as discussed earlier. Patients' symptoms range from an asymptomatic 'clunk' of the wrist joint to localized tenderness over the lunocapitate and triquetrohamate joints as well as weakness of handgrip. Midcarpal joint laxity can be assessed by the following test:

- Lichtman test/midcarpal shift test: This test is performed by slightly flexing the wrist, and with the forearm pronated, the wrist joint is brought from radial into ulnar deviation. Obvious patient discomfort and a palpable clunk indicate midcarpal instability. The cause or pattern of the palpable clunk depends on the type of midcarpal instability. In the anterior type of midcarpal instability, a palpable clunk is due to sudden extension and rotation of a flexed proximal carpal row toward the end of the ulnar deviation movement of the wrist. However, in posterior type midcarpal instability an audible clunk is heard due to dorsal subluxation then realignment of the capitate.

SUMMARY

The selection of correct examination technique largely depends on individual surgeon's experience and the understanding of disease pathogenesis. By performing the tests described earlier, a surgeon would be able to reach the correct diagnosis or narrow the list of disease differential diagnosis. It should also be stated that most of the hand examination techniques have various degrees of sensitivity and specificity; however, a positive test should prompt the surgeon to further investigate the cause of patients' discomfort (e.g. electromyography, ultrasonography, X-ray, computed tomography, or magnetic resonance imaging) or perform further diagnostic interventions such as arthroscopy to reach the final diagnosis.

SUGGESTED READING

Mondelli M, Passero S, Giannini F. Provocative tests in different stages of carpal tunnel syndrome. Clin Neurol Neurosurg 2001; 103:178–183.
A prospective controlled study evaluating the diagnostic accuracy of provocative tests (Tinel, Phalen, reverse Phalen, and Durkan test) to diagnose CTS. Results showed limited efficiency of the provocative tests to distinguish between patients with CTS and the control group.

Parvizi J, Wayman J, Kelly P, Moran CG. Combining the clinical signs improves diagnosis of scaphoid fractures. A prospective study with follow-up. J Hand Surg Br 1998; 23:324–327.
A prospective study evaluating the efficacy of four clinical signs, namely, tenderness in the anatomical snuff box, tenderness over the scaphoid tubercle, pain on axial compression of the thumb, and the range of thumb movement that are commonly performed by physicians to evaluate the presence of scaphoid fractures. The study results show that these clinical signs are inadequate indicators of scaphoid fracture when used alone and should be combined with imaging studies to accurately assess the presence of a scaphoid fracture.

Priollet P, Vayssairat M, Housset E. How to classify Raynaud's phenomenon. Long-term follow-up study of 73 cases. Am J Med 1987; 83:494–498.
A long-term cohort study of patients presenting with stigmata of Raynaud's disease. This study provides the reader with a good understanding of the disease pathogenesis and common presenting symptoms, as well as the difference between primary and secondary disease.

Ruland RT, Hogan CJ. The ECU synergy test: an aid to diagnose ECU tendonitis. J Hand Surg Am 2008; 33:1777–1782.
A novel description of the ECU synergy test and a retrospective study correlating findings of the ECU synergy test with other methods of diagnosis of ulnar wrist pain (MRI and wrist arthroscopy). The ECU synergy test was found to be a useful method of clinical examination to differentiate between intra-articular and extra-articular causes of ulnar wrist pain.

Chapter 20 Congenital disorders

Alphonsus Chong

EMBRYOLOGY

The limb bud appears on the 26th day of development. It then curves, and, by the 31st day, the marginal vessel appears. Two days after this, the hand 'paddle' develops, as do the subclavian–axillary–brachial axial arteries. Subsequently, nerve trunks enter the arm. On the 36th day, chondrification of the humerus, radius, and ulna occurs, and the shoulder joint interzone becomes apparent. By the 41st day, digital rays develop within the hand paddle, and chondrification of the metacarpals occurs, after which the ulnar artery appears. Next, the proximal phalanges chondrify, and, on the 44th day, the radial artery appears. At this time, the pectoral muscle mass splits into the clavicular head and the costal head. Three days later, the costal head then divides into the pectoralis minor and the sternocostal head of the pectoralis major. In the hand, the middle phalanges are chondrified, the fingers begin to separate, and joint interzones appear. Chondrification of the proximal parts of the distal phalanges and further separation of the fingers occurs by day 50. By the 54th day, the humerus is ossified and the fingers are completely separated.

AXIS DEVELOPMENT

- The limb bud has three axes defined by different regions or zones (**Figure 20.1**)
- The anterior–posterior axis is patterned by the zone of polarizing activity (ZPA)
- The apical ectodermal ridge (AER) directs proximal to distal development and maintains undifferentiated cells in the progress zone

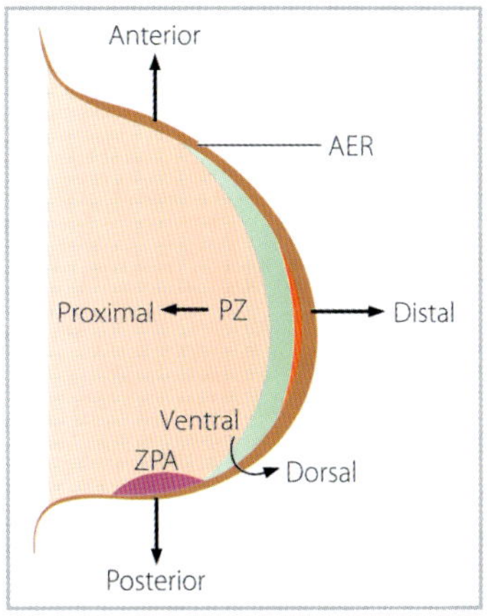

Figure 20.1 The early limb bud has mesenchymal cells surrounded by ectoderm. In the progress zone, which lies just beneath the ectoderm, there are regions that determine the limb development along the anterior–posterior, dorsal–ventral, and proximal-distal axes. AER, apical ectodermal ridge. PZ, progress zone. ZPA, zone of polarizing activity.

- The dorsal–ventral polarity is directed by the dorsal and ventral ectoderms

INTERNATIONAL FEDERATION OF SOCIETIES FOR SURGERY OF THE HAND (IFSSH) CLASSIFICATION

Key features

The IFSSH system is the most widely used and comprehensive classification system. It classifies each limb malformation according to the most predominant anomaly and places it into one of seven categories (**Table 20.1**).

Table 20.1 IFSSH Classification for congenital anomalies of the hand

Main category	Subcategory	Diagnosis (example)
I. Failure of formation (arrest)	Transverse longitudinal	Radial club Cleft hand (typical/atypical) Phocomelia
II. Failure of differentiation (separation)	Soft tissue Skeletal Tumorous	Arthrogryposis Cutaneous syndactyly Camptodactyly Radioulnar synostosis Osseous syndactyly Clinodactyly
III. Duplication	—	Mirror hand Polydactyly
IV. Overgrowth (gigantism)	—	Hemihypertrophy Macrodactyly
V. Undergrowth (hypoplasia)	—	Symbrachydactyly Brachydactyly
VI. Constriction band syndrome	Focal amputation	Constriction band Acrosyndactyly Intrauterine amputation
VII. Generalized	—	Achondroplasia Marfan syndrome

Criticisms of IFSSH classification

Some conditions, such as congenital joint laxity and delta phalanx, are not included in this system. It is also very difficult to classify complex cases in the IFSSH classification. There have been attempts to incorporate etiology into morphologically based classifications (e.g. typical and atypical cleft) to improve the system.

RADIAL LONGITUDINAL DEFICIENCY

Radial longitudinal deficiency, also known as radial club hand, is characterized by a spectrum of tissue deficiencies on the radial side of the forearm and hand. The deficiency can vary from mild hypoplasia to total absence of the bones (radius, radial carpus, and thumb ray), muscles, tendons, ligaments, nerves, and blood vessels. As a result of this deficiency, the whole forearm is shortened and bowed (**Figure 20.2**), and the thumb is often hypoplastic. The incidence of this rare, but serious anomaly is approximately 1 in 55,000 live births.

Assessment

When assessing a patient who presents with radial longitudinal deficiency, a medical history must be taken and associated anomalies noted. These may include vertebral, anal, cardiac, tracheoesophageal, renal, and limb anomalies, Holt-Oram syndrome, or thrombocytopenia absent radius syndrome. The degree of forearm bowing and shortening and elbow stiffness must be assessed, as must the presence of thumb and other finger anomalies. In the Bayne and Klug Classification system, a total absence of the radius (type IV) is recognized as the most common type of radial deficiency.

Treatment

- Early treatment should correct elbow stiffness and wrist deformity. This can be accomplished by stretching and massaging or splinting and casting. It is important to do this from the beginning, because elbow motion is necessary before surgery can be performed. Likewise, a supple wrist will help subsequent centralization, which should be performed by about 1 year of age
- External fixation for distraction may also be used to help with correction before definitive surgery
- For wrist reconstruction, centralization may be achieved by releasing soft tissues, repositioning the carpus, transferring tendons for better balance, and performing corrective osteotomies of the ulna to straighten it.
- Soft tissue distraction followed by microvascular metatarsophalangeal joint transfer to stabilize the wrist and prevent recurrence of the deformity has shown promising long-term results

THUMB HYPOPLASIA

Thumb hypoplasia encompasses a spectrum from small to absent thumb and is often associated with radial longitudinal deficiency. The Blauth classification system (**Table 20.2**) is widely used to help guide treatment of thumb hypoplasia. Assessment of the thumb's carpometacarpal (CMC) joint stability is important to determine the appropriate surgical treatment for thumb hypoplasia. In children who have stable CMC joints (Blauth types I, II, and IIIA), the goals of surgery are to preserve the existing thumb and to augment deficient soft tissue elements, including the first web space, thenar muscles, and the ulnar collateral ligament of the MCP joint. If the CMC joint is unstable or absent (Blauth types IIIB, IV, and V) (**Figure 20.3**), any remnants of the existing thumb should be ablated and reconstruction should proceed by pollicizing the index finger. In older children with an established maladaptive compensatory side-to-side pinch between the index and middle fingers, pollicization may not be useful.

SYNDACTYLY

Syndactyly is a condition where the normal interdigital space of the hands or feet is reduced or eliminated. Syndactyly can exist in isolation or in association with other abnormalities. Isolated syndactyly most commonly occurs between the middle and ring fingers and is often inherited via autosomal dominance. See **Figure 20.4** for syndactyly classifications. Conditions associated with syndactyly include Poland syndrome, symbrachydactyly, and Apert syndrome.

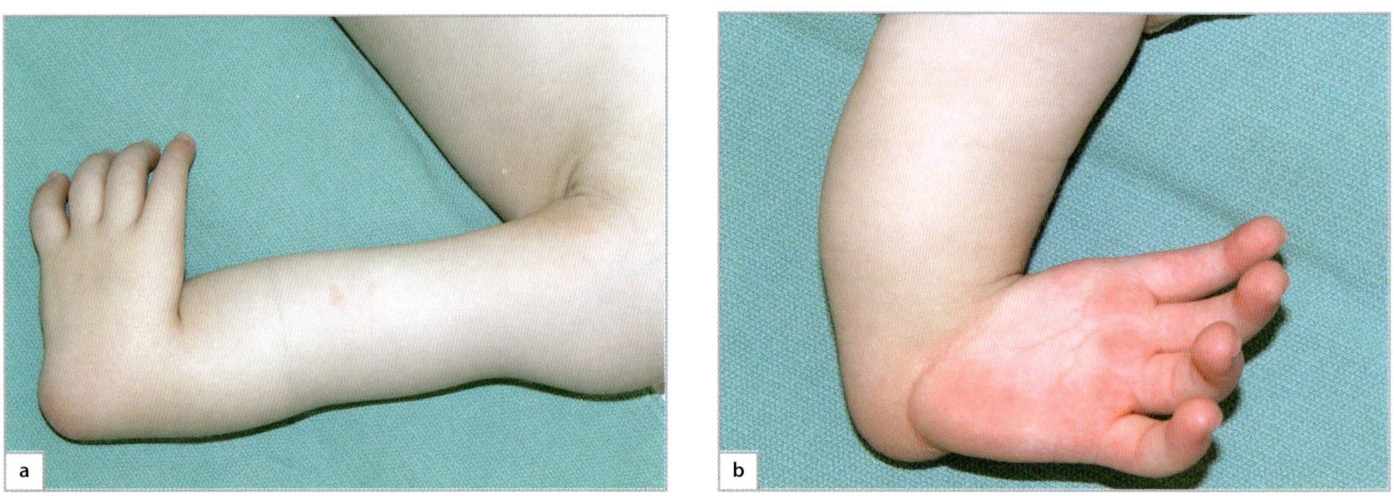

Figure 20.2 Radial club hand with absent thumb.

Table 20.2 Modified Blauth classification of thumb hypoplasia and appropriate surgical treatment

Type	Findings	Treatment
I	Minor generalized hypoplasia	Augmentation
II	Absence of intrinsic thenar muscles	Opponensplasty (typically with abductor digiti mini)
	First web space narrowing	First web release UCL reconstruction
	Ulnar collateral ligament (UCL) insufficiency	UCL reconstruction
III	Similar findings as type II plus:	A: Reconstruction
	Extrinsic muscle and tendon abnormalities	B: Pollicization
	Skeletal deficiency	
	A: Stable carpometacarpal joint	
	B: Unstable carpometacarpal joint	
IV	Pouce flottant or floating thumb	Pollicization
V	Absence	Pollicization

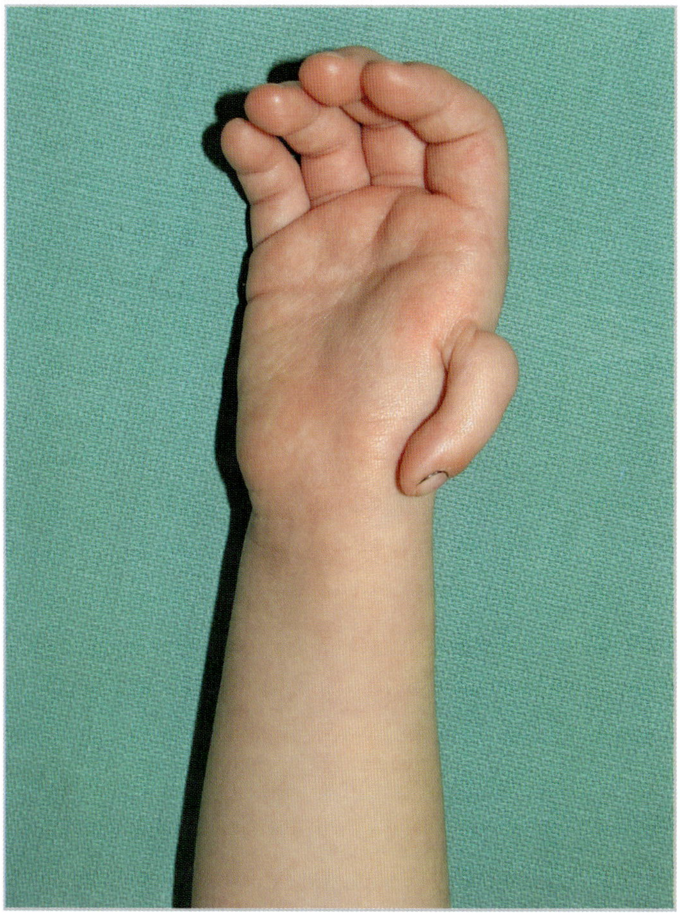

Figure 20.3 Blauth type IV hypoplastic thumb with an unstable carpometacarpal joint and a floating thumb (pouce flouttans).

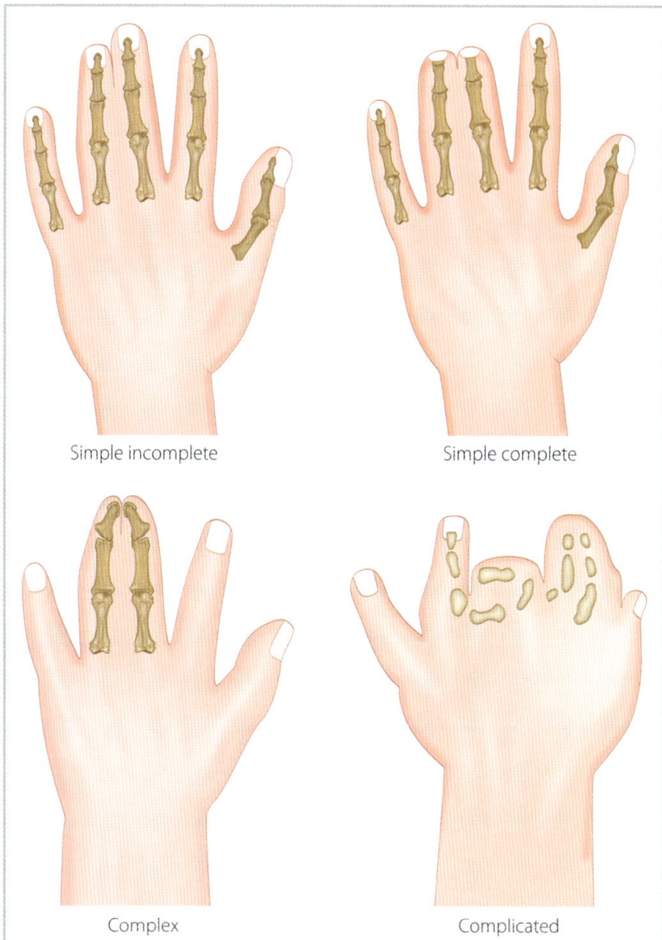

Figure 20.4 Classification of syndactyly. It is based on extent (complete vs. incomplete), and types of tissue involved (simple, complex, complicated).

Treatment

Treatment for syndactyly aims to create a normal web commissure and to prevent recurrence. Many techniques have been published for the treatment of syndactyly. These include various commissure designs and flap design techniques, some of which involve skin grafting. The author's preferred technique is shown in **Figure 20.5**. Although there are a variety of procedures, they are all based on similar principles:

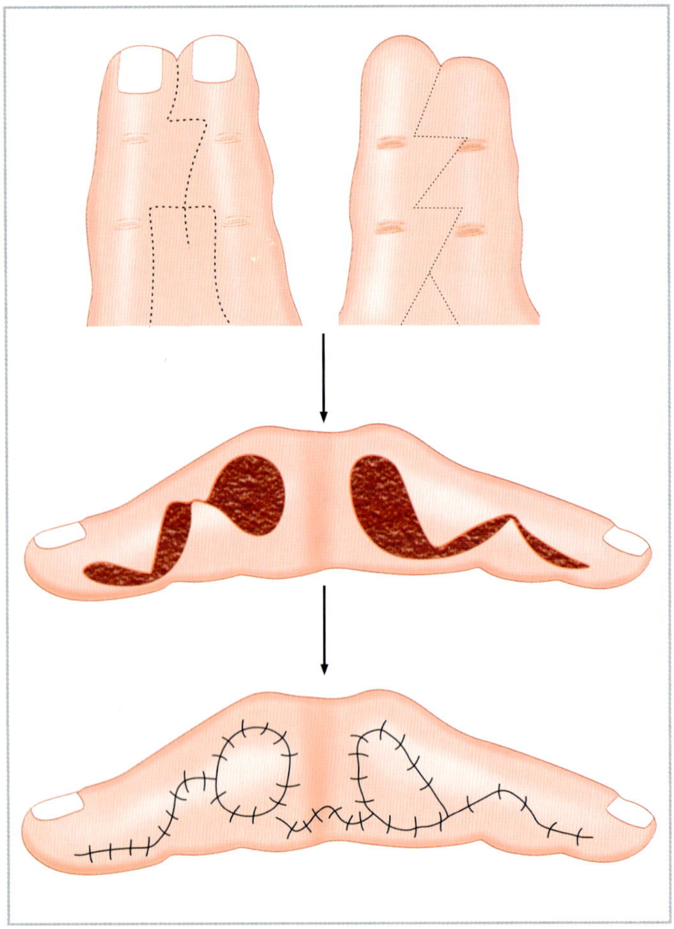

Figure 20.5 A technique for syndactyly separation. The web space is reconstructed using a dorsal rectangular and palmar triangular flap. Interdigitating zigzag incisions are made to prevent contracture of the side of the fingers. Residual defect is skin grafted.

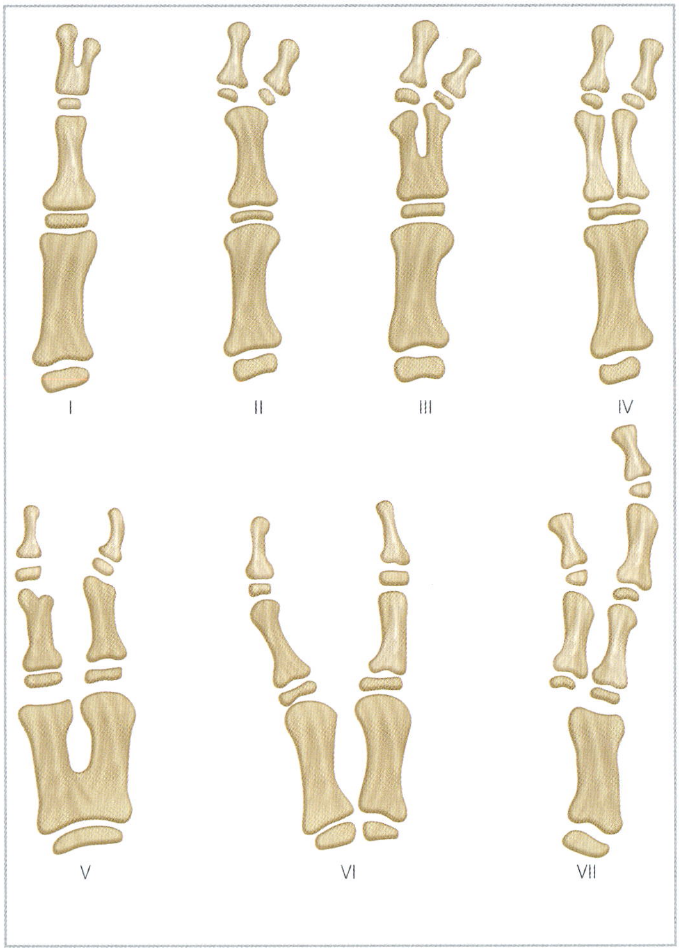

Figure 20.6 The Wassel classification for thumb duplication. I, bifid distal phalanx; II, duplicated distal phalanx; III bifid proximal phalanx; IV, duplicated proximal phalanx; V, bifid metacarpal; VI, duplicated metacarpal; VII, triphalangism.

- Skin flaps are used for commissure reconstruction. The use of the 'best' skin ensures that the most natural looking flap and has the least risk of recurrence (e.g. web creep)
- Incisions for the web division are nonlinear. This reduces the risk of contracture of the scar along the sides of the fingers and subsequent secondary deformity
- The skin graft or primary closure is chosen to avoid compromising circulation in the digit. The relative shortage of skin can be overcome by defatting the skin and bringing more skin into the syndactylized digit by local flap advancement

THUMB DUPLICATION/ POLYDACTYLY

Thumb duplication is one of the most common forms of polydactyly in the hand. Wassel classification, which is based on radiological appearance (**Figure 20.6**), is widely used. However, this classification system is incomplete. Roughly 20% of polydactyly conditions are omitted. For example, floating type conditions do not fit into the Wassel classification system. The most common form of polydactyly in the Wassel classification is the type IV (duplicated proximal phalanx). There are variations of this form based on the size and shape of each duplicate, and these variations affect treatment.

Treatment

- Treatment for thumb duplication aims to better position the thumb, improve the patient's psychosocial well-being, and improve function. There are several surgical procedures, although treatment of this condition is not urgent
- Surgery can be performed on patients as early as age 1 or 2. Typically, excision of the smaller radial duplicate is performed at the same time as reconstruction. Reconstruction entails radial collateral ligament reconstruction, abductor pollicis brevis reinsertion, tendon reconstruction, and occasionally web widening or metacarpal osteotomy
- The Bilhaut-Cloquet surgical technique combines two duplicates to form one larger thumb. It is used for small, symmetrical thumbs. Common complications include nail deformity or late deformities. This technique is normally reserved for cases where reconstruction of one thumb will not produce a thumb of suitable size and stability. The reconstructed thumb should have a nail at least as large as the index finger nail

CAMPTODACTYLY

Camptodactyly refers to flexion deformities of the proximal interphalangeal (PIP) joints. The etymology of camptodactyly is Greek: *campto* meaning 'bent' and *dactylos* meaning 'finger.' It is typically a nontraumatic, congenital disorder that affects the little finger. However, other fingers, or multiple fingers, can be affected. Camptodactyly can be inherited autosomal dominantly or be the result of spontaneous mutation.

Clinical assessment

Camptodactyly may be simple or complex. Simple camptodactyly occurs when it is the only condition present, whereas complex camptodactyly occurs in conjunction with other conditions, such as clinodactyly or syndactyly. Camptodactyly may present early in childhood or late in adolescence and may be a flexible or fixed deformity. The degree of deformity is categorized by the angle of flexion. Angles < 30° are considered mild. If the angle is between 30° and 60°, the condition is classified as moderate. Angles >60° are severe.

The pathoanatomy of camptodactyly may include volar skin tightness, tight fascial bands, abnormal flexor digitorum superficialis or lumbrical tendon, contracted volar PIP joint capsule and/or collaterals, or deficient extensor tendons.

Treatment

- Conservative treatment (i.e. splinting) requires high compliance over a long period of time. Conservative treatment produces better results with <60° of extension lag than surgical intervention
- Surgical treatment should only be offered when conservative treatment has failed, because it can cause stiffness and loss of flexion. The optimal age for surgery has not been determined. Multiple procedures may be required to release skin and fascial tightness, divide or excise aberrant tendons, or release tendon sheaths, joint capsules, and collateral ligaments. The extensor mechanism may also need augmentation or reconstruction

CLINODACTYLY

Clinodactyly is the radioulnar deviation of the finger (**Figure 20.7**). The name has Greek roots: *kliner* meaning 'to bend' and *dactylos* meaning 'fingers.' It is common for the little finger to be turned toward the ring finger, which is often caused by a triangular or trapezoidal middle phalanx. Clinodactyly may be associated with other syndromes and usually does not result in functional problems.

Treatment

- If the deviation is severe (>20°), corrective osteotomy can be considered to close, open, or reverse a wedge. If length is not an issue, closing wedge osteotomy is the easiest and most reliable option. Opening and reversing osteotomies preserve length, but they are more complicated to perform
- Due to the risks of surgery, it should only be performed if the deviation affects function and after skeletal maturity

MACRODACTYLY

Macrodactyly is a very rare condition involving overgrowth of all tissues (**Figure 20.8**). It differs from isolated enlargement due to bone hypertrophy or tumor growth. Nerve territory-oriented macrodactyly is the concept that enlargement follows the path of a particular digital nerve. There are three types of macrodactyly: true (i.e. isolated) macrodactyly, secondary macrodactyly (e.g. vascular malformation), and syndromic macrodactyly (e.g. Klippel–Trenaunay–Weber and neurofibromatosis). There are two types of isolated macrodactyly: static and progressive. Static macrodactyly is present at birth and grows proportionately. Progressive macrodactyly is more common; the onset is in childhood and the affected digit(s) increases in size until skeletal maturity and epiphyseal closure. Clinical features of progressive macrodactyly include large, divergent fingers that are hypertrophic in all aspects.

Treatment

- Treatment may proceed with amputation or reconstruction. Reconstruction must treat all tissues
- Epiphysiodesis or fusion may be used to inhibit longitudinal growth, but it will not affect circumferential growth

TRIGGER THUMB

Trigger thumb usually presents with a flexed thumb interphalangeal (IP) joint. It rarely involves the 'clicking' or 'triggering' that is characteristic of trigger finger in adults. There is often no antecedent history,

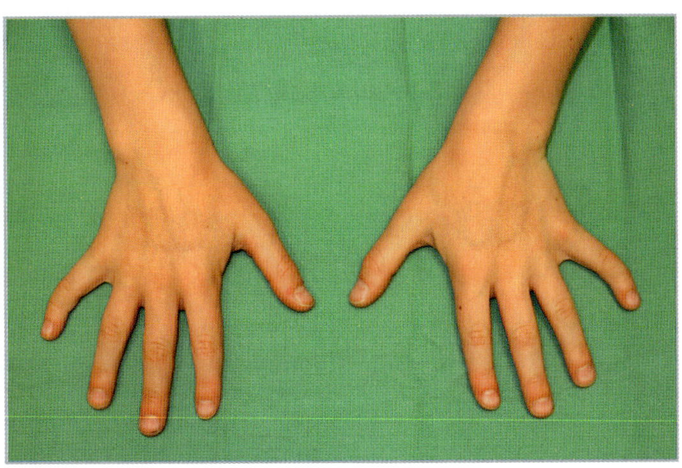

Figure 20.7 Clinodactyly of the little finger.

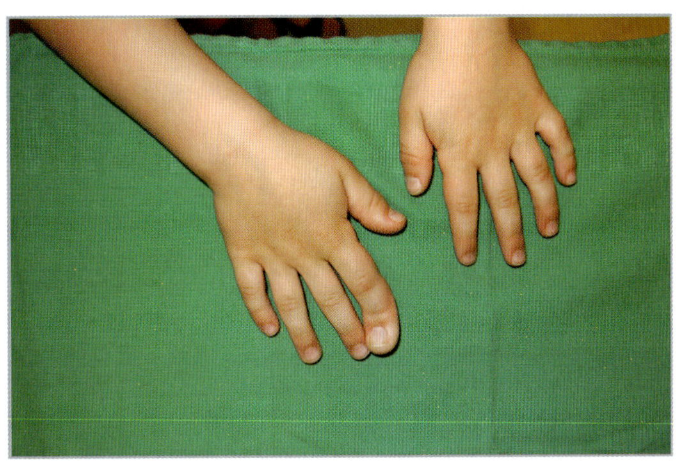

Figure 20.8 Appearance of macrodactylous digits.

and in roughly 30% of cases the condition is bilateral. Trigger thumb may initially go unnoticed, because it is painless and the presentation is often delayed.

Examination will reveal a fixed, flexed IP joint of the thumb. The flexion deformity may be partially or completely ameliorated by the MCP joint flexion. The thumb may or may not allow passive flexion. A Notta nodule will also be present over the region of the A1 pulley.

Treatment

- One study found that most cases recovery spontaneously without treatment
- Conservative treatment involves splinting with a removable thumb spica type splint combined with passive stretching exercises that can be completed by the parents
- Surgical treatment involves the release of A1 pulleys as is done in adults

TRIGGER DIGITS (OTHER THAN THUMB)

Trigger digits are much less common than trigger thumbs and are usually associated with other anomalies in the digit, specifically the flexor tendon.

Treatment

- Conservative treatment by observation may be attempted. If conservative treatment yields no improvement, surgery is indicated
- Release of the A1 pulley alone is often insufficient
  - More extensive exploration of the flexor tendons and flexor sheath is needed
  - Excision or release of abnormalities or abnormal connections between these structures may be necessary to correct the trigger

CONSTRICTION RING SYNDROME

Constriction ring syndrome is also known as amniotic band syndrome, amniotic disruption sequence, and Streeter disease. Constriction ring syndrome presents variably from constriction rings (in digits of the hand, foot, or limb) to amputations and acrosyndactyly (**Figure 20.9**). There are two theoretical etiologies for constriction ring syndrome. The first is intrinsic, where a local problem occurs with mesodermal development. The other is extrinsic, in which the amniotic membrane traps the developing hand or causes vascular damage. Currently, the extrinsic etiology is considered to be more probable. Constriction ring syndrome is associated with club feet and congenital vertical talus. Treatment involves the release of constriction with band excision and Z-plasty, syndactyly release should be performed if there is associated syndactyly.

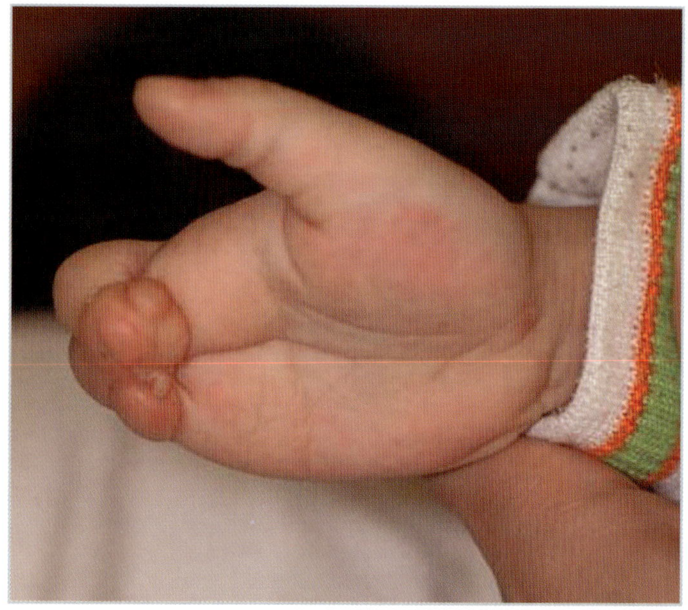

Figure 20.9 Acrosyndactyly in constriction ring syndrome.

CLEFT HAND

There are typical and atypical types of cleft hand. The typical type is bilateral and usually presents with foot involvement, with the hand forming a central, V-shaped cleft. Cleft hand is mostly autosomal dominantly inherited but may be sporadic. Atypical cleft hand is known as symbrachydactyly) and presents unilaterally with a U-shaped cleft and remnant digits. Atypical cleft hand usually occurs sporadically.

Symbrachydactyly

Symbrachydactyly usually presents unilaterally. The word comes from Greek origins: *syn* meaning 'joined' or 'fused,' *brachy* meaning 'short,' and *dactyl* meaning 'digits.' When treating symbrachydactyly, Poland syndrome (deficiency or absence of the pectoralis major muscle) should be considered. If Poland syndrome is suspected, a careful musculoskeletal and systemic assessment should be made, as there are other associated anomalies, some of which may require treatment. Many patients with symbrachydactyly do not proceed with surgical treatment because the other hand is functionally sufficient and the patient can adapt.

Symbrachydactyly classification

Types

- Short finger
  - Often good function, divide syndactyly
- Cleft type
  - Good thumb and small finger
  - Distraction lengthening, free phalanx transfer, toe transfer for tripod pinch
- Monodactylous
  - Normal thumb only; nubbins for fingers
  - Free phalanx transfer, toe transfer
- Peromelic
  - No digits
  - Check to determine if patient can cup palm. If so, it is possible to perform multiple free toe transfers to achieve opposable digits

RADIOULNAR SYNOSTOSIS

Radioulnar synostosis is a rare anomaly and may be an isolated condition. Radioulnar synostosis may also present as part of another syndrome or with associated anomalies such as fetal alcohol syndrome, trisomies 13 or 21, or radial longitudinal deficiency. Proximal radioulnar synostosis is more common. Type I radioulnar synostosis is isolated and complete, whereas type II radioulnar synostosis is partial and associated with radial head dislocation. There is often delayed presentation because of shoulder and wrist compensation.

Treatment

Treatment is determined by the position of the forearm:

- If prosupination is < 20°, then the arm is usually functionally acceptable
- If prosupination is ≥ 60°, the arm tends to interfere with activities of daily living, especially extreme pronation and bilateral involvement. In these cases, surgery is strongly recommended
- If prosupination is between 20° and 60°, then the treatment will depend on individual needs

Surgical options

- Derotation osteotomy for surgical correction
  - This treatment does not add motion
  - This treatment is recommended if the condition is unilateral and the patient can achieve 10°–20° degrees of supination
  - This option is also considered if the condition is bilateral and one side is able to achieve 30°–40° of pronation
- Another surgical treatment option is resection of synostosis. This usually yields poor results with little motion

SUGGESTED READING

Baek GH, Kim JH, Chung MS, et al. The natural history of pediatric trigger thumb. J Bone Joint Surg Am 2008; 90:980–985.
In this study, a cohort of 71 trigger thumbs was prospectively followed up to see their natural history. No treatment was instituted and 63% of the triggers resolved spontaneously. The median time to resolution was 48 months.

Bayne LG, Klug MS. Long-term review of the surgical treatment of radial deficiencies. J Hand Surg Am 1987; 12:169–179.
A classic paper that introduces the classification of radial deficiencies. The authors also review their series of 64 patients with 101 deficiencies.

Littler JW, Cooley SG. Opposition of the thumb and its restoration by abductor digiti quinti transfer. J Bone Joint Surg Am 1963; 45:1389–1396.
This is a practical and useful description of the surgical technique for transfer of the abductor digit minimi muscle for thumb opposition in thumb hypoplasia.

Siegert JJ, Cooney WP, Dobyns JH. Management of simple camptodactyly. J Hand Surg Br 1990; 15:181–189.
The authors reviewed the treatment and results of 57 patients with camptodactyly. They suggest that conservative treatment is the best for digits with less than 60° of extension deficit. Surgery should be reserved for failed conservative treatment, but there is risk of loss of finger flexion.

Teoh LC, Lee JY. Dorsal pentagonal island flap: a technique of web reconstruction for syndactyly that facilitates direct closure. Hand Surg 2004; 9:245–252.
The authors introduce a technique for recreating a web in syndactyly release that obviates the need for skin grafting.

Chapter 21 Chronic infections of the hand and upper extremity

Oluseyi Aliu, Kevin C. Chung

GENERAL PRINCIPLES

Diagnosing chronic hand infections is often challenging, because they are generally not common and the offending organisms are difficult to identify. Diagnosis requires heightened suspicion especially under the following circumstances: (1) Chronic lesions of the hand and upper extremity involving the skin, subcutaneous tissue, tenosynovium, joints, bones, and nerves. (2) Chronic lesions in patients with compromised immunity (history of organ transplant, long-duration steroid treatment, HIV/AIDS, malnourishment, chronic kidney disease, chemotherapy treatment, etc.). (3) Chronic lesions in patients with poor tissue perfusion (chronic venous insufficiency, history of radiation, peripheral vascular disease, etc.).

Bacteria, fungi, mycobacteria, protozoa, and viruses alike can cause chronic infections. Hence, accurate identification of causative organisms depends on adequate culture techniques, appropriate stains, and diligent histological examination. Involve infectious disease specialists early to provide knowledge about presumptive causative organisms and the conditions and media required for culture. Many of the causative organisms are fastidious, slow growers and are thus difficult to identify.

Tissue biopsy with adequate specimen is paramount to diagnosis. A standard workup must include Gram stain for bacteria, acid-fast stain (AFB) for mycobacteria, and potassium hydroxide (KOH) preparation for fungi. Sometimes, specialized stains are needed for identifying organisms and tissue manifestations of infection by histological examination [e.g. Giemsa, periodic acid–Schiff (PAS), Gomori methenamine silver, hematoxylin and eosin (H&E)]. Ensure that the biopsied specimen is sufficient in quantity as to prepare multiple sections for histological examination and improve diagnostic accuracy. Conduct cultures for aerobic, anaerobic, mycobacterial (typical and atypical), protozoal, and fungal organisms.

Other specimens such as abscess contents, drainage from lesions, and synovial fluid may also be obtained when possible and tested similarly to biopsied tissue. Drug susceptibility tests are crucial to ensure appropriate pharmaceutical treatments and to monitor drug resistance. Laboratory tests such as complete blood counts with differential, erythrocyte sedimentation rate, and radiographic tests should be adjuncts to diagnosis by culture and histological examination.

Begin empirical broad spectrum antimicrobial therapy based on suspected organism or results of initial workup and then adjust treatment after definitive culture and sensitivity results are available. Steroid treatments such as for patients with rheumatoid arthritis before establishment of diagnosis often worsens the manifestation of chronic infections and could increase morbidity for patients.

BACTERIAL INFECTIONS

Actinomycosis

Epidemiology/biology

Actinomycosis is caused by endogenous microaerophilic, AFB (−) organisms found in the oral cavity and alimentary tract. The most common organism that causes this infection is *Actinomyces israelii*. The patient's clinical history should be probed for traumatic inoculation, e.g. from a human bite or closed fist contact with teeth. Untreated infections progressively spread through tissue planes and can persist for many years. The infection invariably begins in the skin and can spread deep enough to involve underlying bone if it goes untreated.

Presentation/appearance

Patients with chronic actinomycosis have persistent firm swelling (woody edema) of the involved extremity with restricted motion. There are also multiple small painful nodules and several sinuses. These sinuses produce intermittent purulent drainage that contains yellow granules commonly described as 'sulfur granules.'

Diagnosis/workup

Specimens for staining, histological examination, and culture may be obtained from tissue biopsy of the nodules or from the sinus drainage including the 'sulfur granules.' Staining and histological examination are much more diagnostic than culture because the organism is very fastidious. However, all three tests (staining, histology, and culture) should be performed. In addition, plain radiographs must be obtained to investigate spread of disease to the bone.

Treatment

Actinomyces spp. are widely susceptible to beta-lactams and beta-lactamase inhibitors, (e.g. penicillin), which are first line treatments. The duration of treatment is usually prolonged for effectiveness and hence must be guided by an infectious disease specialist. Surgical debridement (debulking and excision of sinus tracts) is necessary if there is no response to antibiotic treatment or if the infection recurs.

Mycetoma (actinomycetoma and eumycetoma)

Epidemiology/biology

'Mycetoma' literally means fungal tumor. However, mycetomas can be caused by bacteria (actinomycetoma) or fungi (eumycetoma). Causative bacterial organisms are exogenous aerobic, weakly AFB (+), actinomycetes found in soil. Fungal organisms are also found in soil, and they cause disease less often than bacteria. Causative organisms are usually specific to different parts of the world (**Table 21.1**). Infection usually results from inoculation of skin breaks with contaminated soil or parts of woody plants. If left untreated, infection in the upper extremity can spread to involve underlying bone, the axilla, and chest wall as well. Men are mostly affected by the disease and age range is from 20 to 60 years of age.

Presentation/appearance

The presentation of this infection is dependent on the stage of infection. Early on, there is a painless firm subcutaneous nodule. The nodule progresses to a draining abscess, interconnected sinuses, and fistulas. The drainage contains characteristic granules (**Table 21.1**, **Figure 21.1a and b**). If there are no granules, it is not a mycetoma. In late presentation, there is gross enlargement of the involved limb with edematous induration and deformity. As a result, the disease is often mistaken to be a malignancy (**Figure 21.1c**).

Diagnosis/workup

Effective treatment depends on distinguishing between bacterial and fungal causes. Specimens for staining, histological examination, and culture should be obtained by tissue biopsy. Sinus discharge and granules are less ideal specimens. It is imperative to have stains and culture media for both bacteria and fungi.

Clinical features of the infection can also help with diagnosis. The color of the granules gives clues to the offending organism. For example, black granules always indicate a fungal mycetoma (**Table 21.1**). In addition, the size of the granules under the microscope can narrow choices down to a bacterial (usually smaller) versus a fungal cause. Imaging tests may be necessary to determine the extent of bone and soft tissue involvement. Plain radiographs do show bone changes and sonography shows extent of soft tissue disease. However, computed tomographic scan and magnetic resonance imaging are superior modalities. Serological antibody detection tests exist but not widely available.

Treatment

For actinomycetoma, first line treatment is pharmaceutical and antibiotics, which should be used depending on the specific offending organism (**Table 21.2**). Surgical treatment is rarely needed.

For eumycetoma treatment is primarily pharmaceutical (**Table 21.2**), but the treatment is used to limit the extent of the disease rather than cure it. Surgical resection can be used to eliminate disease limited by pharmaceutical treatment. In addition, it may be used to debulk large lesions to improve response to the pharmaceutical treatment. Either way, resection must include uninfected tissue margins to decrease the risk of recurrence. Amputation may be required if disease is unresponsive to pharmaceutical treatment and not controlled by limited debridement.

Syphilis

Epidemiology/biology

The causative organism for syphilis is *Treponema pallidum.* A primary infection requires direct contact of the hand or upper extremity with an infectious syphilitic lesion. Congenital syphilis is syphilis transmitted from mother to child during pregnancy or childbirth. Primary, secondary, and tertiary stages of syphilis are defined by the time, since infection and each stage has distinct symptoms. Primary disease manifests as a chancre at the site of contact approximately 3

Table 21.1 Common organisms that cause mycetoma

Granule color	Organism	Mycetoma type	Where found
Black			
	Madurella mycetomatis	Eumycetoma	Worldwide
	Madurella grisea	Eumycetoma	Central/South America, India
	Leptosphaeria senegalensis	Eumycetoma	Africa
	Leptosphaeria tompkinsii	Eumycetoma	Africa
	Pyrenochaeta romeroi	Eumycetoma	South America
	Pyrenochaeta mackinnonii	Eumycetoma	South America
Pale (white-yellow)			
	Pseudallescheria boydii	Eumycetoma	North America
	Aspergillus spp.	Eumycetoma	Worldwide
	Acremonium spp.	Eumycetoma	Worldwide
	Fusarium spp.	Eumycetoma	Worldwide
	Neotestudina rosatii	Eumycetoma	Africa
	Polycytella hominis	Eumycetoma	North America
	Actinomadura madurae	Actinomycetoma	Central/South America, India
	Nocardia spp.	Actinomycetoma	Central/South America, India
Yellow-brown			
	Streptomyces somaliensis	Actinomycetoma	Africa/Middle East
Red-pink			
	Actinomadura pelletieri	Actinomycetoma	Africa

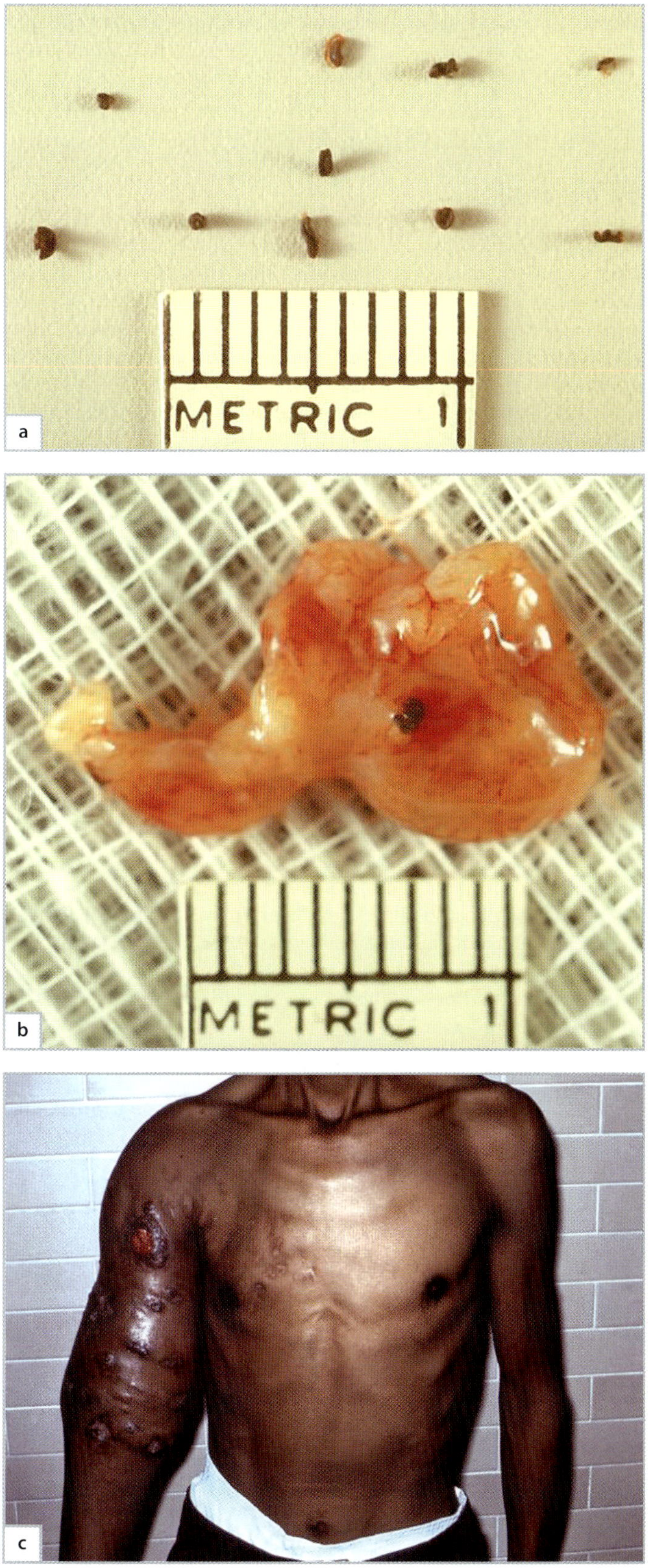

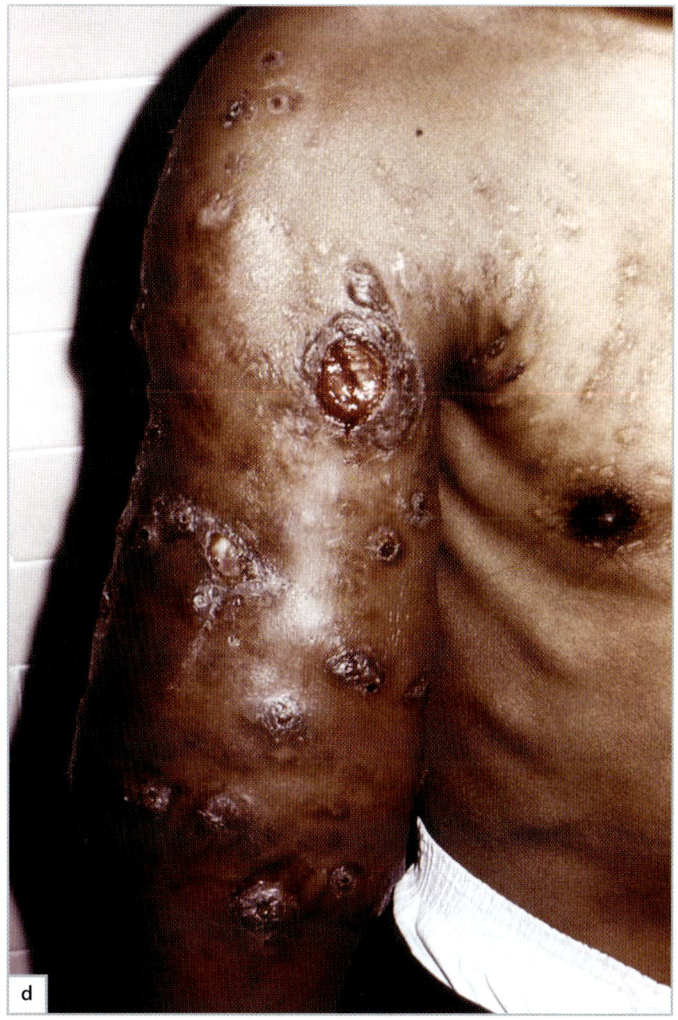

Figure 21.1 (a) Example of black granules of the fungus *Madurella grisea*. (b) Black granule within adipose tissue. (c) and (d) Oblique and frontal views of an upper extremity with late mycetoma. There is gross enlargement of the limb with draining sinuses. At this stage, the disease is often mistaken for a malignancy. With permission from Dr Libero Ajello and the Centers for Disease Control and Prevention.

weeks after infection. Secondary disease is usually manifest as lesions of the skin, mucus membranes, or lymph nodes 1–3 months after primary disease manifestation. Tertiary syphilis manifests as disease of several organ systems including the musculoskeletal system an average of 15 years after initial infection.

Presentation/appearance

Primary syphilis presents as a firm painless ulcer with raised edges and serous drainage (**Figure 21.2a**). This lesion is known as a chancre and is usually accompanied by regional lymphadenopathy. In the upper extremity, this usually occurs on the finger. Secondary syphilis affecting extremities usually presents as dactylitis, which is a painful inflammatory swelling of an entire digit. Tertiary syphilis presents as chronic inflammatory nonmalignant growths (gummas) involving tissues from skin to bone (**Figure 21.2b**). Congenital syphilis also presents as dactylitis that may be accompanied with pathological fractures causing pseudoparalysis.

Diagnosis/workup

Diagnosis is usually established with serological tests. Fluorescent treponemal antibody-absorption test (FTA-Abs) detects antibodies to *Treponema pallidum.* It is a treponemal test with high specificity, and hence, it is used as a confirmatory test for positive venereal disease research laboratory test (VDRL) and rapid plasma regain tests (RPR). VDRL and RPR are both nontreponemal tests with lower specificity. They are generally used to monitor treatment response and as initial tests for diagnosis. Dark-field examination of serous discharge under microscope will show *Treponema pallidum* and is usually confirmatory. Plain radiographs show characteristic bone changes of secondary syphilis, which include diaphyseal expansion with evidence of endosteal destruction similar to 'spina ventosa' findings in mycobacterial osteomyelitis. Pathological fractures of metacarpals or phalanges may be present.

Treatment

Congenital, primary, secondary, and tertiary syphilis are all treated pharmaceutically (**Table 21.2**) with dosing depending on the stage. Hence, infectious specialists must be involved to direct therapy. Protective splinting and occupational therapy for dactylitis and pathologic fractures are the purview of the hand surgeon.

FUNGAL INFECTIONS

General

Fungal infections may involve skin and subcutaneous tissues or deep tissues such as tenosynovium. Skin manifestations such as dermatophysis are the most common fungal infections and are mostly seen by primary care physicians. Hand and upper extremity subcutaneous and deep tissue infections require specialist attention.

Fungal isolates in cultures of lesions from patients with compromised immunity should never be dismissed as contaminants. In addition, if a lesion does not respond to broad-spectrum antibiotics, a fungal infection should be suspected. Several antifungal drugs, such as ketoconazole and itraconazole, have serious hepatotoxic side effects and significant drug interactions. Hence, hand and upper extremity surgeons must be vigilant for signs of drug side effects when treating patients with chronic fungal infections.

Chronic paronychia

Epidemiology/biology

Chronic paronychia is an infection of the subcutaneous tissues around fingernails, and the most common causative organism is *Candida albicans.* Notably, some soft tissue malignancies mimic chronic paronychia. Persistent exposure of the hand to moisture is a strong risk factor (e.g. dishwashing, laundering, habitual thumb sucking in children). This persistent moisture causes maceration of the skin making the infection possible. Women are three times more likely than men to be affected. Patients can have secondary bacterial infection of the proximal nail fold usually caused by *Pseudomonas aeruginosa.* Antimicrobial treatment of this secondary infection does not treat the underlying paronychia.

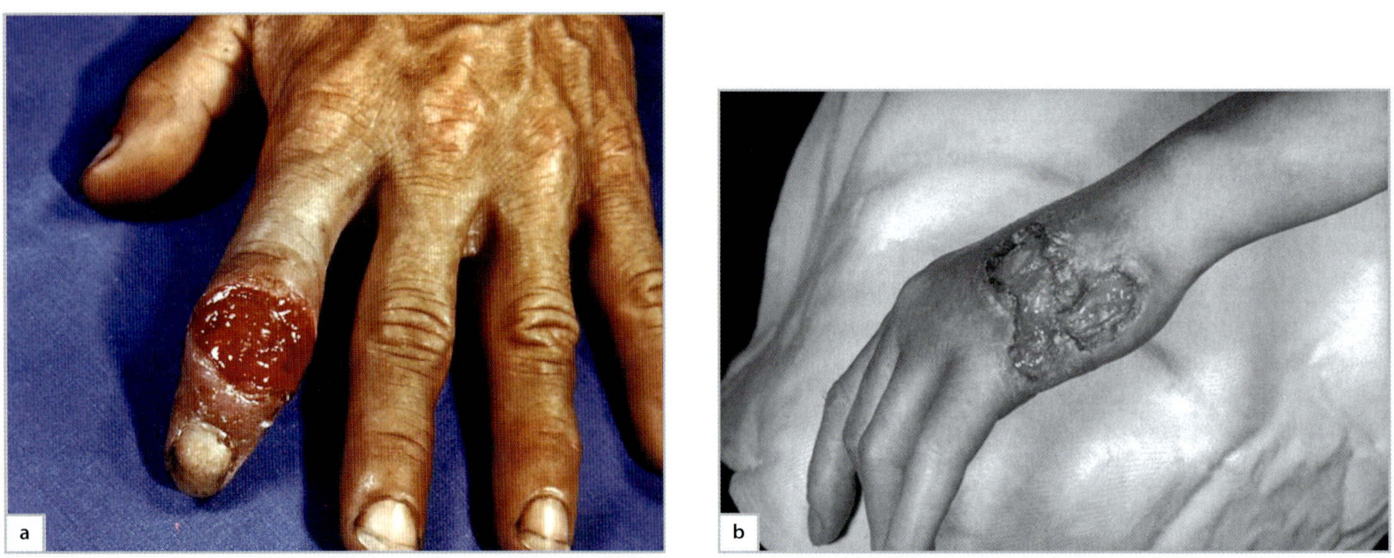

Figure 21.2 (a) Primary syphilitic lesion known as chancre on dorsum of the index finger. (b) The nonmalignant lesion in the figure is a 'gumma,' a manifestation of tertiary syphilis in the upper extremity. With permission from Susan Lindsey and the Centers for Disease Control and Prevention.

Presentation/appearance

Initially, there is local inflammation with erythema and tender swelling of the nail fold without an abscess (**Figure 21.3a**). Overtime the eponychium becomes retracted and indurated with tense skin. Eventually, without adequate treatment, the eponychium thickens and the nail becomes discolored and disfigured with ridges (**Figure 21.3b**).

Diagnosis/workup

Diagnosis is usually based on patient history (exposure to moisture) and signs at presentation. Scrapings of involved tissues should provide adequate specimen for KOH preparation. Biopsy is not necessary; however, tissue biopsy to investigate soft tissue malignancies may be considered for disease that is unresponsive to appropriate treatment.

Treatment

For mild cases, avoidance of moisture is important. Prolonged treatment with topical antifungal preparations is the first line pharmaceutical treatment. Oral antifungal preparations are indicated in severe cases (**Table 21.2**). If infection is persistent despite pharmaceutical treatment, surgical treatment with eponychial marsupialization is indicated (**Figure 21.3c**).

Sporotrichosis

Epidemiology/biology

Sporotrichosis is caused by *Sporothrix schenckii*, an organism that is plentiful in soil. Infection usually results from traumatic inoculation with plant thorns. Because of this, infection is an occupational hazard for people that work with plants, e.g. gardeners, florists, and horticulturists. The hand and upper extremity are most commonly affected. The disease usually manifest as lymphocutaneous infection but can also cause deep tissue infection in patients with immune compromise. Sporotrichosis is not an opportunistic infection.

Presentation/appearance

Lesions begin as painless nodules that appear up to 10 weeks after inoculation (**Figure 21.4a**). Nodules eventually form a firm ulcer with raised borders and seropurulent discharge. The ulcerated nodules multiply linearly and proximally along lymphatic channels going through the same evolution from nodule to ulcer (**Figure 21.4b**). Regional lymphadenopathy is usually present.

Diagnosis/workup

Deep tissue biopsy is necessary for culture and histological examination with special stains (PAS). Identifying the organism is very difficult and multiple sections must be examined. The caregiver may use seropurulent drainage or aspirate for culture and stains but deep tissue biopsy is superior. Serological tests using polymerase chain reaction (PCR) techniques exist but are not widely available.

Treatment

Treatment of lymphocutaneous sporotrichosis is pharmaceutical (**Table 21.2**), and the lesions generally heal without the need for surgical intervention.

Table 21.2 Pharmaceutical treatments for chronic hand and upper-extremity infections

Hand/upper-extremity chronic infection	Pharmaceutical treatment
Bacterial	
Actinomycocis	IV penicillin + subsequent PO penicillin/amoxicillin Alternatives (penicillin allergic): tetracycline/ erythromycin/clindamycin
Actinomycetoma	Streptomycin + dapsone/trimethoprim-sulfamethoxazole
Syphilis	IM benzathine penicillin Alternative (penicillin allergic): doxycycline
Fungal	
Eumycetoma	Depends on specific organism (**Table 21.1**): ketoconazole/itraconazole/fluconazole
Candidiasis (paronychia)	Topical clotrimazole/PO fluconazole
Sporotrichosis	PO itraconazole Alternatives: SSKI/terbinafine/fluconazole
Aspergillosis	Amphotericin B Alternative (localized lesion): itraconazole
Mucormycosis	Amphotericin B
Extracutaneous sporotrichosis	Amphotericin B Alternatives: itraconazole/fluconazole
Protozoal	
Leishmaniasis	Topical paromomycin/intralesional sodium stibogluconate
Viral	
Human orf	Immunocompromised patients: intralesional injection/topical cidofovir Immunocompetent patients: topical imiquimod

IM, intramuscular; IV, intravenous; PO, per ostium (by mouth); SSKI, saturated solution of potassium iodide.

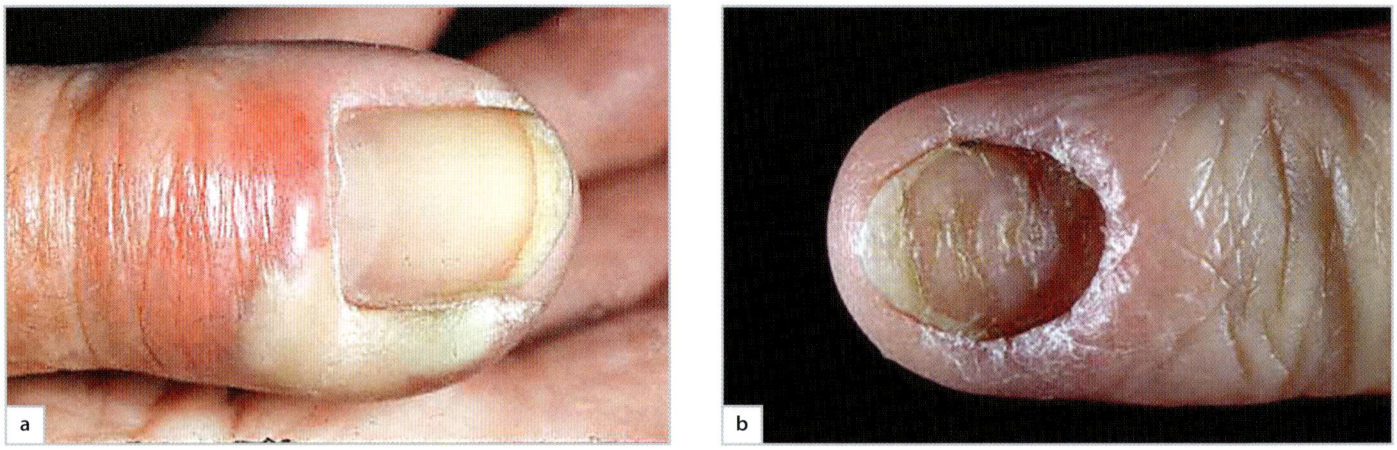

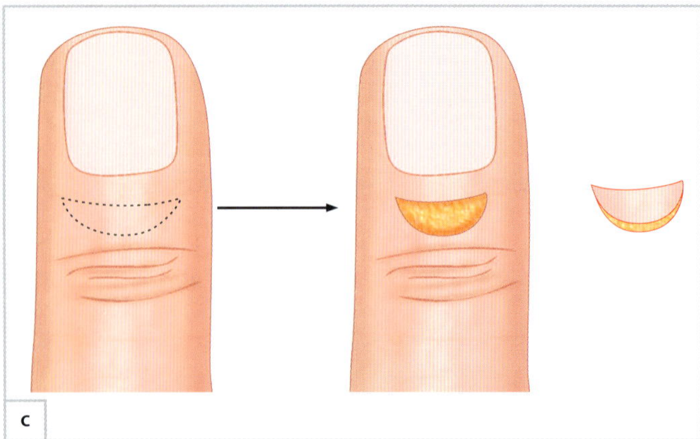

Figure 21.3 (a) Local erythema and swelling of the nail fold in early fungal paronychia. (b) The figure demonstrates findings in chronic fungal paronychia including a tense indurated eponychium with disfiguration of the nail. (c) Eponychial marsupialization for the treatment of chronic fungal paronychia not responsive to pharmaceutical treatment.

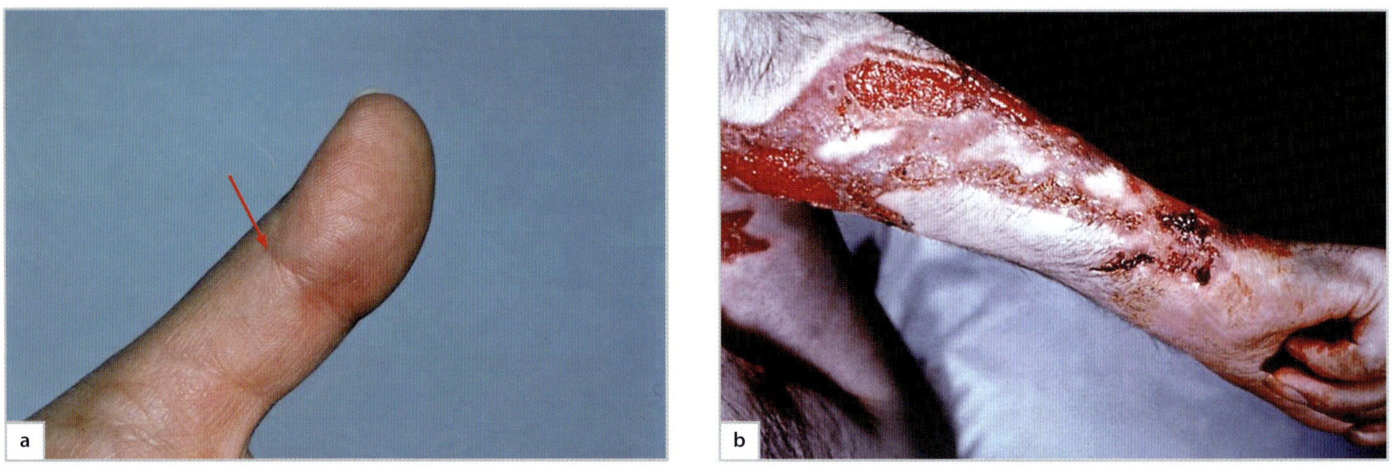

Figure 21.4 (a) Sporotrichosis lesions begin insidiously as painless nodules at the point of inoculation. With permission from Dr William Kaplan and the Centers for Disease Control and Prevention (CDC) (red arrow at the interphalangeal joint crease of the thumb in the figure). (b) Eventually sporotrichosis lesions ulcerate and track proximally along lymphatic channels. With permission from Dr Lucille K. Gorg and the Centers for Disease Control and Prevention.

Extracutaneous sporotrichosis

Epidemiology/biology

This infection is also caused by *Sporothrix schenckii* in patients with compromised immunity. The organism causes a pneumonia that spreads hematogenously to deep tissues of the upper extremity including bones, joints, and tenosynovium. Hand and wrist joints are most commonly infected.

Presentation/appearance

For extracutaneous sporotrichosis, the characteristic lesions of lymphocutaneous sporotrichosis along lymph channels are absent. Joint infections present with swelling and erythema over the affected joint with a draining sinus. Osteomyelitis also presents with swelling and a draining sinus to the infected bone. There is commonly a concomitant arthritis with osteomyelitis. Tenosynovial disease presents with boggy swelling similar to the tenosynovitis of rheumatoid arthritis. Patients may present with carpal tunnel and median nerve compression symptoms if flexor tendons are affected. Patients may also present with compromised range of motion from extensor tendon rupture.

Diagnosis/workup

Diagnosis is very difficult because sporotrichosis is a rare cause of arthritis, osteomyelitis, or tenosynovitis. Antecedent pneumonia in the patient's history may provide a clue, and in that case, an etiology for compromised immunity must also be investigated. Definitive diagnosis requires culture from tissue biopsy, joint aspirate, or drainage from sinus (less desirable). Rice bodies may be found during biopsy and sent for culture. Plain radiographs should be obtained to assess joint and bone disease for treatment planning.

Treatment

Treatment for extracutaneous sporotrichosis involves concomitant pharmaceutical and surgical treatment. Pharmaceutical treatment is more aggressive than for lymphocutaneous sporotrichosis, and infectious disease specialists must be involved in directing therapy (**Table 21.2**). Surgical drainage and irrigation of infected joints and debridement of infected bone are necessary for control of infection. Amputation may be necessary in stubborn infections. Arthrodesis may be needed for reconstruction after treatment of joint disease.

Aspergillosis

Epidemiology/biology

This infection is commonly caused by *Aspergillus fumigatus*. This is an opportunistic infection, and hence, severely immunologically compromised patients are most at-risk. Patients with hematological malignancies and those on cytotoxic drugs are particularly at-risk. It is a deep tissue angioinvasive infection that causes necrosis of tendons, joints, and neurovascular tissues. In addition, the infection can disseminate rapidly and is often fatal. Upper-extremity infection usually results from iatrogenic inoculation such as from venipunctures or use of contaminated dressing supplies in susceptible patients. Hematogenous spread is also possible in cases of disseminated disease from primary respiratory aspergillosis.

Presentation/appearance

Lesions begin as erythematous or violaceous firm papules that progress to hemorrhagic blisters or necrotic ulcers.

Diagnosis/workup

Tissue biopsy of the lesion for KOH wet preparation, histological examination after special stains (PAS or Gomori methenamine silver), and culture. It is a relatively fast growing fungus.

Treatment

Concomitant pharmaceutical and surgical treatment is required. This is a deadly infection in patients with compromised immunity; hence, both forms of treatment must be expedient. Infectious disease specialists must direct pharmaceutical treatment (**Table 21.2**). Surgical treatment involves radical debridement of necrotic/infected tissues to control the infection. Amputation may be required in disease unresponsive to the pharmaceutical treatment.

Mucormycosis

Epidemiology/biology

Causative organisms of mucormycosis are fungi of the order *Mucorales* and *Rhizopus* spp. are the most common isolates. They are ubiquitous organisms found in most soil and decaying matter. Many cases of soft tissue mucormycosis result from soil contamination of traumatic wounds and transmission from contaminated dressings. The organisms invade blood vessels and cause tissue destruction by thrombosis and subsequent necrosis. Mucormycosis is an opportunistic infection and patients with immunological compromise including those with poorly controlled diabetes mellitus are at the highest risk. The infection can affect superficial or deeper tissues of the upper extremity; however, most hand and upper-extremity infections are superficial (cutaneous and subcutaneous). Progression to deep tissues is not uncommon. Mucormycosis is a highly destructive and very aggressive infection with a significant mortality rate (up to 15% for cutaneous disease).

Presentation/appearance

Infection begins as a cellulitis that rapidly progresses to dermal necrosis that advances equally rapidly (it behaves like necrotizing fasciitis). The presence of black purulent material and an advancing black eschar is characteristic of mucormycosis, and thus a good clinical clue for diagnosis (**Figure 21.5**).

Diagnosis/workup

Expedient diagnosis is paramount because of the destructive nature of the infection and its high mortality rate. Clinical signs noted in the presentation/appearance can provide clues, e.g. black pus, advancing dermal necrosis with cellulitis. Diagnosis requires deep tissue biopsy for specialized stains (H&E, Gomori methenamine silver or PAS), histological examination, and cultures. To expedite a presumptive diagnosis, frozen sections may be sent for analysis during the biopsy procedure if mucormycosis is suspected. Histological examination will show the characteristic vascular invasion. This is a fast growing fungus in cultures with the right media and adequate specimen (from tissue biopsy). The culture helps isolate the offending species.

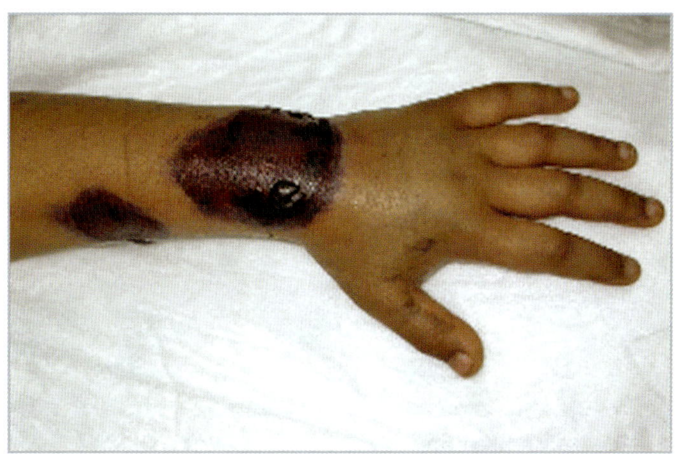

Figure 21.5 The black eschar shown in the figure above is characteristic of mucormycosis. The eschar advances in a similar fashion to necrotizing fasciitis.

Treatment

The underlying cause of immunological compromise must be addressed (e.g. aggressive management of poorly controlled diabetes, cessation of cytotoxic drugs, weaning immunosuppressive drugs). Management for this infection includes expedient and concomitant surgical and pharmaceutical treatment. Surgical treatment requires radical surgical debridement of infected and necrotic tissue. Amputation may be required for control of the infection. Resection may be extensive enough to subsequently require reconstruction with grafts/ flaps. An infection specialist must direct pharmaceutical treatment (**Table 21.2**).

PROTOZOAL INFECTIONS

Leishmaniasis

Epidemiology/biology

Leishmaniasis is caused by the organisms *Leishmania* spp., and the disease is very common in the tropics and subtropics (Africa, South America, Mediterranean, Middle East, and Asia). The vector for this disease is the sand fly. Leishmaniasis is transmitted with a bite from the sand fly. Reservoirs for the protozoa include canines, rodents, and infected humans. Cutaneous manifestation has a propensity for exposed body parts including extremities, where the sand fly settle and bite. The lesion usually heals without treatment in patients with competent immune systems. Healing can take up to 15 months and may result in a disfiguring morbid scar, especially with large lesions.

Presentation/appearance

The lesion begins as papule at the insect bite site that evolves into a painless ulcer over several weeks to 6 months. The ulcer has indurated edges, a necrotic base with a thick adherent crust (**Figure 21.6**). Multiple ulcers are possible in patients with immunological compromise or those bitten by multiple sand flies at once.

Diagnosis/workup

One may perform a tissue biopsy from the ulcer edge for a bloodless tissue impression smear and Giemsa stain to identify the protozoa under oil immersion microscopy. The specimen may be obtained from scrapings of the lesion's crust. Diagnosis by culture of the organism is very difficult because it takes up to 1 month to grow. PCR is the gold standard for diagnosis, although it is not widely available.

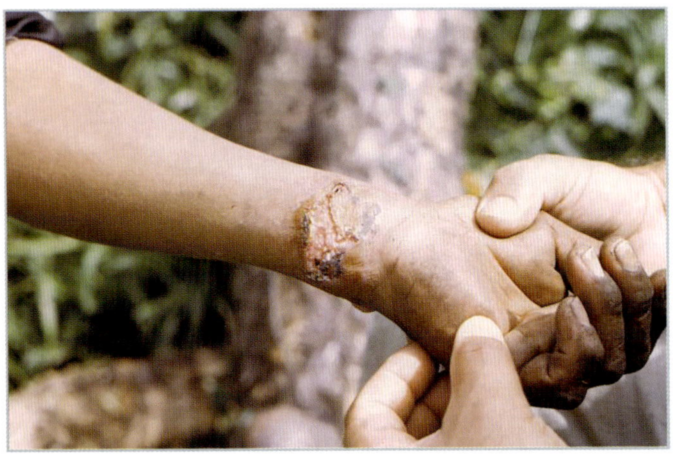

Figure 21.6 Cutaneous leishmaniasis ulcer. The ulcer in the figure has the characteristic heaped up edges and crusty base. With permission from Dr AJ Sulzer and the Centers for Disease Control and Prevention.

Treatment

The disease has a self-limited course in immune competent patients that takes up to 15 months. Treatment is pharmaceutical (**Table 21.2**) and is primarily intended to prevent highly morbid disseminated disease, devastating secondary infections, and the disfigurement of untreated large lesions.

VIRAL INFECTIONS

Human orf (ecthyma contagiosum)

Epidemiology/biology

This infection is caused by the *Parapoxvirus* orf virus, an organism that is primarily endemic in shee and goats, although it has also been reported in deer and domestic pets. This virus can survive on fomites for long periods of time (several months). The disease mostly affects individuals that have contact with infected sheep and goats or contaminated products from them. The infection occurs through inoculation of old wounds or traumatic inoculation of new wounds on exposed body parts such as the upper extremity (the most affected anatomical region). Viral transmission may also occur from contaminated fomites and human-to-human by physical contact.

Presentation/appearance

Lesions begin as a firm papule that progress into pustule-appearing nodules called contagious purulent dermatitis. In fact, the lesion is not at all purulent. These nodules weep serous fluid and eventually crust over. Black dots are seen beneath the crust. In the final stages of the lesion's evolution, it develops papillomatous projections from its surface before resolution. Multiple localized lesions are not uncommon, and the lesions may assume very large proportions in patients with compromised immunity. Generally, patients do not have any systemic symptoms.

Diagnosis/workup

Examination of a suspension prepared from specimen under electron microscope is the quickest method of presumptive diagnosis; however, it cannot distinguish the orf virus from other members of the *Parapoxvirus* genus. Diagnosis is hence generally made clinically from patient's history of exposure to sheep or goats and appearance of the lesion. One can perform tissue biopsy or use specimens of crust or fluid from nodules for cultures, although this takes up to 1 month. Only PCR can definitively identify the offending organism as *Parapoxvirus orf virus.*

Treatment

In patients with competent immunity, the disease course is self-limiting (6–8 weeks). Pain control, protective immobilization, and local wound care are helpful. Patients may benefit from topical proinflammatory preparations to shorten disease course (**Table 21.2**). In patients with compromised immunity, complete excision of large lesions and reconstruction with grafts or flaps may be indicated. There are scant reports of successful treatment with antiviral preparations (**Table 21.2**).

SUGGESTED READING

Ahmed AO, van Leeuwen W, Fahal A, et al. Mycetoma caused by Madurella mycetomatis: a neglected infectious burden. Lancet Infect Dis 2004; 4:566–574.

Amadio PC. Fungal infections of the hand. Hand Clin 1998; 14:605–612.

Barros MB, de Almeida Paes R, Schubach AO. Sporothrix schenckii and sporotrichosis. Clin Microbiol Rev 2011; 24:633–654.

Hoyen HA, Lacey SH, Graham TJ. Atypical hand infections. Hand Clin 1998; 14:613-634.

Reithinger R, Dujardin JC, Louzir H, et al. Cutaneous leishmaniasis. Lancet Infect Dis 2007; 7:581–596.

Spellberg B, Ibrahim AS. Recent advances in the treatment of mucormycosis. Curr Infect Dis Rep 2010; 12:423–429.

Chapter 22 Tendinopathy and work-related upper-limb disorders

Yirong Wang, Evan J. Kowalski, Kevin C. Chung

INTRODUCTION

Tendinopathy of the hand is a common upper-extremity disorder. More specifically, it can refer to tenosynovitis, tenovaginitis, and tendinosis.

- Tenosynovitis: Inflammation in the synovial lining of the tendon
- Tenovaginitis: Constriction of a tendon by a tight covering or sheath
- Tendinosis: The progressive degeneration of a tendon due to age, poor blood supply, friction, or overuse
- These three conditions may occur independently or in combination with one another

TRIGGER FINGER

Trigger finger is a common hand condition characterized by an initial painless click in the finger that gradually becomes painful over time. In advanced cases, the digits can be locked in flexion or extension, and the digits must be forcibly unlocked to bring them into a normal position. The ring finger is most commonly involved, followed by the thumb, the middle finger, the index finger, and then the small finger. In the diabetic population, trigger finger is documented to be more common in females, presenting bilaterally and in multiple digits more often than in nondiabetic patients.

There are two main types of trigger finger: primary trigger finger and secondary trigger finger.

- Primary (idiopathic) trigger finger
  - The vast majority of trigger digits are primary idiopathic trigger finger or thumb
  - Occurs more frequently in women than in men
  - Usually occurs between the fourth to sixth decades of life
- Secondary trigger finger is associated with rheumatoid arthritis, diabetes mellitus, gout, amyloidosis, and mucopolysaccharidoses

Adult trigger digit

Pertinent anatomy and pathology

The finger flexor tendon sheaths consist of a bilayer synovial lining, enclosed by five annular and three cruciate pulleys. The thumb flexor sheath is enclosed by two annular pulleys and one oblique pulley (**Figure 22.1a**). The A1 pulley is the most commonly affected structure involved in trigger digits. Located at the metacarpophalangeal (MCP) joint, it attaches to the volar aspect and base of the proximal phalanx. A narrow fibro-osseous tunnel is formed by a groove in the palmar surface of the A1 pulley and metacarpal neck, allowing the flexor tendons of the fingers and thumb to enter the finger. Trigger digits occur due to a disproportion between the digital retinacular sheath and the flexor tendons and synovial sheath. The digital finger nerves course along the sides of the A1 pulley. However, the radial digital nerve for the thumb crosses the A1 pulley and is at risk for injury during trigger thumb release (**Figure 22.1b**).

Histological analyses of diseased A1 pulleys and superficialis tendons show fibrocartilaginous metaplasia. The normal inner gliding layer of the A1 pulley is characterized by spindle-shaped fibroblasts and ovoid cells. If these cells transform and develop properties more like that of chondrocyte cells, the A1 pulley may triple in thickness. A flexor tendon will catch when attempting to glide through a sheath that is stenotic, resulting in an inability to smoothly flex or extend the digit.

Clinical appearance and diagnosis

Patients present with a clicking or locking of the interphalangeal (IP) joints during flexion and extension. They often feel a gradual tenderness and pain on the palm, MCP joints, or proximal IP (PIP) joints. Locking in flexion and pain at the PIP joint is the most common complaints associated with this disorder. Persistent locking of the finger may lead to a fixed flexion contracture at the PIP joint, and occasionally, the finger may become locked in an extended position. A significant clicking of the digits during active extension must be observed to assure a correct diagnosis of this condition, because other conditions can cause similar symptoms of pain. The flexor sheath should be palpated for a discrete nodule or diffuse tenosynovitis, because this finding may have important prognostic and treatment implications.

Treatment

Treatments include activity modification, nonsteroidal anti-inflammatory drugs, splinting, steroid injection, and surgical release. Mild triggering may resolve spontaneously and therefore does not require treatment.

- One study showed that the MCP joint blocking splint, worn continuously for 6 weeks, was effective in 77% of subjects
  - The splint extends from the palm across the MCP joint and includes a ring around the proximal phalanx and is designed to allow flexion of the PIP joint.
- Many authors recommend corticosteroid injection without splinting as the initial treatment.
  - Injection at the A1 pulley with a 0.5 mL solution of 50:50 mixed with Kenalog 10 and 1% lidocaine
  - Injection of the involved flexor tendon sheath was found to provide long-term symptom relief in 60–92% of affected digits, using up to three injections

- Corticosteroid injection treatments do not show significant improvement for patients with nodular trigger digits, diffuse stenosing tenosynovitis, multiple digit involvement, symptoms lasting >6 months, or diabetes mellitus
- A1 pulley release is the standard surgical treatment for trigger digits
  - Incisions are made at the proximal edge of the A1 pulley exactly over the tendon sheath (**Figure 22.1c**)
  - The A1 pulley should be incised with scissors (**Figure 22.1d**) or a no. 15 blade
  - Caution should be taken to protect the neurovascular bundles, especially because the radial neurovascular bundle of the thumb navigates in an oblique direction from the ulnar to radial aspect across the MCP joint crease

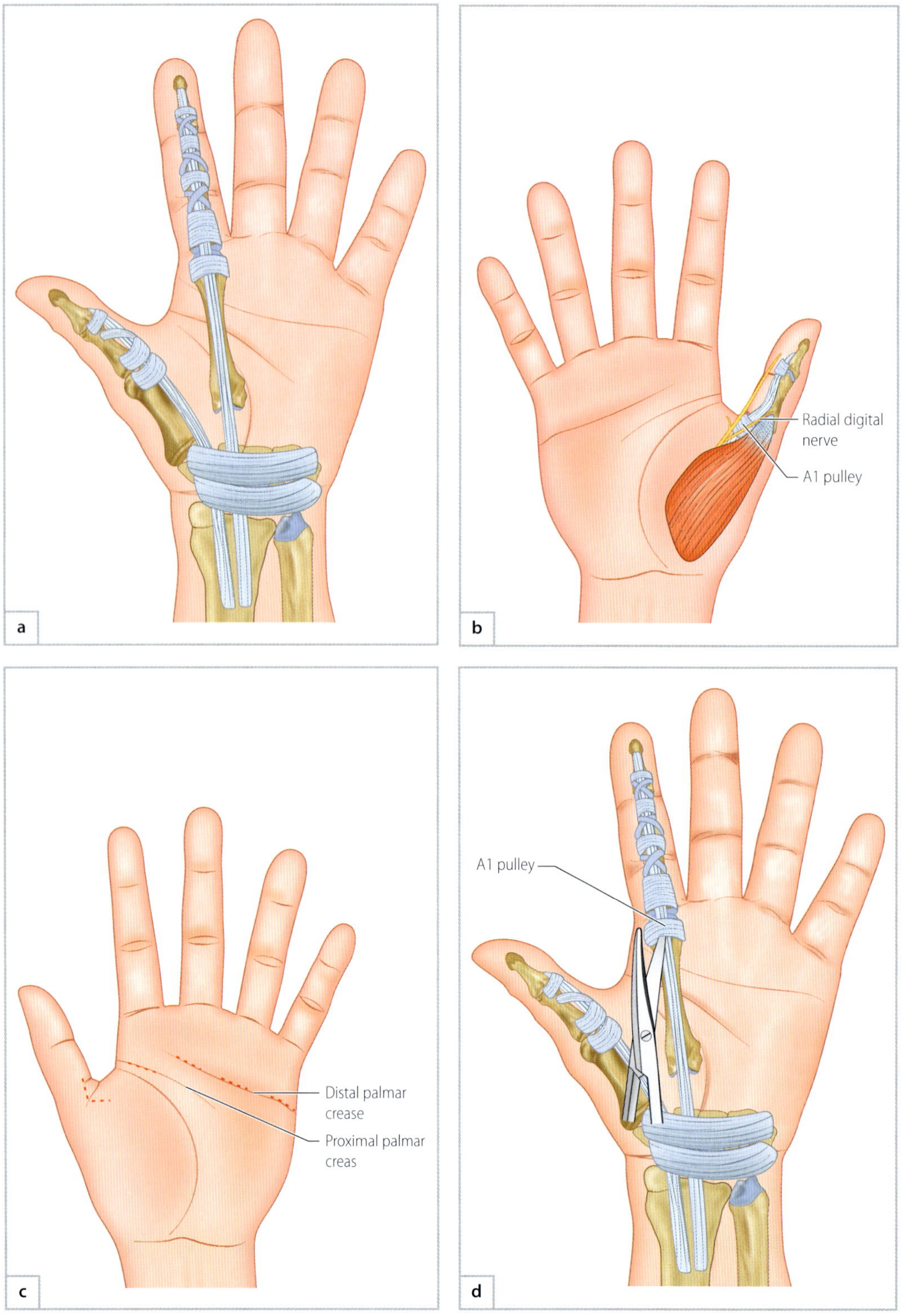

Figure 22.1 (a) Anatomy of the finger flexor tendon pulleys. (b) The radial digital nerve of the thumb courses directly over the thumb A1 pulley, making it susceptible to damage during surgery. (c) Incisions for trigger finger release should be made at the proximal edge of the A1 pulley. (d) The A1 pulley can be released with a no. 15 blade or scissors.

Pediatric trigger digit

In contrast to adult trigger digits, pediatric trigger digits usually only show involvement with the thumb, although it may affect any digit. Pediatric trigger thumb represents about 2% of all upper-extremity abnormalities in children, with a reported incidence between 0.5 and 3 per 1000 children. A number of studies support the notion that pediatric trigger thumb is an acquired condition and not congenital.

Etiology

At present, the exact etiology remains unknown. Fundamentally for trigger thumb, triggering is caused by a disproportion between the flexor tendon and retinacular sheath. Pathologically, in infants, the disease progression generally involves a nodule (Notta node) within the flexor pollicis longus tendon, but with no hypertrophy of the A1 pulley. Upon evaluation with electron microscopy, tendon nodules, and sheaths acquired from children experiencing pediatric trigger thumb exposed large quantities of fibroblasts and mature collagen but demonstrated no degenerative or inflammatory changes.

Triggering of digits other than the thumb can have a unique etiology, with many different variables to blame, such as

- An abnormal relationship of the profundus and sublimis tendons
- A more proximal decussation of the flexor digitorum superficialis (FDS) tendon
- Nodules in either the FDS or flexor digitorum profundus tendon
- A thickened A2 pulley
- A tight A3 pulley

Diagnosis

Pediatric trigger thumb presents as a fixed partially flexed thumb IP joint or an inability to flex the extended thumb. Physical examination usually demonstrates a thumb IP joint flexion contracture and a palpable nodule near the MCP joint. Trigger thumb in a child must be distinguished from congenital clasped thumb, spasticity, or arthrogryposis. In trigger thumb, the MCP joint has no involvement, whereas congenital clasped thumb involves flexion contractures at both the IP and MCP joints of the thumb. Pediatric trigger finger patients present with a palpable mass (Notta node), triggering, or the presence of a fixed flexion contracture.

Treatment

- Treatment options include observation, splinting, and open surgical release of the A1 pulley
- For pediatric trigger thumb, release of the A1 pulley has been advocated as a quick, safe, and effective procedure. However, trigger thumb in children may have spontaneous resolution, and therefore, the optimal timing of surgery is controversial
  - Surgery is generally recommended for patients presenting with one or both of the following symptoms:
    - After 1 year of age
    - With persistent triggering
  - Surgical release outcomes are generally favorable in children
- Due to the wide range of causal elements for trigger finger, an A1 pulley release alone sometimes will not correct the triggering
  - Additional treatments, such as resection of one FDS tendon slip or an A3 pulley release, may be required
  - The success rate of surgical treatment can be increased with an understanding of the contributing factors for this condition and a willingness to investigate the entire flexor mechanism

de QUERVAIN SYNDROME

de Quervain syndrome presents as a gradual onset of radial wrist pain and painful thumb movements. The pain sometimes can be sharp and severe and may be exacerbated by grasping, thumb abduction, and ulnar deviation of the wrist, often associated with repetitive tasks involving the thumb and wrist. The incidence of de Quervain tenovaginitis is approximately 0.93 per 1000 person-years. Women have been shown to be at significantly higher risk than men for this condition, as demonstrated by the adjusted incidence rate ratio of 4.45. Typically, de Quervain disease is seen in the age ≥40 but is also common in pregnant and lactating women. Those of African descent are also at high risk for the occurrence of de Quervain tenosynovitis.

Pertinent anatomy and pathology

The de Quervain syndrome is a stenosing tenovaginitis of the first dorsal compartment of the wrist (**Figure 22.2a**). The first dorsal compartment is approximately 2-cm-long and is located over the radial styloid proximal to the radiocarpal joint, containing the abductor pollicis longus (APL) and extensor pollicis brevis (EPB) tendons. The anatomy of the first dorsal compartment is highly variable among individuals. The EPB tendon has a rounder and smaller shape than the APL tendon, with approximately 5–7% of individuals lacking this tendon. Inserting at the base of the proximal phalanx, the EPB functions to extend the MCP joint and to weakly abduct the thumb. The APL usually has two or more tendon slips (up to seven slips) that may insert onto the base of the thumb metacarpal, trapezium, volar carpal ligament, opponens pollicis, or abductor pollicis brevis. The primary function of the APL is to abduct the thumb and assist with radial deviation of the wrist. The most frequent deviation in tendon anatomic configuration consists of one EPB tendon with two APL tendon slips.

Approximately 40% of individuals have the first dorsal compartment divided into two separate fibro-osseous tunnels via a septum. In this configuration, the ulnar-sided tunnel contains the EPB tendon, and the radial-sided tunnel contains the multiple APL tendon slips. It should be noted that the radial sensory nerve runs along the sheath of the first dorsal compartment and must be gently retracted during any procedure (**Figure 22.2b**).

Although the exact etiology for de Quervain syndrome remains unclear, the condition is thought to be the result of repetitive or sustained tension on the tendons of the first dorsal compartment. The tension then stimulates fibroblastic changes that lead to thickening and swelling or inflammation of the surrounding extensor retinaculum and extensor tendons.

Diagnosis

The clinical presentation of de Quervain syndrome remains fairly consistent. Patients present with radial wrist pain, and exacerbation of symptoms is caused by grasping and raising objects with the wrist in neutral rotation. Physical examination will demonstrate localized inflammation and tenderness above the first dorsal compartment that reaches approximately 1–2-cm proximal to the radial styloid process.

- The Finkelstein test is a classic examination performed to diagnose de Quervain disease:
  - It is performed by grasping the patient's thumb and quickly deviating the hand and wrist ulnarly
  - A positive test reproduces the pain

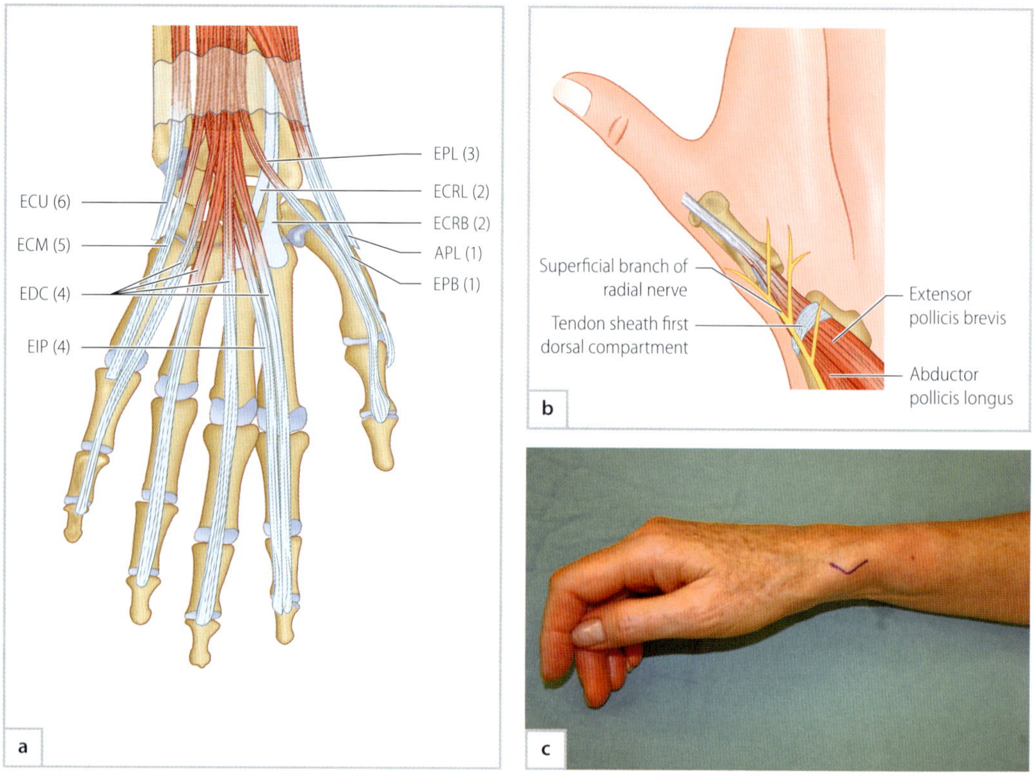

Figure 22.2 (a) These are the six compartments for the extensor tendons at the wrist: (1) Extensor pollicis brevis and abductor pollicis longus; (2) extensor carpi radialis longus and brevis; (3) extensor pollicis longus; (4) extensor digitorum and indicis; (5) extensor carpi; (6) extensor carpi ulnaris. (b) The superficial branch of the radial nerve courses along the first compartment, and care must be taken not to injure the nerve during surgery. (c) To expose the first compartment, a V-shaped or transverse incision is made over the radial styloid during surgical treatment of de Quervain syndrome.

- The Eichoff maneuver is another test useful for diagnosing de Quervain disease:
  - The test is designed to provoke a pain response by deviating the wrist ulnarly while holding the thumb in the palm beneath the flexed fingers
- The differential diagnosis includes intersection syndrome, radial styloid fracture, scaphoid fracture, or instability or basilar arthritis of the thumb:
  - Intersection syndrome results from tendinopathy between the APL and second compartment and typically presents with symptoms more proximal (4 cm) to the wrist
  - Radial styloid fractures, scaphoid fractures, instability, or basilar arthritis of the thumb can be distinguished through radiographs and a positive grind test
  - A grind test on the thumb carpometacarpal joint performed with axial compression, flexion, extension, and circumduction will cause crepitus and pain

Treatment

- Nonsurgical treatments include:
  - Corticosteroid injections
  - Nonsteroidal anti-inflammatory drugs
  - Thumb-spica splinting
  - Therapeutic modalities including
    - Stretching
    - Strengthening
- Splinting alone was found to be the least successful treatment option
- Corticosteroid injection is often used as an initial treatment
  - The success rate ranges from 62% to 93% with injections into the first compartment depending on the corticosteroid formulation
- Some studies have demonstrated that pregnancy-related de Quervain disease is self-limiting, and symptoms may resolve spontaneously after cessation of breast feeding. Corticosteroid injection is especially recommended for this type of patient to provide pain relief.
  - The injection consists of 0.5–1 mL of corticosteroid with 0.5–1 mL of a local anesthetic
  - The needle is directly inserted into the first extensor compartment at the level of the radial styloid
  - With a correct injection, the solution should be felt spreading proximally and distally inside the sheath
- During surgical treatment, care must be taken to protect and avoid excessive dissection of the superficial radial nerve and its branches. The majority of complications involve traction or trauma to this nerve, leading to persistent pain above the incision. Complete release of all subcompartments within the first dorsal compartment is crucial to a successful surgery
- The surgical steps should proceed as follows:
  - A V-shaped or transverse incision is made over the radial styloid (**Figure 22.2c**)
  - After the skin flap is elevated and the radial sensory nerve is gently dissected free and retracted, the tendon sheath is incised along its course
  - Complete release of both the APL and EPB sheaths
  - Theoretically, one should release the sheath more dorsally to retain parts of the volar sheath to prevent volar subluxation of the tendons
  - The wound should then be closed
- Approximately, 90% of patients can be expected to have a satisfactory outcome after surgical release, but relief of symptoms may take a few weeks

INTERSECTION SYNDROME

Intersection syndrome is a relatively uncommon condition characterized by pain, variable swelling, and tenderness of the dorsal forearm in the area where the extensor carpi radialis longus (ECRL) and extensor carpi radialis brevis (ECRB) tendons are crossed by the APL and EPB muscles. The muscles and tendons cross around 4-cm proximal to the wrist joint, on the radial aspect of the forearm. In severe cases, crepitus may be noted on palpation. This syndrome is frequently associated with repetitive wrist activity and is possibly the only tendon condition that is distinguished by a consistent association of overuse.

Pertinent anatomy and pathology

On the dorsal aspect of the wrist are six discrete compartments for the extrinsic extensor tendons:

- The first dorsal compartment contains the APL and EPB tendons
- The second dorsal compartment is located on the radial side of the Lister tubercle and contains the ECRL and the ECRB
- The ECRL inserts on the base of the second metacarpal, and the ECRB inserts on the base of the long finger metacarpal
- The two tendons are powerful wrist extensors that also cause radial deviation
- The APL and EPB muscle bellies cross the ECRL and ECRB tendons between 3.5 and 4.8 cm (mean 4.18 cm) proximal to the Lister tubercle (**Figure 22.3**)

The exact pathophysiology of this disorder remains unclear. Initially, it was believed that the condition was due to friction between the muscle bellies of the APL and EPB with the tendon sheath enclosing the ECRL and ECRB. In 1985, data demonstrated that tenosynovitis of the second dorsal compartment was to blame. It remains controversial as to which of these mechanisms is directly causative or if both contribute to the clinical syndrome.

Diagnosis

Patients present with pain, swelling, tenderness, and crepitus at the intersection area. Some research has reported that this disorder has been known to be associated with occupational wrist overuse, eventually revealed by some form of hand trauma.

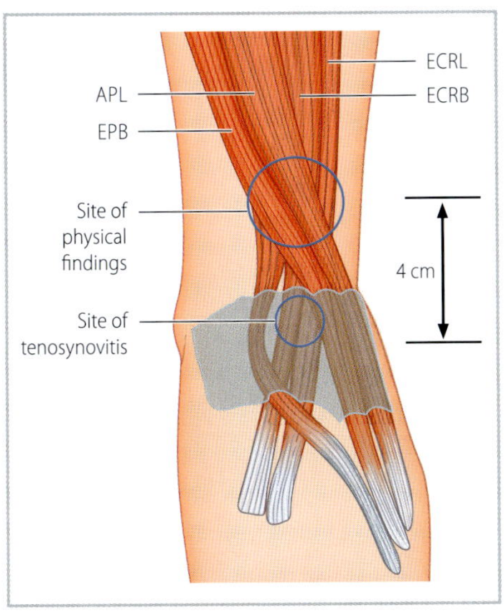

Figure 22.3 The abductor pollicis longus and extensor pollicis brevis bellies cross the extensor carpi radialis longus and brevis tendons approximately 4-cm proximal to Lister tubercle.

Treatment

- The conservative treatment includes rest, modification of work activities, prescription of nonsteroidal anti-inflammatory medication, and immobilization with thumb spica or wrist in slight extension
- For persistent symptoms, a steroid injection at the site of greatest tenderness may provide relief
  - Most patients improve and remain asymptomatic
- Patients indicated for surgical intervention are treated with a longitudinal incision over the radial wrist extensor, followed by release of the second dorsal compartment
  - The wrist should be splinted in moderate extension for about 2 weeks for comfort and to minimize the potential for extensor tendon bowstringing

EXTENSOR POLLICIS LONGUS TENOSYNOVITIS

Tenosynovitis of the extensor pollicis longus (EPL) tendon occurs rarely and is usually associated with rheumatoid arthritis, an old Colles' fracture, or rarely from overuse.

Pertinent anatomy

The EPL curves around the Lister tubercle in the third extensor compartment. As the tendon slides through an osseous groove in the radius, the Lister tubercle serves to alter the tendon's initial course to an oblique axis leading toward the thumb (**Figure 22.4**). The EPL inserts on the base of the distal phalanx of the thumb, using the Lister tubercle of the radius as a fulcrum to power extension of the distal phalanx.

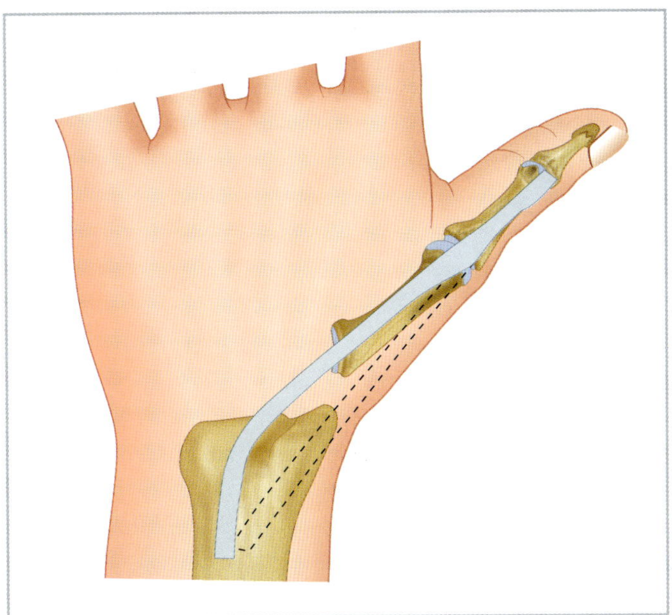

Figure 22.4 The extensor pollicis longus runs parallel to the axis of the forearm until it is diverted toward the thumb by Lister tubercle.

Clinical appearance and diagnosis

The EPL tenosynovitis usually presents as pain and swelling just distal to the Lister tubercle, where the tendon changes direction, or along the course of the tendon. Precise localization of maximum tenderness from the inflammation is the key to diagnosis.

Treatment

- Once the diagnosis is made, early surgical release is advocated because this tendon is prone to rupture if left untreated, especially in patients with rheumatoid arthritis
- Rerouting of the tendon radial to its anatomic tunnel is recommended
  - After the initial skin incision is made over the Lister tubercle, the EPL tendon should be identified and then opened along its entire length
  - The EPL should then be transplanted subcutaneously over the extensor retinaculum
  - After transplantation, the tunnel is ready for closure to prevent relocation of the tendon back into the groove

EXTENSOR CARPI ULNARIS TENDONITIS

Extensor carpi ulnaris (ECU) tendonitis is a common disorder that must be included in the differential diagnosis of ulnar-sided wrist pain.

Pertinent anatomy

The sixth dorsal wrist compartment contains the tendon of the ECU, originating from the ECU muscle approximately 6–7-cm proximal to the wrist. The ECU is encompassed by a deep fibro-osseous sheath that is separated from the band holding the extensor tendons together in the extensor retinaculum. The tendon occupies approximately 90% of the space of the fibro-osseous sheath. Over the distal ulna it curves ulnarly passing into a groove between the ulnar styloid process and the ulnar head (**Figure 22.5a**) before inserting onto the dorsal base of the fifth metacarpal.

The ECU subsheath is part of the triangular fibrocartilage complex (TFCC) of the wrist (**Figure 22.5b**), a structure spanning the length of the distal radioulnar joint (DRUJ). The TFCC serves as support to stabilize the DRUJ and ulnar carpus while providing a cushioning effect to the ulnar wrist. The ECU tendon plays a significant role in the stability of the DRUJ, allowing for unrestricted forearm rotation due to its relationship with the extensor retinaculum.

The ECU is predisposed to tendonitis due to its deep fibro-osseous tunnel and the angulation of the tendon itself. Damage can be caused to the ECU by forceful:

- Wrist supination
- Flexion
- Ulnar deviation

The destructive forces acting upon the ECU have the potential:

- To injure or even rupture the ECU tendon sheath
- To lead to volar subluxation of the tendon out of the distal ulnar groove within a redundant sheath

Clinical appearance

A traumatic twisting incident is usually the inciting event. Patients usually present with increasing pain and swelling on the ulnar side of the wrist. Sleep may be affected when all motions of the wrist cause severe pain. Some patients will complain of dorsal hand paresthesias because the dorsal sensory branch of the ulnar nerve courses over the distal ulna and the ECU. For patients experiencing tendon subluxation, an audible snap may be apparent as the supinated wrist moves from extension to ulnar deviation and flexion.

Diagnosis

Patients presenting with chronic dorsal ulnar-sided wrist pain can be considerably difficult to diagnose, due to the complicated structural anatomy in this small space and the possible presence of concomitant pathology.

- Radiographs are helpful to rule out other conditions that can cause ulnar-sided wrist pain including:
  - DRUJ arthritis
  - Ulnar styloid fractures
  - TFCC injuries
  - Ulnocarpal impaction syndrome
- Magnetic resonance imaging (MRI) can help identify inflammation surrounding the ECU

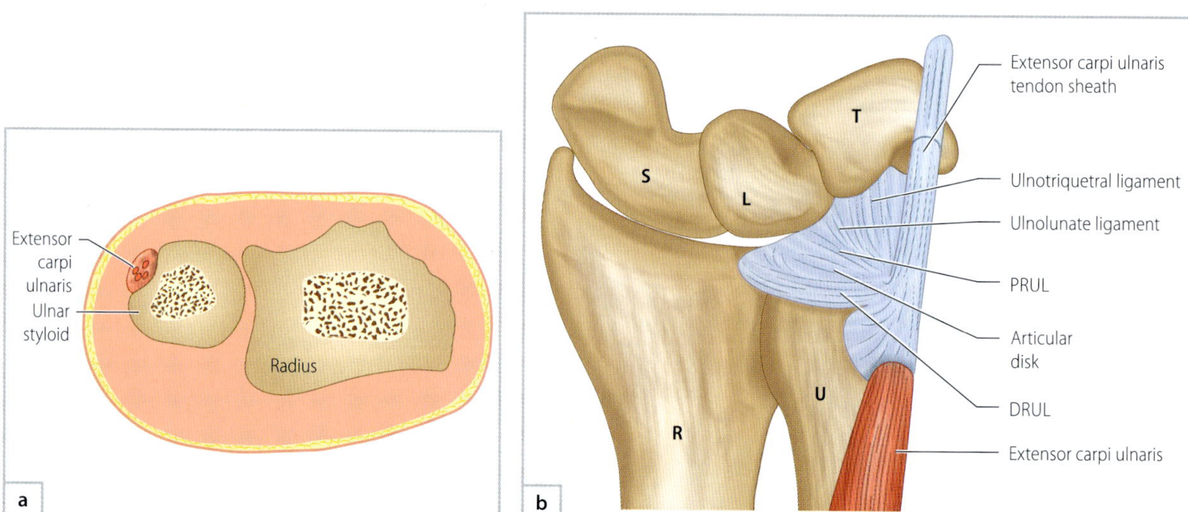

Figure 22.5 (a) In this cross section of the distal radius and ulna, arrows show the extensor carpi ulnaris as it courses between the ulnar styloid (S) and the ulnar head (H). (b) The sheath of the extensor carpi ulnaris is part of the triangular fibrocartilage complex.

- Complete relief of pain after a lidocaine injection confirms the diagnosis, differentiating the process from an intra-articular injury
- Dynamic ultrasound is able to quickly and accurately make the ECU tendon subluxation diagnosis

Treatment

- Conservative treatment generally provides relief of the symptoms, including
  - Activity modification
  - Splinting (in slight extension)
  - Anti-inflammatory medications
  - Physical therapy
- Corticosteroid injection is helpful when conservative treatments have failed
- With persistent pain or painful subluxation or dislocation is noted, surgical intervention is indicated. Operative treatment involves complete incision of the fibro-osseous canal of the sixth dorsal compartment:
  - A dorsal incision is made over the ECU tendon
    - The dorsal cutaneous branch of the ulnar nerve is identified and protected
  - The tendon sheath and the tunnel should be released longitudinally
  - The tendon subsheath can be reconstructed if a patient experiences painful ECU tendon subluxation or dislocation

FLEXOR CARPI RADIALIS TENDONITIS

Flexor carpi radialis (FCR) tendonitis is an uncommon cause of radiovolar pain in the wrist. The condition typically affects individuals in their fifth decade and is more often diagnosed in women.

Anatomy

The musculotendinous segment of the FCR tendon originates approximately 15-cm proximal to the radiocarpal joint, and the muscular fibers end an average of 8-cm proximal to the wrist. The synovial sheath extends from the origin to the insertion of the FCR, and the tendon itself is enclosed by dense fibers from the antebrachial fascia, 4–5 cm proximal to the radiocarpal joint. The tendon enters a 17-mm-long fibro-osseous tunnel bordered radially by the body of the trapezium, palmarly by the trapezial crest and the transverse carpal ligament, ulnarly by a retinaculum septum that separates the tendon from the carpal tunnel, and dorsally by the insertion of this septum onto the trapezial body (**Figure 22.6**). The tendon occupies approximately 90% of the space inside the tunnel, maintaining direct contact with the surface of the trapezium.

As the FCR crosses the trapezial ridge, it angles sharply dorsally. In most patients, the FCR tendon is inserted at three locations:

1. A small slip is connected to the trapezial crest or tuberosity
2. Eighty per cent of the remaining tendon is inserted on the base of the second metacarpal
3. Twenty per cent on the base of the third metacarpal

The deep palmar arch is located 2–3 mm distal to the insertion of the tendon

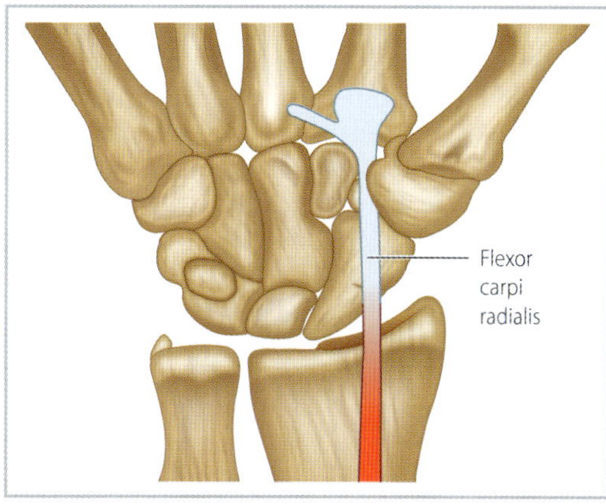

Figure 22.6 The flexor carpi radialis tendon occupies approximately 90% of the fibro-osseous tunnel that is courses through. The tunnel is bordered radially by the body of the trapezium, palmarly by the trapezial crest and the transverse carpal ligament, ulnarly by a retinaculum septum that separates the tendon from the carpal tunnel, and dorsally by the insertion of this septum onto the trapezial body.

Pathology

The FCR tunnel sits adjacent to the trapezium, scaphoid, radius, and palmar arch, predisposing it to tenosynovitis, either with or without some form of trauma. Primary tenosynovitis may develop due to overuse. It can also be secondary to pathology in the surrounding structures, including scaphoid fractures, scaphoid cysts, osteoarthritis of the carpometacarpal joint of the thumb, scaphoid–trapezium–trapezoid joint arthritis, and ganglion cysts.

Clinical appearance and diagnosis

The patient usually complains of pain and tenderness over the FCR tendon proximal to the scaphoid tubercle and trapezoid crest. Pain increases with resisted wrist flexion and radial deviation. Radiographs can recognize adjacent osseous structure pathology, and MRI may help rule out cysts and ganglions. A successful lidocaine injection in the offending sheath confirms the diagnosis.

Treatment

- Nonoperative treatment is generally effective for primary tendonitis and includes activity modification, anti-inflammatory medications, physical therapy, splinting preventing wrist flexion, and corticosteroid injection
  - Corticosteroid injections are preferably administered from the volar side over the site of tenderness
- Nonoperative treatment in secondary cases should not be prolonged due to the potential for fraying and rupture of the tendon
- Surgical intervention should proceed as follows:
  - Exposure of the tendon is performed through a 3–4-cm longitudinal incision over the course of the FCR starting proximal to the wrist crease and extending to the base of the thenar eminence
  - Care must be taken to avoid injury to the palmar cutaneous branch of the median nerve, which lies just ulnar to the FCR
  - At the distal end of the incision, the thenar branches of the radial sensory nerve and terminal branches of the lateral antebrachial

cutaneous nerve course above the thenar eminence, and care must be taken not to damage these structures
- The sheath should then be opened just proximal to the fibrous tunnel and dissection performed distally only until slightly past the trapezial tubercle
- Frayed fibers of the tendon should be excised, and the trapezial groove removed using a rongeur after inspection for spurs or sharp edges
- After debridement, the sheath should not be closed
  - A conforming dressing is applied for 10–14 days

MISCELLANEOUS

Saddle syndrome

Saddle syndrome refers to post-traumatic interosseous-lumbrical adhesions that produce intermetacarpal pain during intrinsic contraction by impingement on the deep transverse metacarpal ligament (TML).

Anatomy and pathology

The second, third, and fourth lumbrical muscles insert into the extensor hood mechanisms, only after coursing radially beside the long, ring, and small fingers while remaining volar to the deep TML along their path. The second dorsal and second and third palmar interosseous muscles follow a similar path beside the long, ring, and small fingers. However, these interosseous muscles course dorsal to the TML and insert at the base of the proximal phalanx in addition to the extensor hood mechanism (**Figure 22.7a**). Trauma to the hand, such as a crush, direct blow, fall, or torqueing stress can result in adhesions (**Figure 22.7b**) between the interosseous and lumbrical muscles, with subsequent painful impingement on the TML during intrinsic contraction. If these adhesions also develop between the intrinsic muscles and the deep TMLs or MCP capsule, discomfort may be produced by stretching of the intrinsic tendons.

Clinical appearance

Patients present with pain in the distal intermetacarpal space, most frequently associated with stressful and prolonged use of the hand, especially from gripping objects. A catch during full flexion may be observed that corresponds with pain. Other less frequent symptoms are night pain, swelling, and limited range of motion. Upon physical examination, the patient will demonstrate tenderness of the intermetacarpal space.

Treatment

- After a severe crush injury to the intermetacarpal area, the proper splint and early full mobilization may serve to reduce the incidence of saddle deformity. The intrinsic plus position is often ideal (MCP joint at 90° and IP joints at 0°), as it allows for the intrinsic muscles to be at resting length while enabling maximum overlap of the TML
- Surgical treatments include release of these adhesions, partial resection of the ligament, and early mobilization, which can result in a significant improvement

SECRETAN DISEASE

Secretan disease is a rare and self-inflicted traumatic edema and/or hemorrhage of the dorsum of the hand. The disease involves a chronic phase coupled with recurrent episodes, possibly resulting in chronic edema, fibrosis, and prolonged disability.

- There are two general categories of patients who deceitfully injure themselves:
  - One is malingerers, who usually do so with the hope of monetary gain
  - The other group is composed of patients with deep-seated psychiatric disorders

Clinical appearance

Patients usually experience trauma that is not severe enough to produce a fracture and present with swelling or a wound of the dorsal hand. All observed problems persist beyond the usual resolution time. Physical examination and laboratory evaluation demonstrate no abnormalities. A rapid resolution usually is seen after a plaster cast or splint is placed on the involved extremity, but symptoms will recur without extremity protection. A malingerer will often utilize the intermittent application of some form of tourniquet to propagate a constant and unexplained edema. The physical damage is increased with each episode. Repetitive blunt trauma will cause increasingly severe peritendinous fibrosis of the digital extensor tendons. Of course, this gross pathological condition mechanically restricts range of motion.

Treatment

- Injury that is self-inflicted or perpetuated must be considered whenever the events following injury:

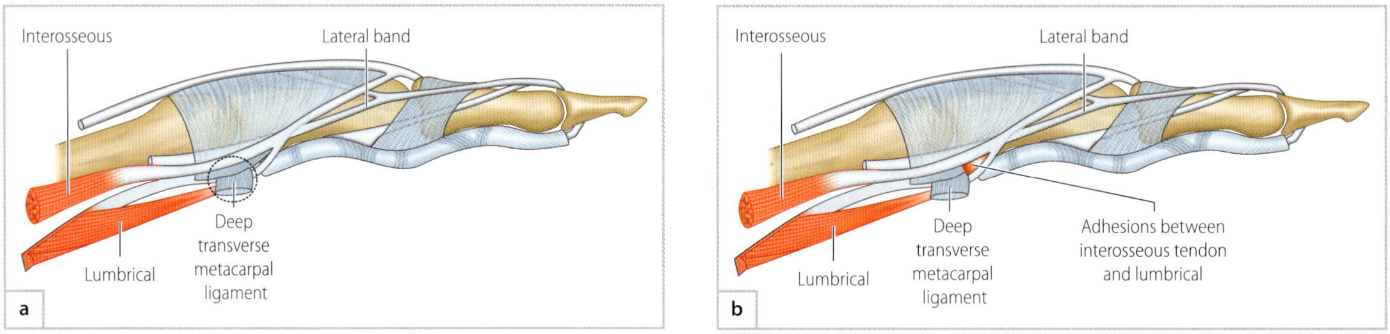

Figure 22.7 (a) This demonstrates the path of the lumbrical muscles and intraosseous muscles into the extensor hood. The transverse metacarpal ligament can be found between the lumbrical and intraosseous muscles. (b) Adhesions between the lumbrical muscles and intraosseous muscles can be caused by trauma to the hand.

- Fail to take the predicted course with no clear explanation
- Keep mysteriously recurring
- Early diagnosis and intervention, within 5 months of onset of symptoms, seems to be associated with a better prognosis
- For patients with psychiatric disorders, psychiatric treatment and wound management must be given, as well as additional plaster or other protective devices. For patients returning to work, psychotherapy without direct attempts at insight is the suggested course of treatment

WORK-RELATED UPPER-LIMB DISORDERS

Work-related upper-limb disorders (WRULDs) are among the most common disorders seen by general practitioners and occupational physicians and have become one of the most significant and costly health problems in the working population. These disorders consist of both specific and nonspecific causes of work-related arm pain:

- Specific conditions include hand-arm vibration syndrome and soft tissue syndromes (fascia, tendon, or nerve) with definitive diagnostic findings
- Nonspecific WRULD is effectively a diagnosis by exclusion, also referred to as
  - Nonspecific arm pain
  - Overuse syndrome
  - Repetitive strain injury and repetitive strain disorder
    - Cumulative trauma disorder

Risk factors

Epidemiologic studies have identified several combinations of personal factors, work factors, and psychosocial factors related to upper-extremity musculoskeletal disorders. Personal factors include age, prior history of upper-extremity musculoskeletal disorders, diabetes, and obesity. The main work-related factors of upper-extremity musculoskeletal disorders are a high level of physical demand, high repetitiveness of the task, use of vibration tools, rapid work pace, insufficient recovery time, heavy lifting, forceful manual exertion, sustained awkward posture of the wrists, elbows, or shoulders, and mechanical pressure concentration. Psychosocial factors include job stress, and these factors clearly play some part in all cases.

Approach to WRULD patients

There are four basic areas to be taken in patients suffering from WRULDs:

- Step 1: Evaluation of the patient
  - Using evidence to assess a patient's current symptoms and definitively verify the presence of a disorder
- Step 2: Investigation of the work environment and activities of daily living
  - Examining a patient's work environment and work assignments to reveal any possible inciting agents
  - Ergonomic factors
    - Monitor and evaluate the tools and equipment a patient uses while at work
    - Determine if it is possible to modify or replace the current tools and equipment so that it would decrease stress on affected areas
  - Evaluate the patient's requirements for activities of daily living
- Step 3: Analysis of a patient's psychosocial behavior
    - Determine if there are any psychological factors that may be contributing to the patient's condition
- Step 4: Treatment and therapy protocol
  - Anti-inflammatory medication coupled with a muscle strengthening and stretching therapy program should be employed during the initial phase of treatment
    - Treatment should begin early to avoid aggravation of symptoms into more serious conditions

SUGGESTED READING

Ahuja NK, Chung KC. Fritz de Quervain, MD (1868-1940): stenosing tendovaginitis at the radial styloid process. J Hand Surg 2004; 29:1164–1170.
The study introduces Fritz de Quervain, MD, the first surgeon that described and treated de Quervain syndrome and his contributions to medical science. The history and management of this condition is also described.

Cardon LJ, Ezaki M, Carter PR. Trigger finger in children. J Hand Surg 1999; 24:1156–1161.
In this retrospective study, the authors reviewed the results of the surgical treatment for pediatric trigger finger and reported the associated etiology in the flexor mechanism. The study indicated that trigger fingers in children have variable causes and are different from trigger thumbs. A1 pulley release alone will not always correct the triggering.

Chicarilli ZN, Watson HK, Linberg R, Sasaki G. Saddle deformity. Posttraumatic interosseous-lumbrical adhesions: review of eighty-seven cases. J Hand Surg 1986; 11:210–218.
The study describes the pathological anatomy of saddle syndrome and the relationship between pathological anatomy, clinical appearance, and treatment decision making. The authors reviewed 87 cases of lumbrical adhesions and found that all patients except 3 were able to resume or continue their current occupation. In addition, 58% of patients were found to have excellent results and a complete resolution of symptoms, whereas 29% experienced good results and only mild symptoms after extended use of the hand.

MacLennan AJ, Nemechek NM, Waitayawinyu T, Trumble TE. Diagnosis and anatomic reconstruction of extensor carpi ulnaris subluxation. J Hand Surg 2008; 33:59–64.
This study describes the treatment for extensor carpi ulnaris subluxation. The paper indicates that ultrasound is an effective and noninvasive method of diagnosing ECU tendon subluxation. In addition, a new technique for anatomic ECU tendon sheath reconstruction is described and evaluated.

Roquelaure Y, Ha C, Rouillon C, et al. Risk factors for upper-extremity musculoskeletal disorders in the working population. Arthritis Rheum 2009; 61:1425–1434.
In this study, the authors assessed the risk factors for upper-extremity musculoskeletal disorders in the working population. The main risk factors, including personal, work-related, physical, and psPychosocial factors, have been shown to be strongly associated with clinically diagnosed upper-extremity disorders. The relatively high rate of occurrence of this condition in workers necessitates physicians to understand the associated risk factors and symptoms of this disorder to provide effective treatment.

Chapter 23 Nerve disorders

Ellen Y. Lee (23.1–23.4), Aymeric YT. Lim (23.1–23.4),
Sandeep J. Sebastin (23.4), Ter Chyan Tan (23.5), Martins Kapickis (23.6)

23.1 NERVE INJURY AND REPAIR

NERVE ANATOMY

Microanatomy

The neuron is made up of a cell body and an axon (**Figure 23.1**). In the peripheral nervous system, the cell bodies are found in the anterior horn cells of the spinal cord (motor nerves) or at the dorsal root ganglion (sensory nerves). The cell bodies communicate with the end organ by relaying electrochemical signals up and down axons. The axons can be either myelinated or nonmyelinated. Myelinated nerves are those covered with a myelin sheath produced by the Schwann cells and conduct impulses at a faster rate than nonmyelinated fibers. Ultimately, the propagated impulses reach their final destination, the end organs. An end organ can be a muscle fiber, a free nerve ending, specialized group of sensory receptors in the skin or mechanoreceptors in muscles, tendons, or joints.

Apart from the motor and sensory fibers, peripheral nerves also carry autonomic fibers originating from ganglion cells of the sympathetic chain. The autonomic nerve fibers supply the skin of the hand and generally have the same distribution as the sensory fibers.

Studying the cross-sectional anatomy of a nerve fiber (**Figure 23.2**), it is evident that individual fibrils are surrounded by an endoneurium, and the nerve fibrils are grouped into fascicles surrounded by a perineurium. Fascicles are then grouped into a single nerve fiber, which is surrounded by an epineurium ('endo,' 'peri,' 'epi'). Within the nerve, the nerve fibers are arranged according to their distribution whether motor or sensory fibers, i.e. proximally located fibers are mixed fibers (motor and sensory), whereas distally the fascicles are grouped into a separate motor or sensory branches as they leave the nerve bundle to reach out to their specific targets cells, e.g. in skin or muscles.

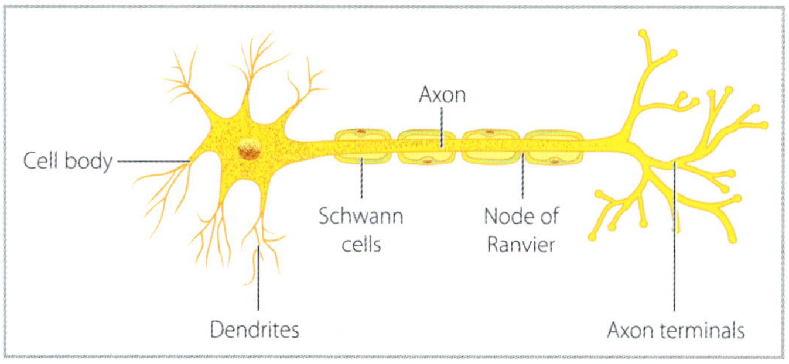

Figure 23.1 Basic anatomy of a nerve cell.

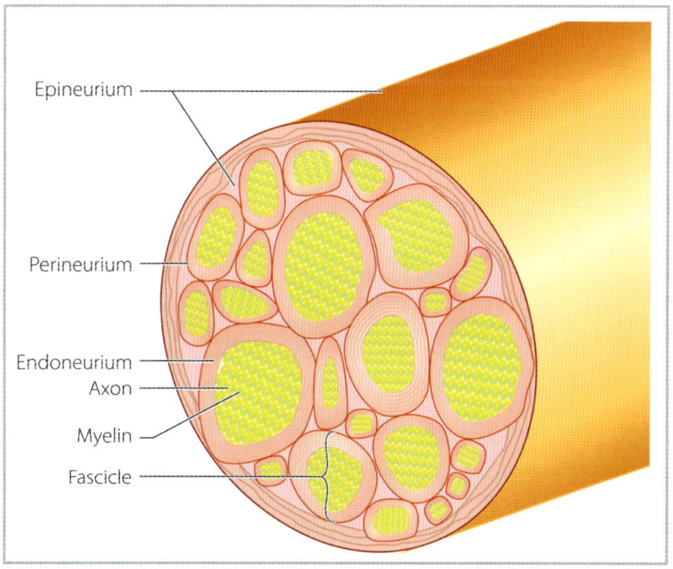

Figure 23.2 Cross section of a nerve trunk.

Macroanatomy

The motor and sensory innervation of the upper limb is supplied via the branches of the brachial plexus. The brachial plexus is a complex network of peripheral nerves originating from cervical spinal roots 5, 6, 7, 8 and T1. Occasionally, the brachial plexus would receive contributions from the spinal roots C4 and T2. Muscles are generally grouped according to the peripheral nerve innervations or by myotomes (the dominant cervical root supplying the nerve branch). For example, proximal muscle groups are supplied by the cranial roots (C5, 6 to shoulder), whereas distal muscle groups are supplied by the caudal roots (C8 and T1). Similarly, sensory territories are categorized based on their peripheral nerve innervation or by dermatomes (territory supplied by each cervical root), with C5 supplying the shoulder proximally and T1 supplying the most distal part and medial aspect of the forearm. Lastly, there is a coronal arrangement of the brachial plexus in such a way that the anterior or ventral division fibers produce prehension (flexion, internal rotation, and pronation), and the posterior or dorsal division fibers are responsible for opposite movements (extension, external rotation, and supination).

PHYSICAL EXAMINATION

Assessment of motor function

Gross manual neurological examination is used to assess the motor function. Testing motor function is reported using the British Medical Research Council (MRC) grading system as shown in **Table 23.1**.

Table 23.1 British Medical Research Council motor grading

MRC grade	
0	No visible or palpable contraction
1	(+) palpable contraction, no motion seen
2	Motion with gravity eliminated. Cannot move against gravity
3	Motion against gravity
4	Motion against gravity and some resistance
5	Motion again resistance, same as contralateral uninjured side

MRC, Medical Research Council.

Assessment of sensory function

The sensory function of an injured nerve can be assessed using techniques that involve testing the patient's ability to recognize, identify, and localize a stimulus. Assessment of sensory function traditionally includes evaluation of light touch, pinprick and two-point discrimination (2PD). For an area supplied by an injured nerve, the recovery of sensation usually follows a consistent pattern after nerve regeneration or restoration of nerve function. Pain is the first to return followed by perception of touch and finally by the ability of 2PD. The dermatomal distribution of sensory nerves of the upper limb to be tested is shown in **Figure 23.3**. Sensory recovery can be reported using the Highet scale, also part of the British MRC grading system (**Table 23.2**).

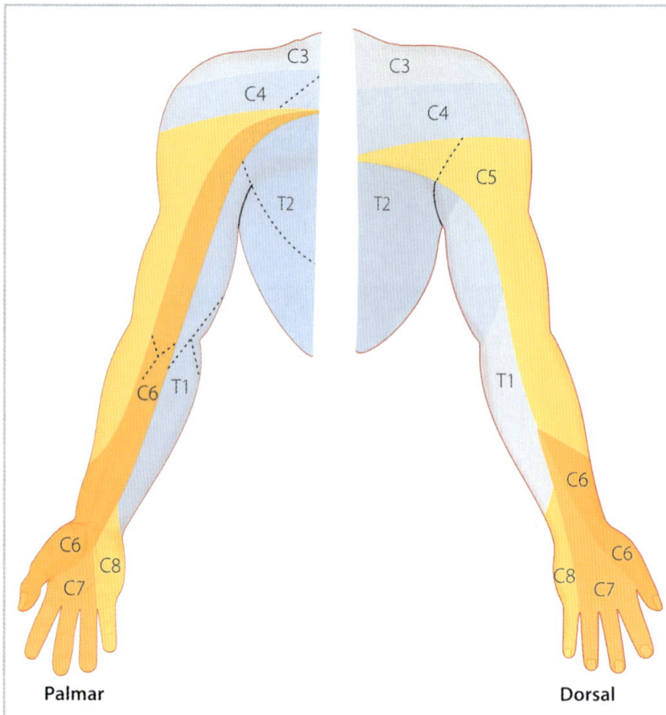

Figure 23.3 Sensory dermatomes.

Table 23.2 British Medical Research Council sensory grading/Highet scale

MRC grade	
S0	No sensation
S1	Deep cutaneous pain in autonomous area of the nerve
S2	Superficial cutaneous pain and some tactile sensitivity
S3	Superficial cutaneous pain and some touch without over-response
S3+	Superficial cutaneous pain and some touch without over-response AND recovery of some two point discrimination (2PD <15 mm)
S4	Normal sensation

MRC, Medical Research Council; 2PD, two-point discrimination.

NERVE INJURY

A nerve injury can affect the nerve fiber itself or one or more of its coverings (**Figure 23.4**).

Myelin sheath

If only the myelin sheath is affected and the axon is physically intact, the injury is called neurapraxia ('apraxia' means 'nonaction' in Greek) or Sunderland type 1 injury. A conduction block occurs. Transient blocks last only for a few hours and show no overt pathological changes. Moderate and severe blocks can persist for > 4 weeks. There is usually an inflammation around the compressed segment and demyelination changes. However, these are temporary rather than permanent changes. There will be a complete recovery once the myelin sheath has regenerated. Neurapraxia is often seen with external compression such as in prolonged tourniquet compression.

Axon

If the nerve fiber itself is affected with a loss of axonal continuity, the injury is called axonotmesis ('tmesis' means 'cutting' in Greek). Once an axon is severed, Wallerian degeneration and regeneration of the nerve fiber takes place, as follows (**Figure 23.5**):

1. Distal to the severed fiber, there is fragmentation of the myelin sheath and axon. Initially, the proliferating Schwann cells and macrophages clear debris resulting from trauma or nerve injury
2. The Schwann cells then line up in bands of Bungner along the endoneurial tubes
3. The cell body swells, the nucleus migrates toward cell periphery and subsequently alters RNA and protein metabolism of the nerve cell
4. Sprouts from the axonal stump start to grow into longitudinal tubes. Eventually, a single sprout will connect with a target organ
5. Recovery is expected if there is a complete regeneration of the axon and surrounding connective tissue. With mild injury, complete regeneration of the axon and endoneurial covering results in favorable outcomes
   a. Higher grades of nerve injury are seen when the three coverings of the nerve are affected (endoneurium, perineurium, and epineurium) as described by Sunderland. The greater the injury the more nerve disruption and hence the poorer prognosis that often require a surgical repair.
6. End organ degeneration: Distal to the nerve injury, atrophy, and fibrosis of the denervated muscles becomes significant at 6 months after injury.

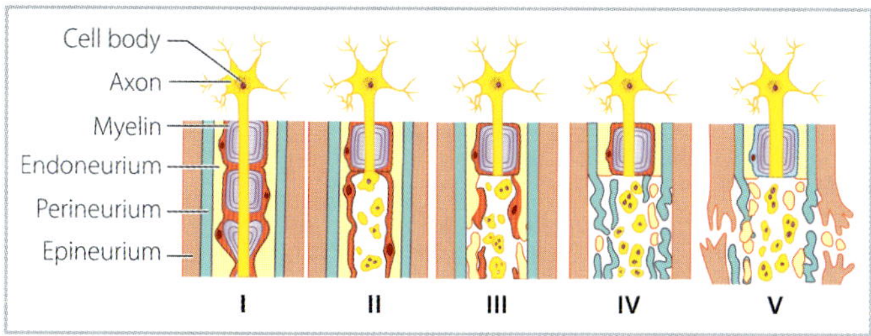

Figure 23.4 Sunderland grading of nerve injuries.

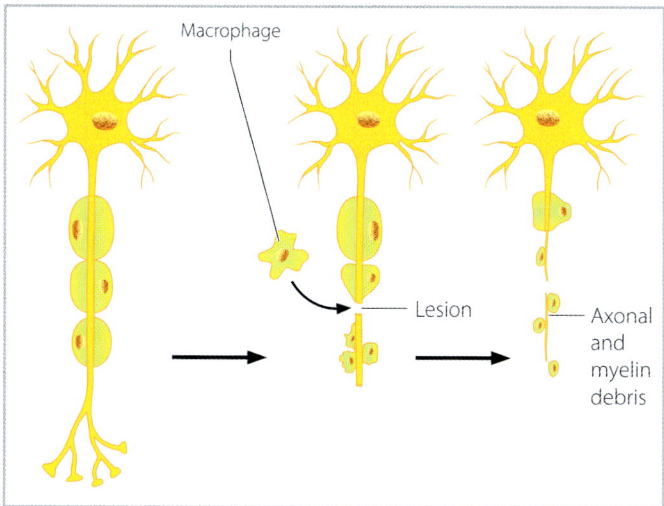

Figure 23.5 Wallerian degeneration.

TREATMENT OF NERVE INJURIES

Nonsurgical treatment

For closed injuries or in cases of suspected neuropraxia (temporary loss of motor and sensory), simple observation is usually sufficient while awaiting a spontaneous nerve recovery. There are no proven measures or medications that can hasten nerve regeneration.

Surgical treatment

Timing

Early exploration and repair is indicated for open injuries such as laceration injuries. It is technically easier to repair severed nerves with end-to-end repair at the time of injury when the stumps are still fresh and have not contracted. For closed injuries such as traction injuries, an early nerve repair or transfer provides better outcomes than late reconstruction. The indication for exploration and repair of closed nerve injuries is when there is no clinical or electrophysiological evidence of recovery after 6 weeks to 3 months after the initial insult.

Principles of nerve repair

Dissection causes trauma, and all efforts must be made to handle the nerves gently and with care. When exploring a wound, it is important not to start looking for nerve stumps in a scarred or highly disorganized traumatized tissue. Dissection should proceed from a region of normal tissue to the zone of injury. Once the ends of the severed nerve are identified, one should try to match each fascicle to its counterpart. Tissue loss in crush injuries complicates matters, and the alignment can be obtained by matching extrinsic nutrient vessels on the surface of the nerves or by using topographic nerve maps drawn by Sunderland or Zancolli. Excessive tension at a nerve repair site results in local ischemia and should be avoided. Tension in a repair is just right if the stumps can be held together with a fine 10-0 sized suture without suture snapping. Flexion of the extremity to make nerve ends come together is a maneuver that is usually not recommended. For instance, when the ulnar nerve is severed in the arm or in the proximal forearm, anterior transposition of the nerve to gain additional length can avert the need for grafting by minimizing the gap between the two ends.

Nerve suturing should always be performed under magnification. All suture materials incite an inflammatory reaction. Hence, minimal fine interrupted sutures, enough to lightly oppose the nerve ends, are preferred (8-0 sutures are used for larger nerves and 10/0 for smaller ones). Tissue glue can also be used to hold nerve stumps together. A group fascicular repair is indicated when the topography of the motor and sensory nerves can be identified as in the ulnar nerve at the wrist. A strong perineurial repair should be performed to provide a scaffold for the growing fascicles (**Figure 23.6**). In all other situations, epineurial repair is indicated (**Figure 23.7**).

Nerve grafting

Nerve grafts derive their nutrition from the wound bed before an ingrowth of vessels from the proximal and distal ends of the nerve, which usually takes 3–4 days after nerve grafting. Nonvascularized nerve grafts of > 10 cm do poorly. Therefore, with nerve defects > 10 cm, other methods of reconstruction such as nerve transfers should be considered. However, when using a nerve graft to repair a nerve defect, the graft should be reversed (distal to proximal) prior to use.

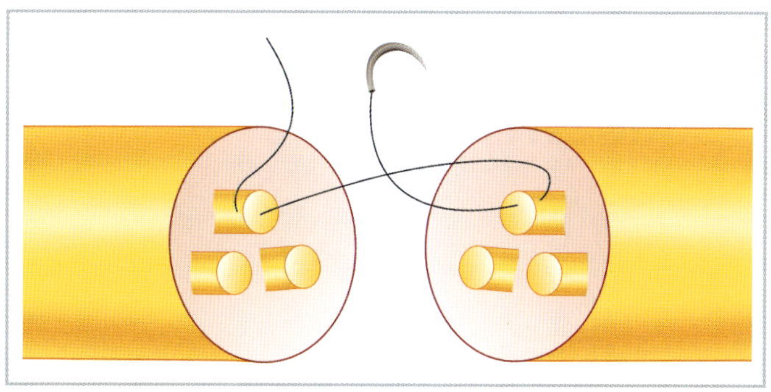

Figure 23.6 Fascicular repair.

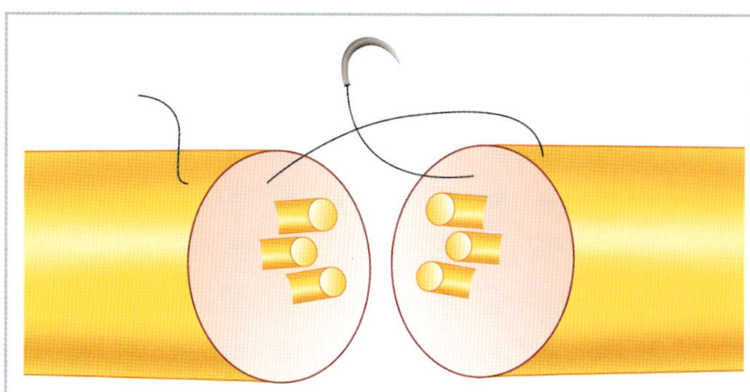

Figure 23.7 Epineurial repair.

In theory, this prevents scattering of regenerating nerve fibers down the diverging fascicles of the graft.

When choosing a donor nerve, one should consider donor site morbidity and the caliber of the nerve graft, the defect, and the length of nerve available. Cutaneous nerves are the most commonly utilized nerves for grafting, especially the sural nerve. Other suitable donor nerves are the medial or lateral antebrachial cutaneous (LABC) nerves.

Prior to harvesting a nerve graft, first the affected nerve should be prepared by refreshing nerve edges (excising scarred ends). Then the nerve defect is measured and matched to the donor site. Once the graft is harvested, the nerve graft should be placed parallel to the defect to match corresponding fascicles. When a good end-to-end alignment is achieved, epineurial sutures secure the graft in the same way described above for primary nerve repair. Occasionally, fibrin glue may be used to connect the nerve fascicles.

Nerve transfer

Nerve transfer involves transferring a branch or some of the fascicles of a functioning donor nerve to a nonfunctioning injured nerve. This is indicated in situations when the nerve defect is large (>10 cm) or when there is no proximal nerve stump available for grafting. A detailed discussion of nerve transfer indications and techniques is explained in the brachial plexus injuries chapter.

Neurolysis

Neurolysis is the process of freeing the nerve from its surrounding tissues by releasing the adhesions and resecting scar tissue around or within the nerve. Neurolysis is generally indicated in the following situations:

- To relieve pain caused by adhesions or constrictive scar tissue
- To hasten recovery in cases where progression of recovery has suddenly plateaued
- When early exploration reveals a nerve in continuity but surrounded by scar

PROGNOSIS AND REHABILITATION OF NERVE INJURIES

Factors affecting outcome of nerve repair

1. Patient factors: Young patients do better than older patients
2. Mechanism of injury: A cleanly transected nerve (glass, knife cut) will recover better than a crushed, avulsed (wood saw, ring avulsion), ruptured (blast injury) nerve after repair
3. Timing: There is a general decline in recovery when the interval between injury and repair is > 6 months
4. Type of nerve injured: Pure motor or sensory nerves have a better rate of recovery than mixed nerves
5. Level of injury: Lower and more distal nerve repairs have better outcomes than proximal nerve injuries
6. Method of repair: End-to-end tension-free sutures give the best results. For the reasons previously mentioned, shorter nerve grafts have better outcomes than longer grafts
7. Quality of surrounding tissue: A repair done in a scarred or granulating bed will contribute to a poorer result

Objective evidence of recovery is noted with an advancing Tinel sign, presence of tender muscle sign, and increasing muscle strength or sensory discernment. Re-exploration of a repaired nerve is indicated when there is an acute and exquisitely tender spot at the site of the repair (suture line rupture) or when there are no signs of recovery within 6–9 months.

Rehabilitation after nerve repair involves maintaining the denervated areas in the best possible condition pending re-innervation. Once there is some motor and sensory recovery, the patient can be started in re-education programs. An integral part in supervised therapy is to train the patient to persevere and practice on his/her own.

SUGGESTED READING

Aird RB, Naffziger HC. The pathology of human striated muscle following denervation. J Neurosurg 1953; 10:216–227.
Timeline for muscle fibrosis and atrophy post-denervation was defined after studying 134 muscle biopsy specimens. At 2 months post-denervation, percentage incidence of moderate or advanced atrophy and fibrosis starts increasing. By 11-month post-injury, 50% of denervated muscles already had moderate to advanced atrophy and fibrosis. This gives credence to perform early nerve repair or reconstruction, such that the time to reinnervation of distal muscles will be shorter than time to significant muscle fibrosis.

Dellon AL, Curtis RM, Edgerton MT. Evaluating recovery of sensation in the hand following nerve injury. Hopkins Med J 1971; 130:235–243.
A consistent pattern of sensory recovery was seen for 15 injured median or ulnar nerves at the elbow or wrist. Pin-prick sensation was always first to return and is generally followed by perception of 30 cps vibration, moving touch, constant-touch, 256 cps vibration, and finally Weber's two-point discrimination.

Lundborg G, Rydevik B. The effects of stretching the tibial nerve of the rabbit. A preliminary study of the intraneural circulation and the barrier function of the perineurium. J Bone Joint Surg 1973; 55B:390–401.
Using in vivo rabbit tibial nerves, the authors showed that stretching the nerve to 8% of its length caused 50% reduction in venous outflow. Stretching the nerve to 15% of its length caused complete cessation of blood flow. If this stretch is maintained for half an hour then released, intraneural blood flow will be restored with no increase in vessel permeability. Perineural barrier is maintained.

MacAvoy MC, Green DP. Critical reappraisal of Medical Research Council muscle testing for elbow flexion. J Hand Surg 2007; 32A:149–153.
The MRC grading scale defines varying degrees of weakness well (grades 0,1,2,3); however, the degree of strength regained is not as well defined (grade 3,4,5). This is illustrated in a cadaveric experiment showing that what is labeled as MRC 4 (joint held in position against less than maximal resistance) represents 96% of the entire spectrum of potential strength. The implication is that an MRC 4 grade does not automatically indicate a good outcome.

Waller A. Experiments on the section of the glossopharyngeal and hypoglossal nerves of frogs, and observations of the alterations produced thereby in the structure of their primitive fibers. Phil Trans R Soc Lond 1980; 140:423–429.
Dr Augustus Waller described microscopic alterations seen when nerves are sectioned. These findings are now often referred to as 'Wallerian degeneration.'

23.2 NERVE COMPRESSION SYNDROMES

The major nerves of the upper limb are the median nerve, radial nerve, and the ulnar nerve, and their major branches, namely, the posterior interosseous nerve (PIN), anterior interosseous nerve (AIN), and the deep motor branch, respectively. These nerves are vulnerable to compression along their course from proximal to distal. This compression may arise from normal anatomical structures, variations in normal anatomy, or due to other pathology. Some causes of upper limb nerve compression include

- Fibro-osseous tunnels - Carpal tunnel (median nerve)/cubital tunnel (ulnar nerve)
- Fibro-muscular tunnels - Arcade of Frohse (posterior interosseous nerve)
- Variant anatomy - Gantzer muscle - accessory muscle of flexor pollicis longus (FPL) (AIN)
- Synovitis - Rheumatoid arthritis (median nerve at carpal tunnel)
- Space occupying lesions - Ganglion (radial nerve at the elbow, ulnar nerve at the wrist)
- Pathological anatomy - Humeral shaft fracture (radial nerve), distal radius fracture (median nerve), cubitus valgus deformity (ulnar nerve)

PATHOLOGY

Compression leads to nerve ischemia causing a failure of conduction. Venous congestion of extra and intraneural vessel networks causes a vicious cycle wherein poor oxygen delivery to nerve fibers increases capillary permeability and jeopardizes the blood nerve barrier. This causes something akin to a closed compartment syndrome, with increased endoneurial fluid pressure and development of intrafascicular edema, making the nerve even more hypoxic. Prolonged edema along the nerve fibers eventually results in adhesion formation and fibrosis that further constricts the nerve. Nerve compression syndromes are not caused by pure external compression on the nerve. Often, longitudinal traction on the nerve compounds the problem.

A clinically silent pre-existing lesion (such as cervical root compression) increases the susceptibility of the peripheral nerve to dysfunction at another level (median nerve in carpal tunnel). The proximal lesion interferes with axon transport along the nerve rendering it more vulnerable distally, referred to as a double crush syndrome. A similar condition is one wherein a metabolic neuropathy renders a nerve more susceptible to compression injury, as seen in the association between diabetes mellitus and carpal tunnel syndrome (CTS).

CLINICAL PRESENTATION

Peripheral nerves have three functions - autonomic, sensory, and motor. Nerve compression leads to nerve dysfunction that manifests as alterations in these three functions in the anatomic domain of the nerve affected.

- Autonomic dysfunction manifests as loss of sweating
- Sensory dysfunction manifests as
  - Pain
  - Paresthesia (abnormal sensation: burning, tingling, pins, and needles)
  - Hypoesthesia
  - Anesthesia
- Motor dysfunction can manifest as
  - Clumsiness
  - Weakness
  - Atrophy

In the clinical assessment of patients with nerve compression, the history focuses on sensory and motor symptoms, and the examination focuses on objective documentation of the deficit. This objective assessment includes

- Sensory function: Ten test, 2PD and Semmes-Weinstein monofilament testing
- Motor function: MRC grade
- Provocative tests: These tests increase the pressure on the nerve in areas of compression by changing the position of the joint or tightening the muscles to reproduce the symptoms
- Tinel sign: There is often a positive Tinel sign at areas of compression

The diagnosis of nerve compression is clinical with electrophysiological tests as adjuncts. In general, the treatment of any nerve compression is rest and activity modification to avoid activities that provoke the symptoms, followed by surgical decompression when there is no improvement or when there are permanent sensory deficits or when there is objective muscle weakness.

MEDIAN NERVE

The anatomy of the median nerve has been detailed in **Figure 23.8**. The nerve may be compressed at the following points along its course:

- Above the elbow: The ligament of Struthers links a supracondylar process to the medial epicondyle and creates a fibro-osseous tunnel in 1% of the population
- Below the elbow (**Figure 23.9**)
  - The lacertus fibrosus
  - The fibrous arch between superficial and deep pronator heads
  - The arch of the flexor digitorum superficialis (FDS)
- There are three zones of the flexor retinaculum that make up the carpal tunnel roof (**Figure 23.10**). They are the proximal portion

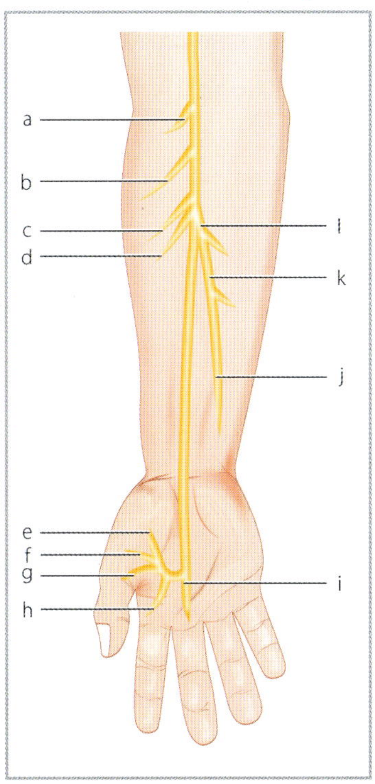

Figure 23.8 Median nerve and its branches. a. Prontor tetes branch; b. Flexor carpi radialis; c. Palmaris longus; d. Flexor digitorum superficialis; e. Abductor pollicis brevis; f. Flexor policis brevis; g. Opponens pollicis; h. First lumbrical; i. Second lumbrical; J. Pronator quadratus; k. Flexor digitorum profundus; l. Flexor pollicis longus

(distinct from antebrachial fascia); middle portion (transverse carpal ligament); and the distal portion (thick aponeurosis between thenar and hypothenar muscles. These should be divided for complete surgical release.

The following compression syndromes are associated with the median nerve:

Pronator tunnel syndrome

Symptoms/signs

This results from compression of the median nerve around the elbow. Patients present with pain in the anterior aspect of the distal arm or proximal forearm with repetitive pronation and supination, with or without paresthesia or diminished sensation in median nerve-innervated fingers. Symptoms disappear during sleep. There are usually no motor symptoms.

Clinical signs for this syndrome include altered or diminished sensation in median nerve distribution of the hand. Also, patient will have weakness in both extrinsic and intrinsic median nerve innervated muscles.

Investigations

Electrodiagnostic studies do not contribute to diagnosis.

Provocative tests

Provocative tests for pronator tunnel syndrome include

- Resisted elbow flexion with supinated forearm tightening the lacertus fibrosus
- Resisted pronation with elbow extended and wrist flexed tightening the pronator teres (PT)
- Resisted flexion of the proximal interphalangeal joint (PIPJ) of the middle finger tightening the FDS arcade
- Resisted flexion with elbow in 120°–130° flexion to detect compression by ligament of Struthers
- Positive Tinel sign at proximal edge of PT in chronic cases

Management

Nonoperative management involves immobilization, physical therapy, and anti-inflammatory medication. Anti-inflammatory medication will help those with occasional symptoms arising from increased physical activity.

For surgical management, check if there is a concomitant CTS. If CTS is present, consider performing a carpal tunnel release first. Patients with persistent pain would benefit from surgical release of all possible points of compression at the elbow.

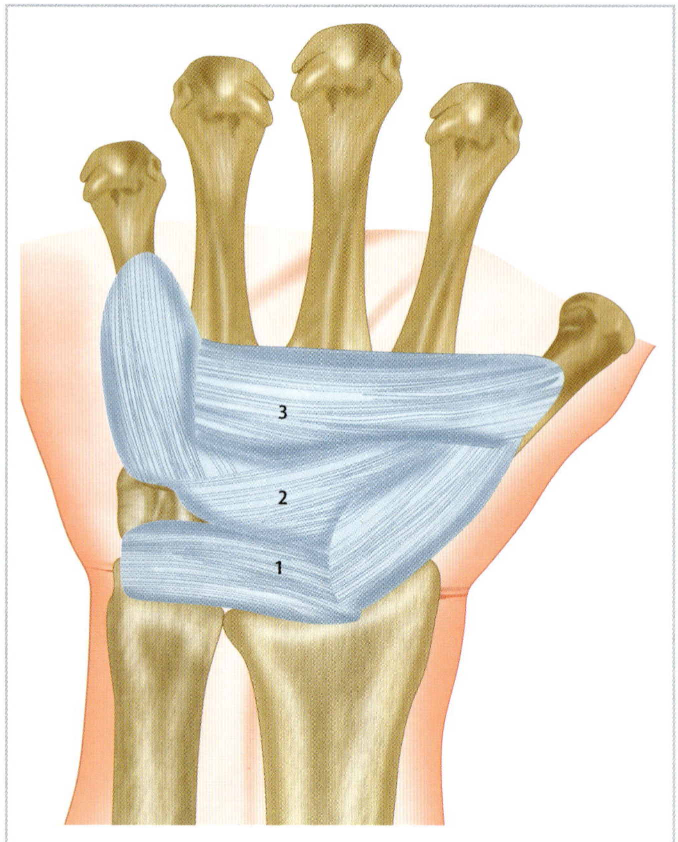

Figure 23.10 Parts of flexor retinaculum. 1, proximal portion; 2, middle portion; 3, distal portion.

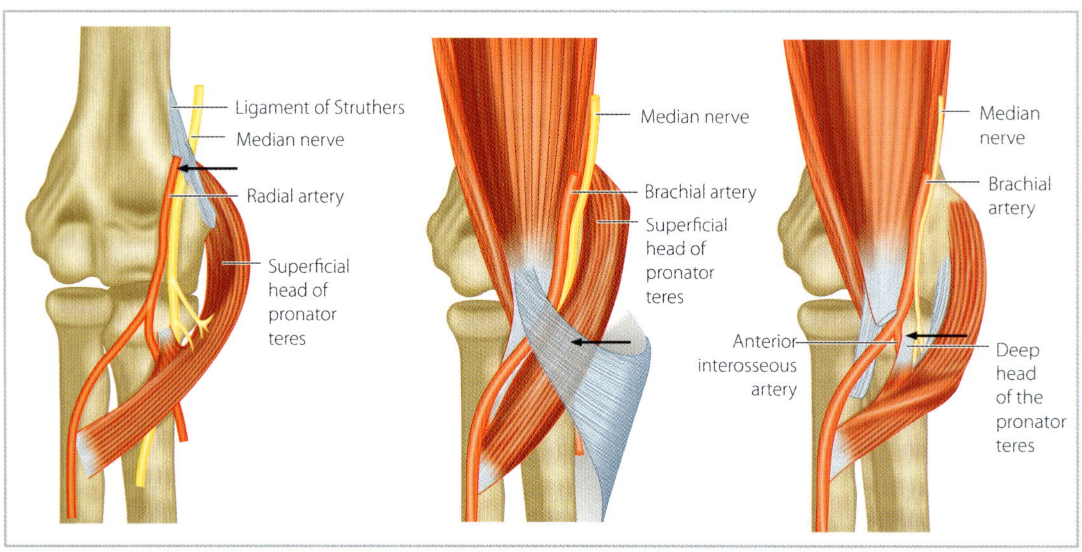

Figure 23.9 Median nerve points of compression (arrows) at the elbow.

AIN syndrome

Symptoms/signs

Patients present with unrelenting deep pain in the volar proximal forearm. There is no paresthesia or numbness. Patients may complain of altered handwriting, due to weakness of flexor digitorum profundus (FDP) of the index and FPL, if the dominant hand is involved.

Signs include an inability to make an 'O' sign (**Figure 23.11**). The patient will have weak resistance to forced supination with a fully flexed elbow (to eliminate one head of PT) compared with the normal side. Magnetic resonance imaging (MRI) is indicated if compression by a space-occupying lesion (anomalous muscle of Gantzer, cysts or vascular malformation, or nerve tumor) is suspected. Electromyography (EMG) can confirm motor weakness of FDP index and FPL but is not necessary for diagnosis.

Management

Patients who do not have a definite cause of compression are observed for 3 months, especially when they show signs of recovery. Surgical management involves release of all possible points of compression at the elbow, particularly the lacertus fibrosus, deep head of the PT, the FDS arcade, and excision of anomalous muscle of Gantzer if present.

Carpal tunnel syndrome

Symptoms/signs

Carpal tunnel syndrome is caused by compression of the median nerve under the transverse carpal ligament. A common early complaint is nocturnal pins and needles that disturb sleep. The patients are often > 40 years of age who wake up massaging or shaking their hands. As the syndrome progresses, paresthesia occurs during the day when patients read the newspaper, drive a car, or talk on the phone too long because these activities required prolonged flexion of the wrist, which causes increased pressure in the carpal tunnel that is akin to the Phalen test. It is common for patients to report that the entire palm is involved. They may report clumsiness in buttoning clothes, as well as weakness in opening bottle caps. In advanced disease, thenar atrophy is noticed by the patient.

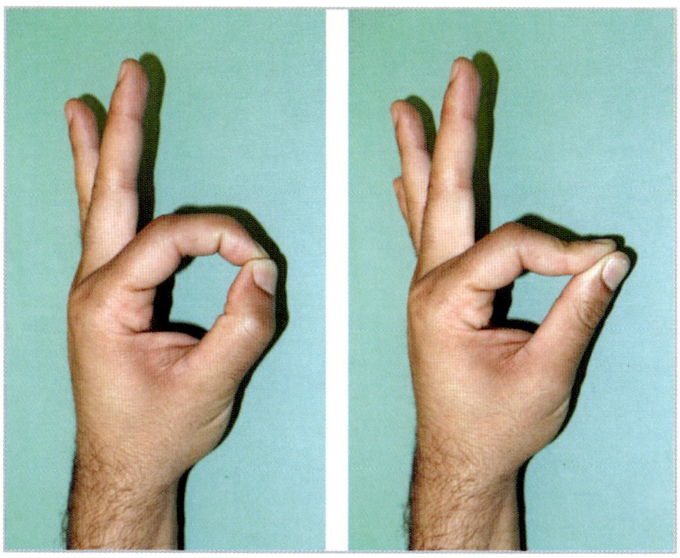

Figure 23.11 Square pinch of AIN syndrome.

Sensory deficit should be marked out in a hand diagram using the ten test or 2PD. The ten test requires patients to describe the sensation in the area being tested as a fraction of 10 compared with the same area in their normal hand. This test shows good correlation with Semmes–Weinstein monofilament testing and is sensitive even in the earliest stages of sensory loss. Abductor pollicis brevis (APB) strength is tested by asking the patient to hold the thumb in palmar abduction, as the examiner tries to break the pose or by asking patient to palmar abduct the thumb while applying resistance. APB strength of <50% of ipsilateral index finger flexion is 98% specific for diagnosing advanced CTS.

Provocative tests

- The Phalen test is the most sensitive (up to 87% reported). It involves asking the patient to rest his elbows on the table and holding both forearms vertically, allowing both hands to drop into flexion at the wrist
- Tinel sign at the wrist has consistently high specificity of up to 97% and allows surgeons to identify the point of maximal compression
- Carpal tunnel compression test is also specific. This has the advantage of being easier to perform in patients with limited wrist range of motion

Investigations

Investigations are ordered only in specific circumstances. Radiographs should only be ordered when there is suspicion of bony deformity as cause of nerve compression, such as distal radius fracture, perilunate dislocation, fractured hook of hamate. MRI should only be ordered when there is suspicion of a space-occupying lesion, such as a nerve tumor, as cause of compression within the carpal tunnel. High-resolution ultrasound is helpful in determining the area of incomplete release in persistent or recurrent CTS. Electrodiagnostic studies can be normal. They are not necessary before surgery when clinical history and examination are typical of CTS. They are ordered when one is considering more proximal sites of median nerve compression or presence of polyneuropathy.

Management

General success rate of early medical treatment of CTS is 52% at 3 months.

Nonoperative treatment involves wrist splinting and anti-inflammatory medication, with or without local steroid injection. Nonoperative treatment has a poor success rate in the presence of following factors: age <50 years, positive Phalen test in <30 seconds, constant paresthesia, duration >10 months, stenosing flexor tenosynovitis. Sixty-six percent of patients are relieved with above treatment when none of the above factors are present. Local steroid injection has short-term success rate of 80% when combined with splinting. This decreases to 22% at final follow-up from 6 months onward. It does not matter what type of steroid you use or where in the carpal tunnel you inject the steroid.

Surgery is indicated if there is incomplete relief from nonsurgical treatment, constant sensory symptoms, or weakness/atrophy of the APB. Eighty percent of patients have complete symptom relief in 3 months, 90% have complete relief in 18 months.

Mini-incision open release involves a 1-cm palmar curvilinear incision over the distal edge of the transverse carpal ligament. It gives the benefit of endoscopic release without the cost or the risk. The distal edge of the transverse carpal ligament is approximately 2 mm proximal to the palmar fat pad. Seeing the palmar fat pad during carpal tunnel release signals that the end of distal dissection is near.

The pattern of recovery is as follows: Nocturnal symptoms, mechanical paresthesia resolve within days. Pillar pain generally resolves in 3–4 weeks, in some patients it lasts a maximum of 9 months. If there is permanent digital anesthesia preoperatively, there will be partial resolution of anesthesia with recovery of protective sensation. Grip and pinch strength return to preoperative levels in 3 months.

ULNAR NERVE

The anatomy of the ulnar nerve has been detailed in **Figure 23.12**. The nerve may be compressed at the following points along its course (**Figure 23.13**).

- Around the elbow
  - The arcade of Struthers is formed by the thickened deep investing fascia of the arm, the medial intermuscular septum, and the muscle fibers from the medial head of the triceps. It is present in 68% of adult arms
  - The medial intermuscular septum causes compression only when the nerve is subluxing or when transposed anteriorly
  - The roof of the cubital tunnel is formed by the cubital tunnel retinaculum proximally and Osborne fascia distally. The cubital tunnel retinaculum extends between the medial epicondyle of the humerus and the olecranon. The distance between these two points of insertion lengthens during elbow flexion, effectively decreasing tunnel volume by 55%. Osborne fascia is a band of fibrous tissue bridging the two heads of the flexor carpi ulnaris (FCU)
  - The flexor pronator aponeurosis is an inconsistent fascial connection between the humeral head of the FCU and the muscles of the flexor pronator mass. It is present as a significant band in 45.8% of cases
- At the wrist
  - Guyon canal (**Figure 23.14**): Guyon canal is a fibrous and aponeurotic space with no rigid boundaries, unlike the carpal tunnel. The canal extends from the transverse carpal ligament at the proximal edge of the pisiform bone to the origin of the hypothenar muscles just distal to the hamate. It is triangular proximally becoming ovoid distally
  - Roof and radial border:
    - Proximal – antebrachial fascia
    - Middle – adipose tissue
    - Distal – palmaris brevis
  - Floor: transverse carpal ligament, pisohamate ligament, hypothenar muscles
  - Ulnar border:
    - Proximal – pisiform
    - Distal – junction of hypothenar muscles and roof
  - The course of the ulnar nerve within the Guyon canal can be divided into three zones (Gross and Gelberman, 1985)
    - Zone I – mixed motor and sensory nerve seen proximal to the pisohamate ligament
    - Zone II (deep motor branch to intrinsic muscles)
    - Zone III (sensory to ulnar one and a half of fingers) are in parallel zones distal to the pisohamate ligament

The following compression syndromes are associated with the ulnar nerve;

Cubital tunnel syndrome

Symptoms/signs

Patients with cubital tunnel syndrome report activity-induced or nocturnal paresthesia, with or without numbness along the ulnar border of hand, aggravated by elbow flexion. Complaints regarding motor function include difficulty in using chopsticks or turning a key. When ignored, patients present late with guttering of intermetacarpal spaces. Sensory deficit in the ulnar nerve distribution should be marked out in a hand diagram using the ten test or 2PD. The affected area includes

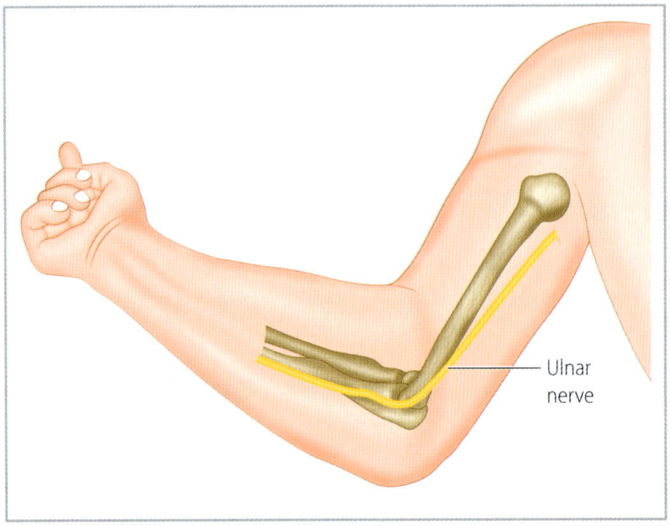

Figure 23.12 Ulnar nerve and its branches.

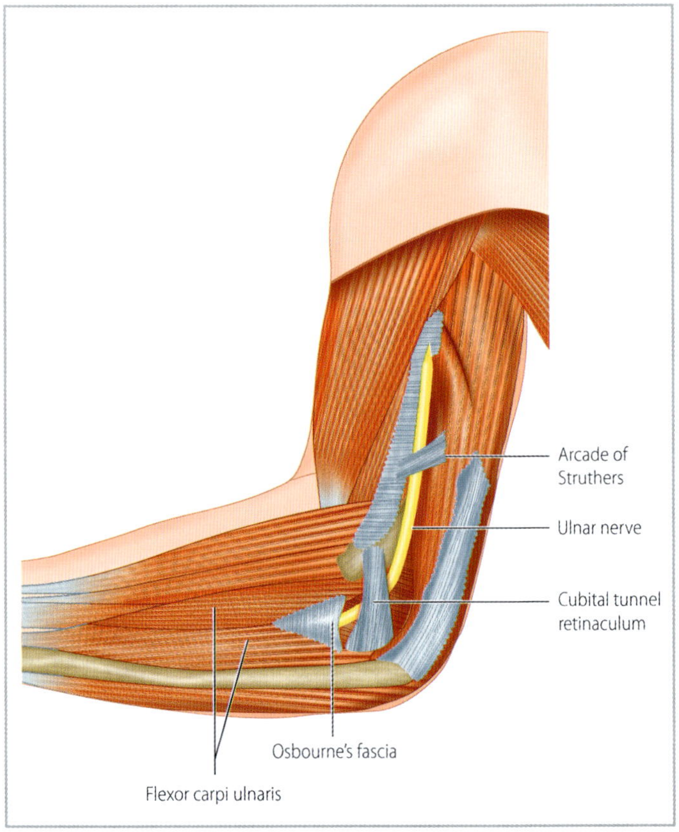

Figure 23.13 Points of compression of the ulnar nerve at the elbow.

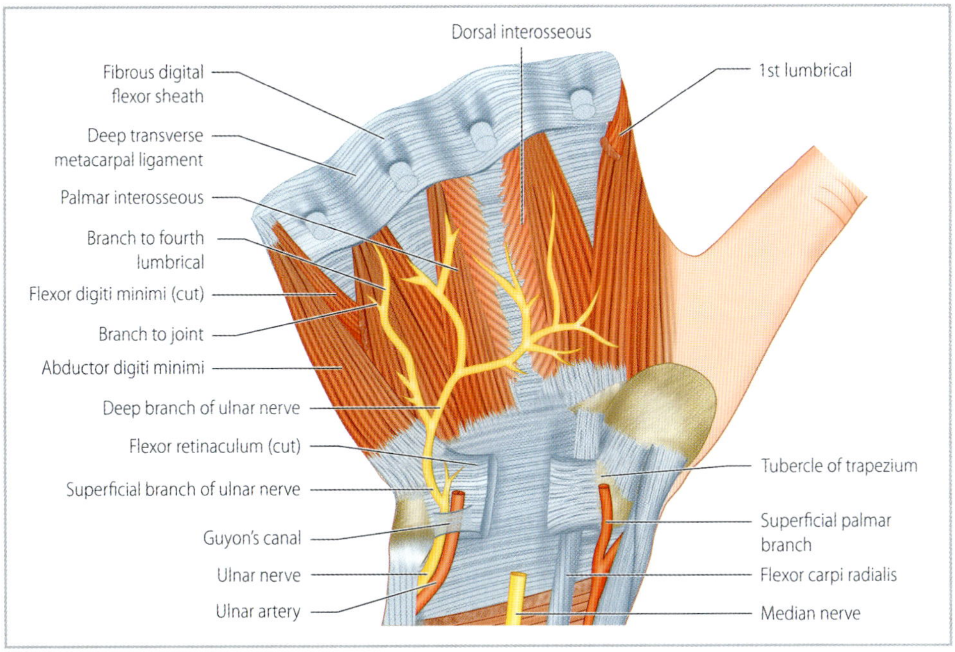

Figure 23.14 Anatomy of the ulnar nerve in the wrist and palm.

the dorsal ulnar border of the hand. The clinician should conduct manual muscle testing of the following muscles:

- FDP 5 /Pollock sign
- Abductor digiti minimi
- Middle finger interossei/Pitres-Testut sign
- Adductor pollicis/Froment sign

Provocative tests

Provocative tests for cubital tunnel syndrome include combined elbow flexion and pressure test. The Tinel sign also helps localize the exact site of compression. Diagnosis involves eliciting a combination of symptoms, objective findings, and provocative tests that defines the probability of disease. There is no consensus reference standard for diagnosis.

Investigations

Radiographs or MRIs are ordered only in the presence of an elbow mass or deformity. High-resolution ultrasound can reliably diagnose nerve subluxation. Electrodiagnostic studies are needed when considering another level of compression [e.g. thoracic outlet syndrome (TOS)].

Management

Nonoperative management involves night splinting with elbow in slight flexion, nerve gliding exercises, and avoiding postures that trigger symptoms. These measures are successful in 89% of patients with symptoms only. History of elbow trauma was associated with worse outcome with conservative treatment.

Surgical management is indicated if there is a lack of symptomatic improvement or worsening symptoms. Presence of intrinsic guttering or clawing affecting activities of daily living. Surgical techniques include:

- Simple in situ decompression (endoscopic or open): In situ decompression involves less dissection and is proven to be effective with acceptable complication rates (subluxation in <10% of cases). Endoscopic decompression has similar or better results when compared with open in situ decompression with recurrence rates of 0.02–5.24%. The advantages include less scar discomfort or elbow extension deficit post surgery. Hematoma is a common complication of endoscopic release. Open decompression is indicated in a previously operated elbow or when there is recurrence from endoscopic release
- Anterior transposition: This is indicated if the nerve subluxes on elbow flexion preoperatively, in the presence of post-traumatic cubitus valgus causing tardy ulnar nerve palsy, or when there is symptomatic subluxation of the nerve after in situ decompression
  - Subcutaneous
  - Intramuscular
  - Submuscular
- Medial epicondylectomy

Results are not significantly different in terms of clinical scores or nerve conduction studies. All modalities work well in grade 1 compression. In grade 3 compression, patient satisfaction rates decrease significantly regardless of surgical modality used and recurrence rates increase, with medial epicondylectomy having the highest satisfaction rate (62%).

Guyon canal compression or ulnar tunnel syndrome

Symptoms/signs

The symptoms for Guyon canal compression depend on the area of compression (zone I, zone II, or zone III). Paresthesia or variable numbness over the little finger and ulnar half of the ring finger is the common complaint in zone I or III compressions. Acute periodic severe pain over the ulnar aspect of the hand with obvious ischemic changes that spontaneously resolves within a few minutes points to hypothenar hammer syndrome, caused by compression of the nerve in this area by thrombosed ulnar artery. Clumsiness, persistent abduction of little finger, clawing of ulnar fingers, and intermetacarpal guttering are common complaints in late stages. Motor deficits are not present in zone III compressions.

Clinical signs include a visible or deep palpable mass, as the most common cause of compression in this area is a ganglion. Sensory deficits are seen in zone I and III compressions. Sensation over the ulnar dorsal border of the hand is spared. Search for tender areas especially around the hook of hamate or pisiform to rule out fractures as cause of compression, especially in patients with a history of recent trauma or in patients involved in activities that cause repetitive trauma to the hypothenar region. Map out the sensory deficit over the volar surface of the little finger and half of ring finger in a hand diagram using ten test or 2PD. Motor deficits are seen in zone I and II compressions. Intact FDP 4 and 5 cause obvious clawing of ulnar 2 fingers. Inability to adduct the little finger (Wartenberg sign) is present in zone I compression. Zone II compression spares hypothenar muscles. Flexion of thumb interphalangeal joint (IPJ) during forceful thumb adduction due to FPL compensates for weakness of the thumb adductor and first dorsal interosseous muscle (Froment sign).

Provocative tests

1. A positive Tinel sign helps localize the area of compression
2. The Allen test will help detect ulnar artery thrombosis as cause of compression, as in hypothenar hammer syndrome
3. Check for concurrent CTS

Investigations

Investigations help shed light on etiology of compression and influence management for this syndrome. High-resolution ultrasound is an inexpensive method to visualize clinically occult lesions, such as a ganglion, in the area. Carpal tunnel view radiographs are ordered if a fracture of the hook of hamate is suspected. MRI may be needed for surgical planning if a vascular lesion is the cause of compression. Electrodiagnostic examination can confirm the site of compression.

Management

Nonoperative management of Guyon canal compression involves wrist immobilization, anti-inflammatory medication, and avoidance of triggering hobbies or work activities. Nonoperative management is recommended for primary nerve compression (no mechanical cause of compression detected) with no objective deficits on examination.

Surgical management involves decompression and excision of mass and is indicated in the presence of a significant mass lesion (large ganglion, tumor, vascular malformation, fracture fragment) causing compression. Decompression is also indicated when there is failure of symptomatic relief with conservative treatment of primary nerve compression or progression of disease with appearance of objective deficits on examination.

RADIAL NERVE

The anatomy of the radial nerve has been detailed in **Figure 23.15**. The nerve may be compressed at the following points along its course.

- Above the elbow
  - Spiral groove – The radial nerve lies in close proximity to the posterior humeral diaphysis for a distance of 8–10 cm till it passes anteriorly through the lateral intermuscular septum. It is vulnerable to compression in spiral or oblique fractures of the humeral shaft or by the accessory fibrous arch of the lateral head of the triceps and the lateral intermuscular septum during forceful elbow extension
- Around the elbow (**Figure 23.16**)
  - Fibrous bands in front of elbow joint

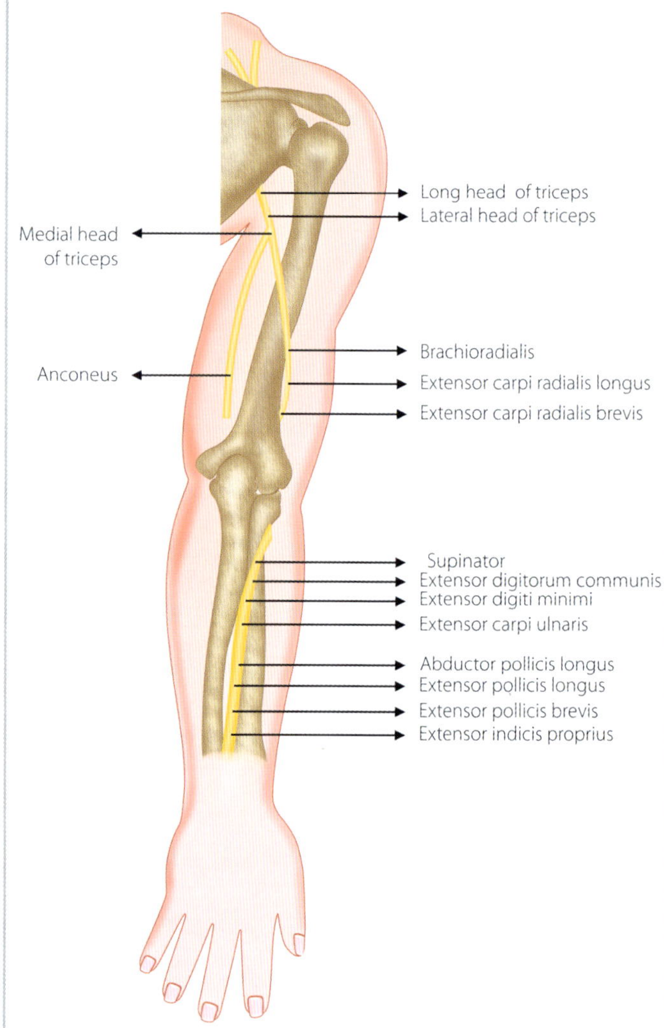

Figure 23.15 Radial nerve and its branches

  - The Leash of Henry (radial recurrent vessels) refers to a network of veins at the level of the radial head, overlying the lower part of the radial tunnel
  - Extensor carpi radialis brevis (ECRB) tendinous origin
  - Arcade of Frohse refers to the fibrous thickening at the margin of the plane between the deep and superficial heads of the supinator where the PIN passes
  - Supinator – distal margin
  - Radial tunnel – This is not a distinct anatomic tunnel. The floor is formed by the capitellum to lower edge of radial head. The upper portion of the tunnel is where the nerve travels anteriorly, bounded by biceps, and brachialis medially and brachioradialis (BR) laterally. In the middle and lower portion, the nerve is bounded anteriorly by brachialis and biceps tendon, laterally by ECRB and by BR medially. It ends when the nerve pierces enters the two heads of the supinator.
- Distal forearm
  - The superficial radial nerve (SRN) running on the deep surface of the BR pierces the antebrachial fascia in between the tendons of the BR and extensor carpi radialis longus (ECRL) at about 7 cm

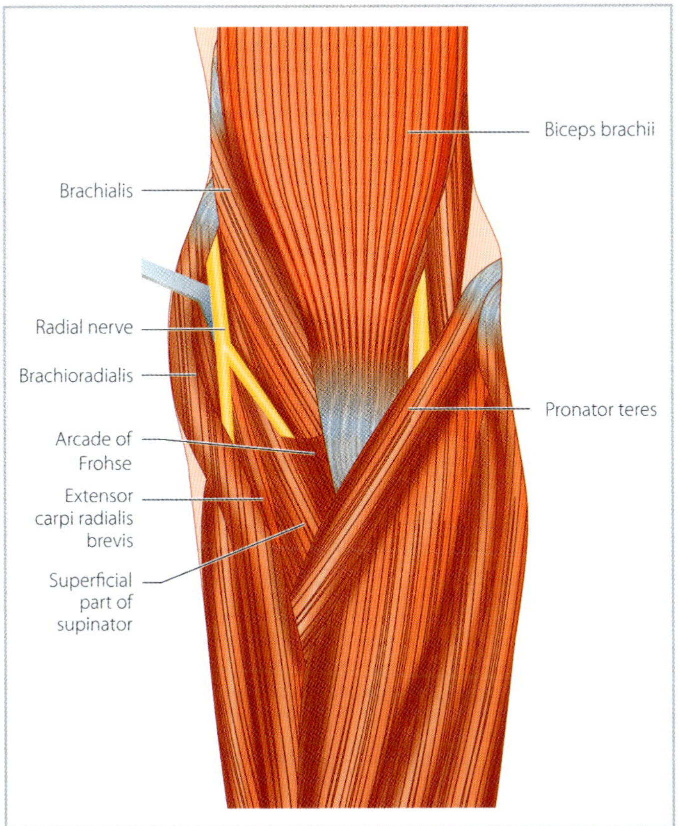

Figure 23.16 Points of compression of the radial nerve around the elbow.

proximal to the wrist to run subcutaneously superficial to the tendons of the first dorsal compartment. The distance between ECRL and BR decreases in pronation and ulnar deviation, compressing the nerve

The following compression syndromes are associated with the radial nerve:

Compression in the spiral groove

Symptoms/signs

Symptoms for compression in the spiral groove include paresthesia and numbness over the posterolateral forearm and radial dorsum of the hand. Wrist drop or inability to extend the wrist and inability to extend the thumb and the metacarpophalangeal joints (MCPJs) of the hand is noted after humeral shaft fracture (reported prevalence of 12%). It is also possible after extrinsic compression of the arm during prolonged coma (Saturday night palsy), prolonged tourniquet application, poor positioning on operating table, or after a history of prolonged and sustained elbow extension in patients with a relatively fixed nerve just distal to the groove.

The clinician should map out the sensory deficit in a hand diagram using ten test or 2PD. Radial nerve deficit is noted over the posterolateral aspect of the forearm, dorsum of the first web space, dorsum of the thumb and index finger up to the middle of the distal phalanx, and dorsum of the middle and ring fingers up to the PIPJ. Patients will exhibit paralysis or weakness of radial nerve innervated muscles.

Provocative tests

The Tinel sign helps localize the level of compression in spontaneous paralysis without history of trauma or extrinsic compression.

Investigations

Regarding investigations, radiographs are needed for fracture management. EMG should be performed after 3 weeks in cases of closed injuries (humeral fracture treated by cast or after extrinsic compression) or spontaneous paralysis can differentiate a neurapraxia from axonotmesis.

Management

Nonoperative management involves a dynamic extension splint, which may be used to support the wrist and hand in a functional position while awaiting recovery. Overall recovery rate of radial nerve palsy associated with humeral shaft fracture during observation is 72–88%, with higher rates for incomplete palsies and closed fractures.

For surgical intervention, the nerve should be explored during open reduction and internal fixation of the humeral shaft fracture. Closed intramedullary nailing is contraindicated in fractures with radial nerve palsy unless the nerve is explored, isolated, and protected prior to nail insertion. After early nerve exploration (within 3 weeks), the probability of recovery is 85%. Exploration and neurolysis are also recommended in cases of conservatively treated fractures, extrinsic compression or spontaneous paralysis that show no signs of recovery by 2 months. For patients with closed humeral fractures managed nonoperatively, the likelihood of recovery after late nerve surgery (> 8 weeks) is 69%.

Radial tunnel syndrome

Symptoms/signs

Symptoms include aching pain over the lateral elbow, accompanied by easy fatigability of the forearm when performing certain actions. This pain can wake patient up at night. Motor weakness reported is usually due to pain.

Clinical signs include a point of maximal tenderness distal to the lateral epicondyle (to differentiate from lateral epicondylitis). No objective sensory deficit can be elicited. Sensation over dorsum of the hand is normal. Motor function should be normal.

Provocative tests

1. Compressing the path of the radial nerve 5 cm distal to the lateral epicondyle can reproduce the characteristic pain
2. Resisted middle finger extension causes radial nerve compression by eliciting ECRB (inserted into the base of the third metacarpal) contraction and compression of the nerve. Elbow extension and supination of forearm against resistance aggravates symptoms

Investigations

Electrodiagnostic tests are often normal. High-resolution ultrasound helps detect dynamic compression or secondary cause of compression by a space-occupying lesion.

Management

For nonoperative management, nonsteroidal anti-inflammatory drug (NSAID), and activity modification will relieve pain albeit temporarily if provocative activities are resumed. Tennis elbow straps exert pressure on the radial nerve and should be avoided in patients with concurrent lateral epicondylitis. Immobilization with wrist extension splints or elbow splints to prevent full extension will enforce rest in manual workers.

Surgical intervention includes decompression, which is indicated when progressive improvement is not achieved with conservative treatment or when symptoms worsen. All possible points of compression are released. Concurrent release of the common extensor origin is recommended in patients with associated lateral epicondylitis.

Posterior interosseous nerve syndrome

Symptoms/signs

Symptoms for PIN include pain prior to onset of weakness. Patients will weakness of grip, difficulty extending the wrist, inability to extend MCPJs.

Clinically, radial deviation of wrist is noted with attempted wrist extension (ECRL intact while rest of extensors are weak). Patients with PIN cannot extend their index to little finger MCPJs (extensor digitorum communis, EDC) when the IPJs flexed. Inability to extend the thumb (extensor pollicis longus, EPL) is noted when the hand is placed flat, palm down on the table. Patients will have intact tenodesis effect. This helps differentiate PIN syndrome from tendon ruptures. Sensory is typically normal.

Provocative tests

The Tinel sign may help localize the area of compression.

Investigations

Electrodiagnostic tests can confirm diagnosis by showing denervation of EDC, extensor indicis proprius (EIP), EDQM, and normal sensory parameters. It is also useful when a double crush syndrome is suspected. MRI can detect secondary causes of compression such as lipoma, synovial cysts, extravasation of synovial pannus.

Management

Nonoperative management includes rest, NSAID, and activity modification. In addition, elbow splints should be tried for 3 months. Surgical decompression is recommended with failure of nonoperative management at 3 months. All possible points of compression near the elbow are released, as in radial tunnel syndrome.

Superficial radial nerve compression or Wartenberg syndrome

Symptoms/signs

Patients present with pain on dorsum of the hand with paresthesia during writing or when performing tasks that require pronation/supination and ulnar deviation. Some would complain of pain on dorsum of the hand due to a tight watch strap. Patients may have no motor symptoms or may be limited by pain on certain motions

Clincially, sensory may be normal or may show deficit over dorsum of first web space, dorsum of the thumb and index finger up to the middle of the distal phalanx, and dorsum of the middle and ring fingers up to the PIPJ. Motor signs are normal.

Provocative tests

1. The Tinel sign helps localize the level of compression. Directly pressing on the nerve at this point will cause the characteristic pain
2. The Finkelstein test is performed to check for concomitant de Quervain tenosynovitis. Patients with only de Quervain disease will have normal sensation over dorsoradial aspect of their hand
3. Characteristic pain is also reproduced by elbow extension, forearm pronation, and wrist ulnar deviation

Investigations

Electrodiagnostic tests can confirm the diagnosis.

Management

Nonoperative management of SRN compression involves activity modification (removal of tight watch band) and wrist splinting. This treatment regimen has a success rate of up to 86%.

Surgical decompression is indicated when there is no relief with conservative management. When the compression is more proximal (as determined by the Tinel sign), a longitudinal incision is preferred. The fascia between the BR and ECRL, as well as a portion of the BR tendon may be excised. When compression is more distal and a concomitant de Quervain tenosynovitis is suspected, a transverse incision allows for both nerve decompression and release of the first dorsal compartment. This minimizes adhesions between the tendons and the nerve.

Digital nerve (Bowler's thumb)

Symptoms/signs

Patients present with pain over the ulnar side of the thumb and hyperesthesia over the distribution of the ulnar digital nerve of the thumb. They may also have overlying callous or atrophy of the ulnar side skin, with or without a palpable sensitive lump. Patients have no motor deficits. Bowling enthusiasts can continue to bowl with thumb guards. Sensory deficit may or may not be present on the ulnar side of the thumb pulp. Motor signs are normal.

Provocative tests

The Tinel sign is strongest over the area of neuroma.

Investigations

Investigations are not necessary.

Management

If diagnosed early, the condition resolves with rest and cessation of aggravating activity. Use of a thumb guard during activity also helps. Most patients respond well to nonoperative treatment.

Surgical exploration and neurolysis is an option for patients who do not improve with 6 months of conservative treatment. Synovectomy may be performed in the same sitting if proliferative synovitis of the FPL is seen compressing the nerve. In recurrent cases, excision of the neuroma and repair of the nerve had been reported with poor results (no or >6 mm 2PD on the pinching side of the thumb).

SUGGESTED READING

Chung KC, Walters MR, Greenfield MVH, Chernew ME. Endoscopic versus open carpal tunnel release: a cost-effectiveness analysis. Plast Reconstr Surg 1998; 102:1089–1099.
Using decision analysis model, endoscopic carpal tunnel release was found to be a cost-effective procedure if median nerve injury can be avoided. Thus, surgeons need to receive adequate training in this method before it can be recommended as a standard procedure.

Gellman H, Gelberman RH, Tan AM, Botte MJ. Carpal tunnel syndrome: an evaluation of provocative tests. J Bone Joint Surg 1986; 68A:735–737.
Sensitivity and specificity of Phalen test and Tinel test were determined by comparing results of these tests in 67 hand with electrodiagnostically proven carpal tunnel syndrome and 50 hands of normal control subjects.

Gerritsen AA, de Vet HC, Scholten RJ, et al. Splinting vs surgery in the treatment of carpal tunnel syndrome: a randomized controlled trial. JAMA 2002; 288:1245–1251.
This randomized control trial compared patient-reported outcomes in splint or surgically treated carpal tunnel patients. More patients who underwent open carpal tunnel release reported better outcomes (completely recovered or much improved) at 3 and 18 months after surgery compared with patients treated with wrist splinting.

Gross MS, Gelberman RH. The anatomy of the distal ulnar tunnel. Clin Orthop Relat Res 1985; 196:238–247.

Katz JN, Keller RB, Simmons BP, et al. Symptoms, functional status, and neuromuscular impairment following carpal tunnel release. J Hand Surg 1995; 20A:549–555.
This prospective cohort study gave detailed information on the pattern and timing of recovery after carpal tunnel release. This is useful information to have when advising patients on what to expect after surgery.

Phalen GS. The carpal tunnel syndrome: seventeen years' experience in diagnosis and treatment of 654 hands. J Bone Joint Surg 1966; 48A:211–228.
This is the often-cited paper of Dr George Phalen's experience with carpal tunnel syndrome. It gives a comprehensive history of the condition, as well as an extensive discussion of clinical findings, pathogenesis, and treatment. Interesting to note is that only 40% of Dr Phalen's 439 patients required surgery. Carpal tunnel release almost always resulted in immediate relief of pain and paresthesia. Seventy-eight per cent regained normal sensation and 67.9% regained normal thenar muscle power 6-month to 1-year post surgery.

Szabo RM, Slater RR, Farver TB, et al. The value of diagnostic testing in carpal tunnel syndrome. J Hand Surg 1999; 24A:704–714.
By comparing findings in three groups, Dr Szabo and colleagues found that if a patient has an abnormal hand diagram, abnormal sensation by SW monofilament testing, positive carpal compression test, and night pain, the probability of that patient having carpal tunnel syndrome is 0.86. Adding electrodiagnostic testing did not increase the diagnostic power of the four clinical test.

Zlowodzki M, Chan S, Bhandari M, et al. Anterior transposition compared with simple decompression for treatment of cubital tunnel syndrome. A meta-analysis of randomized controlled trials. J Bone Joint Surg 2007; 89A:2591–2598.
This meta-analysis showed that simple decompression is a reasonable treatment option in cubital tunnel patients with no prior trauma or surgery on the affected elbow. The authors found no significant difference in clinical outcome scores (3 studies, $n = 261$) and postoperative motor nerve conduction velocities (2 studies, $n = 100$) between the two procedures.

23.3 NERVE PALSY

The options available for reconstruction of a patient with nerve palsy include nerve repair, nerve transfer, and tendon/muscle transfer. The selection of the appropriate option is determined primarily by the time since the injury. Nerve repair is done in the acute situation, whereas nerve transfer is done in the acute or subacute situation (<6 months post injury), and tendon/muscle transfers are considered in the chronic setting.

NERVE TRANSFER

Indications

- Acute situations wherein there is a questionable chance of recovery from nerve repair. For example, in long segment crush injuries requiring long nerve grafts
- Subacute stage (<6 months post injury), wherein time to reinnervation of distal denervated muscles from the time of surgery (nerve transfer) is < 11 months post injury

Principles

- Proximity to target muscle: The shorter the distance, the shorter the time required for the regenerating nerve to reinnervate the muscle, and the better the outcome
- Primary axon type (motor, sensory, or mixed): Choose a motor nerve donor for a motor nerve recipient. Motor nerve fascicle can be dissected free from a mixed nerve with guidance from electrical stimulation
- Donor muscle should be expendable or have multiple points of innervation
- Donor–recipient nerve size match
- Donor nerve must have adequate axons
- Synergism between donor nerve muscle and recipient muscle: Lesser need for cortical reorientation and easier postoperative rehabilitation

Technique

- The recipient nerve should be assessed by electrical stimulation to avoid sacrificing a recovering nerve
- The donor nerve should be assessed before and after dissection of the fascicle to check function and quality of donor fascicle, as well as remaining function of the donor nerve without the cut fascicle. It is acceptable to use a recovered donor nerve when there is limited donor availability
- Motor nerve transfers should be performed in a direct end-to-end fashion
- Critical sensory transfers should also be performed directly end-to-end if donor nerve is available. End-to-side transfers, in their best results, can give only protective sensation
- Site of transfer must be planned at the same level as recipient nerve branch to minimize nerve regeneration distance. Ensure direct tension free nerve repair without the need for postoperative immobilization by dissecting adequate length distally for the donor nerve and proximally in the recipient nerve

TENDON TRANSFER

Tendon transfer surgery is an operative procedure that restores balance to the hand by redistributing the remaining motor power in the forearm and hand so that the patient will be able to actively control their hand.

Indications

- Failure of nerve repair or transfer
- Inadequate functional recovery after nerve repair or transfer
- Used primarily in late presentation (long duration between injury and surgery) wherein the denervated muscle would have already undergone fibrosis
- Used for patients whose deficit is caused by demyelinating neuropathy like leprosy or Charcot–Marie–Tooth disease
- Can be used primarily in patients who can afford only one surgery due to poor general health condition

Principles

- Suitable recipient site/soft tissue equilibrium:
  - Skin – Not swollen nor warm. Soft pliable scars. Resurface first if necessary
  - Bone and joints – Fractures well aligned and securely fixed. Involved joints must have good passive range of motion
  - Nerves – Intact sensation in critical areas such as thumb pulp
  - Vessels – adequate inflow and outflow
- Suitable muscle:
  - Expendable: Loss of donor muscle action should not increase patient's morbidity
  - Adequate strength: Choose a donor with enough strength to balance the rest of the working muscles to enable more efficient use of the hand
  - Adequate excursion: Excursion refers to the distance through which tension can be maintained by the muscle. In adults, wrist flexors and extensors have approximately 33 mm of excursion, whereas extrinsic finger extensors and finger flexors have approximately 50 and 70 mm, respectively. If excursion of transferred muscle is inadequate, patients compensate by using tenodesis effect. Excursions can also be limited by adhesions, but this can be addressed by therapy
  - Synergistic: Wrist extensors (radial nerve) make good donors for finger flexors (median nerve) because in normal grasp, they actively contract together on opposite sides of the wrist joint to produce equal torque on each side, forming a stable post for grasp
  - Straight line of pull from origin to intended insertion is most efficient
  - One tendon – one function: Transferring one tendon for one action is most effective; however, this may not be an option when you have limited available donors. One muscle can be used to move multiple joints in parallel producing one action [e.g. flexor carpi radialis (FCR) to EDC], but it is important to set all insertions at the same distance to allow equal excursion. If not, the transfer will only move the joint to which it is more closely attached. It has been proven that splitting a bipennate muscle like FCU up to 80% of its distal length creates two independently

contracting unipennate submuscle units. This increases the number of potential donor muscles, especially when donors are limited due to combined nerve injuries.

Technique

1. Help patients identify the donor muscle and strengthen it with exercise before the surgery. This will help them apply the transferred tendon more easily after the transfer
2. Tensioning of the transferred tendon is performed by securing donor to recipient with one trial suture and observing the tenodesis effect of the transfer. Other adjuncts include marking the donor muscle length with sutures before cutting the tendon and pulling the muscle back to length during inset
3. Transferred tendon is attached to recipient by at least three Pulvertaft weaves. This involves weaving the donor into the recipient tendon in 90° angles and securing each weave with strong nonabsorbable sutures
4. Attach/reinsert transferred muscle at a slightly greater tension. Patients will feel a sense of discomfort that helps them identify the transferred muscle and its new action. This also compensate for postoperative stretching of repair site
5. Most transfers wound require total postoperative immobilization for at least 4 weeks with another 2 weeks of intermittent mobilization to allow for tendon healing

Management of individual nerve palsies

It is useful to make a table that answers the following questions to determine the best plan for a given nerve palsy.

1. How long has it been since the injury?
2. What is needed? Which muscles are not working?
3. What is available? Which muscles are working?

Radial nerve palsy

High radial nerve palsy

1. What is needed?
   a. Sensory: dorsum of first web space
   b. Motor: Wrist extension, finger MCPJ extension, and thumb extension
2. What is available?
   a. Nerve transfers (**Table 23.3**): It is advisable to perform nerve transfer to restore protective sensation even when motor nerve transfers are no longer viable options
   b. Tendon transfers (**Table 23.4**): Early end-to-side PT to ECRB transfer during time of nerve repair was advocated by Burkhalter for the following reasons:
      i. Transfer works as an internal splint while awaiting nerve regeneration. It is a working substitute if ECRB does not recover
      ii. It adds power to wrist extension should reinnervated muscle recover
      iii. The FDS to EDC transfer (Boyes transfer) is recommended in patients with a fused wrist

Low radial/PIN palsy

1. What is needed?
   a. No sensory deficit
   b. Motor:
      i. Finger extension (EDC)
      ii. Thumb extension (EPL)
2. What is available?
   a. Nerve transfer (**Table 23.3**)
   b. Tendon transfer (**Table 23.4**)
      i. FCR to EDC transfer is preferred as the ECRL and ECRB are intact, and the extensor carpi ulnaris (ECU) more commonly is not. Using the FCU would cause a static radial deviation deformity. This is performed together with a palmaris longus (PL) to EPL transfer
      ii. If PL is absent, the Boyes set of transfers is recommended

Median nerve palsy

High median nerve palsy

1. What is needed?
   a. Sensation in radial three fingers, especially thumb and index finger tip
   b. Motor: Thumb opposition, thumb to index finger pinch
      i. Opposition: Involves abduction, flexion, and pronation of the thumb
      ii. Finger flexion: All the FDS tendons, the index and middle finger FDP, and FPL affected

Table 23.3 Summary of available nerve transfers for peripheral nerve palsy

Deficit	Donors: motor				Donors: sensory	
Radial nerve	Median branch to FDS (FDP intact) to radial branch of ECRB	Median branch to FCR (FCU intact) and PL to PIN	Ulnar branch to FCU (FCR intact) to PIN		Lateral antebrachial cutaneous (LABC) to radial sensory (SRN)	
Median nerve	Anterior interosseous nerve (AIN) (PQ) + graft to recurrent motor branch to thenar muscles	Radial ECRB branch or radial supinator branch to AIN (FDP2 & FPL)	Radial ECRB or ulnar FCU or MCN branch to brachialis (biceps intact) to median PT	MCN branch to brachialis (biceps intact) to AIN (FDP2 & FPL)	Ulnar common digital nerve to fourth web space to median common digital nerve to first web space and radial digital nerve thumb	SRN to median common digital nerve to first web space and radial digital nerve thumb
Ulnar nerve (UN)	AIN (PQ) to ulnar deep motor branch				LABC to dorsal sensory branch of UN	Median third web space fascicle to ulnar sensory branch to palm

ECRB, extensor carpi radialis brevis; FCR, flexor carpi radialis; FCU, flexor carpi ulnaris; FDP, flexor digitorum profundus; FDS, flexor digitorum superficialis; FPL, flexor pollicis longus; MCN, musculocutaneous nerve; PIN, posterior interosseous nerve; PL, palmaris longus; PQ, pronator quadratus; PT, pronator teres.

Table 23.4 Common tendon transfers for radial nerve palsy

Function (recipient)	Tubiana	Brand/Starr	Boyes
Finger extension (EDC)	FCU	FCR	FDS IV (through interosseous membrane IOM)
Thumb extension (EPL)	PL	PL	FDS III to EPL & EIP (through IOM) FCR to APL & EPB
Wrist extension (ECRB)	PT	PT	PT

EDC, extensor digitorum communis; ECRB, extensor carpi radialis brevis; EIP, extensor indicis proprius ; EPB, extensor pollicis brevis; EPL, extensor pollicis longus; FCR, flexor carpi radialis; FCU, flexor carpi ulnaris; FDS, flexor digitorum superficialis; PL, palmaris longus; PT, pronator teres.

iii. FCR and PT also affected but wrist flexion and pronation still possible with FCU and pronator quadratus (PQ)

2. What is available?
   a. Nerve transfer (**Table 23.3**): To restore sensation for pinch. Musculocutaneous nerve (MCN) or radial nerve ECRB or supinator branches transfer to AIN for flexion of thumb and index fingers
   b. Tendon transfer (**Table 23.5**):
      i. For thumb to index pinch:
         (a) Index flexion: ECRL to FDP II transfer. Tenodesis of FDP II to FDP III and IV at flexor zone V
         (b) Thumb flexion: BR to FPL. Tension is set such that wrist extension will cause the desired flexion of the thumb and the thumb pulp will touch the radial side of the index middle phalanx
      ii. Opposition:
         (a) Is a composite of thumb abduction, flexion, and pronation
         (b) The trajectory of transfer changes depending on prioritized motion.
            1. Transfers proximal to pisiform allow more abduction (moves thumb out of the plane of the hand) than flexion or pronation
            2. Transfers near or distal to the pisiform allow more thumb flexion and pronation than abduction
         (c) Four common transfers for opposition:
            1. Burkhalter: EIP to APB insertion
            2. Royles: FDS IV to EPL and APB
            3. Camitz: PL to APB
            4. Huber: Abductor digiti minimi to APB

Low median nerve palsy

1. What is needed:
   a. Sensation in the three radial fingers
   b. Motor: Thumb opposition
2. What is available?
   a. Nerve transfer (**Table 23.3**)
      i. To restore sensation for pinch
      ii. If intact, AIN to the PQ branch can be used to power recurrent motor branch to the thenar muscles
   b. Tendon transfer (**Table 23.5**)
      i. Opposition: As in high median nerve palsy
      ii. Adjuncts: Littler neurovascular island flap from ring finger (RF) for sensate thumb tip

Ulnar nerve palsy

High ulnar nerve palsy

1. What is needed?
   a. Sensory: Ulnar border and dorsum of the hand, little finger pulp
   b. Motor:
      i. Ring finger and long finger distal interphalangeal joint (DIPJ) flexion (FDP IV and V): Absence of which may delay or mask a claw deformity
      ii. Pinch: Thumb adduction (adductor pollicis) and index abduction (first dorsal interosseous)
      iii. MCPJ stabilization/claw correction (third and fourth lumbricals, all interossei)
         (a) The claw deformity (Duchenne sign) progressively develops as a result of the unopposed action of long extensor on the MCPJ when the intrinsic muscles are paralyzed. The disability arises due to the inability of the index to little fingers to sequentially flex from the MCPJs first then the PIPJs and lastly DIPJs. The IPJs will flex first. Hyperextension of the MCPJs will push the object out of the hand instead of allowing it to grasp the object (**Figure 23.17**)
         (b) Bouvier maneuver (**Figure 23.18**):
            1. If the patient can actively extend his PIPJs with MCPJ stabilization (Bouvier negative), procedures to stabilize the MCPJ would be sufficient.

Table 23.5 Common tendon transfers for median nerve palsy

Function	Donors	Alternatives
Opposition		
Abduction (APB) Abduction & pronation (APB & EPB)	PL (Camitz)	ADM (Huber)
	EIP (Burkhalter) if PL absent	FDS IV (Royles)
Thumb IPJ flexion (FPL)	BR	
Finger flexion		
FDP II	ECRL	Tenodesis with FDP III & IV
FDP III	Tenodesis to FDP IV at flexor zone V	

APB, abductor pollicis brevis; BR, brachioradialis; ECRL, extensor carpi radialis longus; EIP, extensor indicis proprius; EPB, extensor pollicis brevis; FDP, flexor digitorum profundus; FDS, flexor digitorum superficialis; FPL, flexor pollicis longus; IPJ, interphalangeal joint; PL, palmaris longus.

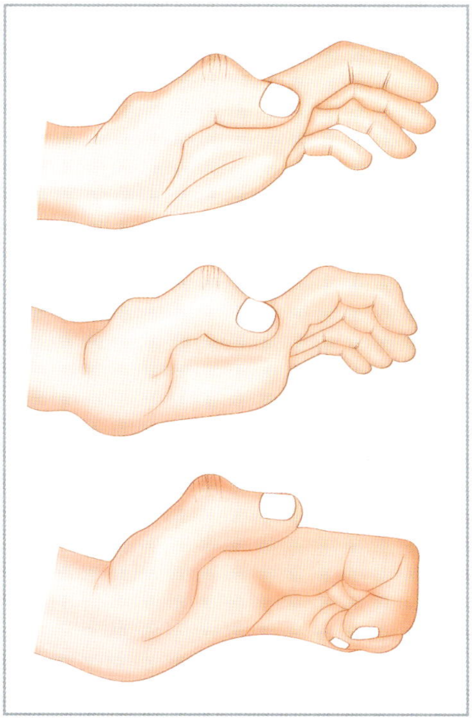

Figure 23.17 Claw disability.

a. These include static procedures to produce MCPJ flexion (dermodesis, Zancolli capsulodesis, combination of both or bone block). Static correction corrects the deformity but does not restore sequential finger flexion. It also stretches out with repeated stress and time. They are useful when extrinsic extensors are weak or when there are not enough donor tendons available for rebalancing the hand
b. Dynamic procedures such as ECRL or FDS III/IV to A1 pulley are required in patients who need a strong grip. Tendon transfers correct the deformity and the disability and hence are recommended when there are normal extrinsic muscles available as donors

2. If patient cannot extend PIPJs with MCPJ stabilized (Bouvier positive), check whether there is a PIPJ flexion contracture.
   a. If the PIPJ can be passively extended, then one can proceed with dynamic procedures and insert the donor tendon slips to the lateral bands (extensor hood) to augment extrinsic extension force and allow PIPJ extension. If a stronger motor is needed, use ECRL with grafts
   b. If there is fixed flexion contracture, correct the contracture first by splinting or surgical release.
   c. It is recommended include all four fingers when performing transfers for claw correction because of the progressive nature of the deformity

iv. Little finger (LF) adduction (third palmar interosseous): Wartenberg correction
v. FCU: Wrist flexion is still possible if FCR (median nerve) is intact

2. What is available?
   a. Nerve transfer (**Table 23.3**)

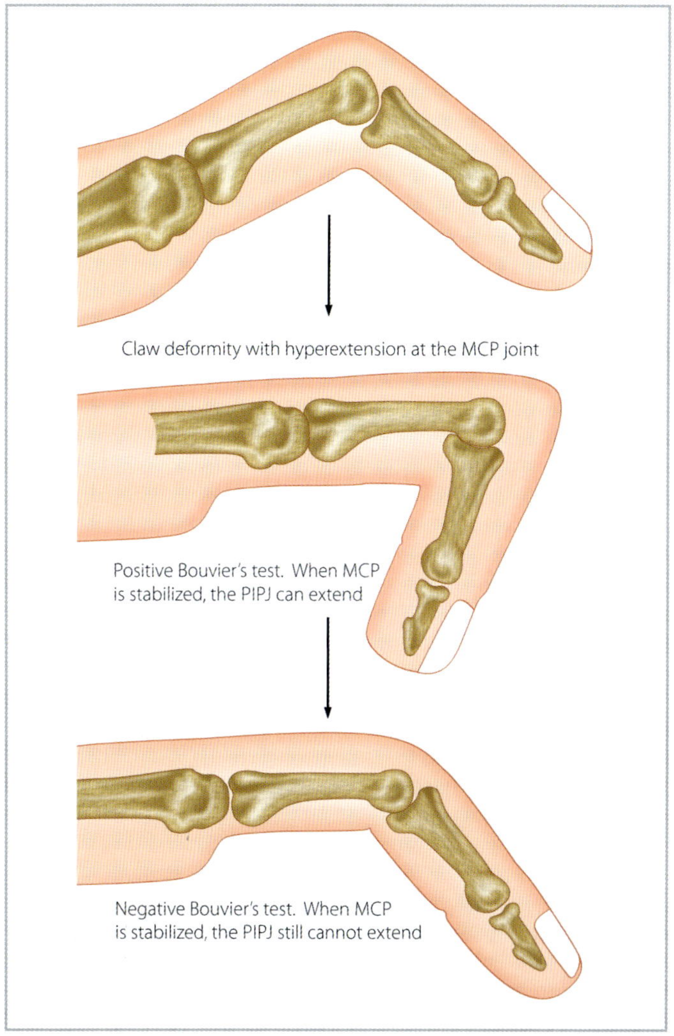

Figure 23.18 Bouvier maneuver. (a) Claw deformity with hyperextension at the MCPJ. (b) Positive Bouvier test. When MCPJ is stabilized, the PIPJ can extend. (c) Negative Bouvier test. When MCPJ is stabilized the PIPJ cannot extend.

      i. Provides sensation
      ii. Primary transfer of AIN (PQ) to deep motor branch of the ulnar nerve for intrinsic muscle function is advised if injury is near or above the elbow
   b. Tendon transfer (**Table 23.6**)
      i. For ring and little finger flexion: Tenodesis of FDP IV&V to FDP III with horizontal mattress sutures at the wrist (flexor zone V). This is performed with the wrist in neutral and the fingers held approximating a normal cascade
      ii. Restoration of pinch
         a. For thumb adduction
            1. Smith: ECRB transfer: Preserves FDS for finger flexion
            2. Abreu: EIP transfer: The distal harvest of EIP results in extension lag of the PIPJ/MCPJ
         b. For index abduction
            1. If the extensor hood is not repaired adequately
               a. Bunnell: EIP
               b. Bruner: extensor pollicis brevis (EPB)
      iii. For correction of claw deformity
         a. Remember to address any joint contracture first

Table 23.6 Common tendon transfers for ulnar nerve palsy

Function	Donors /motors			
RF & LF DIPJ flexion				
FDP IV & V	Tenodesis to FDP III proximal to carpal tunnel (flexor zone IV) in high ulnar nerve deficit			
Pinch				
Thumb adduction (AdP)	Smith ECRB + tendon graft for high ulnar deficit	Littler FDS IV for low ulnar deficit	Abreu EIP	
Index finger abduction (1st dorsal interosseous)	Bunnell EIP	Bruner EPB		
MCPJ stabilization /claw correction				
A1 /A1+A2a pulley	FDS III for high ulnar and FDS IV for low ulnar deficit (Zancolli)		Brand ECRL + tendon graft	
Lateral band	FDS III for high ulnar and FDS IV for low ulnar deficit (Stiles –Bunnell)		Brand ECRL + tendon graft	
LF adduction				
3rd palmar interosseous	Ulnar half EDC IV to intrinsic expansion (radial side) of LF extensor hood		Ulnar half of EDM to radial collateral ligament of MCPJ LF	

DIPJ, distal interphalangeal joint; ECRB, extensor carpi radialis brevis; ECRL, extensor carpi radialis longus; EDC, extensor digitorum communis; EIP, extensor indicis proprius; EPB, extensor pollicis brevis; FDS, flexor digitorum superficialis; FDP, flexor digitorum profundus; MCPJ, metacarpophalangeal joint.

b. Static
  1. Dermodesis: Involves excising 1.5-cm ellipse of skin over the palmar crease and creating a surgical flexion contracture
  2. Zancolli capsulodesis: Distally based U flap of volar plate is advanced proximally and secured with mini Mitek suture anchor at the neck of the metacarpal
  3. Metacarpal head dorsal bone block – for long established intrinsic minus hand. Usually performed after dorsal capsulotomy of the MCPJ in patients with fixed hyperextension deformity
  4. MCPJ fusion with plates or *Kirschner* (K)-wires.

c. Dynamic
  1. FDS III for MCPJ stabilization. Named according to insertion described:
     (a) A1 pulley/A1 and A2a pulleys – Zancolli
     (b) Lateral bands – Stiles – Bunnell
     (c) Proximal phalanx – Burkhalter (technically demanding and acts as a pure MCPJ flexor)
     (d) Complications of FDS transfer include the following:
        i. Swan neck deformity – 15%
        ii. Isolated mallet deformity – 29%
        iii. PIPJ flexion contracture – 26%
        iv. Insufficient finger flexion – 18%
  2. Brand transfer – ECRL + tendon graft to A1 pulley or lateral bands
  3. Both flexor and extensor routes are described. Extensor route is prone to adhesions as tendons pass through the interosseous membrane but is useful if there is extensive scarring and tissue loss on the flexor side of the forearm

iv. For long finger adduction:
  a. Ulnar half EDC IV to intrinsic expansion (radial side) of long finger extensor hood
  b. Ulnar half of extensor digiti minimi (EDM) cut and dissected 2–3 cm proximally, passed under EDM and EDC V to phalangeal attachment of the radial collateral ligament of MCPJ

Low ulnar nerve palsy

1. What is needed?
   a. Sensory: little finger pulp
   b. Motor:
      i. Pinch: Thumb adduction (adductor pollicis) and index abduction (first dorsal interosseous)
      ii. MCPJ stabilization/claw correction (third and fourth lumbricals, all interossei)
      iii. Long finger adduction (third palmar interosseous): Wartenberg correction
2. What is available?
   a. Nerve transfer for sensation (**Table 23.3**)
   b. Tendon transfer (**Table 23.6**)
      i. Restoration of pinch
         (a) For thumb adduction
            1. Littler: FDS IV is recommended since FDP IV is intact
            2. Smith: ECRB + tendon graft
         (b) For index abduction
            1. Bunnell: EIP
            2. Bruner: EPB
      ii. For correction of claw deformity
         (a) Static
            1. Zancolli capsulodesis ± dermodesis
         (b) Dynamic
            1. FDS transfer – FDS IV is the preferred donor when FDP IV is intact because FDS III contributes to strength of a chuck grip
            2. Brand transfer – ECRL + tendon graft to A1 pulley/lateral bands is recommended for patients with supple fingers
      iii. For long finger adduction:
         (a) Half EDC IV to intrinsic expansion of LF extensor hood
         (b) Ulnar half of EDM to RCL of MCPJ LF

Combined nerve palsies

Same prerequisites apply. There are limited donor muscles. Additional muscle units can be freed as donors by fusing joints.

Ulnar and median deficit

High ulnar and median deficit

1. What is needed?
   a. Sensory – palmar sensation: Because of abnormal palmar sensation, this hand will not be used for precision activities. Focus should be on improving simple grasp and pinch. First web space span should be maintained with splints
   b. Motor – thumb and index pinch (AdP and first dorsal interosseous, FPL and FDP), long finger adduction (third palmar interosseous), thumb abduction (APB), sequential finger flexion (lumbricals, interossei, and FDPs, FPL) and wrist flexor (FCU).
2. What is available? Only radial nerve powered muscles and their nerves are available. MCN branch to brachialis can also be used for transfer.
   a. Nerve transfer
   b. Tendon transfer (**Table 23.7**)
      i. Sensory: LABC nerve to dorsal branch of the ulnar nerve, SRN to median nerve common branch to first web space, and radial digital nerve to thumb
      ii. Motor: Radial ECRB branch to median PT, radial supinator branch to median AIN

Low ulnar and median deficit – most common combined palsy

1. What is needed?
   a. Sensory: Palmar sensation for pinch
   b. Motor: Thumb and index pinch (adductor pollicis and first dorsal interosseous, FPL and FDP2), long finger adduction (third palmar interosseous), claw correction (lumbricals and interossei), thumb abduction (APB)
   c. Keep first web space open with splints
2. What is available?
   a. Nerve transfer
      i. Sensory: SRN to median nerve common branch to first web space and radial digital nerve to thumb. Dorsal cutaneous branch of the ulnar nerve may also be used as donor
      ii. Motor – AIN (PQ) to deep motor branch of ulnar nerve
   b. Tendon transfer (**Table 23.7**)

Radial and ulnar deficits

1. What is needed?
   a. Sensory: Long finger pulp, ulnar border, radial dorsum of hand
   b. Motor: Wrist and finger extension (ECRB, EDC, EPL), thumb and index pinch (adductor pollicis), claw correction (lumbricals and interossei), ring and little finger flexion (FDP IV and V)
   c. This has better function because significant palmar sensation is preserved. However, reconstruction involves restoring antagonistic actions like finger extension and flexion. Staged surgery is recommended, restoring extension first, then flexion (claw correction, ring and long finger flexion)
2. What is available?
   a. Nerve transfer
      i. Sensory: LABC to SRN or dorsal sensory branch of ulnar nerve and median third web space fascicle to ulnar sensory branch to palm
      ii. Motor: Median branch to FCR (FCU intact) and PL to PIN and AIN (PQ) to deep motor branch of ulnar nerve
   b. Tendon transfer (**Table 23.8**)

Median and radial nerve deficits

The most difficult to treat.

1. What is needed?
   a. Sensory: Palmar sensation for pinch
   b. Motor: Wrist and finger extension (ECRB, EDC, EPL), thumb abduction (APB), thumb, index, and middle finger flexion (FDP II, III, FPL)
   c. This hand functions like a biological prosthesis. There are not enough available donor muscles
2. What is available?
   a. Nerve transfer
      i. Sensory: Ulnar common digital nerve to fourth web space to median common digital nerve to first web space and radial digital nerve thumb
      ii. Motor: MCN branch to brachialis (biceps intact) to AIN, ulnar branch to FCU to PIN with wrist fusion
   b. Tendon transfer (**Table 23.9**)
      i. Given lack of donor muscles, split FCU transfer is most useful

Table 23.7 Summary of tendon transfers for combined median and ulnar nerve palsy

Function (recipient)	High palsy donor	Low palsy donor
Thumb adduction (AdP)	Smith ECRB + tendon graft	Littler FDS IV
Index finger abduction (1st dorsal interosseous)	Bruner EPB	Bruner EPB
MCPJ stabilization (claw correction)	Tenodesis with graft (deep transverse metacarpal ligament to extensor apparatus) or Zancolli capsulodesis or ECU + tendon graft transfer if wrist is fused	Brand ECRL + tendon graft or FDS IV
LF adduction (3rd palmar interosseous)	Ulnar half of EDM to radial collateral ligament of MCPJ LF	Ulnar half of EDM to radial collateral ligament of MCPJ LF
Opposition (APB)	EIP	EIP
Thumb flexion (FPL)	BR + MCPJ fusion	Intact
Finger flexion (FDP x4)	ECRL	Intact
Wrist flexion (FCU)	None /fuse	Intact

BR, brachioradialis; ECRB, extensor carpi radialis brevis; ECRL, extensor carpi radialis longus; ECU, extensor carpi ulnaris; EDM, extensor digiti minimi; EIP, extensor indicis proprius; EPB, extensor pollicis brevis; FCU, flexor carpi ulnaris; FDP, flexor digitorum profundus; FDS, flexor digitorum superficialis; FPL; flexor pollicis longus; MCPJ, metacarpophalangeal joint.

Table 23.8 Summary of tendon transfers for combined radial and ulnar nerve palsy

Function (recipient)	Donor	Alternative
Wrist extension (ECRB)	PT	
Finger extension (EDC)	Boyes FDS III	FDS II
Thumb extension (EPL)	PL	FDS III
Thumb adduction (AdP)	Littler FDS IV + MCPJ fusion	
MCPJ stabilization (claw correction)	Zancolli capsulodesis or tenodesis with graft (deep transverse metacarpal ligament to extensor apparatus) or	PL to A1/A2a pulleys or lateral bands or
Finger flexion (FDP IV & V)	Tenodesis to FDP III at flexor zone V	
Wrist flexion (FCU)		PL to FCU insertion

ECRB, extensor carpi radialis brevis; EDC, extensor digitorum communis; EPL, extensor pollicis longus; FCU, flexor carpi ulnaris; FDP, flexor digitorum profundus; FDS, flexor digitorum superficialis; MCPJ, metacarpophalangeal joint; PL, palmaris longus.

Table 23.9 Summary of tendon transfers for combined radial and median nerve palsy

Function (recipient)	Donor	Alternative
Wrist extension (ECRB)	Wrist fusion	
Finger extension (EDC)	Split FCU	
Thumb extension (EPL)	Split FCU	
Opposition (APB)	Huber AdM	
Thumb flexion (FPL)	Tenodesis of FPL across IPJ or Thumb IPJ fusion	FDP V
Finger flexion (FDP II, III)	Tenodesis to FDP IV & V at flexor zone V	
Forearm pronation	Biceps rerouting around radius	

ECRB, extensor carpi radialis brevis; EDC, extensor digitorum communis; EPL, extensor pollicis longus; FCU, flexor carpi ulnaris; FDP, flexor digitorum profundus; IPJ, interphalangeal joint.

SUGGESTED READING

Brandsma JW, Ottenhoff-de Jonge MW. Flexor digitorum superficialis tendon transfer for intrinsic replacement. Long term results and the effect on donor fingers. J Hand Surg 1992; 17B:625–628.

The authors reviewed 127 hands that underwent FDS transfer and documented donor finger deficits encountered. They also discussed in detail possible causes of these deformities.

Lim AYT, Kumar VP, Pereira BP, Hua J. Independent function in a tendon transfer of the split flexor carpi ulnaris. Plast Reconstr Surg 1999; 104:1739–1741.

Independent thumb and finger extension was described in a patient who had a split FCU transfer after loss of extensor muscles in an avulsion injury of the forearm.

Pereira BP, Kumar VP, Lim AYT, Tan JAC, Tan BL. Properties of the two neuromuscular compartments in a split bipennate muscle. J Orthop Res 2004; 22:1325–1330.

This experiment on in situ FCU muscles of monkeys showed that once split distally into humeral and ulnar components, each unit was capable of independent contraction upon stimulation of their innervating nerve branch.

23.4 NEONATAL BRACHIAL PLEXUS PALSY

Neonatal brachial plexus palsy (NBPP) has a frequency of 0.63–2.6 per 1000 live births. The incidence of NBPP has remained relatively stable despite awareness of the problem and improved obstetric techniques. NBPP can be divided into two broad groups based on the age at presentation. One group includes children who present in infancy (early NBPP) and are suitable for microsurgical nerve reconstruction surgery. The other group presents later in life with sequelae or deformity (late NBPP). These patients are no longer suitable for nerve reconstruction procedures, and treatment consists of secondary procedures to improve or enhance shoulder, elbow, forearm, and hand function.

EARLY NBPP

Risk factors

The risk factors include macrosomia, multiparous pregnancies, previous deliveries resulting in NBPP, prolonged labor, breech delivery, assisted delivery (vacuum or forceps), cephalopelvic disproportion, gestational diabetes, and shoulder dystocia.

Classification

The severity of the NBPP can range from a neurapraxia type of injury, which may resolve without any deficit within 3 weeks, to an avulsion of the nerve root that has no potential for spontaneous recovery. Narakas and others have graded NBPP into four groups, with each succeeding group representing a more severe injury. Groups 1 and 2 account for 73% of NBPP patients, whereas groups 3 and 4 account for 20–25% of patients.

- Group 1 infants have involvement of the C5 and C6 roots and represent the classic Erb-Duchenne palsy. The important muscles that derive their innervation solely from the C5 and C6 roots include abductors and external rotators of the shoulder (supraspinatus, infraspinatus, and deltoid), flexors of the elbow (biceps brachii, brachialis, and coracobrachialis), and the supinator muscle. Therefore, infants with Erb palsy lack shoulder abduction and external rotation, elbow flexion, and forearm supination. However, they have good hand and wrist function
- Group 2 infants have involvement of the C7 root in addition to the C5 and C6 (extended Erb palsy). This leads to paralysis of the subscapularis, teres major, clavicular fibers of the pectoralis major, BR, ECRL and ECRB, and occasionally the ECU and EDC. These infants have good flexion of the wrist and digits but lack extension. These deficits combined with the impairment caused by the C5 and C6 palsy leads to the classic 'waiter's tip' posture, which results from loss of bicep function to flex the elbow and to supinate the forearm
- Group 3 infants have involvement of all roots (C5–T1) and present with a flail extremity
- Group 4 infants have, in addition to involvement of all roots, injury to the second-order preganglionic sympathetic fibers. These fibers exit the spinal cord at the level of the T1 and enter the cervical sympathetic chain, where they are in close proximity to the lower roots of the brachial plexus (C8, T1). This results in a constellation of signs (ptosis, myosis, enophthalmos, and anhydrosis) on the ipsilateral side of the face, better known as Horner syndrome (**Figure 23.19**) after Johann Friedrich Horner, the Swiss ophthalmologist who first described the syndrome in 1869

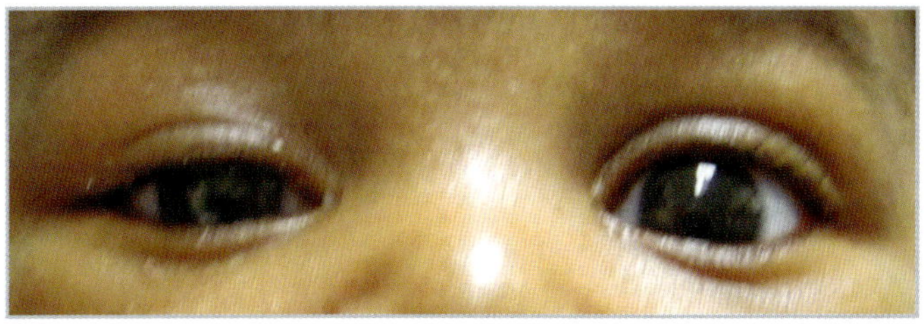

Figure 23.19 Horner syndrome

Rarely, only the lower roots (C8–T1) may be involved (Klumpke palsy). These infants have good shoulder and elbow function but poor hand function.

Natural history

The potential for recovery decreases with an increase in extent and severity of the injury. A detailed prospective study by Gilbert and Tassin reported the following results:

- Group 1 NBPP: Ninety percent of patients progressed to full spontaneous recovery if there were clinical signs of recovery (presence of elbow flexion with elbow, wrist, thumb, and finger extension) before 2 months of age
- Group 2 NBPP: Sixty-five percent of patients recovered fully, but the remainder had persisting defects in shoulder and elbow movement. The timing of recovery of this group of patients is delayed with clinical signs of recovery not evident until 3–6 months of age
- Group 3 NBPP: Less than 50% recover fully spontaneously, with the majority of patients disabled by significant deficits of movement throughout the arm; in approximately 25% of patients, even wrist and finger extension remain functionally compromised
- Group 4 NBPP: Patients have little if any chance for a full spontaneous recovery and most will have a complete neurologic deficit of motor and sensory function in the affected arm

Clinical evaluation

History

A detailed maternal, obstetric, and perinatal history is required, inquiring about the following: previous pregnancies and deliveries, history of any systemic illness, such as maternal diabetes, duration of labor as well as the method of delivery. The history should also include information regarding the child's early postnatal period (birth weight, any respiratory difficulties or intensive care treatment, feeding ability, fractures, presence of paralysis or neurological disorders (e.g. Horner syndrome), and signs of recovery from neurological symptoms if present).

Examination

The aim of the initial examination in early NBPP is to answer the following questions:

1. Does the child have any other pathology other than the affected arm?
2. Is there Horner syndrome?
3. What group is the injury (Group 1–4)?

The initial examination should include

- Examination of the head, neck, trunk, lower limbs, and unaffected upper limb

  - Head: Shape and size
  - Eyes: Conjugate movements, Horner syndrome
  - Neck: Control in supported sitting and prone positions, range limitations actively or passively, pseudotumor (it is a palpable mass in the sternocleidomastoid (SCM) associated with an abnormal head posture and restricted neck movements. It is one of the differential diagnoses for congenital muscular torticollis, and one hypothesis suggests birth trauma as a causative factor)
  - Chest: Respiratory pattern, chest movement symmetry
  - Abdomen: Symmetrical diaphragmatic movement
  - Legs: Range of motion, tone, movement pattern
  - Unaffected arm: Range of motion passively and actively, strength
- Examination of the affected upper limb
  - Resting position (attitude)
  - Appearance
    - Shorter and thinner arm with extra skin folds
    - Deep axilla that may indicate a possibility of shoulder subluxation
    - Check for fractures by palpating the clavicles, humerus, and ribs
    - Palpate the humeral head in the posterior soft spot under the acromion to check for glenohumeral subluxation or dislocation
  - Active range of motion in supine and sitting or supported sitting position. The baby should be encouraged to reach for toys while lying on the side, supine, and sitting. It is important to compare the active range of motion of the injured with the noninjured arm
  - Passive range of motion: This should be performed at the end of the examination as the child may cry with manipulation of his/her arm and refuse to cooperate with the rest of the clinical examination
  - Strength: In a young child or an infant, manual muscle testing is not feasible because it requires voluntary cooperation. The MRC scale for measuring muscle strength has a limited application in infants who cannot follow commands to produce voluntary actions. The active movement scale proposed by Curtis allows assessment of motor function in infants. The Mallet score is useful in the assessment of shoulder and elbow function in children >3 years of age. The Raimondi scale can be used for evaluation of hand function
  - Evidence of pain (look for scars or wounds over the affected extremity that may signal the inability of the child to feel pain)
- Examination of infant reflexes: Absent or inadequate infantile reflexes on one side in infants (<3–4 months) suggest a disorder of the motor system such as a brachial plexus palsy or hemiplegia
  - Moro reflex: It is characterized by abduction of the arms followed by adduction and crying in response to a sudden loss of support
  - Asymmetric tonic neck reflex: When the face is turned to one side, the arm and leg on that side extend and the arm and leg on the contralateral side flex
- Observation of feeding: Sucking, swallowing
- Observation of interaction with environment: Vision, hearing, and touch

Once the severity of the injury has been established, the aim of the follow-up examinations is to determine the extent of recovery (if any) of muscle function. This will aid in surgical decision making. The recovery of biceps function is usually used as an indicator of likelihood of spontaneous recovery. The 'cookie test' can be used to assess biceps function in 6–9-month-old infants with NBPP. A cookie is placed in the child's hand on the affected side and the child's affected arm should be gently held adducted against the trunk to isolate elbow flexion. The test is considered normal if the cookie can reach the toddler's mouth with <45° of neck flexion.

Investigations

Radiographic imaging

- X-rays: Radiographic imaging is used in the first days postpartum to exclude fractures in the shoulder region and the presence of a diaphragmatic asymmetry caused by phrenic nerve paresis. It can also be used to check for evidence of shoulder subluxation, as there is an 8% prevalence of posterior shoulder dislocation with NBPP before the age of 1
- Computed tomographic (CT) scan: It is not useful in the acute stage. In babies who do not show sufficient neurological recovery by the third month, a CT-myelogram can be performed to exclude root avulsions
- MRI: Similar to the CT scan. It can show pseudomeningoceles that signal root avulsion and is less invasive than a CT-myelogram. However, a child would still need sedation for an MRI or a CT study to be completed. MRI is also useful for evaluating glenohumeral joint congruency and the degree of subluxation to direct further shoulder management

Ultrasonographic and electrodiagnostic investigations

- Ultrasonography: Helps in evaluating the position and congruency of an unossified shoulder joint that cannot be otherwise evaluated by standard radiographs. In addition, it allows dynamic evaluation of the shoulder to assess whether the subluxation is reducible. It can also help in the diagnosis of entrapment of the radial nerve in an associated humeral shaft fracture
- Electrodiagnostic studies: These are not necessary in the acute setting. It may have a role in estimating the prognosis of a child's neurological and functional recovery. It is important to remember that sensory and motor nerve responses (amplitudes and distal latencies) in an infant are approximately 50% of that of an adult

Treatment

Nonsurgical treatment

- Therapy: The parents and caregivers should be the child's primary therapist. The goal is to maintain a full passive range of motion at all joints, especially shoulder external rotation (in both abduction and adduction) and forearm pronation and supination. The child is encouraged to use the involved arm by restraining the unaffected arm to promote cortical recognition and integration of the affected limb
- Splints: Splinting is used during sleep and to protect floppy joints. An intrinsic plus splint is indicated in patients with involvement of the lower roots

Surgical treatment

- Indications
  - Group 4 infants (flail arm with Horner syndrome)
  - Group 3 infants (flail arm) with no recovery of biceps by 3 months
  - Group 1 and 2 infants with no recovery of shoulder external rotation and elbow flexion/forearm supination by 4–6 months
- Reconstructive priority: Unlike adult brachial plexus injury, in which the priority for primary reconstruction is elbow flexion,

followed by shoulder function, and finally hand function, restoration of hand function is the primary priority in NBPP. This is because of the shorter distance for nerve regeneration, superior neuroregenerative capacity, and central nervous system (CNS) plasticity in infants. The order of priority in NBPP includes

- Hand grasp
- Elbow flexion
- Shoulder function
- Elbow, wrist, and finger extension

- Surgical options: The treatment options available for early NBPP include excision of neuroma and interpositional nerve grafting, neurolysis of neuroma, and nerve transfers (intraplexal and extraplexal). The most common lesion seen in NBPP is a neuroma in continuity, and the preferred treatment is an excision of the neuroma and interpositional nerve grafting (± an intraplexal nerve transfer). The usual source for nerve grafts are the sural nerves that may be required to be harvested bilaterally. A neurolysis is considered in patients with partial recovery who show some fascicular continuity within the neuroma. An extraplexal nerve transfer is considered in infants with avulsion of the proximal roots. Depending on the severity of the injury, different combinations of procedures are possible.
  - Group 1 and 2 infants (C5, C6 ± C7): A neuroma in continuity of the C5 and C6 roots is the most common presentation in NBPP. This is usually treated by excision of the neuroma and connecting multiple sural nerve grafts from the proximal end of the C5 and C6 roots to the suprascapular nerve (SSN) (intraplexal transfer) and the anterior and posterior divisions of the upper trunk (**Figure 23.20**). If the proximal roots are not available due to an avulsion type injury, an extraplexal nerve transfer can be considered. These include the transfer of the spinal accessory nerve (SAN) to the SSN; medial pectoral nerve to the MCN; or the Oberlin transfer (ulnar nerve fascicle to MCN)
  - Groups 3 and 4 (C5–T1): The usual injury pattern is a rupture of the C5 and C6 roots and avulsion of the C7, C8, and T1 roots. Sural nerve grafts are used to bridge the proximal C5 and C6 roots to the middle and lower trunks to restore hand function. Extraplexal nerve transfers are used to restore elbow flexion (intercostal nerves to MCN) and shoulder function (SAN to SSN).

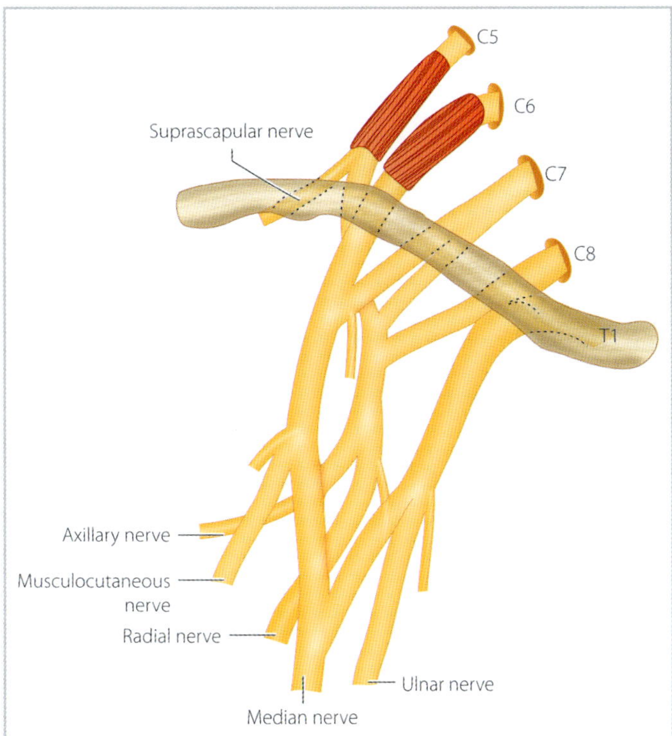

Figure 23.20 Sural nerve grafting after excision of C5-C6 neuroma in continuity.

LATE NBPP

Etiology

- Degree of muscle recovery: This contributes to the development of secondary deformities. Three types of muscle impairment can be seen after recovery: (1) paresis (incomplete recovery with weak motor strength), (2) paralysis (no recovery with atrophy), and (3) cocontraction (simultaneous contraction of different muscles - coactivation by simultaneous nerve inputs). Cocontractions can cause functional impairment, if these muscles are antagonistic. Although paresis and palsy are seen both in the adult and obstetric plexus lesion, cocontraction is a problem limited to late NBPP
- Associated bone, joint, and soft tissue injuries
  - Epiphysiolysis of proximal humerus, fracture of the clavicle
  - Anterior subcoracoid dislocation of the shoulder
  - Fibrosis of the shoulder girdle muscles/SCM/Biceps after birth trauma
- Poor initial treatment
  - Forced manipulation to correct contractures
  - Casts or splints in exaggerated position of abduction and external rotation
  - Delay in surgical correction of muscular contractures leading to articular deformity and joint displacement

Common secondary deformities

Proximal musculature (shoulder and elbow) recovers earlier and more completely than distal musculature (forearm and hand). Therefore, deformities and contractures due to muscle imbalance and aberrant reinnervation are more common in the shoulder and elbow compared with the forearm and hand. Based on a relatively large series of 148 patients, Zancolli et al. listed the following as common secondary deformities following NBPP.

- Internal rotation contracture of the shoulder (72%)
- Flexion contracture of the elbow (62%)
- Supination contracture of the forearm (69%)
- Pronation contracture of the forearm (29%)
- Ulnar deviation of the wrist (27%)
- Varying types of finger paralysis

Pathogenesis

- Internal rotation contracture of the shoulder: This results from an imbalance between the strength of the relatively unaffected internal rotators, which are the latissimus dorsi, subscapularis, teres major and teres minor, and the paralytic external rotators (infraspinatus)
- Elbow flexion contracture: The pathophysiology of the elbow flexion contracture is poorly understood. It is believed to be a combination of muscle imbalance (biceps recovery with weak or

absent triceps), postural secondary to a shoulder internal rotation contracture where the patient stands with a slightly abducted shoulder with resultant flexion of the elbow, or due to trauma during birth and subsequent biceps fibrosis.

- Forearm supination contracture: These contractures result from unopposed action of the supinator muscles, namely, the biceps (C5,6) and supinator (C5,6) in the presence of paralytic pronators, namely, the PT (C6,7), and PQ (C7,8T1). It is seen in NBPP groups 2, 3, and 4, who have had recovery of their C5,6 function.
- Forearm pronation contracture: This results from unopposed action of the pronators in the presence of paralytic supinators. It is seen in NBPP group 1 (Erb palsy) children, who have had no or partial recovery of their C5,6 roots.
- Ulnar deviation of the wrist: The ulnar deviation of the wrist results from muscle imbalance produced by paralysis of the ECRB and ECRL (C6,7), FCR (C6,7) in relation to the unopposed activity of the ECU (C7,8), and the FCU (C8T1)

Clinical evaluation

The aims of clinical evaluation in late NBPP are:

- To identify the deformities
- To determine the severity of the deformities (flexible or fixed)
  - Active and passive range of motion
  - Condition of soft tissues (skin and musculotendinous units)
  - Condition of joints [enlocated/subluxed/dislocated (reducible/irreducible)]
- To determine the strength of active muscles
- To understand the goals and concerns of the child and the family

The clinical examination of the upper limb should include

- Shoulder
  - Attitude
  - Range of motion (active and passive)
    - Shoulder abduction, flexion, and extension
    - Internal and external rotation in abduction and adduction while stabilizing the scapula
  - Muscle strength grading (shoulder abductors/internal and external rotators)
  - Muscle tightness
    - Subscapularis (measure scapulohumeral angle in abduction with scapula stabilized)
    - Pectoralis, latissimus dorsi, and teres (palpation of muscle in abduction and external rotation)
  - Presence of cocontraction
    - Between shoulder abductors and adductors
    - Between elbow flexors (biceps) and shoulder abductors (deltoid) (Trumpet sign)
  - Presence of scapular winging
  - Glenohumeral joint: Look for posterior humeral head dislocation (loss of external rotation between examinations; if reducible, range of external rotation improves with reduction)
- Elbow
  - Attitude
  - Range of motion (active and passive)
    - Flexion and extension
  - Muscle strength grading (biceps and triceps)
  - Muscle tightness (biceps, brachialis, and triceps)
  - Presence of cocontraction (between elbow flexors and extensors)
  - Assess elbow joint: Look for subluxation/dislocation of the proximal end of the radius/ulna
- Forearm
  - Attitude
  - Range of motion (active and passive)
    - Pronation and supination
  - Assess proximal and distal radioulnar joints and look for subluxation/dislocation
- Wrist and hand
  - Attitude
  - Range of motion (active and passive)
    - Wrist flexion and extension
    - MCPJ (Thumb and fingers)
  - Muscle strength
    - FCU/FCR/ECU/ECRL and ECRB

Investigations

The MRI is the best imaging modality for the assessment of secondary deformities in infants and young children, especially the predominantly cartilaginous shoulder. MRI allows assessment of glenohumeral congruency, deformity of the glenoid, and muscle mass. It allows early detection of shoulder deformities; however, it requires sedation in young children. A CT scan can be considered after puberty. Plain radiographs are adequate to assess secondary deformities around the elbow and wrist joint and to detect subluxation of the radial head or distal radioulnar joint.

Treatment

Nonsurgical treatment

- Therapy
  - Passive range of motion and stretching exercises
  - Myofascial release (osteopathic manipulative technique)
  - Promote leisure and activities of daily living
  - Constraint induced movement therapy (constrain uninvolved arm to encourage use of involved arm)
  - Splinting: Depending on the deformity, appropriate splinting can be considered. Splints include shoulder supports, pronation and supination splints, and intrinsic plus splints
- Pain management: Children with late NBPP do not have neuropathic pain. The absence of pain when the injury is distal to the dorsal ganglion has been attributed to the delayed maturation of peripheral nerves, especially at the nodes of Ranvier, leading to slower sensory and motor conduction velocities in infants (<50% of normal values at birth, progressing to normal values at ~2 years of age), and the excellent plasticity of the CNS in infants
- Botulinum toxin: There have been a number of anecdotal reports of the use of botulinum toxin type A (BTX-A) in the treatment of cocontractions. It is a reversible neurotoxin with a half-life of approximately 3 months. It is injected into the target antagonistic muscle at a total dose of 2–4 units/kg divided between multiple sites along the muscle under surface EMG guidance. It acts presynaptically by blocking the release of acetylcholine at the neuromuscular junction. The injections are repeated two or three times every 4–6 months. Good results have been reported in children with triceps cocontraction, and these results have persisted beyond the pharmacological effect of BTX-A. However BTX-A injections into the biceps, deltoid, latissimus dorsi, and pectoralis major muscles have not yielded the same success as triceps injections. It must be kept in mind that BTX-A injections may require anesthesia, present risks even with precise administration, and provide a temporary result with risk of permanent muscle weakness if the drug is administered repeatedly

Surgical treatment

- Timing: The best age for the reconstruction of late NBPP deformities is at age ≥ 4. These children are easier to evaluate, do not have severe contractures, and are able to cooperate in rehabilitation. The optimal age for shoulder and elbow reconstruction is during the preschool years (4–6 years), whereas the optimum age for forearm and hand reconstruction is during the school going years (6–13 years)
- Correction of shoulder deformities
  - Reducible glenohumeral joint
    - Release (or lengthening) of tight subscapularis, pectoralis, and anterior capsule of shoulder
    - Transfer of latissimus dorsi and teres major into rotator cuff insertion of supraspinatus to improve external rotation and abduction (**Figure 23.21**)
    - Trapezius transfer to humerus (deltoid insertion) to improve abduction
  - Incongruous/dysplastic glenohumeral joint
    - Derotation osteotomy of the humerus
- Correction of elbow deformities
  - Flexion contracture (>60°) with congruous joint
    - Release of antecubital fascia, lacertus fibrosis, and anterior capsule
  - Z-lengthening of biceps tendon, partial release of brachialis and BR, and fractional lengthening of flexor pronator mass (**Figure 23.22**)
  - Weak elbow flexion
    - MRC grade 0–1 (Steindler flexorplasty, if wrist extension and finger flexion is good; pedicled bipolar latissimus dorsi transfer or free-functioning muscle transfer, if wrist extension and finger flexion is poor)
    - MRC grade 2–3 (triceps to biceps, if triceps cocontraction present; deltoid to biceps, if deltoid cocontraction present; pectoralis major transfer or Steindler flexor plasty, if no cocontraction)
- Correction of forearm deformities
  - Supination deformity
    - Elbow joint or wrist joint congruent (biceps rerouting ± interosseous membrane release)
    - Elbow joint or wrist joint incongruous (radial head excision/Sauve-Kapandji procedure)
- Correction of wrist and hand deformities
  - Ulnar deviation deformity of the wrist:
    - FCU to ECRL transfer
    - ECU to ECRL or ECU to abductor pollicis longus transfer
    - Weak or absent wrist or finger extension:
    - Flexor to extensor transfer
    - Extensor tenodesis or application ± wrist arthrodesis
  - Weak or absent finger flexors:
    - Extensor to flexor transfer
    - Free functioning muscle transfer for FDP
  - Thumb instability:
    - Opponensplasty with FDS IV or EIP
    - Claw deformity:
    - Zancolli Lasso procedure or capsulodesis

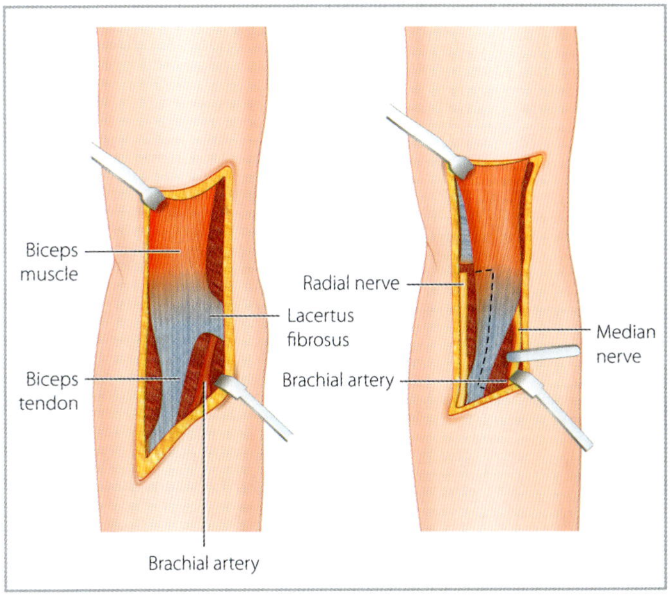

Figure 23.22 Steps in release of an elbow flexion contracture.

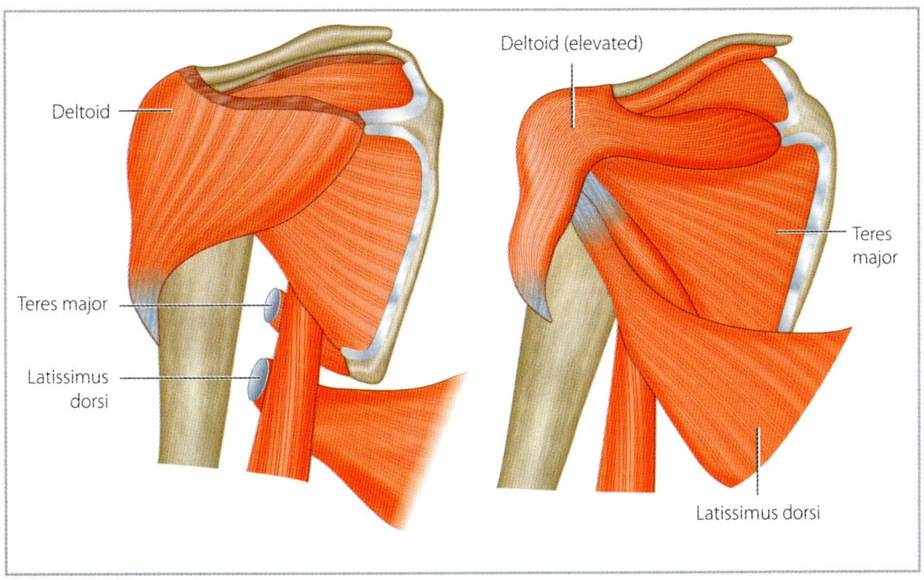

Figure 23.21 Steps in transfer of latissimus dorsi and teres major to greater tuberosity of humerus.

- Sensory reconstruction: In general, sensory disturbance of the forearm and hand does not seem to be a significant problem in most children with late NBPP. The change of limb dominance, where the injured side becomes nondominant and the excellent recovery of sensation in NBPP has been attributed to CNS plasticity in infants. Sensory neurons have a better survival rate than motor neurons and are less dependent on trophic factors from target cells for survival. In the young, sensory neurons always project to several spinal segments, in contrast to motor neurons, which are restricted to 2–3 segments. However, one must be aware that the denervated limb is at risk for self-mutilation and contact burns due to decreased sensibility and poor motor control

SUGGESTED READING

Capek L, Clarke HM, Curtis CG. Neuroma-in-continuity resection: early outcome in obstetrical brachial plexus palsy. Plast Reconstr Surg 1998; 102:1555–1562.
The authors showed that there is no significant loss of upper extremity motion after resection of neuroma-in-continuity (NIC) in obstetric palsy patients (mean age of 9 months). They did this by comparing limb motion scores of 26 patients who underwent resection and interpositional nerve grafting with 17 patients who underwent neurolysis alone at 3-, 6-, and 12-month postsurgery. Resection of NIC did result in functional loss at 3 months but both groups had improved motion scores by 6-month postsurgery.

Ezaki M, Malungpaishrope K, Harrison RJ, et al. Onabotulinum toxin A injection as an adjunct in the treatment of posterior shoulder subluxation in neonatal brachial plexus palsy. J Bone Joint Surg 2010; 15A:2171–2177.
Use of Botox to help shoulder joint reduction was shown in a cohort of 35 neonatal plexus palsy infants with posterior subluxation or dislocation of the shoulder. The infants were treated with Botox injection and casting at a mean age of 5.7 months and followed up for a minimum of 1 year (range 12–80 months). Shoulder reduction was maintained in 24 (69%) patients. There were no complications reported.

Nikolaou S, Peterson E, Kim A, Wylie C, Cornwall R. Impaired growth of denervated muscle contributes to contracture formation following neonatal brachial plexus injury. J Bone Joint Surg Am 2011; 93:461–470.
Using a mouse model (C5-C6 nerve root excised), the authors showed that after 4 weeks, the denervated subscapularis, biceps, and brachialis muscles were fibrotic with reduced cross-sectional area and longitudinal growth, causing obvious joint contractures.

Smith NC, Rowan P, Benson LJ, Ezaki M, Carter PR. Neonatal brachial plexus palsy. Outcome of absent biceps function at three months of age. J Bone Joint Surg 2004; 86A:2163–2170.
Twenty-eight babies with no biceps function at 3 months of age were followed until a mean age of 11 years. Biceps function was present by 6 months in 71% (20 babies), including all upper trunk type patients. Children who regained biceps function between 3 to 6 months of age had better shoulder abduction, hand to neck, and hand to back scores than those who regained biceps function after 6 months.

Waters PM. Comparison of the natural history, the outcomes of microsurgical repair, and the outcome of operative reconstruction in brachial plexus birth palsy. J Bone Joint Burg 1999; 81A:649–659.
In this 97 patient series by a single surgeon, outcomes were analyzed by grouping patients according to the month biceps recovery was noted. Infants who recovered biceps function on the 4th, 5th, and 6th month did not have complete neurologic recovery. Shoulder abduction, external rotation, hand-to-mouth, and hand-to-neck scores worsened with longer delay in biceps recovery.

23.5 THE SPASTIC UPPER LIMB AND TETRAPLEGIA

This topic covers a wide range of conditions, which present as a spectrum from flaccidity to spasticity with an admixture between. The spastic upper limb is classically associated with a child who has cerebral palsy (CP), but there are multitudes of patients with similar physical presentation who suffer from other conditions, such as a stroke. In a similar manner, the tetraplegic patient is typically associated with a flaccid upper limb who is wheelchair bound. However, with advances in spinal cord care and the rapidity of modern treatment strategies, the tetraplegic patient has a substantially higher survival rate and may present with a narrower zone of injury or an incomplete lesion of the cord. As a result, the interplay of both a flaccid and spastic component is now a more common presentation. For both these conditions, though the etiology and pathophysiology differ somewhat, the examination and assessment together with surgical principles are broadly similar. The surgical armamentarium is vast but has similar backgrounds for both conditions. It is imperative to have the patient intimately involved in the process of review, selection of the appropriate surgical procedure, and rehabilitation for these conditions, to make it a tailored patient outcome directed process.

THE SPASTIC UPPER LIMB

Spastic upper limb is a motor disorder that can lead to major disability, influencing a patient's rehabilitation, interfering with function, and limiting independence. It is a common disorder of the arm and hand, and physiological consequences of several causes, including:

- Stroke (cerebral vascular accident)
- Traumatic brain injury
- CP
- Cervical spine injury

A CNS injury is the common link between these conditions that causes an upper motor neuron paresis or palsy.

Incidence

Traumatic brain injury

- A traumatic brain injuries most commonly seen in patients <40 years old are mainly caused by:
  - Motor traffic accidents
  - Industrial injuries (fall from height)

Stroke

- Affects one in 1000 individuals each year
- Spastic hemiplegia most common

Cerebral palsy

- Secondary to ischemic CNS injuries in the perinatal period
- Complex and multifactorial etiology: an interplay of several risk factors, including maternal problems and infant characteristics
- Affects two children per 1000 live births and 10% of premature children with a low birth weight
- Monoplegia, hemiplegia, diplegia, triplegia, and quadriplegia. All have a single final common pathway: spasticity in the hand.

Pathophysiology

Upper motor neuron disorder secondary to the above conditions result in

- A loss of normal inhibitory control of tone, presenting peripherally as spasticity
- Muscle spasticity causing imbalance across the joints
- Loss of hand function

Cerebral palsy has the added complexity that a central nervous injury occurs during the perinatal period, and therefore, the effect of the muscle imbalance on an immature skeletal system has to be factored in as well.

Spasticity is defined by five characteristics:

1. Selective: predominant in flexor and adductor muscles
2. It is elastic. Attempts at stretching the involved muscles are met with resistance and resistance increase with the amount of strength applied. If force is applied for long enough, the muscles might yield – clasp knife spasticity
3. Present at rest and exaggerated by voluntary movements, emotion, fatigue, and pain
4. Osteotendinous reflexes are exaggerated, brisk, and diffuse
5. Synkinesis: A phenomenon wherein paralyzed muscles incapable of a certain voluntary movement attempt to execute this movement in association with contraction of accompanying intact muscles

Clinical presentation in the upper limb

- Shoulder adduction and internal rotation spasticity
  - The pectoralis major and the subscapularis are usually the main deforming forces
- Elbow flexor spasticity
  - Brachioradialis and biceps muscle are mainly responsible for the spastic forces to cause elbow flexion
- Forearm pronation
  - Spasticity is more involved in the pronator muscles, such as the PT and PQ, than the weak supinators
- Wrist flexion and ulnar deviation
  - Spastic flexors have more power than the extensors, and the ulnar deviators are more powerful than the radial deviators
- Thumb-in-palm is a common deformity caused by multiple muscles and is associated with great functional impairment
- Finger swan-neck deformity
  - Can be caused by intrinsic spasticity or extrinsic finger flexors
- Clenched fist deformities
  - The pattern and severity depends on the extent of the central nervous insult

Spasticity alone is not the norm. There can be spasticity, flaccidity, or athetosis. The mixture of these conditions must be recognized to apply the appropriate management.

History taking

- The history is dependent upon the cause of the spasticity:
  - Stroke, comorbidities, and density of stroke
  - Traumatic brain injury, multiple trauma patient with other cognition issues
  - CP
    - Most common form of spasticity of the hand
    - Associated with low birth weight and prematurity
    - Associated with seizures and mental retardation

- Developmental delays need to be assessed
- Overall use of the upper limb should be quantified from the history, parents/caregiver, and by direct observation
- The principles of assessment and physical examination for spastic conditions are similar irrespective of the etiology

Physical examination

The detailed physical examinations allow the surgeon to determine the balance between the spastic and weakened muscles. It is of crucial importance to identify the specific offending muscle by palpation and use of anatomic landmarks, or EMG and muscle stimulation. The dynamic positioning of the shoulder, elbow, forearm, wrist, fingers, and thumb in grasp, release, and pinch functions should be noted (**Figure 23.28**). These measurements can serve as the references for decision making before any treatments, because they have a direct impact on how a possible reconstruction will function. Physical examination also includes:

- Observation as to the extent of use of the upper limb by the patient
- Passive range of motion of the shoulder, elbow, forearm and wrist, and hand
- Active range of motion. Specific muscle testing of voluntary motor control of antagonist muscles because these can be used for a tendon transfer
  - Example: FCU or FCR for wrist extension
  - Pictures of the spastic hand and arm should be obtained in different views
  - Video recording of serial examination of the upper limb should be performed. This enables the recording of progress in the course of treatment
- Muscle tone: Passive range of motion must be performed slowly so as to overcome muscle spasticity in a gentle and sustained manner
- Joint contractures are also noted: If full passive range of motion is present for the muscle and joints, there is no contracture. However, if there is a loss of range of motion of joints unaffected by a change of position of the wrist, there is a contracture
- Voluntary movement and sensory deficit, intelligence and parental comprehension, and expectations

Hand function evaluation and classifications (CP)

Hand functional evaluation can be performed using two classifications:

1. A 0–8 scale of upper extremity functional level was described by House in 1981 (**Table 23.10**) and can be used to evaluate functional assessment.
2. The universally adopted classification of Zancolli (**Table 23.11**) can be used to assess hand and wrist function.

The history and examination should be reviewed and questions asked regarding the suitability of surgery. These are similar to questions posed for tendon transfer procedures.

- How old is the patient?
- What is the patient's overall limb function? (Use classifications)
- What muscle is spastic and causing joint imbalance leading to limb dysfunction?
- What muscles are flaccid of poor motor control leading to joint imbalance and limb dysfunction?
- What muscles are volitional and available for transfer?
- Is there significant athetosis or dyscoordination?

Multidisciplinary team management

- Involve or consult a
  - Rehabilitation physician/physiatrist
  - Neurologist and neurosurgeon
  - Team of therapists (occupational, hand, and cognitive)
  - Dedicated nursing staff
- Ideal for a multidisciplinary team organized into a 'spasticity management team'

Treatment

Treatment includes nonsurgical treatment and surgical treatment. The goal of treatment is to improve muscle balance to maximize hand function while preserving voluntary control.

- Primary lesions in the CNS are not treated
- No full normalization of the hand will be achieved, but instead the goal is to improve joint position so as to enable the hand to take on an assistive role
- Identify the specific offending muscle by palpation and the use of anatomic landmarks, or EMG and muscle stimulation

Treatment of upper arm spasticity should be managed with a global approach and defined clearly in advance. Shoulder and elbow deformi-

Table 23.11 Zancolli assessment of wrist function

Group 1	Complete extension of the fingers with neutral extension of the wrist
Group 2a	Finger extension with wrist flexion Active extension of the wrist with the fingers flexed
Group 2b	Finger extension with wrist flexion No active extension of the wrist with the fingers flexed
Group 3	No active extension of the fingers even with maximal wrist flexion

Table 23.10 Upper extremity functional use classification (House)

Class	Designation	Activity level
0	Does not use	Does not use
1	Poor passive assist	Uses as stabilizing weight only
2	Good passive assist	Can hold onto object placed in hand
3	Good passive assist	Can hold onto object and stabilize it for use by other hand
4	Poor active assist	Can actively grasp and hold it weakly
5	Fair active assist	Can actively grasp object and stabilize it well
6	Good active assist	Can actively grasp object and then manipulate it against the other hand
7	Spontaneous use, partial	Can perform bimanual activities easily and occasionally uses the hand spontaneously
8	Spontaneous use, complete	Uses hand completely independently without reference to the other hand

ties should be treated to achieve important results for personal hygiene, and the treatment of the proximal sites is a critical step to provide a releasing effect on the distal joints.

Nonsurgical treatment

Nonsurgical treatments are mainly used in the early stages of the disease, including casting, splinting, muscle training, and rehabilitation, as well as botulinum toxin injection. Soft splints can be used in mild deformities and assist in maintaining the hand while permitting some movement. Tone reducing medications and injection of botulinum toxin into the spastic muscle may aid in the management of spastic posturing.

- Tone reducing medications: Diazepam, baclofen
- Tone reducing injections: intramuscular injection of botulinum toxin can be indicated for the correction of spastic posturing in the absence of a fixed deformity
  - Botulinum Toxin A injection is one of the mainstream techniques in the management of the spastic upper limb
  - It allows for better functional assessment of the antagonistic muscles with the reduction of tone of the spastic muscles
  - Reversible and lasts on average 3–4 months
  - Therapy during the period of action allows for better functional use of the hand and increased stretch of the spastic muscle
  - Diagnostic adjuncts to treatment: Nerve blocks with local anesthetic agents such as marcaine/lignocaine can be used to correct, albeit temporarily, a deformity
  - Differentiate spasticity from fibrous contractures in muscle groups
  - Allow assessment of individual muscles after abolishing spasticity of antagonists and cocontractions of adjacent muscles:
  - Within a muscle group it differentiates between spastic and normal ones
  - This aids the surgeon in projecting the result of surgery
  - Therapy interventions such as splinting and stretching programs
- Tone reducing neurosurgery treatment
  - Selective dorsal rhizotomy

Surgical treatments

Surgery is mainly for patients in the later stages of a spastic disorder with a fixed deformity, and it should be undertaken only after careful consideration. Indications for surgical treatment include

- If the patient is not a candidate for the previously described conservative treatments
- If the above treatments do not resolve the condition adequately

The key concept in surgical treatment is to rebalance the deformed forces by decreasing the deforming forces, augmenting the weakened muscles, and stabilizing the joint.

Techniques available

- There are a multitude of surgical treatment options for each type of deformity in a spastic upper limb. It is difficult to specifically describe one technique to reconstruct one of these deformities, because the pathology and preoperative hand function between patients varies so widely.
- The techniques available follow the surgical treatment principles of
  - Soft tissue releases, e.g. fractionation procedures for muscles, a surgical technique that involves the lengthening of a myotendinous unit, by a single or multiple tenotomies, at the myotendinous junction
  - Tendon transfers to augment weak or flaccid muscles
  - Bone and joint stabilization
    - Bony fusions, e.g. wrist fusions
- Elbow flexor lengthening can be performed to treat flexor spasticity at the myotendinous junction, and the biceps can be fractionally lengthened at the distal biceps tendon, or the branchioradialis can be lengthened at the myotendinous junction
- Surgery for wrist flexion deformities and finger flexion deformities can be performed at the same time as correction of a pronation deformity. The FCU can be transferred to the ECRB to provide wrist extension and some extent of supination. The FDS and FDP can be lengthened at the myotendinous junction. If the fractional lengthening is not adequate to correct the flexion, FDS to FDP transfer is performed
- For thumb-in-palm deformity, it is difficult to reconstruct the 3 digits or 2 digits pulp pinch. The objective for correction of thumb-in-palm deformity is to obtain lateral or key pinch grip between the middle phalanx of the index finger and the thumb during grasping activities and thumb abduction and extension during release

Outcomes and results

Outcomes are difficult to assess due to the diverse levels of functional use, varying CNS involvement and varying degrees of spasticity. Van Heest and House (1999) have reported that patients with fair to good voluntary control had the greatest functional improvement.

SUMMARY
The spastic upper limb has many causes, but the common final pathway is a dysfunctional spastic hand and arm
Surgery is not indicated for all patients, and physicians and therapists play an important role in the care of the spastic hand and arm
Careful evaluation and follow-up of the patient with a spastic upper limb will enable the surgeon to select the most appropriate combination of procedures to correct the deformities, to allow for an assistive hand and arm
Surgery for severe deformity is beneficial, improving both the appearance and ease of management for caregivers

TETRAPLEGIA

Definition

- Paralysis of all four limbs

History and evolution

- Earliest records with a reference to spinal cord injury (SCI) are found in the Edwin Smith Papyrus, circa 2500–3000 BC.
  - Classified as 'an ailment not to be treated'
- Much has changed over the centuries, but most of what we know about these injuries today comes from the mid 20th century. In the last 50 years, there has been an advancement in the understanding and treatment of these injuries due to the increasing survival rates after SCI, the possibility of community reintegration, and many quality of life improvements
- The 1920s popularized the flexor hinge splints, which culminated in the 1950s with the finger-driven flexor hinge hands (Nickel 1963)
- Sterling Bunnell in 1948, 'Surgery of the Hand'
  - 'When you have nothing, something is a lot'
- J. N. Wilson in 1956 highlighted the concept of not recommending wrist fusion preserves the wrist flexor tenodesis effect
- Pioneers from the 1970s to 1998, such as Lipscomb, Freehafer, Lamb, Moberg, and Zancolli crystallized what we have to practice with today, although their initial operations were unpredictable,

with some authors (Guttmann 1976) even suggesting that < 5% were suitable for hand surgery

- Erik Moberg in 1975 postulated four philosophies:
  - Apart from the brain, the hand represents the most important residual resource, 'tetraplegics walk on their hands'
  - There are three roles of hands, grip, feeling, and human contact
  - Surgery should be reversible
  - Key grip and elbow extension are essential
- First International Congress on Tetraplegia was a gathering in 1978 in Edinburgh, Scotland.
  - Conferences facilitated the progress of surgical rehabilitation of the tetraplegic patient
  - There have been 11 conferences (circa 2013)

Epidemiology and etiology of SCI

- The United States has 40 new cases per million people
- A total of 11,000 cases per year, with a predominance in the active age group of 20s–40s
- Male preponderance (**Figure 23.23**)
- Common cause: vehicular accidents and falls.

Concept of the injured metamere

This concept was coined by B Coulet in 2002. In tetraplegic patients with an SCI at the same level, there is a varying degree of neurologic deficit. This is determined by both direct physical neuronal damage and the amount of secondary swelling from edema, venous stasis, spinal venous infarction, compromise of the arterial blood supply, and release of noxious substances such as lipases, free radicals, and excitotoxins. The initial direct physical neuronal damage does not immediately produce the full scope of the eventual neurological impairment. In fact, secondary changes may cause most of the damage to the spinal cord, which explains the high variability of clinical presentations encountered. The injured metamere can be classified into short (I), long (II), or intermediary types (III).

Assessment of the tetraplegic patient

This evaluation involves the assessment of the hand, the overall patient, and the psychological makeup of the patient.

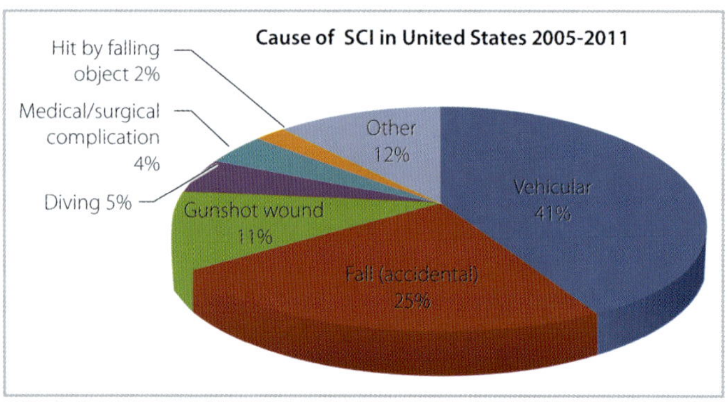

Figure 23.23 Cause of spinal cord injuries in the United States 2005–2011. Based on data from Chen et al. Causes of spinal cord injury. Top Spinal Cord Inj Rehab 2013; 19:1–8.

Assessment of the tetraplegic hand (tangible evidence)

The hand assessment is of great importance and is correlated to the International Classification for Surgery of the Hand in Tetraplegia (ICSHT) to look for tangible evidence of motor and sensory recovery. In patients with tetraplegia, the evaluation is mainly focused on elbow extension and hand grip. Testing includes subjective muscle testing and using MRC grading, whereas functional testing includes tests for abductor pollicis longus (i.e. Sollerman test).

Other considerations (intangible evidence)

- Must have achieved neurological and psychological stability
- Motivated and intelligent
  - The 'Quad' as described by Hentz is different
    - Has limited functional resources
    - Aware of precarious position
    - Big emotional impact on surgery
    - Lifelong problem with lifelong commitment
- No surgery in painful conditions

Key questions in the assessment of the tetraplegic patient

- How does the patient accomplish tasks of daily living?
  - Dependent or independent bed mobility?
  - Does the patient use an electric wheelchair?
  - Any use of adaptive devices for grooming, dressing, and feeding?
  - If reconstructive surgery is performed, are there adequate resources to tide the patient over the period of greater functional dependence, i.e. a caregiver?

Treatment preferably based on a dedicated team

- Team-based decision-making process
- Team members include
  - Patient
  - Surgeon
  - Rehab physician
  - Therapist
  - Family
- Why a team?
  - It is a shared responsibility with a major commitment on all parties. It avoids the 'its someone else's patient' conundrum
  - It requires a sizable dedication of resources based in a community hospital or a spinal injury center
  - The team will then be consulted with the patient based on a decision-making algorithm

Indication of surgery

- The surgery is both reconstructive and rehabilitative
- The indications based on anatomic and remaining muscles only indicate what can be done, not what should be done
- Cannot be solely based on experience as the numbers are small and needs years to arrange for necessary expertise
- Questions fielded include
  - When can we do it?

- Who to do it on?
- What to do?

When?

- Surgery should be performed as early as possible, before the patient adapts to their condition. Surgery is still possible, however, in patients who present late. For patients presenting late, a few more new adjustments have to be made. There are no absolute contraindications as long as the patient is willing
- Surgery can be performed between 12–18 months and can be as short as 7–8 months after the SCI
- After the tetraplegia has stabilized, with spasticity and hygiene issues sorted and able to sit in the wheelchair

Who?

The well-motivated, well-informed patient, in a stable psychological condition is a good candidate for surgery. The patient should have precise and realistic goals for rehabilitation. Other factors include age, profession, education, and family support. It has been noted that unsatisfactory results occasionally occur due to an error in patient selection.

What?

What to do is based on whatever the well-informed patient desires, not what the surgeon wishes to accomplish. The surgical techniques and tools are based on the level of tetraplegia, as classified by the ICSHT. Surgical treatment involves conventional techniques used in hand surgery, such as arthrodesis, tenodesis, and tendon transfers.

The elbow

The return of function of the normal elbow is the goal of surgery for the tetraplegic patient. The positioning of the hand in space, which affects activities such as overhead reach, functions of the activity of daily living such as hygiene, eating, and driving, are all affected by a good elbow. The stability afforded by a functioning elbow allows for wheelchair mobility, pressure relief, and also in transfer from bed to chair and commode. All of the above require shoulder control.

The wrist

The wrist tenodesis effect is important in the reconstruction of hand grip (**Figure 23.24**).

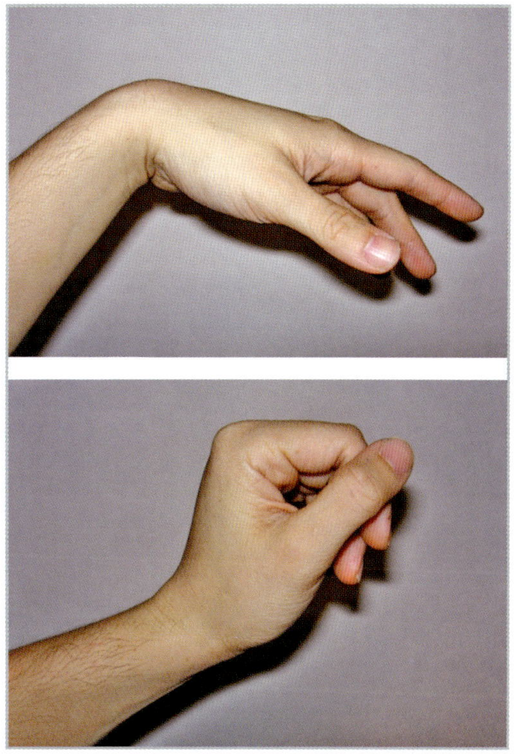

Figure 23.24 The wrist tenodesis effect.

Surgical reconstruction

The strategy for surgery and what can be offered to the patient in procedures are summarized in **Table 23.19**. The general guidelines for reconstruction include

- Arthrodesis to permit stabilization of joints that lack muscle stabilization
- Tenodesis is performed to stabilize a joint or so that another joint, usually one that controls more proximal movement, will result in the tightening of the fixed tendon and movement of the more distally located joint
- The transfer of the power of a volitional and expendable muscle tendon unit compensates for the absence of function of another muscle tendon unit (i.e. BR transfer to the ECRB for wrist extension and tenodesis effect)
- The types of operations can be broadly classified (using the ICSHT) into:
  - Surgery for elbow extension, which include biceps to triceps transfer and deltoid to biceps transfer
  - Surgery for weaker patients, IC group 0,1,2
    - Grasp, wrist extension, and key pinch
  - Restoring key pinch, IC 2 and some IC 3 patients
  - Restoring both grasp and release, IC group 3,4,5
  - Restoring strong grasp and refined pinch, IC group 6.7.8,9
    - Surgery of the paralytic hand only

Functional neuromuscular stimulation

Functional electrical stimulation (FES) using the Freehand system was introduced in 1995 by the Cleveland FES center and was used from 1998 to 2002. This allowed the patient with a high injury to activate and control a preprogrammed sequence of muscle contractions and thus achieve a useful grasp for one hand. The sale of this system was terminated with about 250 patients when it was stopped for commercial reasons in 2002.

SUMMARY

- Carefully chosen reconstructive surgery for the upper limb is useful in properly educated patients and can be both effective and durable
- Functional surgery of the hand and upper limb must be followed by rehabilitation in a rehabilitation center with a team of rehabilitation specialists, physiotherapists, occupational therapists, and social workers

SUGGESTED READING

Spastic hand

Wall SA, Chait LA, Temlett JA, et al. Botulinum A chemodenervation: a new modality in cerebral palsied hands. Br J Plast Surg 1993; 46:703.
This paper introduces the concept of use of Botulinium A as an adjunct for the treatment of spasticity in CP. Botox as it is more commonly known is now a mainstay in the management.

Green WT. Tendon transplantation of the flexor carpi ulnaris for pronation-flexion deformity of the wrist. Surg Gynecol Obstet 1942; 75:337–342.
This classic paper offers an insight into the initial efforts in cerebral palsy surgery. It addresses the common deformity of a spastic upper limb.

Guttmann, L. Spinal cord injuries, comprehensive management and research (2nd edn.). Oxford; Blackwell Scientific Publications, 1976.

Van Heest AE, House JH, Cariello C. Upper extremity surgical treatment of cerebral palsy. J Hand Surg Am 1999; 24:323–330.
A summary on the surgical treatment of cerebral palsy.

Tetraplegia

Nickel VL, Perry J, Garret AL. Development of useful function in the severely paralyzed hand. J Bone Joint Am 1963; 45:933.
The first few attempts in using orthotics to overcome a complex problem. The 'flexor-hinge' hand has since been superseded.

Moberg E. Surgical treatment for absent single-hand grip and elbow extension in quadriplegia: principles and preliminary treatment. J Bone Joint Surg Am 1975; 57:196–206.
Moberg's work on surgical treatment of tetraplegia.

Coulet B, Allieu Y, Chammas M. Injured metamere and functional surgery of the tetraplegic upper limb. Hand Clini 2002; 18:399–412.
This gives an understanding to the limit of damage to the spinal cord in tetraplegia. It introduces the 'metamere' as a distinct entity separate from the classic cervical level reference we use.

23.6 THORACIC OUTLET SYNDROME (TOS)

Thoracic outlet syndrome is an array of disorders that involve injury of neurovascular structures in the cervicobrachial region.

CLASSIFICATION

The TOS is not an anatomical, but rather a functional concept, which assumes that the neurovascular structures exit the upper thoracic area through an outlet. We now understand TOS as three main syndromes according to Wilbourn classification:

1. Neurogenic TOS (most common)
2. Venous TOS (second most common)
3. Arterial TOS

Any of these syndromes can exist alone, but may also occur in combination with one another.

PERTINENT ANATOMY

The thoracic outlet can be divided into of three triangles (**Figure 23.25**):

- Interscalene triangle: The boundaries of the interscalene triangle are formed by the scalenus anterior muscle anteriorly, scalenus medius posteriorly, and the first rib inferiorly. The upper part of the interscalene triangle contains the ventral primary rami of the C3, C4, and C5, which take part in the formation of the phrenic nerve. The lower part of the interscalene triangle contains the upper, middle, and lower trunks of the brachial plexus and subclavian artery, which passes between the scalenus anterior and scalenus medius muscles. The origins and insertions of the scalene muscles are as follows:
  - Scalenus anterior muscle: Arises from the anterior tubercles of the transverse processes of the C3–C6 vertebrae and inserts into the scalene tubercle on the first rib
  - Scalenus posterior muscle: Arises from the posterior tubercles of the transverse processes of the C2–C7 vertebrae and inserts on the superior surface of the first rib behind the groove for the subclavian artery
  - Scalenus minimus muscle: Found in 30–50% of TOS cases. The scalenus minimus muscle is located between the subclavian artery and the T1 root of the brachial plexus. This muscle takes origin from the transverse process of the C6 and C7 vertebrae and insets into a fascial support of the pleura and first rib
- Costoclavicular triangle: The costoclavicular space is a triangular space formed by the medial portion of the clavicle anteriorly, the first rib, insertions of the anterior and middle scalene muscles posteromedially, and the upper border of the scapula posterolaterally. The subclavian vein is the main structure passing through the costoclavicular triangle
- Sub or retropectoral triangle: The boundaries of the retropectoral triangle are the coracoid process superiorly and the insertion of the pectoralis minor muscle anteriorly. However, it is very rare for TOS to occur due to neurovascular compression at this site

ETIOLOGY

The most common cause of neurogenic TOS is a hyperextension neck injury. Vascular (arterial or venous) TOS is more commonly associated with congenital and anatomic anomalies that cause compression of the neurovascular structures within the thoracic outlet:

- Osseous causes
  - Cervical rib (**Figure 23.26**). Bilateral in 50% of cases
  - Rudimentary first ribs

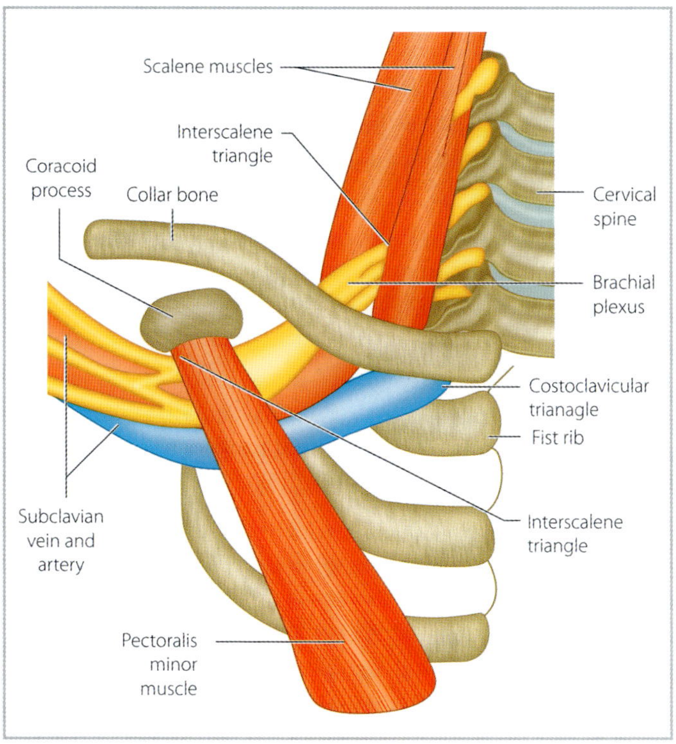

Figure 23.25 Thoracic outlet area. The arrows show sites of potential neurovascular compression.

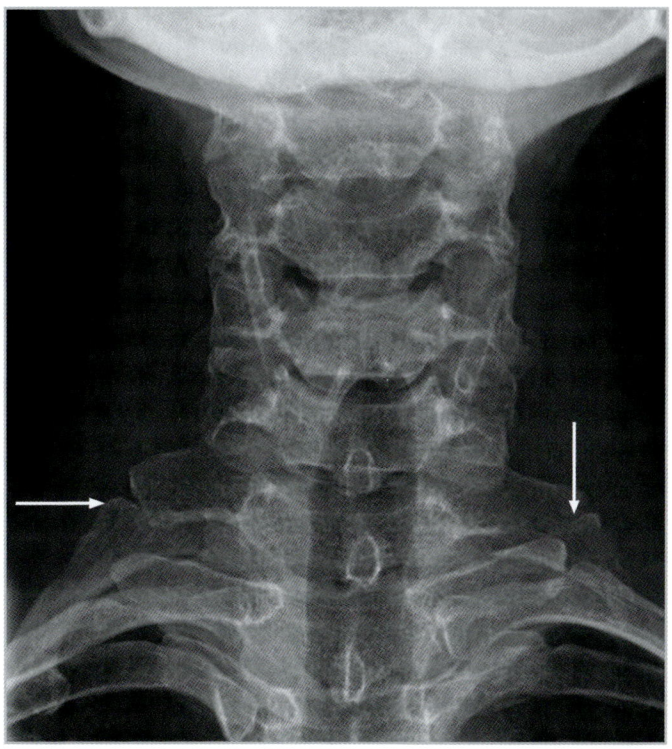

Figure 23.26 Cervical spine X-ray. White arrowheads show bilateral cervical ribs.

  - Fractures of the first rib and subsequent callus formation
  - Narrow costoclavicular space
  - Clavicle pathology (e.g. nonunion/malunion, osteomyelitis, tumor)
- Soft tissue causes
  - Traumatic: Scalene muscle injury
  - Congenital bands and ligaments: For example, people born with a cervical rib are 10 times more likely to develop TOS than people born without a cervical rib. However, even in patients with a cervical rib, it may still require some type of neck injury to induce the symptoms of TOS
  - Anomalous scalene muscle insertions
  - Inflammatory
  - Infections
  - Connective tissue disease
  - Neoplastic, e.g. Pancoast tumor (pulmonary tumor involving the apex of the lung)

CLINICAL PRESENTATION

No single symptom is pathognomonic for TOS. Typically, it is the constellation of symptoms, such as neurological, musculoskeletal, and vascular indications, that defines the condition.

Neurogenic TOS

Neurogenic TOS affects more females than males, with a female to male ratio of 3.5:1, and an age of onset between 20 and 40 years old. Neurogenic TOS can be further subdivided into true neurogenic TOS and nonspecific (occasionally referred to as electrically negative) TOS. In true neurogenic TOS, sensory symptoms are present together with positive findings of objective tests (e.g. EMG), whereas in nonspecific TOS, patients complain of sensory symptoms, but objective tests are often negative. Up to 90% of the cases are associated with a history of trauma, especially neck injuries (whiplash type). Symptoms are predominantly neurologic, which include paresthesia, numbness, and pain of the fingers, most commonly at the ring and little fingers (ulnar nerve cutaneous distribution, C8–T1) as well as symptoms of motor weakness, such as weakness of handgrip. Patients may also complain of a radicular type pain (electric sharp shooting pains) radiating to the neck, shoulder, and arms. Other symptoms are vague and include headaches as well as cold intolerance of the hand due to compression of the sympathetic nerves (e.g. Raynaud phenomenon).

Venous TOS

Venous TOS is known to be more common in male athletes between the ages of 20 and 30 years old. Repetitive movements during exercise compress the subclavian vein and precipitate venous thrombosis. Stress/exercise-induced thrombosis has been described as Paget–Schroetter syndrome (upper extremity deep vein thrombosis that typically occurs in the axillary or subclavian veins). In an acute venous thrombosis, patients complain of a sudden onset of pain, edema, and cyanosis. On the other hand, with intermittent sublclavian vein compression, symptoms are usually less profound (less amount of edema and cyanosis). To compensate for the sluggish venous return caused by a complete or partial venous occlusion, the collateral veins engorge and become visible over the upper arm and breast area.

Arterial TOS

This is the least common type of TOS, affecting males and females equally, between the ages of 20 and 30 years old. Arterial TOS is most commonly associated with osseous anomaly such as a cervical rib or first rib malformation. The subclavian artery becomes compressed against a cervical rib or other bone malformation that leads to arterial stenosis and the formation of aneurysms. The clinical presentation may vary from an acute limb ischemia (pulselessness, pallor, pokilothermia, and limb weakness) due to complete occlusion of the subclavian artery, to relatively mild forms of chronic ischemia due to partial occlusion of the arterial lumen. Patients suffering with partial occlusion of the subclavian artery often experience symptoms of chronic ischemia, which include intermittent claudications, trophic changes, fingertip ulcerations, and gangrene.

Clinical evaluation

The assessment of TOS requires obtaining a thorough patient history and performing a meticulous physical examination together with clinical suspicion. It is often not possible to perform a comprehensive physical examination at a busy hand surgery outpatient clinic. Therefore, it is advisable to segregate all patients suspected for TOS into a specialized TOS outpatient clinic session.

History taking

The surgeon should inquire about the history of a previous trauma. The surgeon should also try to differentiate between neurogenic and vascular TOS based on a patient's symptoms, if possible.

Physical examination

This is the most useful tool for the diagnosis of TOS. The examiner should always follow the same examination pattern. In addition, careful record keeping is paramount to monitor a patient's clinical progression or deterioration. A physical examination consists of the following assessment methods:

- Nerve compression maneuver (e.g. Tinel test): This may reproduce a patient's symptoms and should be performed from distal to proximal, in the following order:
  - Carpal tunnel
  - Pronator tunnel
  - Cubital tunnel
  - Medial aspect of forearm
  - Infraclavicular fossa
  - Supraclavicular fossa over brachial plexus
- Provocative tests: The majority of provocative or stress tests that constitute the physical examination rely on the diminishing pulse of the radial artery after a patient performs different types of maneuvers with his/her upper extremity. However, most of the tests previously described in literature, such as Adson, Wright, and Halstead tests, have been shown to be unreliable with varying degrees of sensitivity and specificity for the diagnosis of TOS and, therefore, will not be discussed further. Nevertheless, the Roos test, also known as the elevated arm stress test, has been found to have the highest predictive value among the provocative tests. The Roos test is performed by externally rotating and abducting a patient's arm to 90°, then the patient is asked to rapidly make a tight fist and then open the hand, and close it again repeatedly for 3 minutes. Most of patients would not tolerate a full 3 minutes of this exercise; however, the reproduction of a patient's symptoms and fatigue is considered a positive test (**Figure 23.27**).

Electrodiagnostic evaluation

The EMG and nerve conduction velocity may help in diagnosing TOS but are usually nonspecific and always dependent upon the experience

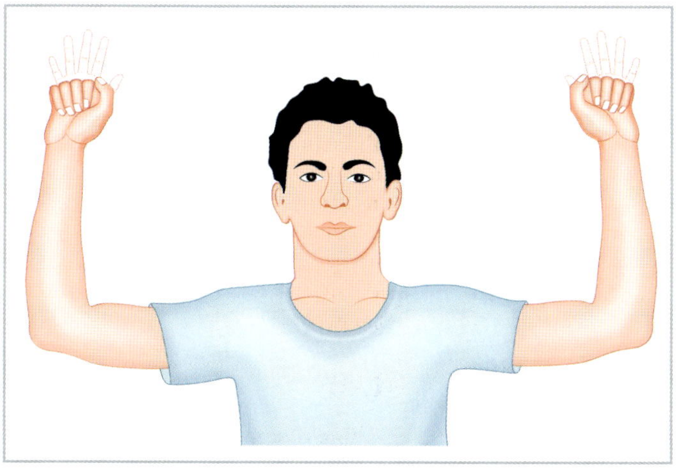

Figure 23.27 The elevated arm stress test, also known as the Roos test, to evaluate thoracic outlet syndrome. The patient holds their arms up as shown and rapidly opens and closes the hands for 3 minutes.

of the EMG specialist. In addition, the majority of patients suffering from neurogenic TOS are of the electrically negative subtype (the most common type). However, abnormal electrodiagnostic studies may occasionally be an early sign of neurogenic TOS or may aid in the diagnosis of other conditions, such as compressive neuropathies (e.g. carpal tunnel or cubital tunnel syndromes).

Radiologic evaluation

Radiographic evaluation should be part of the initial assessment of patients presenting with symptoms of TOS. Neck/chest X-rays (AP, lateral and oblique) should be performed, and osseous anomalies compressing neurovascular structures are visible on plain radiographs. However, if the results of the X-rays are negative and a patient's symptoms are strongly suggestive of TOS, a CT or MRI is warranted. This may reveal a soft tissue cause of TOS or demonstrate a nerve impingement.

Regarding vascular TOS, a duplex ultrasound of the subclavian vessels, may show a vessel stenosis, obstruction, or flow problems. Finally, arteriography and venography may be used to diagnose arterial and venous TOS, respectively; however, these are invasive procedures and should, therefore, be performed only as a last resort.

DIFFERENTIAL DIAGNOSIS

- Nerve compression syndromes: 40–50% of patients with TOS have peripheral nerve compression symptoms
- Subacromial bursitis and/or impingement syndrome: In patients with TOS and suspected associated bursitis, a guided triamcinolone injection is recommended
- Cervical spine strain/strain (radiculopathy)
- Cervical disk disease and cervical arthritis
- Spinal stenosis
- Brachial plexus injury
- Temporomandibular joint pathology
- Complex regional pain syndrome.

Treatment

An algorithmic approach for the treatment of TOS is depicted in **Figure 23.28**. The majority of patients suffering from TOS are

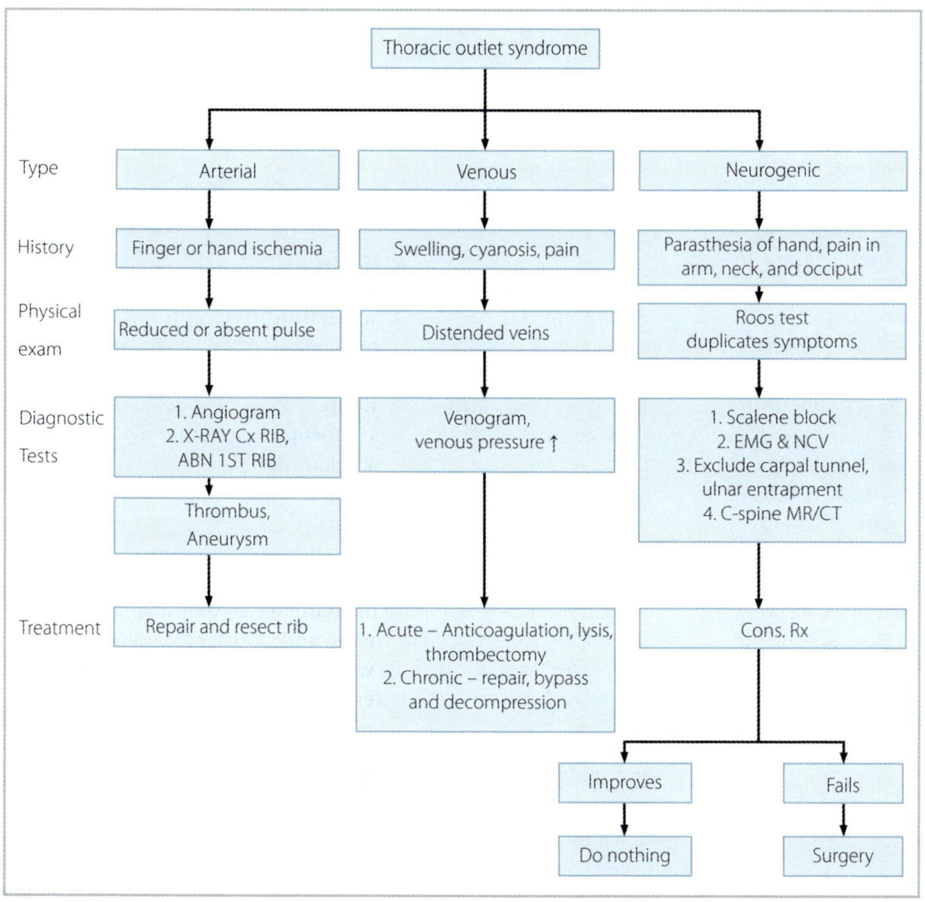

Figure 23.28 Algorithm for the treatment of thoracic outlet syndrome.

successfully treated with conservative measures unless there is significant neural damage or vascular compression.

Conservative treatment

The duration of conservative management should be between 4 and 6 months, after which time a surgical treatment is sought. Conservative treatment aims to relieve pressure caused by external stressors at the different compression points by instituting the following measures:

- Comfortable day/sleeping body habits
- Address ergonomics of work posture
- Reduce weight (occasionally females may require a breast reduction procedure)
- Edema control
- Relaxation exercises

Pain control

Pain is a major cause of patient frustration and discomfort. The following measures help to ease off pain and improve patient compliance with physical therapy:

- Trigger point injections (hydrocortisone and lidocaine): 90–95% of patients with TOS have upper back myofascial trigger points, which can be treated by steroid injections
- NSAIDs
- Muscle relaxants
- Heat (hot showers and heating pads)
- Compression stockings
- Limb massage and biofeedback techniques
- Tricyclic antidepressants and selective serotonin reuptake inhibitors for neuropathic pain, such as gabapentin or pregabalin (the drug of choice)
- Exercises: Tendon gliding exercises, brachial plexus gliding exercises, and nerve gliding exercises.

Surgical treatment

Surgery should be performed immediately if a patient presents with distal muscle atrophy or acute ischemia due to arterial occlusion. Thoracic outlet decompression is also recommended if a patient fails to respond to conservative measures. This includes the following procedures:

- Anterior and middle scalenectomy: Causes decompression of the thoracic outlet. When performing anterior scalenectomy, the phrenic nerve has to be identified and preserved, and 80% of the muscle has to be excised. The long thoracic nerve (LTN) is also prone to injury, because it may run through the middle scalenus muscle. Only when the LTN is identified and retracted may the surgeon proceed to middle scalenectomy. Only 30–50% of the middle scalene should be excised
- Neurolysis: Freeing of the nerves and excision of loose muscle fibers, connective tissue bands, and scalene minimus muscle (if present)
- Resection of the first rib: Some investigators support the opinion that scalenectomy alone will suffice for treatment, as resection of the first rib is associated with higher morbidity and a longer recovery period
- Venous TOS: The surgical treatment here is focused around the removal of external venous compression (decompression) and restoring a patent venous lumen. Restoring venous flow can be accomplished by thrombolysis or thrombectomy, depending on the site and size of thrombosis. Regarding venous decompression, this is achieved by scalenectomy and first-rib resection, which should be performed only after successful thrombolysis or thrombectomy
- Arterial TOS: TOS decompression is usually achieved by performing the above-mentioned procedures (anterior and middle scalenectomy, first-rib resection, or scalenectomy plus first-rib resection). However, in addition, the artery is frequently replaced with a saphenous vein graft or a prosthetic material as the artery is often nonsalvageable
- Sympathectomy: This is currently an infrequently performed operation because of poor outcomes in the first few years after surgery

Complications of surgery

- Apical hematoma: Spontaneously resolves within 7–10 days
- Pneumothorax and hemopneumothorax (10%): For early detection of injury during the course of surgery, the operative field should be flooded with normal saline and the anesthesiologist asked to hyperventilate the lung. Bubbles are observed in minor injuries. Standard placement of a chest tube through second intercostal space in the case of pneumothorax is required
- Injury to the subclavian artery is very rare
- Injury to the subclavian vein is rare but more common in patients with venous compression due to an engorged venous network
- Postoperative subclavian vein thrombosis: More common in patients with venous compression
- Injury to brachial plexus: More common in transcervical first-rib resection. The roots of the plexus are injured more by traction than transaction. It is advisable to use a bipolar diathermy, since monopolar can cause undue muscle twitching pushing brachial plexus roots against the diathermy needle, thus injuring them
- Injury to LTN: The nerve has to be identified and freed before dividing the middle scalene muscle. Injury is caused by cutting one of the three nerve branches resulting in a winged scapula. Full recovery is expected in several months
- Injury to the phrenic nerve: Avoid using a cautery near the nerve and avoid unnecessary traction. Usually, the injury is not permanent, but it may cause dyspnea in the early postoperative period. Incidence of phrenic nerve paresis has been reported to be as high as 12%
- Injury to intercostobrachial nerve in a transaxillary approach: Most injuries are caused by traction. It is more common to cause causalgic pain in the nerve that has been overstretched than in the nerve that has been cut
- Inadequate resection of the posterior portion of the first rib: Not more than 2–2.5 of the posterior portion can remain. The costovertebral joint is the limit
- Injury to the thoracic duct: Recognized by clear/milky fluid leaking into the wound mostly from the left side. Avoid transecting the fat pad, and instead, elevate or retract it as a flap. Rarely, re-exploration is necessary for persistent leaks

Postoperative rehabilitation

- Start a gentle range of motion in the first postoperative day
- Adequate pain control helps increase the range of motion and decrease possibility of the brachial plexus tethering to scar tissue
- Continue conservative modalities of treatment as necessary

Treatment outcomes

It should be noted that clinical improvement is a subjective parameter. It is not easy to compare outcome results in the literature because authors use different grading systems and assessment measures. However, in general, supraclavicular scalenectomy with/without first-rib resection yields approximately 70% clinical improvement of patients' symptoms, whereas combined surgical procedures yield higher than 80% improvement. It is also worth noting that work-related injuries are associated with higher treatment failure rates than road traffic accidents.

Recurrent TOS

The long-term results show that recurrence of symptoms may develop in 15–20% of patients who undergo surgery and 80% of the recurrences seen are within the first 2 years postoperatively.

Common causes of treatment failure include:

- Contraction of scar
- Scalenotomies performed instead of scalenectomies
- Retention of the long-posterior first-rib stump
- Intractable upper back myofasciitis

Treatment of these causes includes performing the following corrective procedures:

- Removal of the remaining posterior portion of the first rib if >1 cm is present
- External neurolysis of the brachial plexus
- Scalenectomy (excision of 80–90% of the anterior and 40–50% of the middle scalene muscles) if the primary procedure was scalenotomy
- Sympathectomy in patients with sympathetic overactivity

SUGGESTED READING

Braun RM, Sahadevan DC, Feinstein J. Confirmatory needle placement technique for scalene muscle block in the diagnosis of thoracic outlet syndrome. Tech Hand Up Extrem Surg 2006; 10:173–176.
This article offers a simple clinical method to assess needle placement in the scalene muscle before an injection of local anesthetic, which, if properly placed, weakens the scalene muscle and often leads to temporary relief of symptoms associated with neurovascular compression.

Fugate MW., Rotellini-Coltvet L., Freischlag JA. Current management of thoracic outlet syndrome. Curr Treat Options Cardiovasc Med 2009; 11:176–183.
This article shows follow-up data indicating that appropriately selected patients benefit from surgical intervention. To prevent recurrence, patients must undergo first rib resection and anterior scalenectomy, as well as resection of any rudimentary or cervical ribs. Regardless of the type of TOS encountered, proper treatment requires a multidisciplinary approach.

Roos DB. Experience with first rib resection for thoracic outlet syndrome. Ann Surg 1971; 173:429–442.
Classic and historical article of first rib resection using the axillary approach for operative relief of the outlet syndrome are presented, and extension of the axillary technic to (1) cervical rib resection, (2) thoracic sympathectomy, (3) axillary-subclavian subclavian vein thrombectomy, and (4) thoracoplasty is described. Complications encountered means of avoiding them and general results in a series of 276 cases are discussed.

Sanders RJ., Hammond SL., Rao NM. Diagnosis of thoracic outlet syndrome. J Vasc Surg 2007; 46:601–604.
Diagnosis of different types of thoracic outlet syndrome is discussed in detail. Stress tests are evaluated critically. Authors emphasize that physical examination is most important and several provocative maneuvers are described in the article.

Sanders RJ, Rao NM. The forgotten pectoralis minor syndrome: 100 operations for pectoralis minor syndrome alone or accompanied by neurogenic thoracic outlet syndrome. Ann Vasc Surg 2010; 24:701–708.
Pectoralis minor syndrome (PMS) commonly accompanies NTOS and frequently exists alone. Its recognition is important as many patients with suspected NTOS can be treated successfully with a simple, essentially risk-free PM tenotomy. Should this fail, thoracic outlet decompression can always be performed at a later date.

Chapter 24 Vascular disorders of the hand

Yirong Wang, Evan J. Kowalski, Kevin C. Chung

INTRODUCTION

A vascular disorder refers to a weakening or decrease in the structure or functional capacity of the vasculature (**Figure 24.1**) of the hand. These disorders should be treated promptly to relieve painful symptoms that would decrease work productivity and avoid ischemia that could lead to loss of digits or portions of the extremity due to untreated sequelae.

ASSESSMENT

History

Many vascular disorders are directly linked to an injury. Acute or chronic trauma, including vibration exposure, has the potential to damage arteries and veins, causing a vascular disorder. Other causes include congenital processes and systemic illnesses such as atherosclerosis, diabetes, or connective tissue disorders because vessels are more susceptible to trauma in patients with systemic diseases. Patients who smoke or whose occupation is associated with vibrating tools have a predisposition to vascular disorders.

Clinical examination

The clinical examination is essential to appropriately diagnose and treat a vascular disorder. Careful evaluation is critical, because the symptoms of vascular disorders can easily be confused with symptoms of other illnesses.

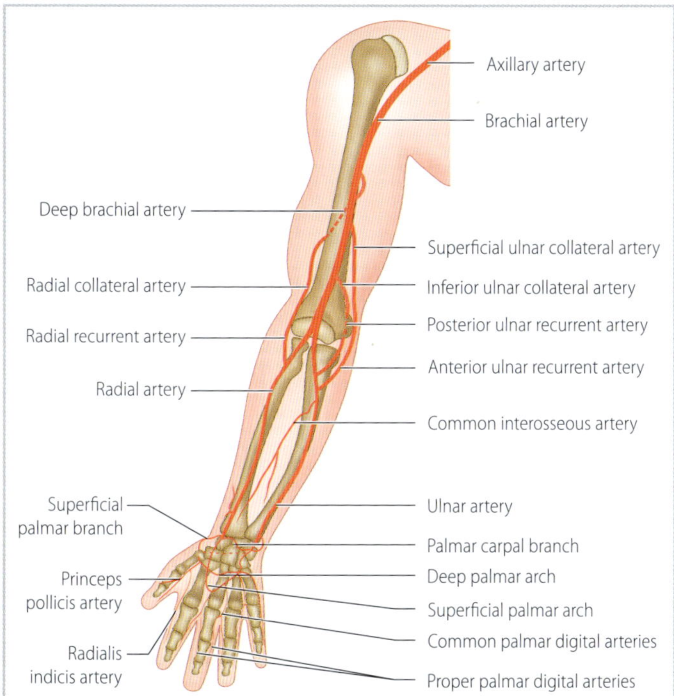

Figure 24.1 The vascular anatomy of the upper extremity.

Symptoms

- Ischemic symptoms
  - Cold sensitivity
  - Pain
  - Tingling
  - Swelling
  - Sensory change
  - Nonhealing ulceration
  - Necrosis
  - Vascular anomalies

Evaluation

A pale color and coolness of the skin indicate a loss of arterial blood flow, whereas a blue color may indicate venous stasis or congestion. Skin integrity should be evaluated, including symptoms such as ulceration and Gangrene (**Figure 24.2**). A sensation examination will help determine if there is nerve involvement. Two-point discrimination (2PD) is used to test the nerve innervation of an area of the skin and has two distinct testing modalities: Static 2PD and dynamic 2PD.

- Static 2PD
  - The test is used to determine the minimum distance between two distinct points that can be distinguished by the patient
  - A therapist uses special calipers to touch the area being tested
  - The static 2PD of digits should approach 6 mm
- Dynamic 2PD should be 3 mm
  - The caliper is moved longitudinally from proximal to distal in a linear fashion along the surface of the finger

Capillary refill time is a measure of collateral circulation and should occur in <2 seconds, with >2 seconds possibly indicating ischemia. The radial and ulnar pulses are palpable in three distinct areas:

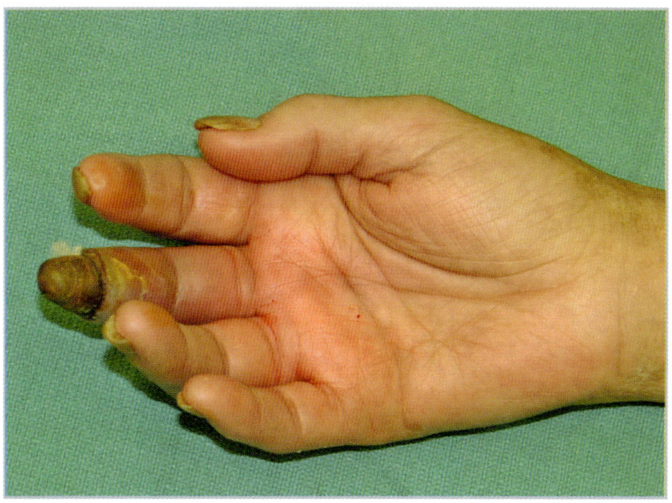

Figure 24.2 Gangrene of the finger results in loss of digit.

1. The radial wrist groove
2. The anatomical snuffbox
3. The radial side of the pisiform in the distal aspect of the wrist

An Allen test is useful to determine the function of the artery in the hand (**Figure 24.3a–c**). Before the examination, the examiner's fingertips should be placed over the patient's radial and ulnar arteries in the wrist. The test begins as the patient is asked to clench the fist, squeezing the blood out of the hand. The examiner should then occlude the radial and ulnar arteries, turning the hand white. Upon release of the ulnar artery, the examiner should note the time taken for the color to return. The same steps are then repeated for the radial artery.

- Rapid fill is < 6 seconds
- Delayed fill is 6–15 seconds
- Absent fill is no refill after 15 seconds
  - A delayed or absent fill might indicate an occlusion

Investigation

There are a variety of tools that can be used to investigate the vascular status of the hand. Doppler ultrasound and pulse echo ultrasound are used to assess vascular anatomy or the blood flow in a vessel. Digital plethysmography (pulse volume recording, PVR) analyzes changes in the volume of limbs or digits to measure blood flow. Volume changes are converted to analog tracings, and normal, stenotic, and occluded vessels show different characteristic tracings.

A digital-brachial index (DBI) can be calculated with a segmental arterial pressures examination:

- Average normal DBI is 0.97, with the lower limit of normal being 0.75
- DBI > 0.7 suggests adequate vascular flow

Color duplex imaging provides a visual interpretation of blood flow and can be used to verify if a mass is vascular and determine the exact location of stenosis. Thermography is useful to accurately conduct temperature measurements over large areas of skin surface. Magnetic resonance imaging (MRI) and magnetic resonance angiography (MRA) can be used to image vascular malformations of the hand and provide detailed information regarding the extent, local tissue involvement, and flow characteristics of lesions. Although angiography will delineate the vascular anatomy of the hand with great precision, it is an invasive procedure, using potentially harmful contrast agents and radiation. Nevertheless, it remains the reference standard for vascular evaluation, providing the best anatomic detail and structural information on upper-extremity vasculature.

VASCULAR OCCLUSIONS

Vascular occlusions of the upper extremity can lead to ischemia symptoms. Localized vascular occlusions generally include thrombosis, aneurysm, embolism, or tumor. Smoking can affect distal segment circulation.

Hypothenar hammer syndrome

Physiology

This disorder is common in patients who utilize the hypothenar aspect of the hand as a hammer. The superficial nature of the ulnar artery at the Guyon space, covered only by the superficial aponeurosis, palmaris brevis muscle, subcutaneous tissue, and skin predisposes the artery to this condition (**Figure 24.4**). As it courses directly over the hook of the hamate, the hard surface provided by the hamate gives even a low-energy repetitive trauma the potential to damage the ulnar artery (**Figure 24.5**). As a result of the impact, a thrombosis of the ulnar artery develops, with secondary distal embolization of the digital arteries. In rare occurrences, a repetitive injury will lead to the formation of an aneurysm or pseudoaneurysm. Severe cases of thrombosis may include the involvement of adventitia, and reflex vasospasm may result as the blockage affects the periarterial sympathetic fibers, further decreasing adjacent collateral flow.

Diagnostic criteria

- Often include an occupational history of repetitive hand and wrist trauma
- A history of smoking

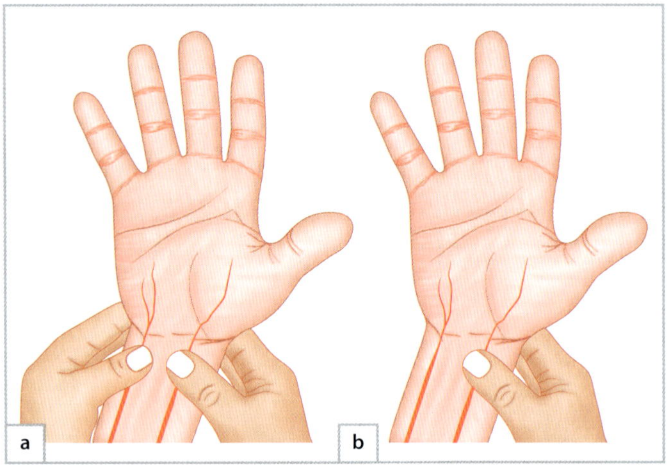

Figure 24.3 The Allen test measures the functional capacity of the arteries in the hand. (a) The examiner should occlude both the radial and ulnar arteries and has the patient clench the hand into a fist several times until the hand turns white. (b) The ulnar artery is released, and the time taken for color to return should be noted. The process is repeated, but this time the radial artery is released, and the time taken for color to return is noted.

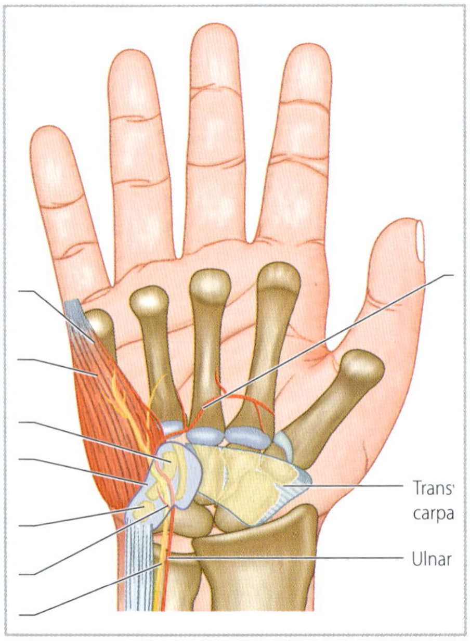

Figure 24.4 Anatomy of the ulnar artery and Guyon space.

- Symptoms of this disorder include cold intolerance, pain, pale skin color, cyanosis, mottling of the digits, ulceration on the ulnar aspect of the hand, and tenderness in the palm (**Figure 24.6**)
- An Allen test can show reduced or no flow through the ulnar artery
- A DBI or PVR can be obtained to evaluate digital perfusion
  - DBI < 0.7 suggests inadequate vascular flow
- Angiography or computed tomography (CT) angiography should be performed to determine whether or not surgery is indicated
  - Angiography can show a detailed length of the ulnar artery thrombosis and emboli of digital arteries
  - CT angiography (**Figure 24.7**) can help verify the presence of occlusions

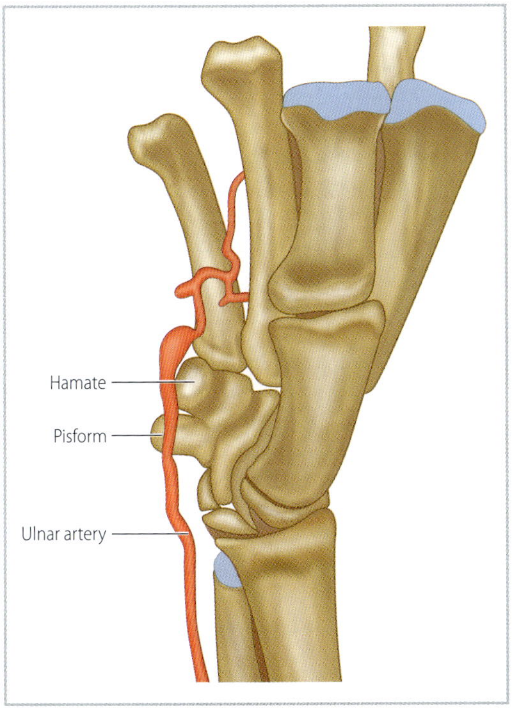

Figure 24.5 This shows the ulnar artery coursing directly over the hook of the hamate, leaving it vulnerable to trauma.

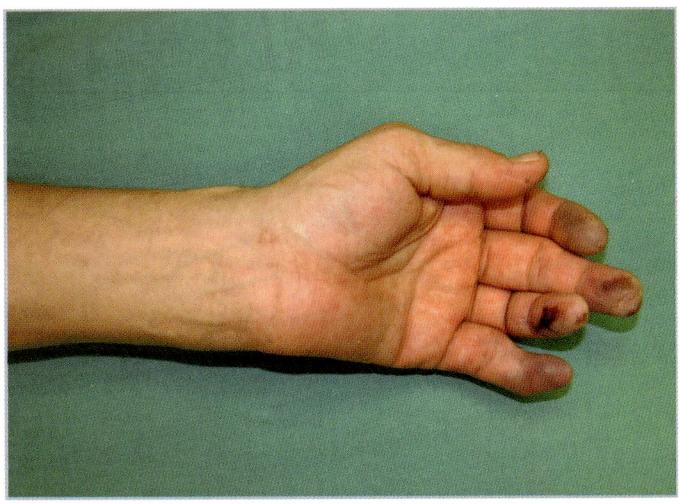

Figure 24.6 Symptoms of hypothenar hammer syndrome, including cyanosis, mottling, and ulceration of the digits.

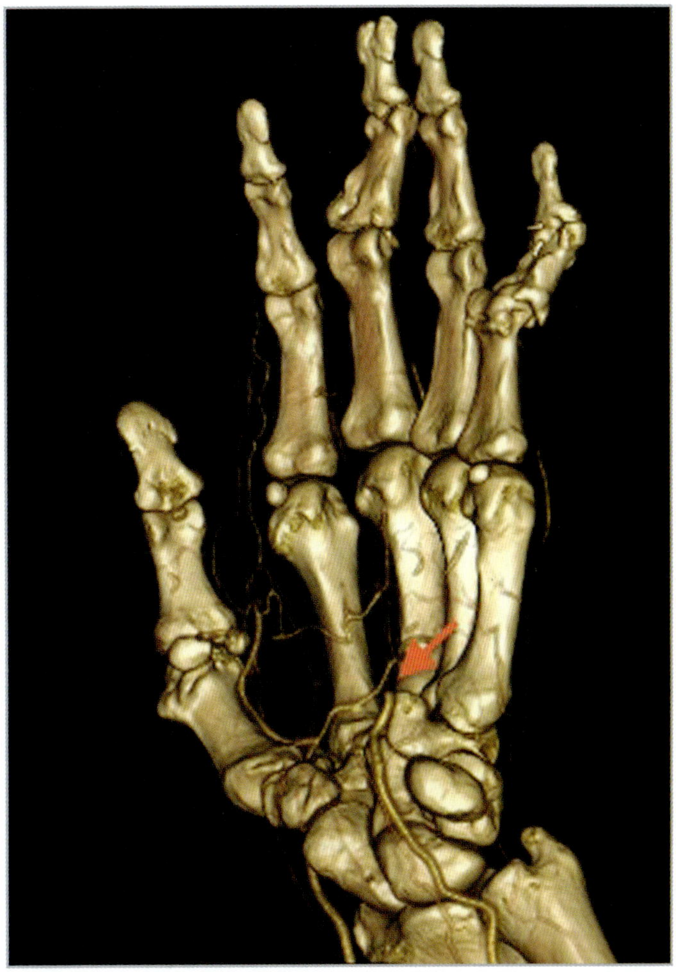

Figure 24.7 Computed tomographic scan of a patient suffering from hypothenar hammer syndrome with an occlusion, shown by arrow, at the hook of the hamate.

Treatment

- In the presence of sufficient collateral circulation, nonsurgical treatment methods can be implemented to treat vasospasms, including smoking cessation, maintenance of the hand in a warm environment, calcium channel blockers, stellate ganglion blockade, oral sympatholytics, vasodilators, and the use of thrombolytic therapy
- In cases of a more advanced disease, such as digital ulceration and chronic pain at rest, surgical intervention may be indicated, including resection of the involved arterial segment and vascular reconstruction
  - For patients who present with inadequate collateral circulation (DBI < 0.7), a reconstructive procedure should be performed using an interposition reversed vein graft
    - Angiography should be used first to determine whether the artery is able to be reconstructed
  - Interposition reversed vein graft:
    - Remove or bypass occluded artery (**Figure 24.8a**)
    - Harvest the saphenous vein (**Figure 24.8b**)
    - Suture it to a good pulsatile flow vessel, such as the ulnar artery and distally to an unoccluded superficial palmar arch (**Figure 24.8c**)
    - This procedure requires microsurgery techniques

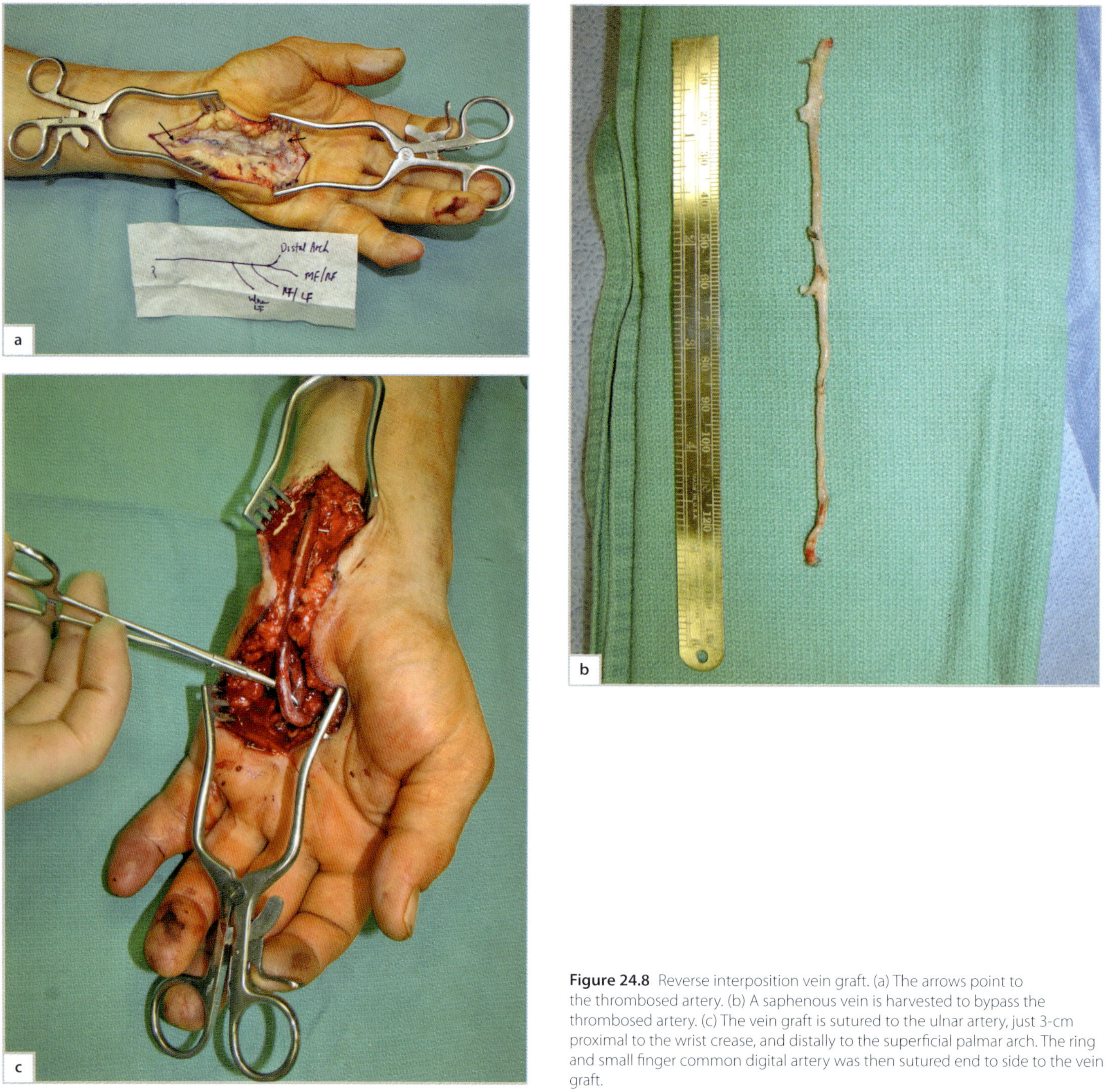

Figure 24.8 Reverse interposition vein graft. (a) The arrows point to the thrombosed artery. (b) A saphenous vein is harvested to bypass the thrombosed artery. (c) The vein graft is sutured to the ulnar artery, just 3-cm proximal to the wrist crease, and distally to the superficial palmar arch. The ring and small finger common digital artery was then sutured end to side to the vein graft.

Aneurysm

Physiology

An aneurysm is defined as a permanent circumscribed dilation of a vessel wall that has increased to over 50% of the expected normal diameter.

- A true aneurysm results from damage to the arterial wall, which causes weakness and gradual vessel wall dilation (**Figure 24.9a**).
  - Histological evaluation will demonstrate that all components of the arterial wall are present, and all three layers of the arterial wall are visible
  - It can be congenital, or caused by blunt trauma, arteriosclerosis, Kawasaki syndrome, metabolic disorders, osteogenesis imperfect, Buerger disease, cystic adventitial, or hemophilia
- A false aneurysm (pseudoaneurysm) usually occurs after a penetrating or crushing injury to the arterial wall (**Figure 24.9b**)
  - A hematoma is formed as blood leaks into surrounding tissue, which later becomes fibrosed
  - Once fibrosed, new canals form through the hematoma, creating a fibrous outpouching of the artery
  - Histological examination will reveal an absence of normal arterial wall elements

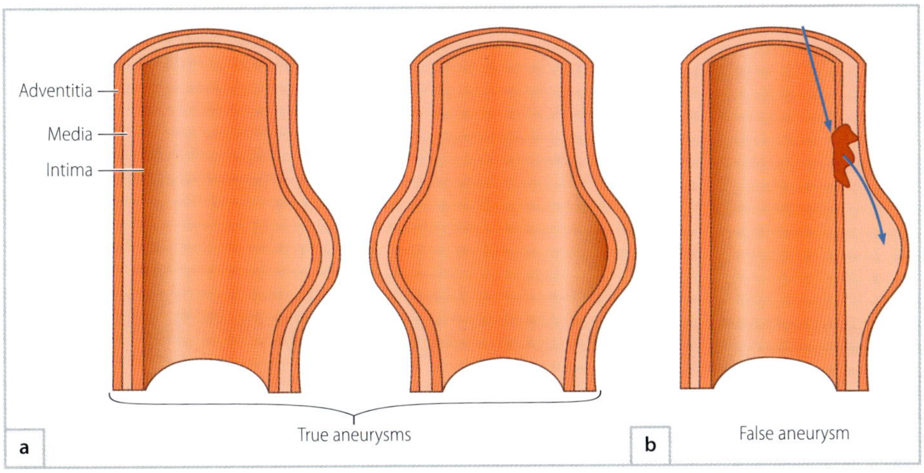

Figure 24.9 Aneurysm. (a) A true aneurysm is characterized by a dilation of all three layers of the arterial wall. (b) In a false aneurysm blood leaks out of the arterial wall creating a hematoma that becomes fibrosed. Once the process is complete, histological examination will reveal that the arterial wall lacks the normal anatomic layers.

Presentation

Patients often present with a painless, warm, palpable mass along the course of an artery, and the progress is usually slow and insidious. Damage of the arterial intima encourages platelet aggregation, which leads to thrombosis formation and production of emboli. The predominant type of aneurism is a false aneurysm, and the most common mechanism is a penetrating injury. Patients can present with signs and symptoms of distal digital embolization, including

- Pain
- Cyanosis
- Pallor
- Coolness
- Recurrent episodes of vasospasm

Diagnosis

Color duplex imaging and MRA can noninvasively show the lesion. Arteriography demonstrates whether the aneurysm is occluded and can define the extent of the lesion and the condition of the downstream digital artery blood flow.

Treatment

Most aneurysms should be treated with excision and ligation before embolization occurs. In the presence of inadequate collateral flow, reconstruction with a vein graft is indicated.

Embolism

Sources

- The most frequent origins of an embolism are the heart, subclavian artery, and the superficial palmar arch
- Seventy percent of all emboli found in the upper extremity are of cardiac origin due to either a recent myocardial infarction or an atrial fibrillation
  - Cardiac emboli usually affect the brachial artery
- The subclavian artery is the most frequent arterial source, secondary to thoracic outlet compression and poststenotic dilatation
  - These emboli usually affect wrist-level and digital-level vessels
- Emboli originating from the wrist and palm usually result from aneurysms or thrombosis
  - These emboli affect the common and proper digital arteries

Presentation

Patients present with symptoms that include acute pain, a pale color to the skin, or pulselessness. In the more proximal aspects of the hand, ischemia may result in muscle paralysis, whereas this effect is not seen in more distal regions. A secondary vasospasm may compromise undamaged collateral flow. Necrosis is common in untreated digits.

Diagnosis

The acute onset of symptoms suggests an embolic event. A segmental pressures examination can determine the extent and location of symptoms. Arteriography, MRA, and duplex Doppler help localize the source and position of the emboli.

Treatment

- To halt the progression of a distal or proximal thrombus from the origin of the embolism, full heparinization should be implemented
- Fogarty catheters and small Fogarty catheters can be used to remove the embolus as far as the superficial palmar arch
- In the hand, embolic events often necessitate surgical resection of the site of origin, accompanied by a subsequent revascularization procedure
- Reperfusion may result in compartment syndrome that must be immediately released

VASOSPASTIC DISEASE

Vasospastic disease refers to episodic attacks leading to small vessel constriction in the distal extremities. These episodes are usually induced by cold or emotional stress. Primary vasospastic disease in the hand, indicating there is no underlying condition, is known as Raynaud disease or primary Raynaud phenomenon. Secondary vasospastic disease found in the hand is termed Raynaud syndrome or secondary Raynaud phenomenon and is typically associated with scleroderma or other disorders.

- Raynaud phenomenon presents as a triple color change of the digits:
  - The fingers initially become white due to ischemia
  - Then they turn blue from limited venous filling
  - The digits turn red from vasodilation and hyperemia as they are warmed, with accompanying dysesthesias, coldness, and pain of the fingers

- Any fingers affected generally exhibit a color change at least twice during an episode, but all of these changes should be completely reversible

Raynaud disease

Raynaud disease is a primary vasospastic condition of the palmar and digital vessels that has no association with other diseases (**Figure 24.10**). It is predominant in females and has a peak incidence between the ages of 20 and 30 years, showing a strong familial association and presenting with symmetrical blanching, sometimes with the toes, nose, and ears also being affected. Ulceration, gangrene, and digit loss do not occur as a result of primary Raynaud disease because these patients have intact vasculature.

Secondary Raynaud phenomenon

Secondary Raynaud phenomenon is a chronic digital ischemia secondary to one of more than 40 primary disorders. It is frequently associated with scleroderma, systemic lupus, rheumatoid arthritis, and occlusive vascular disease. Symptoms are often unilateral and asymmetrical and often associated with heavy cigarette smoking. Patients exhibit symptoms ranging from pain and paresthesia in milder forms of the disease to ulcers and gangrene in more serious manifestations (**Figure 24.11**).

Diagnosis

- Diagnostic testing for primary or secondary Raynaud disease is designed to quantify digital flow in the presence of cold stress and to search for the presence of an underlying obstructive arterial disease
- Cold recovery time is a simple and noninvasive diagnostic technique:
  - A patient's hands are immersed in ice water for 30 seconds and then fingertip temperatures are measured every 5 minutes
  - Vasospastic disease is diagnosed in patients who do not recover baseline digital temperature within 30 minutes
  - This test is not often performed because it is painful for patients with reactive vessels
- If occlusive arterial disease is suspected, arteriography can be performed to demonstrate structural details of the vessels. Arteriography should be obtained on patients with digit threatening vasospastic disease to determine whether they are candidates for revascularization procedures such as arterial bypass

Treatment

Treatment is designed to inhibit an exaggerated vasospasm and enhance the vasodilatory response. Supportive treatments include keeping the hands warm, avoiding cold exposure, and avoiding all caffeine and tobacco use.

- Biofeedback training teaches the skill of self-regulation of skin temperature. For thermal biofeedback, a thermistor is attached to the hand to measure peripheral skin temperature. Patients learn to control the constriction and dilation of their blood vessels during about 20 training sessions. Biofeedback training is most useful in treating:
  - Patients with Raynaud disease
  - Vasospasm from nonneural or nonvascular etiology
  - Raynaud phenomenon with adequate collateral circulation. The results are much less noticeable in patients experiencing inadequate collateral circulation
- Parenteral calcium channel blockers (nifedipine) are useful to reduce the frequency of ischemic attacks
- Palmar or digital periarterial sympathectomies may be helpful when PVRs show improvement after a sympathetic block (**Figure 24.12a** and **b**)
- Other therapies include stellate ganglion nerve blocks, arterial bypass, and amputations for patients with intractable pain or nonhealing ulcers
- Botulinum toxin type A injection into the perineurovascular tissue of the wrist (**Figure 24.13**) or the distal palm or along the digits has recently been reported to treat vasospastic ischemia of the digits
  - The toxin works by inhibiting the release of acetylcholine from the presynaptic membrane
  - This form of chemical sympathectomy inhibits smooth muscle contraction to cause vasodilation, significantly improving pain relief and healing of ulcers

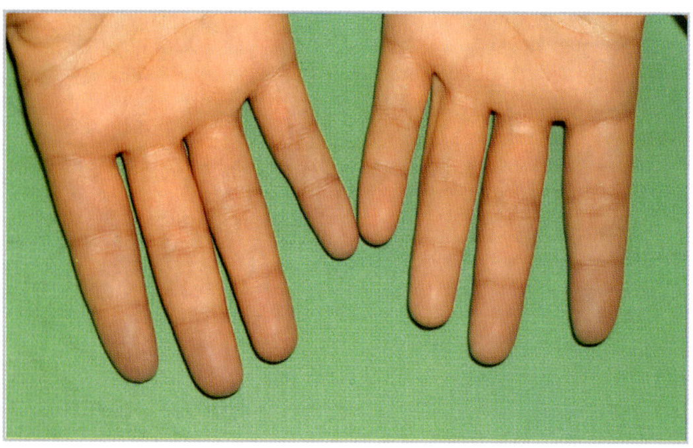

Figure 24.10 Primary Raynaud phenomenon with the characteristic blue color of the digits.

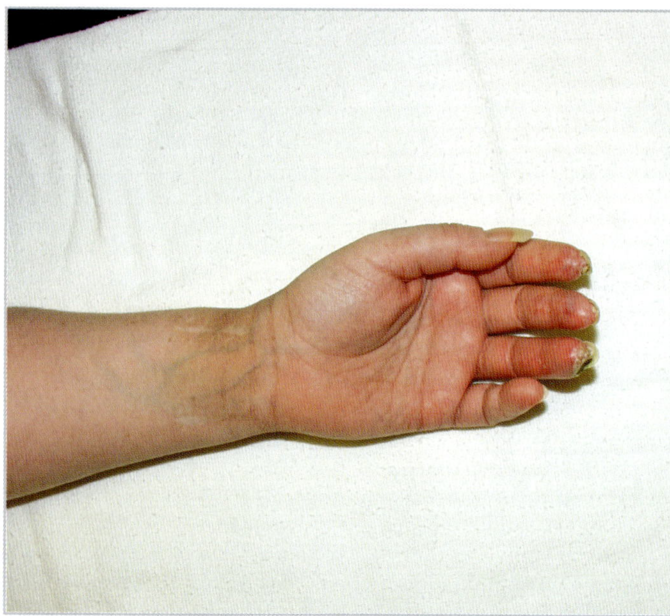

Figure 24.11 Secondary Raynaud phenomenon can cause ulcers that may lead to loss of digit if left untreated.

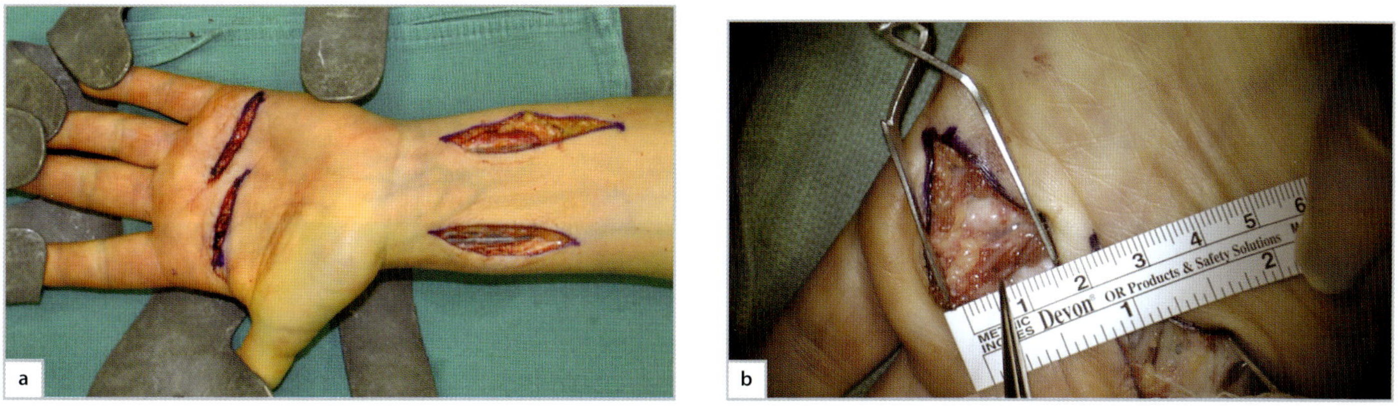

Figure 24.12 Digital sympathectomy for treatment of primary and secondary Raynaud disease. The goal is to increase vessel dilation by interrupting the sympathetic output signals or removing the constriction of periadventitial fibrosis surrounding the arteries. (a) The adventitia of the proper and common digital arteries and the radial and ulnar arteries is excised, to remove the sympathetic fibers. (b) The instrument points to the common digital artery.

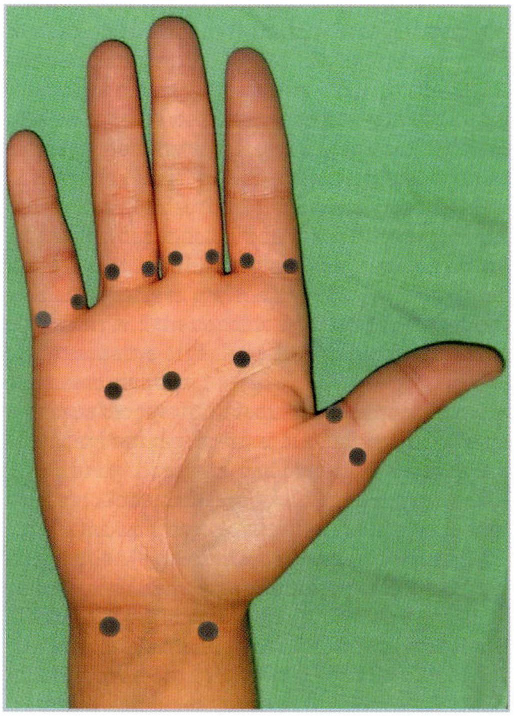

Figure 24.13 The patterns of Botox injection used to treat primary and secondary Raynaud disease.

Hand-arm vibration syndrome

Hand-arm vibration is defined as the transfer of vibration from a tool to a worker's hand and arm. Regular exposure to hand-transmitted vibration can result in symptoms and signs of peripheral vascular, neurological, and musculoskeletal disorders collectively known as hand-arm vibration syndrome (HAVS). This chronic and progressive disorder has the potential to result in lasting disability. HAVS is most common in occupations that require pneumatic drills, grinders, and impact wrenches, where the damage is determined by the length and extent of exposure to vibration.

Symptoms

The vascular component known as 'vibration white finger' presents as periodic blanching of the affected fingers induced by cold weather, followed by pain upon rewarming of the hand. It is usually asymmetrical, initially affecting only tips of one or more fingers temporarily. With time and disease progression, the frequency, duration and severity of the blanching increases. In advanced cases, HAVS may affect all of the phalanges of the fingers with trophic fingertip changes.

Neurological symptoms include numbness, tingling, reduced sensitivity to touch and temperature, and loss of dexterity. Symptoms begin as pain and stiffness in the hands and wrists, caused by damage to the nerve supply and thenar muscles that significantly decrease grip strength. The symptoms are progressive, and advance from intermittent to persistent as the neurovascular structures are increasingly damaged.

The neurological symptoms of HAVS may be similar to carpal tunnel syndrome (CTS). Because early identification of HAVS is critical to treatment, care must be taken to differentiate these two disorders to avoid wrongly labeled CTS. Sensory symptoms relating to CTS are commonly known to wake patients at night, while HAVS symptoms often appear when the hand is exposed to cold and vibration. A patient's vibration exposed occupational history is another important factor that may be helpful to differentiate between CTS and HAVS symptoms.

Investigation

There is no standardized test designed to diagnose HAVS, but several techniques are useful for the assessment of this disease.

- Vascular Doppler and duplex scanning of the upper limbs should be performed to routinely detect a coexisting occlusive disease
- A prolonged rewarm time of finger skin temperature test should be investigated further, as it could be an indication of a vasospasm
  - Although this is a symptom of HAVS, it is not specific to this particular disease
- Neurological tests include 2PD and nerve conduction studies

Treatment

- Prevention is key for this disease, with early identification of at-risk workers, recognition of early symptoms, and avoidance of exposure the mainstay of treatment
- Supportive treatment includes avoidance of cold weather and smoking cessation
- Pharmacological treatments such as calcium channel antagonists, α-antagonists, and prostaglandins have been used, but there is little evidence in the literature that proves the effectiveness of these treatments.

ACUTE VASCULAR INJURIES

Acute vascular injuries can be caused by penetrating or blunt force trauma or iatrogenic injury, such as stab wounds, gunshot wounds, and lacerations. Upper extremity arterial trauma represents 30–50% of all peripheral vascular injuries. Blunt force trauma injuries account for 6–10% of upper-extremity vascular trauma and are often associated with musculoskeletal injuries and neural injuries. Approximately, 90% of acute vascular injuries are the result of penetrating trauma, with the majority involving the brachial artery. These injuries can lead to acute ischemia, delayed thrombosis, or distal embolization, and therefore, restoration of blood flow is essential to prevent distal ischemia and tissue loss.

Diagnosis

- Patients may present with
  - Active bleeding
  - Hematoma
  - Painful, cold, pale, pulseless limb
  - Paralysis
  - Loss of efficient capillary filling
- Most diagnosis can be made by physical examination and Doppler ultrasonography examination
- Angiography may be useful for the assessment of the extent of vascular injury
- The routine use of preoperative angiography is unnecessary in acute open injury because of two main reasons:
  - An evaluation can be made based on the mechanism of injury
  - The time required to obtain angiography can cause a delay in definitive treatment

Operative exploration indication

- Revascularization should be completed within the critical ischemic time:
  - Four hours for proximal injuries
  - Twelve hours for distal injuries
- When open wounds are close to major vessels, operative exploration in a controlled environment is indicated, because the wound is already open and careful exploration will not cause any additional damage. One should not explore the wound for vascular injury in the emergency department when the lights and the instruments are not optimal
- Operative exploration is indicated for closed injuries, persistent pain, paralysis, and loss of capillary filling, as well as cold, pale, pulseless, and numb digits

Treatment

- The first priority is to quickly restore arterial perfusion
  - Critical ischemia requires immediate repair of damaged vessels
  - A reversed interposition vein graft should be used if there is tension during anastomosis (**Figure 24.8a–c**)
- A salvage operation must be performed rapidly, especially for an extremity that contains muscle tissue, because the success rate for salvaging falls significantly after 6 hours of ischemia. A 50% failure rate is expected with a critical vessel injury after only 12 hours without treatment. If intervention has been delayed, fasciotomy and excision of necrotic muscle may be warranted before revascularization is performed
- Noncritical arterial reconstruction is recommended to decrease the risk of development of cold intolerance and to enhance nerve recovery

VASCULAR ANOMALIES OF THE UPPER EXTREMITY

Vascular anomalies can be separated into two main types: vascular tumors and vascular malformations. This system is based on the founding biological investigation of Mulliken and Glowacki published in 1982. Vascular tumors grow by cellular hyperplasia and can regress or persist depending on the type. Vascular malformations are localized defects in the vascular morphogenesis, resulting from an inconsistency in the regulation of the embryogenesis and vasculogenesis pathways. In contrast to vascular tumors, vascular malformations never regress.

- Vascular malformations primarily fall into two categories: high-flow and low-flow vascular malformations
  - Low-flow lesions are much more common than high-flow lesions (7:1 ratio)
  - Low-flow lesions are typically soft, compressible, and diffuse
  - High-flow lesions have the worst prognosis and are the most difficult to treat

Hemangiomas

Hemangiomas are true tumors that occur in 7–10% of infants. Thirty percent are present at birth, whereas 70–90% are apparent by 4 weeks of age, with a female to male ratio of 3:1.

Presentation

Hemangiomas develop in three distinct phases:

1. Rapid growth
2. A static period of no growth
3. A slow involution

The first growth phase involves rapid cellular proliferation, lasting approximately 10–12 months. The second phase, during which the mass appears to grow at a rate proportional to the rest of the child, can last for years, and can exhibit no discernible color change. The involution phase is a slow process of softening, shrinkage, and color change. After involution, telangiectasias, fibrous masses, and inelastic skin commonly remain. By age 5, 50% of the lesions have regressed, and by age 7, 70% of the lesions have involuted. Infantile hemangiomas do not alter the growth of the affected limb and rarely cause functional problems.

Investigation

The diagnosis is made clinically in most cases according to clinical features. MRI may be required in clinically uncertain cases, for guiding therapy, and to evaluate response to treatment. During the initial phase of proliferation, hemangiomas usually present as well-defined lobulated masses. The mass will have a high signal intensity on T2-weighted images and intermediate signal intensity on T1-weighted images, but no perilesional edema should be present. Injection of a gadolinium contrast material is useful to provide intense and uniform enhancement of images. Ultrasound is also useful to evaluate the size and flow characteristics of the mass. Angiography demonstrates a mass with well-circumscribed margins and a blush, but it is usually unnecessary because MRI and MRA provide adequate information.

Treatment

- Treatment of hemangiomas is primarily observational, because most hemangiomas will spontaneously involute
- Symptomatic or persistent lesions may require additional management, with treatment options including intralesional or systemic steroids

- Ulceration occurs in approximately 30% of hemangiomas, typically during the proliferative phase, and can be controlled by local measures
- Surgical management may be indicated in noninvoluting lesions or lesions with severe symptoms. Surgical excision requires meticulous attention to successfully isolate and ligate any feeder vessels, coupled with complete excision of the lesion. After involution, excision of the fibrofatty remnant may be indicated to improve contour and appearance

Venous malformation (VM)

Venous malformations are the most common vascular malformations. They are slow flow and may involve any tissue.

Presentation

Although symptoms typically do not appear until late childhood or early adulthood, VMs are present at birth. They appear as faint blue, soft, easily compressible, and nonpulsatile masses (**Figure 24.14a**). They engorge when dependent and collapse when elevated and are usually more extensive than they appear from the outside. During pregnancy or with oral contraceptives, the lesion can grow rapidly. The lesion can invade bone, muscle, joints, and nerves (**Figure 24.14b**), with symptoms including pain, skeletal deformity, or decreased function due to lesion enlargement. Ulceration is uncommon with this disorder.

Investigation

- An ultrasound will show a hypoechoic, serpiginous and compressible mass
- MRI can be helpful in determining the extent of the lesion
  - Typically show septated lesions with slow gradual filling of contrast material and characteristic nodular enhancement of tortuous vessels on delayed venous phase images
  - Lack of arterial and early venous enhancement
  - Absence of enlarged feeding vessels or arteriovenous shunting
- The presence of small low-signal-intensity foci, called phleboliths, is the best indicator of a VM
- The mass is only partially opacified during the venous phase of angiography, and therefore not fully visible. As a result, angiography alone is not sufficient to evaluate the presence of VMs.

Treatment

- Conservative measures are the mainstay of treatment for this disorder
- Sclerotherapy (injection of caustic substance such as ethanol) has relatively good success in controlling the lesions and also can be used before surgery to decrease blood loss
- A localized mass may be surgically excised

Capillary malformations

Also known as port-wine stains and nevus flammeus are usually low-flow malformations.

Presentation

These lesions typically appear in infants as pink macules. Some of these malformations fade with time, whereas others become darker and thicker. Although these lesions are superficial, they have been known to have an association with a deeper element that may be partly lymphatic in nature. Capillary malformations can also be associated with bone and soft tissue hypertrophy.

Investigation

- The MRI findings may be nondistinguishable from those of VMs
- Dynamic contrast-enhanced MRI can be useful to help distinguish from VM
  - Capillary malformations typically show early homogeneous enhancement
  - The VMs show delayed enhancement

Treatment

- Treatment is usually conservative
- A dye laser can be used to ablate these lesions
- A localized mass may be surgically excised (**Figure 24.14c–e**)

Arteriovenous malformations (AVM)

Arteriovenous malformation is the least common of all vascular anomalies. There are vascular connections between major arteries and the venous system. Blood flows rapidly from the high-pressure arterial to the low-pressure venous system.

Presentation

Patients can present with

- Warmth, soft tissue enlargement
- Extremity pain
- Palpable thrills and bruits
- May lead to bone overgrowth

Distal ischemia ulceration and hemorrhage may be seen in advanced cases. Growth can be negatively impacted if a significant volume of blood flow is redirected toward the malformation. Lesions are hormonally influenced in women.

Investigation

- Doppler scanning provides hemodynamic information
- Magnetic resonance imaging:
  - High-flow malformations
  - Low signal on both T1 and T2 due to the high-flow arteries and arterialized veins
- Angiography:
  - Vital for imaging AVM
  - Demonstrates the arteriovenous shunts, large feeding arteries, and venous outflow
    - Allows for concurrent embolization treatment

Treatment

- Calcium channel blockers may improve blood flow and reduce ischemic pain
- Treatment typically includes compressive dressings, embolization, surgical resection, or even amputation
- Multiple procedures and treatment in stages are often necessary
- Incomplete treatment can lead to recurrence and may stimulate more aggressive growth
- Carefully planned embolization performed in stages before surgery can decrease the size of the lesion and intraoperative blood loss. Surgery should be performed within 2 days of embolization because collateral blood flow can develop quickly
- Surgery can be performed for localized lesions
- Amputation may be the ultimate solution for a life-threatening tumor

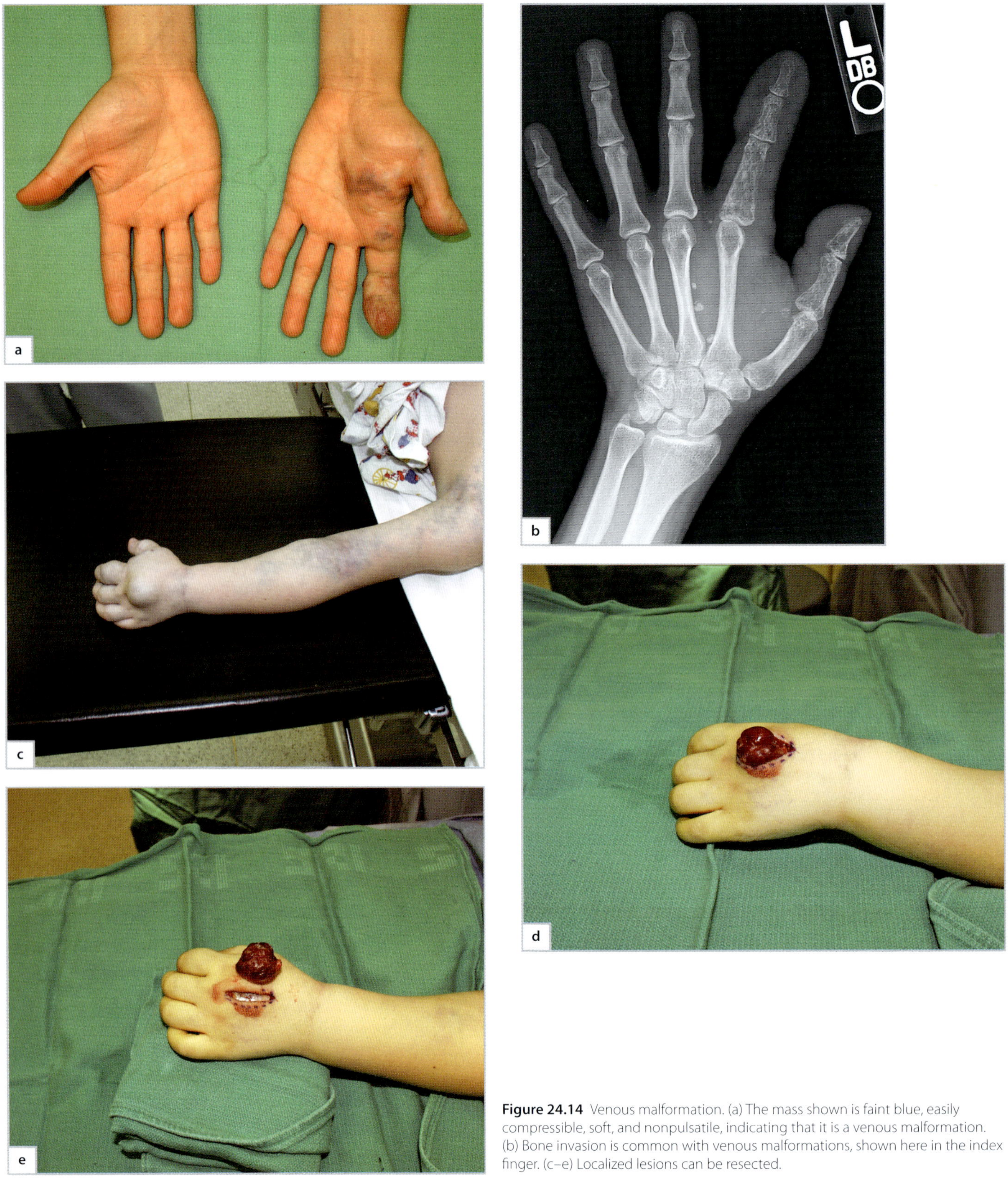

Figure 24.14 Venous malformation. (a) The mass shown is faint blue, easily compressible, soft, and nonpulsatile, indicating that it is a venous malformation. (b) Bone invasion is common with venous malformations, shown here in the index finger. (c–e) Localized lesions can be resected.

SUGGESTED READING

Flors L, Leiva-Salinas C, Maged IM, et al. MR imaging of soft-tissue vascular malformations: diagnosis, classification, and therapy follow-up. Radiographics 2011; 31:1321–1340.

The study demonstrates the imaging diagnosis of different vascular malformation of the upper extremity. This paper demonstrates the various types and degrees of vascular malformations. If available, MRI is an efficient and effective tool for diagnosis of many different vascular malformations.

Fregene A, Ditmars D, Siddiqui A. Botulinum toxin A: a treatment option for digital ischemia in patients with Raynaud's phenomenon. J Hand Surg Am 2009; 34:446–452.

This is a retrospective study that assesses the results of the treatment of recalcitrant digital ischemia with BTX-A. It is also a helpful guide to describing the BTX-A injection procedure and patterns. BTX-A has been proven to significantly improve pain and healing in patients suffering from primary and secondary Raynaud's disease.

Heaver C, Goonetilleke KS, Ferguson H, Shiralkar S. Hand-arm vibration syndrome: a common occupational hazard in industrialized countries. J Hand Surg Eur 2011; 36:354–363.

This study demonstrates the pathogenesis, investigation, and management of hand-arm vibration syndrome. This paper provides an in-depth analysis of the epidemiology, pathogenesis, diagnosis, and treatment modalities available to manage HAVS. It is critical that physicians are able to correctly diagnose this poorly understood disease so as not to confuse it with similar conditions such as carpal tunnel syndrome.

Kotsis SV, Chung KC. A systematic review of the outcomes of digital sympathectomy for treatment of chronic digital ischemia. J Rheumatol 2003; 30:1788–1792.

In this study, the authors conducted a systematic review of digital sympathectomy to determine the effectiveness of digital sympathectomy for treatment of chronic digital ischemia. They reported that the outcomes of digital sympathectomy in the published literature is encouraging, but that the use of this treatment may best be used for patients with severe digital ischemia who have not responded well to other medical treatment.

Lifchez SD, Higgins JP. Long-term results of surgical treatment for hypothenar hammer syndrome. Plast Reconstr Surg 2009; 124:210–216.

It is controversial whether a diseased ulnar artery needs to be reconstructed or merely resected. This study reports the long-term outcomes of patients treated surgically with ulnar artery reconstruction. Ulnar artery reconstruction results in immediate and long-term improvement of measurements of digital blood flow.

Chapter 25 Degenerative osteoarthritis and inflammatory arthritis of the hand and wrist

Jennifer F. Waljee, Kevin C. Chung

DEGENERATIVE OSTEOARTHRITIS

Overview

The term arthritis refers to a generalized process of joint destruction and articular cartilage loss. This joint destruction may result from trauma (secondary), but it is most commonly idiopathic in nature, such as in primary osteoarthritis (inflammatory arthritis will be discussed later in this chapter). There are three specific types of degenerative osteoarthritis: (1) digital osteoarthritis, (2) thumb basal joint osteoarthritis, and (3) Wrist osteoarthritis. Osteoarthritis typically occurs among adults of >50 years of age and most commonly affects the thumb carpometacarpal (CMC) and interphalangeal (IP) joints of the digits. Osteoarthritis is more common among women than among men, and up to 30% of postmenopausal women are afflicted by thumb CMC joint arthritis. Nonsurgical treatment options may alleviate the symptoms of arthritis early in the course of disease, whereas arthroplasty and arthrodesis are often reserved for pain and deformity that significantly impairs hand function.

Pathophysiology

Systemic risk factors for osteoarthritis include ethnicity, age, gender, menopausal status, genetics, bone density, and nutritional deficiencies. Local risk factors include joint injury, occupation, daily activities, joint biomechanics, and instability. Pathologic changes include synovitis and joint effusion, loss of articular cartilage, remodeling of subchondral bone with osteophyte formation, and joint space loss.

Digital osteoarthritis

Clinical presentation

The distal interphalangeal (DIP) joint is the most commonly affected joint in the hand, followed by the proximal interphalangeal (PIP) joint. Patients typically present with painful, stiff, swollen, deformed joints. Clinicians should elicit the patient's history regarding previous trauma and inflammatory conditions [e.g. lupus, rheumatoid arthritis (RA)]. Joint active and passive range of motion should be determined, as well as patient's occupation and demand. In patients with digital osteoarthritis, Heberden nodes and mucoid cysts are commonly seen at the DIP joints, and Bouchard nodes are seen over the PIP joints. Nail plate changes may also be seen with DIP joint arthritis (**Figure 25.1**). The collateral ligaments, extensor apparatus, and joint stability should be assessed to ensure that the joint can support surface replacement arthroplasty (SRA). Otherwise, joint fusion should be performed. Finally, three radiographic views of the hand and involved digit should be obtained to determine joint integrity and bone stock.

Anatomy

The metacarpophalangeal (MCP) joint is a condylar joint stabilized by collateral and accessory ligaments, the joint capsule, and the volar plate. Because of its shape, a condylar joint permits motion in multiple planes, including flexion, extension, adduction, abduction, and circumduction (**Figure 25.2**). In contrast, the PIP and DIP joints are a hinge joint stabilized by the collateral ligaments and volar plate, and allow motion in a single plane (**Figure 25.3**). Stability of the joint depends on the joint capsule, volar plate, articular congruity, and collateral ligaments.

Treatment options

Nonoperative management

Nearly all patients should receive a trial of nonoperative management, and surgical intervention should be reserved for those individuals who fail nonoperative treatment strategies. Although nonoperative strategies can provide excellent functional results and patient satisfaction, they typically do not halt the progression of the disease. Nonoperative treatment strategies include

- Activity modification: Altering activities of daily living to diminish joint stress can minimize the disability due to arthritis
- Splinting: Positional splinting can offload areas of the joint surface that have degenerated and force the joint to rest. Splinting can allow patients to return to activities that were previously not tolerated due to enhanced joint support

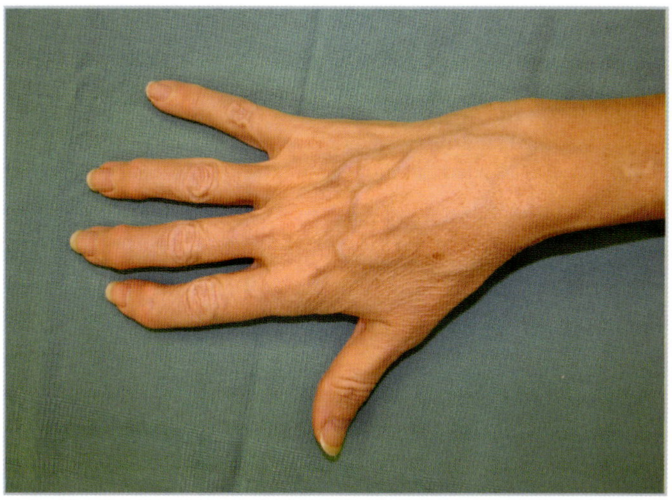

Figure 25.1 Joint deformity related to distal interphalangeal joint osteoarthritis.

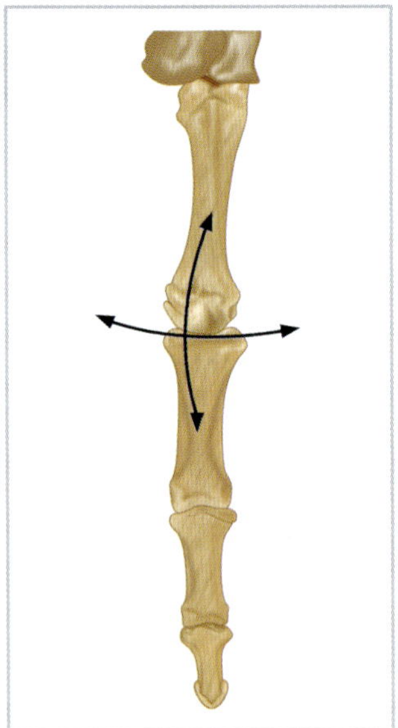

Figure 25.2 Anatomy of the metacarpophalangeal joint.

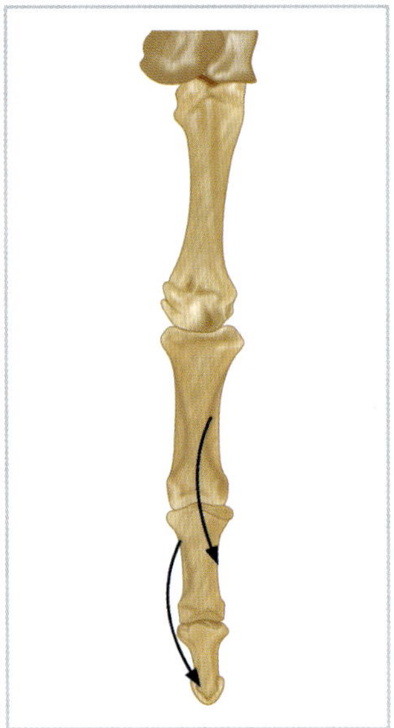

Figure 25.3 Anatomy of the interphalangeal joint.

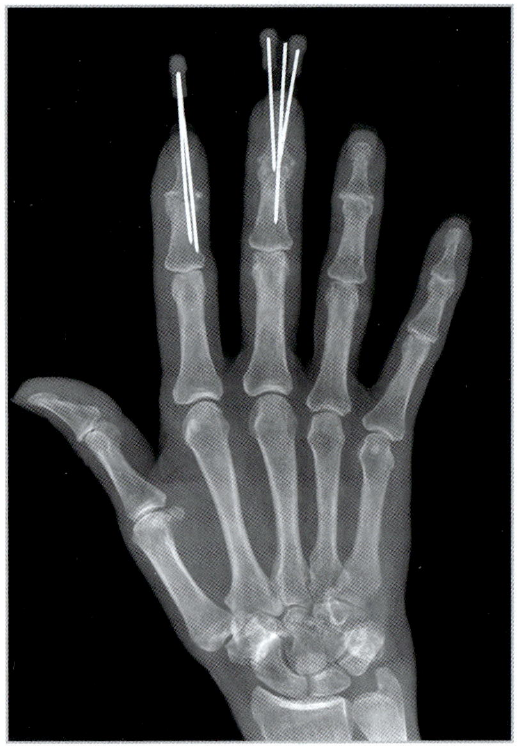

Figure 25.4 Distal interphalangeal joint fusion for osteoarthritis using Kirschner wires.

- Pharmacotherapy: Various medications are available to help treat the symptoms of osteoarthritis, but some may be associated with adverse side effects
  - Nonsteroidal anti-inflammatory drugs (NSAIDs) medications are widely used but may be associated with gastrointestinal, hematologic, and renal adverse effects
  - Topical anti-inflammatory medications (e.g. diclofenac sodium) may alleviate pain without systemic effects
  - Intra-articular corticosteroid injections are well tolerated, but they have only temporary effects. The maximum number of injections that is appropriate is unknown, but their effectiveness often appears to wane over time. Furthermore, repeated injections may compromise the viability of articular cartilage and increase the risk of septic arthritis

Surgical management

Surgical options for osteoarthritis cannot restore full range of motion, and therefore, the goals of surgical intervention are primarily to relieve pain and discomfort. For those patients with inadequate bone stock or joint stability to support an implant, arthrodesis should be considered over arthroplasty. In general, arthrodesis is preferred for radial-sided digits (index) to achieve pain-free pinch stability, whereas arthroplasty is better suited for ulnar digits (middle, ring, and little fingers) to achieve a pain-free grip. Surgical management largely depends on the joint that is affected.

DIP joint

Although silicone implant arthroplasty has been described, DIP joint arthritis is usually managed by arthrodesis and can be performed using a variety of fixation techniques including Kirschner (K)-wire fixation, tension band wiring, or headless screw placement (**Figure 25.4**). A 'T-shaped' approach through the joint is used, and the joint surfaces are prepared to ensure adequate fusion. The DIP joint is typically fused in slight (5°–10°) flexion (**Figure 25.5**).

PIP joint

The PIP joint arthritis can be managed with SRA, silicone arthroplasty, or arthrodesis. Arthroplasty rarely improves arc of motion beyond 60°, but it can relieve pain and improve motion to a more functional position.

- Silicone arthroplasty: Silicone implants have been widely used for arthroplasty since 1966. Complications include reactive synovitis, implant fracture, rotation, and deformation
- SRA: Restores an unconstrained joint surface that is limited by ligamentous support only, but it has a higher rate of complications compared with silicone joint replacement, including implant eroding the bone dislocation, and instability. In contrast, constrained implants are more stable but permit less range of motion. A variety of materials have been used for arthroplasty, including metal polymers (cobalt) and graphite coated with pyrolytic carbon (**Figure 25.6**). Interchangeable proximal and distal components are press fit into the joint using a dorsal approach without the use of bone cement. The collateral ligaments must be preserved to ensure implant stability (**Figure 25.7a and b**)
- Arthrodesis: Can allow for stable and pain-free pinch for radial digits but may significantly limit power grip if performed in ulnar-sided digits. Fusion techniques can include K-wire fixation, tension band wiring, plate fixation, and screw fixation, depending on surgeon's preference (**Figure 25.8a** and **b**). The position of fusion should mirror the digital cascade and range from 40° (index finger), progressing by 5° for more ulnar fingers to 55° (little finger)

MCP joint

Arthroplasty is preferable to arthrodesis for the MCP joint to preserve motion. Arthroplasty options included constrained silicone implants and unconstrained surface replacement implants.

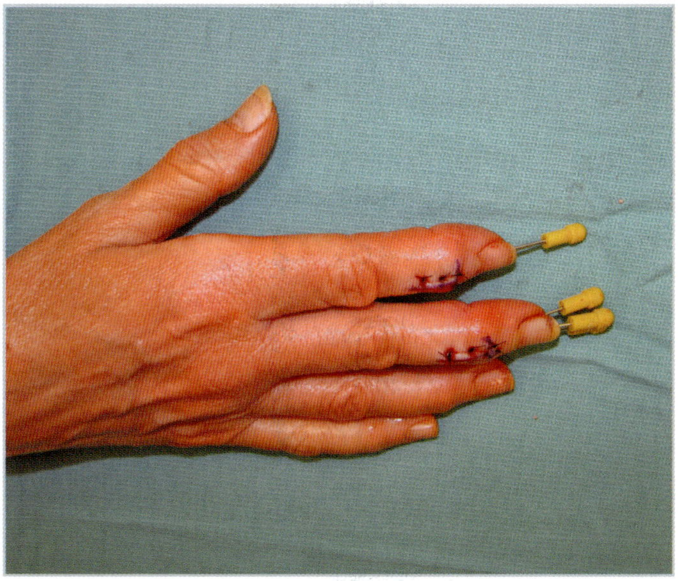

Figure 25.5 Distal interphalangeal joint fusion for osteoarthritis using Kirschner wires.

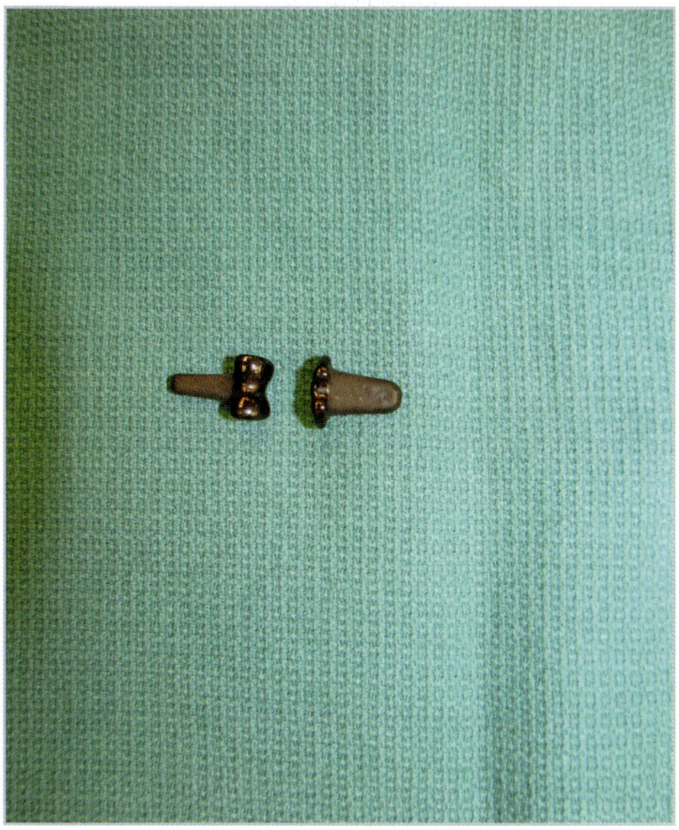

Figure 25.6 Pyrocarbon implant for proximal interphalangeal joint replacement.

- Silicone arthroplasty: Widely used but prone to fracture over time leading to synovitis and osteolysis. Appropriate for patients with severe joint deformities and poor bone stock.
- SRA: The MCP joint is accessed through a dorsal, S-shaped incision, and the proximal and distal pyrocarbon implant is press fit into the medullary canal after osteotomy (**Figure 25.9**). Arthroplasty improves patient reported outcomes including pain and function and increases arc of motion to approximately 60°
- Arthrodesis: This is a salvage option for patients with poorly controlled pain, as fusion at the finger MCP joint significantly limits hand function and is seldom performed at this level, in contrast to the thumb MCP joint that is often fused to achieve thumb stability for stable pinch. Fusion techniques can include K-wire fixation, tension band wiring, plate fixation, and screw fixation, depending on surgeon's preference. Fusion position, if ever needed to be performed, should mirror the normal digital cascade, from 25° at the index finger to 40° at the little finger

Thumb basal joint osteoarthritis

Pathogenesis

Strenuous use over time leads to attrition of the volar beak ligament at the trapeziometacarpal joint, radial subluxation of the CMC joint, and progressive joint instability. In women, it is postulated that hormone-mediated joint laxity predisposes postmenopausal women to CMC arthritis, as well as the anatomic differences in joint congruity, contact surfaces, and joint stresses between men and women.

Clinical presentation

The thumb basal joint is the second most common site of osteoarthritis overall and affects approximately 25% of women and 8% of men. Concomitant scaphotrapeziotrapezoid (STT) arthritis is common among patients with thumb CMC arthritis; however, isolated STT arthritis is rare. Similar to the digital arthritis, patients typically present with the gradual onset of aching pain, stiffness, joint deformity, and swelling. Disease progression is marked by weakness and loss of dexterity. Patients may experience pain with axial loading or rotation and report loss of grip and pinch strength. Patients may also present with a 'zig-zag' deformity due to compensatory hyperextension of the thumb MCP joint, leading to subluxation of the CMC joint and adduction of the metacarpal (**Figure 25.10**). Physical examination findings include focal swelling and tenderness over the involved joint, crepitus with movement due to synovitis, pain with axial loading, and diminished range of motion.

Radiographic staging

Radiographic imaging characteristically reveals diminished joint space, subchondral sclerosis, bony cysts, and osteophyte formation. However, radiographic findings may not necessarily correlate with patient symptomatology. Severity has been classified into four stages:

- Stage 1: Normal radiographs or slightly widened CMC joint space due to synovitis
- Stage 2: Radiographic changes include mild CMC space narrowing and minimal osteophyte formation (<2 mm in diameter)
- Stage 3: Progressive CMC space narrowing and osteophyte formation > 2 mm in diameter
- Stage 4: Advanced CMC arthritis with significant CMC joint space narrowing or obliteration and involvement of the STT joint

Anatomy

The trapeziometacarpal joint is a saddle joint that allows for multiplanar motion (**Figure 25.11**). The palmar beak ligament spans the volar aspect of the thumb metacarpal to the volar aspect of the trapezium. The radial artery runs though the anatomic snuffbox, between the extensor pollicis longus (EPL) and extensor pollicis brevis (EPB) and over the dorsal capsule of the CMC joint. The first

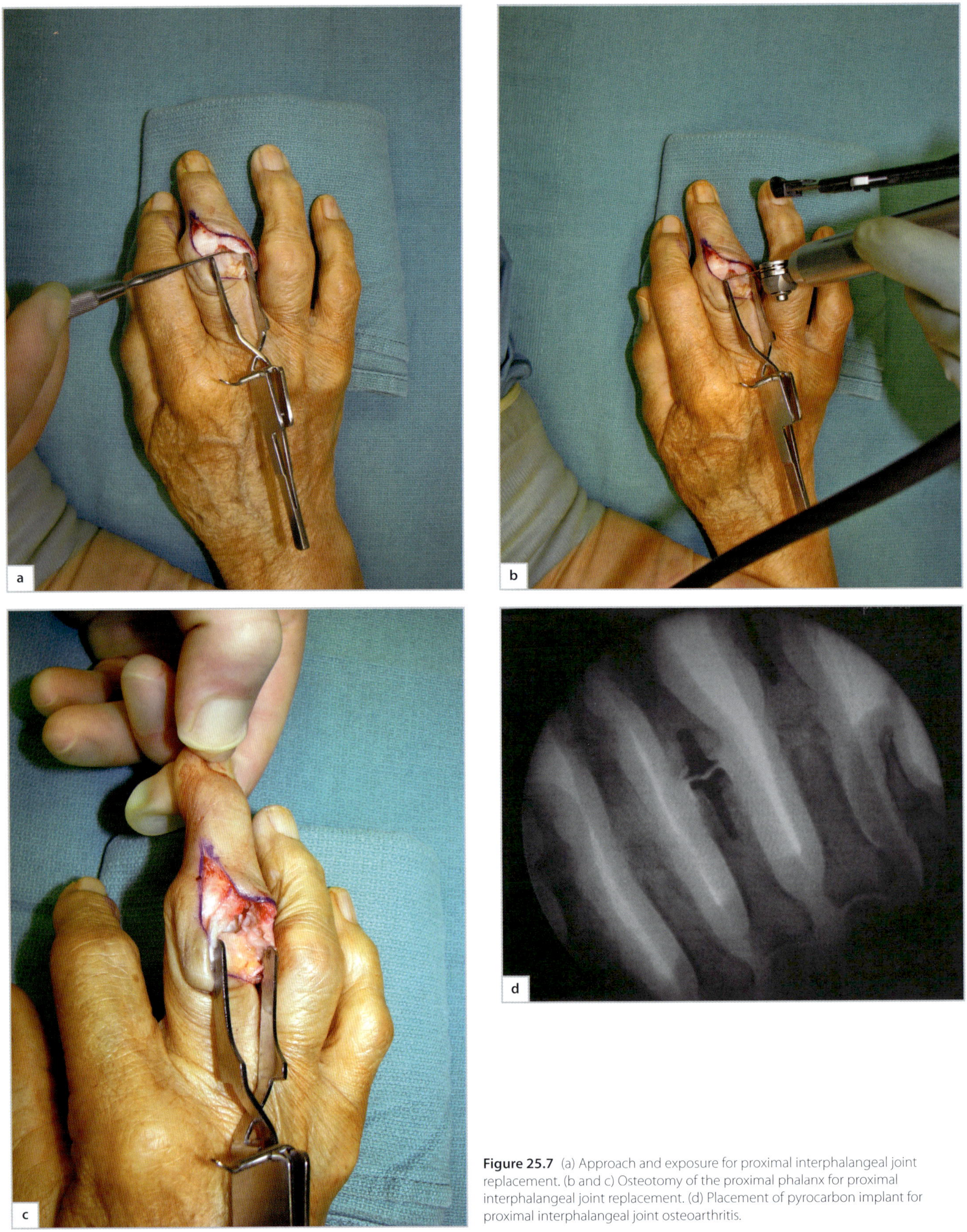

Figure 25.7 (a) Approach and exposure for proximal interphalangeal joint replacement. (b and c) Osteotomy of the proximal phalanx for proximal interphalangeal joint replacement. (d) Placement of pyrocarbon implant for proximal interphalangeal joint osteoarthritis.

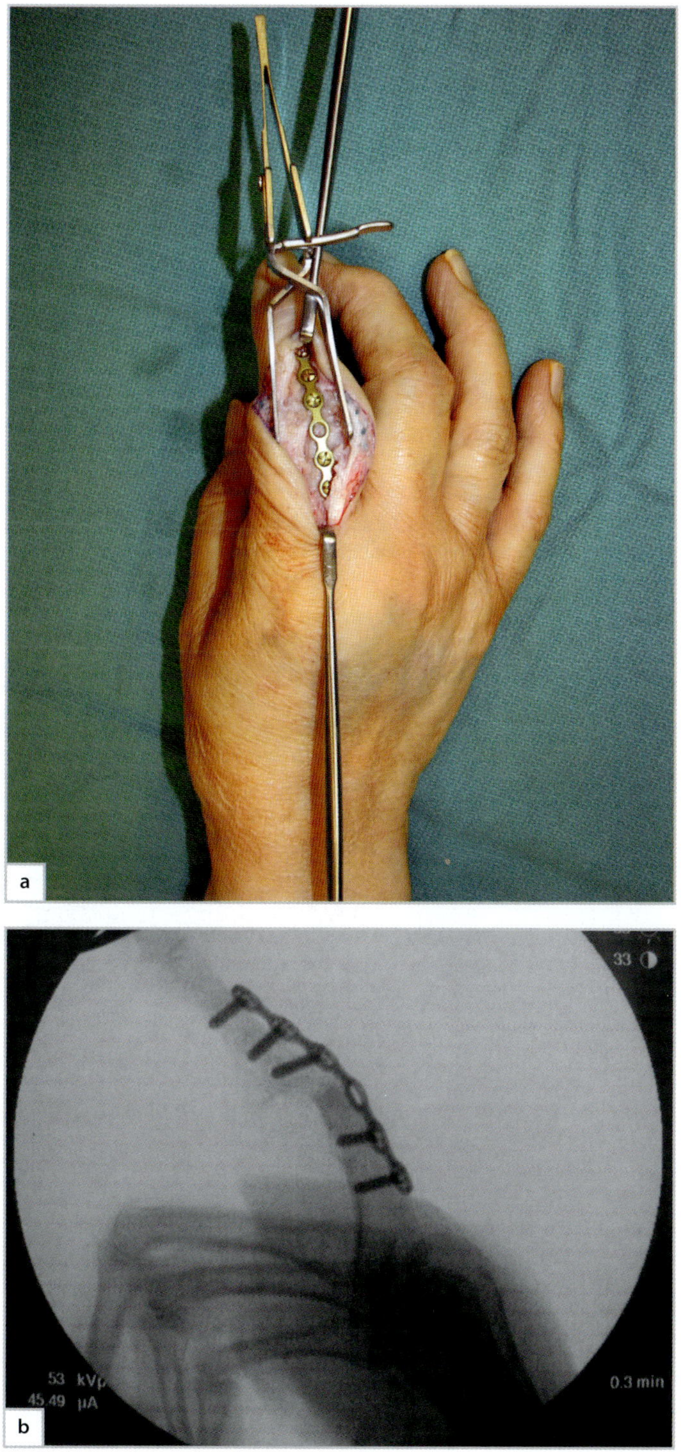

Figure 25.8 (a and b) Proximal interphalangeal joint arthrodesis for osteoarthritis with plate fixation.

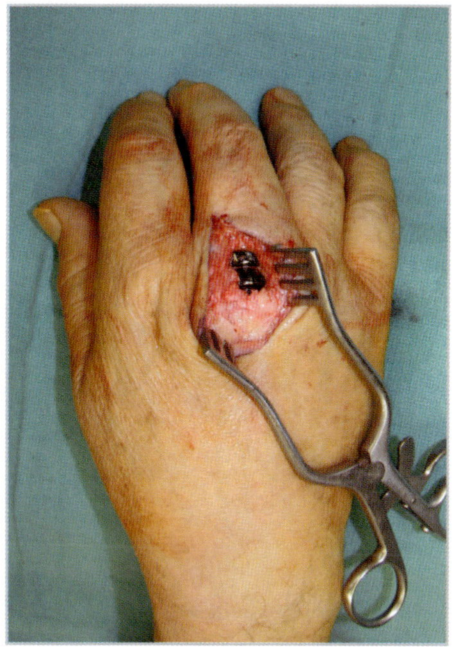

Figure 25.9
Pyrocarbon implant for metacarpophalangeal joint arthritis.

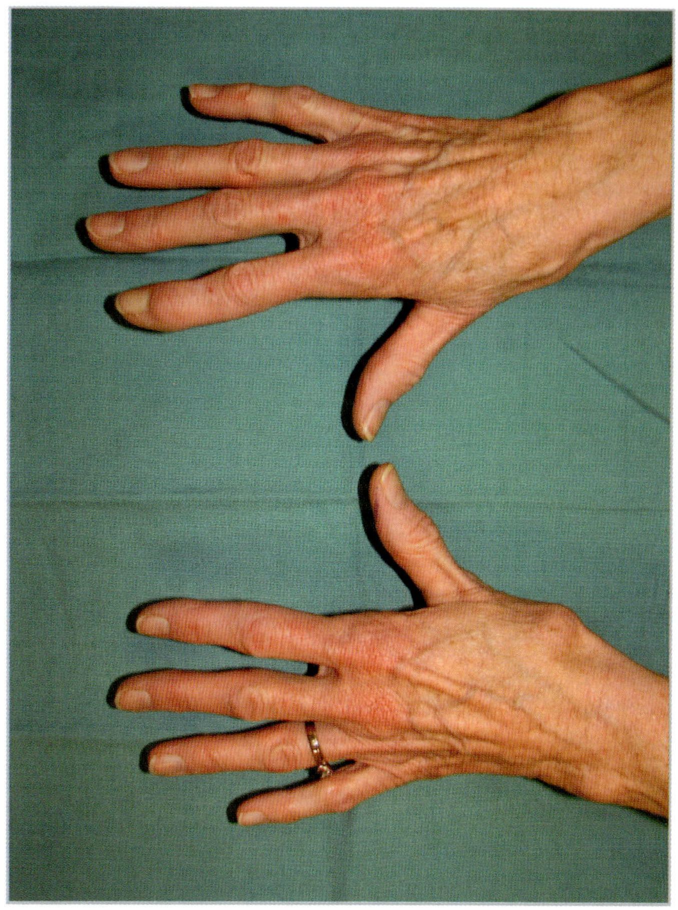

Figure 25.10 'Zig-zag' deformity due to compensatory hyperextension of the thumb MCP joint and subluxation of the CMC joint with adduction of the metacarpal.

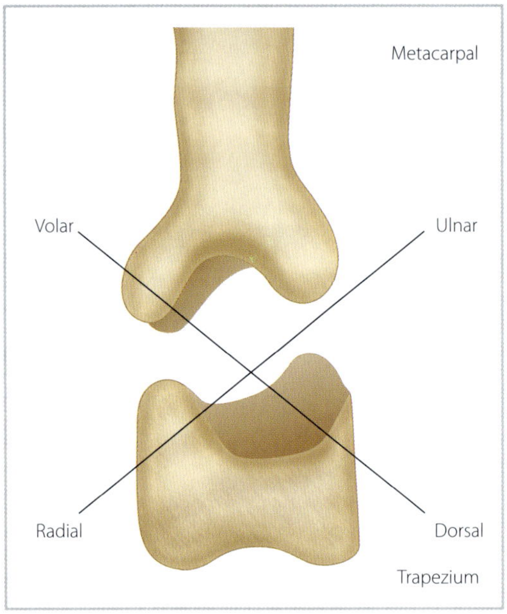

Figure 25.11 Anatomy of the trapeziometacarpal joint of the thumb.

extensor compartment contains the abductor pollicis longus (APL) and EPB tendons. The radial sensory nerve lies in close proximity to the first compartment subcutaneously. The flexor carpi radialis (FCR) tendon lies deep to the trapezium and inserts on the base of the index metacarpal.

Treatment

Nonoperative management

Similar to digital arthritis, patients should receive a trial of nonoperative management prior to surgical intervention. Modalities include splinting, activity modification, NSAIDs, and corticosteroid injections. Intra-articular hyaluronate injections have been used for the treatment of thumb CMC arthritis, although large studies supporting its use are lacking.

Surgical management

The goals of surgical management are to alleviate pain, optimize hand function, and correct joint deformity. Surgical intervention should be reserved for those patients who do not respond to nonoperative measures. Surgical management of thumb basal joint arthritis encompasses a variety of procedures, including trapeziectomy alone, trapeziectomy with ligament reconstruction, and trapeziectomy with ligament reconstruction and tendon interposition. Simple trapeziectomy is one of the earliest and remains one of the most commonly performed procedures for thumb CMC arthritis. Complete trapeziectomy is advocated over partial trapeziectomy due to the progression of arthritis, which will lead to revision. Concerns for metacarpal collapse and diminished grip strength due to a lack of joint stability have prompted the use of various ligamentous reconstructions after trapeziectomy. To date, multiple studies have failed to demonstrate a superior approach, and the decision for surgical technique is primarily based on surgeon's experience and preference.

- Trapeziectomy: The trapezium is excised through a longitudinal incision over the dorsum of the thumb CMC joint, or through a Wagner incision at the junction of the glabrous and nonglabrous skin over the thenar eminence (**Figure 25.12a** and **b**). K-wires can be placed at the base of the thumb metacarpal to the index metacarpal to maintain the joint space for 4 weeks as the joint space fills with organized hematoma
  - To further prevent joint space collapse, tendon grafts may be placed in the joint space after trapeziectomy, including the palmaris longus, APL, and FCR. This may also be performed in conjunction with ligament reconstruction described below
- APL reconstruction (**Figure 25.13**): The radial slip of the APL tendon can be used for suspension through a dorsal incision over the thumb and first extensor compartment after trapeziectomy. The APL tendon slip can be woven through the extensor carpi radialis longus tendon to provide suspension to the thumb metacarpal.
- FCR reconstruction (**Figure 25.14**): Originally described by Eaton and Littler (1973), half of the FCR tendon can be used for volar beak ligament reconstruction. A portion of the tendon is divided proximally and then passed through a tunnel drilled at the base of the thumb metacarpal.
  - Described by Weilby, the FCR tendon may also be used to reconstruct the volar beak ligament by weaving the FCR through the APL and then securing the FCR to the base of the thumb metacarpal, without creating a separate bone tunnel. The APL is then imbricated over the FCR weave.
- CMC implant arthroplasty: Autologous tendon interposition within the CMC joint space after trapeziectomy is commonly performed in conjunction with the ligament reconstruction as described above. Although implant arthroplasty using synthetic materials, such as silicone, metal alloys, and allograft materials, has been described, this technique has been performed much less frequently than autologous tendon interposition due to implant failure and synovitis
- CMC arthrodesis (**Figure 25.15**): Arthrodesis is indicated in younger, higher demand patients with stage 2 or 3 disease. Arthrodesis should not be performed in patients with advanced arthritis, pantrapezial arthritis, or ligamentous laxity without joint destruction (stage 1 disease). The thumb CMC joint can be approached volarly or dorsally, and the base of the metacarpal and distal aspect of the trapezium are denuded with a rongeur to the subchondral bone. The thumb is fused in slight opposition with the distal phalanx of the thumb overlying the index metacarpal when the patient makes a fist. The joint may be fused with either K-wires or a small plate, depending on surgeon's preference, and augmented with a bone graft, harvested from the distal radius if needed. The thumb is then immobilized in a thumb spica cast or splint for 6–8 weeks.
- STT arthritis: For patients with associated STT arthritis, the articular surface of the trapezoid should be inspected during CMC arthroplasty. Surgical options for STT arthritis commonly include distal scaphoid excision, STT fusion with radial styloidectomy, and partial trapezoid excision.

Wrist osteoarthritis

Primary arthritis is relatively rare, and most commonly occurs due to the STT arthritis as described above. More frequently, wrist arthritis results after trauma with resulting instability that leads to carpal collapse and inflammatory arthropathies. Injuries that can result in long-term wrist arthritis include scaphoid fractures with associated nonunion (scaphoid nonunion advanced collapse/SNAC), scapholunate (SL) ligament injuries (scapholunate advanced collapse/SLAC), distal radius fractures, and perilunate dislocations. Rarely, progressive wrist arthritis results from idiopathic causes, such as Kienbock disease (avascular necrosis of the lunate), Preisler disease

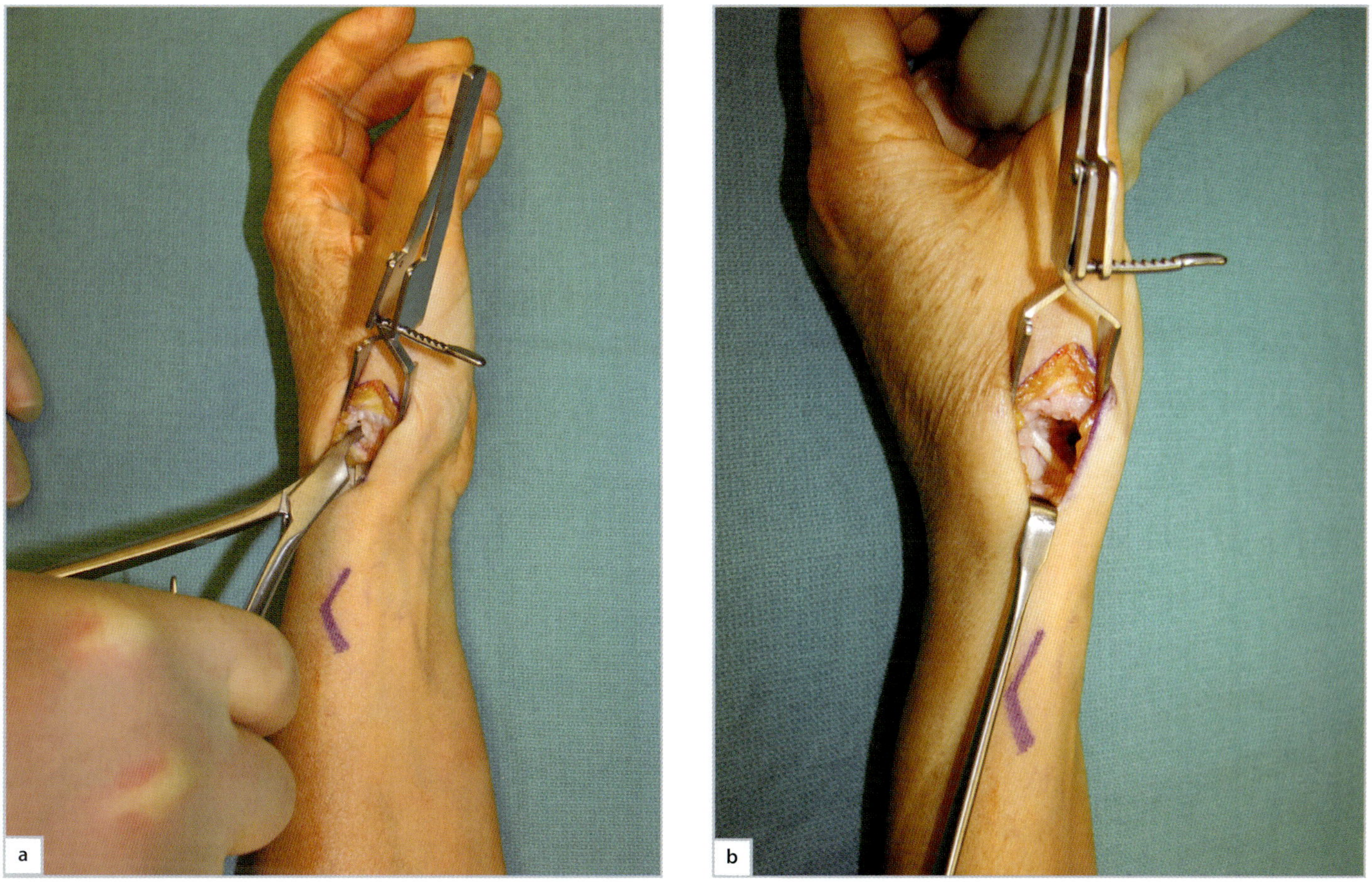

Figure 25.12 (a and b) Trapeziectomy for thumb carpometacarpal joint arthritis.

(avascular necrosis of the scaphoid), or congenital deformities such as Madelung deformity.

Pathogenesis

Traumatic injuries and chronic inflammation result in attenuation of the ligamentous support of the wrist, causing carpal collapse and painful arthritis. For example, in patients with progressive perilunate instability, a predictable pattern of wrist instability and collapse occurs:

- Stage 1: The distal carpal row is hyperextended, and the scaphotrapezoid-capitate ligaments extend the scaphoid. The lunate is held by the short radiolunate ligament. Continued force results in SL ligament injury and disruption
- Stage 2: The scaphoid and distal row dislocates dorsally with respect to the lunate, stressing the radioscaphoid-capitate ligament
- Stage 3: Continued hyperextension results in strain and failure of the lunotriquetral ligament and dorsal dislocation of the triquetrum
- Stage 4: The capitate descends into the radiocarpal space and the lunate dislocates volarly into the carpal canal

In addition, bony fractures or necrosis can result in collapse of the normal bony architecture and subsequent carpal instability and collapse. For example, displaced or proximal pole scaphoid fractures that are unrecognized or fail initial treatment strategies can progress to carpal instability and collapse. Arthritic changes arise at the radial styloid articulation with the distal scaphoid pole and progress to the midcarpal joint causing pancarpal arthritis.

Clinical presentation

Patients commonly present complaining of pain, diminished wrist motion, and wrist deformity. Pain with wrist motion due to arthritis inhibits forearm musculature, leading to weakened grasp. Provocative maneuvers can elicit the etiology and manifestations of arthritis, such as tenderness over the SL interval and radial aspect of the wrist. Plain radiographs can define the carpal architecture and identify patterns of instability and degeneration, and magnetic resonance imaging can be a useful adjunct to identify ligamentous injury and further define degeneration. For example, SLAC and SNAC deformities display a predictable radiographic pattern of wrist progressive arthritis and joint collapse:

- Stage 1: The SL interval is widened, and degenerative changes are seen at the articulation of the radial styloid and distal scaphoid (**Figure 25.16**)
- Stage 2: Degeneration progresses to include the entire radioscaphoid joint, and proximal migration of the distal carpal row occurs (**Figure 25.17a and b**)
- Stage 3: Midcarpal degenerative changes occur, and the scaphoid and lunate may fall into a dorsal intercalated segmental instability deformity (lunate in extension, scaphoid in flexion) (**Figure 25.18**)
- Stage 4: Degeneration progresses to involve the radiolunate articulation, intercarpal joints, and the distal radioulnar joint (DRUJ) (**Figure 25.19**)

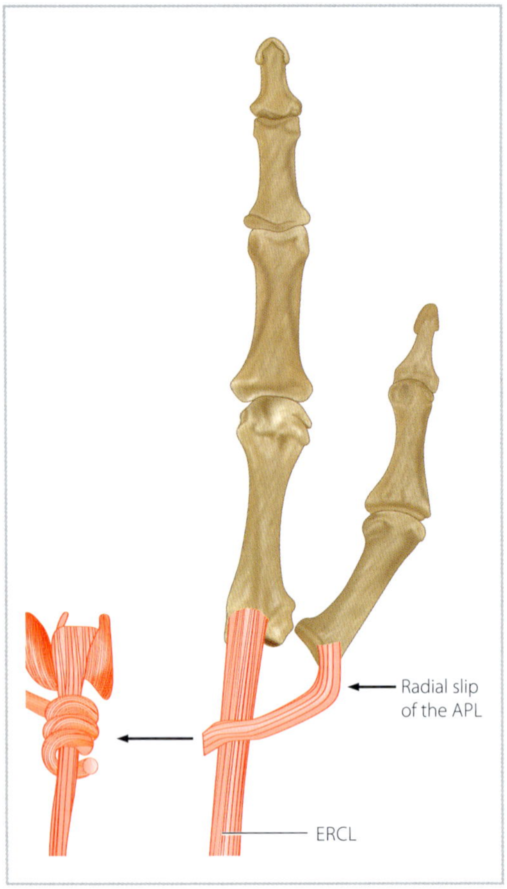

Figure 25.13 Suspension of the trapeziometacarpal joint using a slip of abductor pollicis longus.

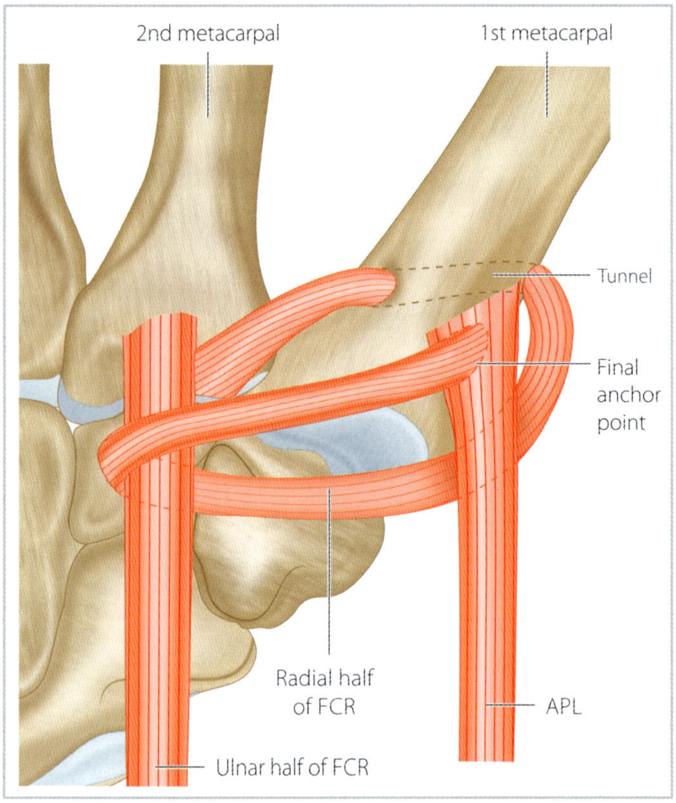

Figure 25.14 Resuspension of the trapeziometacarpal joint using a strip of flexor carpi radialis. APL, abductor pollicis longus; FCR, flexor carpi radialis.

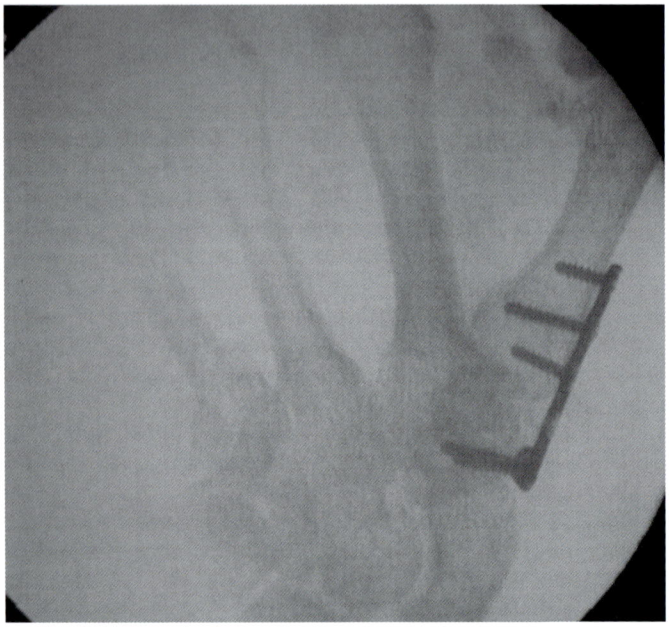

Figure 25.15 Fusion of the thumb carpometacarpal joint with locking plate fixation.

Treatment options

Nonoperative management

As with osteoarthritis of the smaller joints of the hand, patients with wrist arthritis can benefit substantially from conservative measures such as immobilization, splinting, NSAIDs, and corticosteroid injections. Consultation with a hand therapist can identify activity modifications and other modalities that can improve patient symptoms.

Surgical management

Principles of exposure

The wrist is commonly exposed through a dorsal incision in line with the long finger metacarpal. The third compartment is opened, and the EPL is mobilized to be placed in the subcutaneous position during closure so that the swelling in the compartments does not cause avascular necrosis and rupture of the EPL. The wrist capsule is opened between the second and third compartments, and the posterior interosseous nerve can be identified at the base of the fourth compartment. Posterior interosseus nerve neurectomy can be performed at this stage to provide wrist pain relief. The dorsal wrist capsule can be incised longitudinally or transversely, sparing the intrinsic and extrinsic ligaments, depending on surgeon's preference.

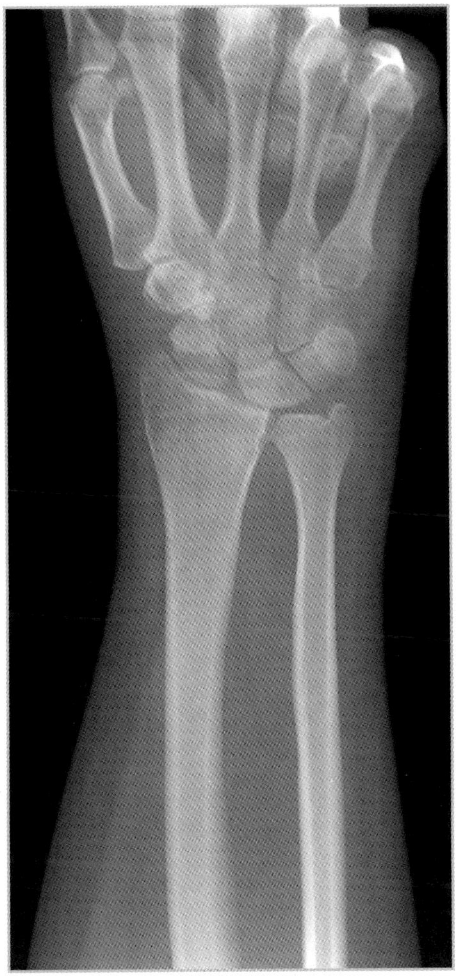

Figure 25.16 Radiographic findings of stage 1 SLAC/SNAC wrist deformity demonstrating widening of the scapholunate interval.

Limited intercarpal fusion

Depending on the area of degeneration, local fusion can be performed to attempt to preserve some wrist motion through the remaining wrist articulations. Complete reduction of carpal instability, fusion using rigid fixation techniques (e.g. headless screws), and augmentation with bone graft harvested from the distal radius will augment fusion rates.

- Radioscapholunate arthrodesis: Indicated for patients who have radiocarpal arthritis with preservation of the midcarpal joint (e.g. after intra-articular distal radius fractures). Fixation is achieved with K-wires or dorsal plating and augmented with a bone graft
- Scaphocapitate arthrodesis: Indicated for patients with chronic SL instability to reduce the scaphoid into an extended position
- Scapholunocapitate arthrodesis with radial styloidectomy: Indicated for patients with SL dissociation and midcarpal degenerative changes but preserved articulation at the radiocarpal joint. The radial styloid is excised to prevent impingement with motion. The SL joint is then reduced, and internal fixation is achieved with K-wires or dorsal plates. Approximately 50% of normal wrist motion is restored with scapholunocapitate fusion and radial styloidectomy
- Four-corner arthrodesis (**Figure 25.20a–c**): Indicated for patients who have SLAC or SNAC wrist arthritis with preservation of the radiolunate joint. The lunate, trapezium, capitate, and hamate are fused with K-wires or circular plates augmented by autologous bone graft harvested from the distal radius or iliac crest. The scaphoid is excised if radioscaphoid arthritis is present, but it should not be used for bone grafting. Four-corner arthrodesis restores approximately 80% grip strength and 60% normal range of motion. Complications include failure of fusion, which may be higher with dorsal circular plate fixation and using the scaphoid for bone grafting
- Proximal row carpectomy (PRC) (**Figure 25.21a and b**): Indicated for patients with radiocarpal arthritis without degenerative changes of the capitate. The scaphoid, lunate, and triquetrum are excised, taking care to preserve the radioscaphocapitate ligament to prevent ulnar translocation of the remaining carpus, as well as the articular surface of the capitate and distal radius. If degenerative changes of the midcarpal joint or lunate facet of the radius are identified, PRC cannot be performed and total wrist fusion should be considered. Prospective studies indicate that 80% of grip strength and 60% arc of motion are preserved with PRC. However, four-corner arthrodesis may preserve greater wrist motion compared with PRC
- Total wrist arthroplasty (**Figure 25.22**): Indicated for low-demand patients with debilitating pain due to pancarpal arthritis, who wish to maintain some range of motion to perform activities of daily living. Patients with bilateral arthritis may choose to have a total wrist fusion over the dominant wrist for stable grip, and a total wrist arthroplasty over the nondominant wrist to preserve some motion for perineal care. The first implant designed for total wrist arthroplasty was the silicone flexible joint spacer, implanted in the distal radius and metacarpal medullary canals. Due to a high rate of implant complications, including implant fracture with synovitis, implant loosening, and bone resorption, these implants are no longer used. Newer designs incorporate intercarpal wrist fusion to improve distal implant stability as well as semiconstrained articular motion to prevent early dislocation
- Total wrist fusion (**Figure 25.23**): Ideal for high-demand patients (e.g. manual laborers) with pancarpal arthritis. Digital range of motion and forearm pronation and supination are preserved, but pain relief is achieved at the expense of wrist flexion and extension. Pain related to DRUJ arthritis or ulnocarpal impaction may not be alleviated by total wrist fusion and should be assessed preoperatively. To achieve total wrist fusion, the wrist is fused with 10–15° of extension. Dorsal plate fixation with an autologous bone graft from the distal radius, proximal ulna, or iliac crest will augment fusion
- Wrist denervation (**Figure 25.24a–c**): This can be considered for patients with chronic wrist pain due to a variety of causes to retain range of motion. A trial of long acting local anesthetic blocks (e.g. bupivacaine hydrochloride and epinephrine injection) of the PIN, anterior interosseous nerve, palmar cutaneous branch of the median nerve, superficial sensory branch of the radial nerve, and dorsal sensory branches of the ulnar nerve can identify patients who will benefit from partial or complete wrist denervation

RHEUMATOID ARTHRITIS

Rheumatoid arthritis is the most common inflammatory joint disease, and it is marked by progressive and persistent synovial inflammation and joint destruction. This joint destruction results from T-cell mediated synovial inflammation and hypertrophy, and approximately 70% of RA patients suffer from joint destruction in the hand and wrist.

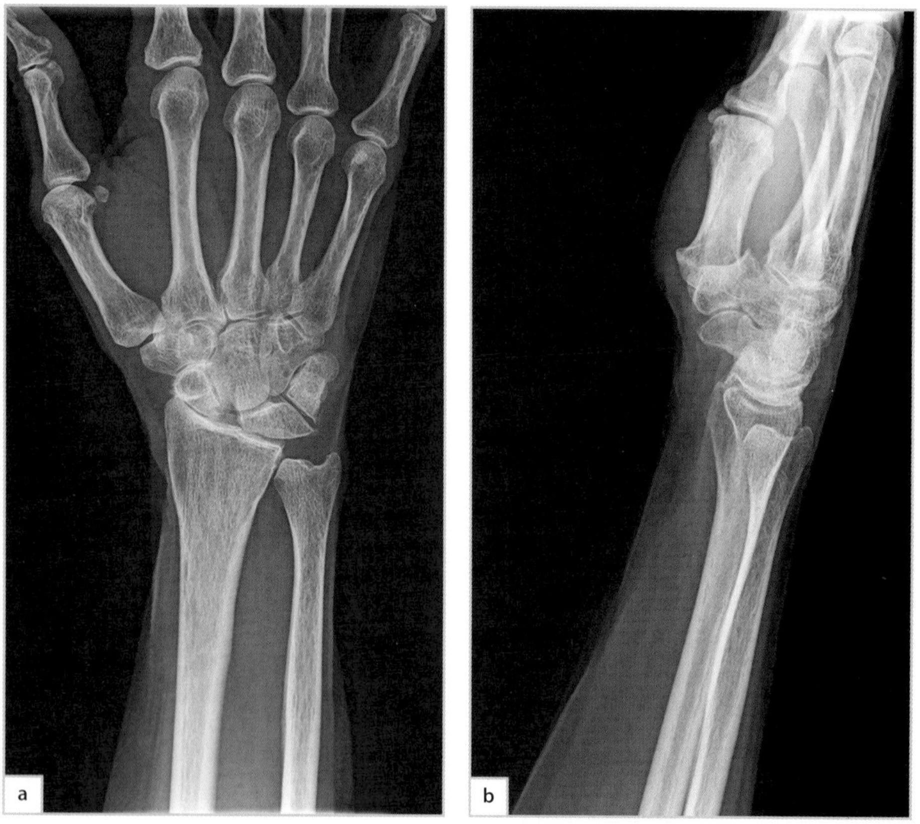

Figure 25.17 (a and b) Radiographic findings of stage 2 SLAC/SNAC wrist deformity demonstrating degeneration of the entire radioscaphoid joint and proximal migration of the distal carpal row.

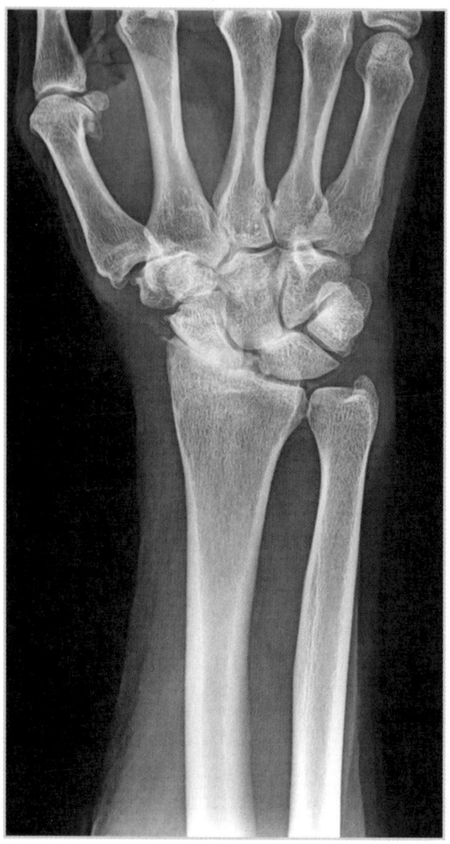

Figure 25.18 Radiographic findings of stage 3 SLAC/SNAC wrist deformity demonstrating midcarpal degenerative changes and dorsal intercalated segmental instability deformity of the scaphoid and lunate (lunate in extension, scaphoid in flexion).

Treatment options

Medical treatment

- NSAIDs: Can improve function by reducing pain and acute inflammation but do not prevent progression of joint destruction
- Corticosteroids: Can reduce inflammation but are limited by systemic effects and do not prevent the progression of disease
- Disease-modifying antirheumatic drugs (DMARDs): Halt the clinical and radiographic progression of joint destruction and induce disease remission. Nonbiologic (e.g. methotrexate) and biologic (medication genetically engineered from human proteins) are DMARDs often used in combination for maximum benefit. Biologic DMARDs include tumor necrosis factor inhibitors and interleukin-1 antagonists

Surgical treatment

The mainstay of therapy for RA is medical treatment, and surgical intervention should be reserved for those patients who have persistent functional limitations despite maximal and optimal medical treatment. Surgical intervention for wrist and hand deformities in general should proceed from proximal to distal, to provide a stable platform for future reconstruction. Joint deformity and destruction may not match the patient's clinical presentation, and many patients can compensate for the effects of RA on the joints of the hand and wrist.

Wrist

Rheumatoid arthritis most commonly affects the wrist, and results in progressive DRUJ laxity and carpal collapse. Laxity of the SL ligament results in flexion of the scaphoid and radial-sided carpal collapse, as

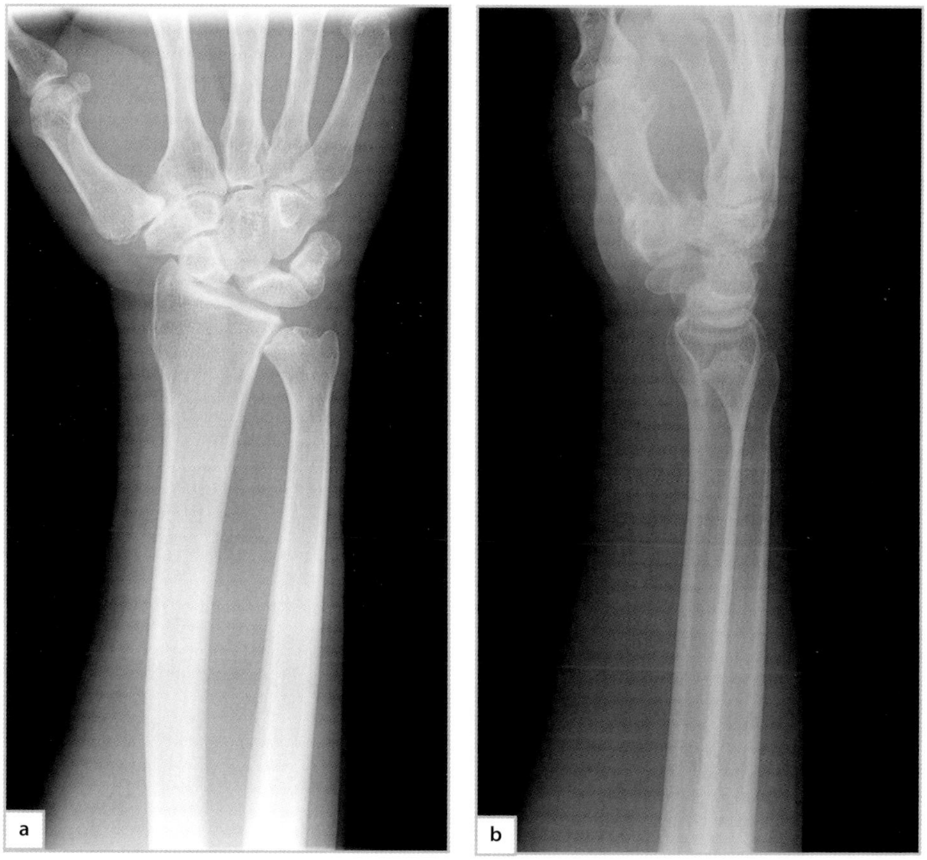

Figure 25.19 (a and b) Radiographic findings of stage 4 SLAC/SNAC wrist deformity demonstrating degeneration throughout the radiolunate articulation, intercarpal joints, and DRUJ.

well as relative lengthening of the distal ulna. The distal radius subluxes volarly, which gives the impression of the ulnar head dislocating dorsally (caput ulna) and results in ulnar-sided carpal impaction. The ulna is a fixed structure that attaches to the elbow and is the stable unit of the forearm, whereas the mobile radius rotates around the ulna. Carpal supination results in difficulty with wrist extension and exacerbation of MCP joint ulnar deviation (**Figure 25.25a** and **b**).

- Limited wrist fusion (e.g. radiolunate fusion, radioscapholunate fusion): Can be considered in patients with carpal subluxation without midcarpal joint destruction to prevent further imbalance and alleviate pain
- Darrach procedure (**Figure 25.26a** and **b**): Distal ulna resection is indicated in patients with DRUJ laxity to alleviate pain and prevent ulnar-sided wrist impaction
  - Can be combined with radiolunate fusion to prevent ulnar subluxation of the carpal bones
  - Ligamentous laxity can result in ulnar translation of the carpus
- Suave–Kapandji procedure: Distal DRUJ fusion with proximal ulna resection can help alleviate pain and improve DRUJ range of motion. This procedure requires adequate bone stock to ensure DRUJ fusion and stability
- Shelf arthroplasty: The distal ulna is excised and rotated, and DRUJ fusion is performed to improve bony contact for fusion (**Figure 25.27a–c**)
- Wrist arthroplasty: Can be considered in patients with bilateral wrist disease to maintain motion. Ligamentous laxity and poor bone stock predispose RA patients to loosening of the implant, implant fracture, periprosthetic bone fractures, and implant wear
- Wrist arthrodesis: Total wrist fusion using plates, K-wires, or pins with bone grafting can reliably alleviate pain among RA patients
  - Fusion position is approximately 10–15° of wrist extension
  - Many RA patients suffer from bilateral disease, and wrist fusion may significantly limit function

MCP joint

Chronic synovitis results in ligamentous laxity at the MCP joint, and MCP deformities due to RA include volar subluxation and ulnar drift. RA joint deformities result in poor grip and pinch and an inability to extend the fingers, as well as an unappealing appearance (**Figure 25.25a** and **b**).

- MCP joint synovectomy, cross-intrinsic transfer (**Figure 25.28a–d**), and extensor tendon centralization: Indicated for patients with early RA and ulnar drift due to ligamentous laxity without significant joint destruction. The lateral ulnar-sided bands are transferred to the radial aspect of the adjacent digit to correct ulnar drift, and the subluxed extensor tendon is reinforced over the central aspect of the MCP joint
- Silicone MCP joint arthroplasty (**Figure 25.29**): Indicated for RA patients with chronic MCP joint subluxation and destruction with adequate bone stock to support an implant. Shortening the metacarpal decreases tension across the extensor tendons, allowing centralization by imbricating the attenuated radial sagittal bands and release of the constricting ulnar sagittal bands and lateral bands. Silicone implants are often used, despite the long-term risk of implant-related complications. SRA with unconstrained implants is not performed due to the risk of implant dislocation resulting from a lack of ligamentous support

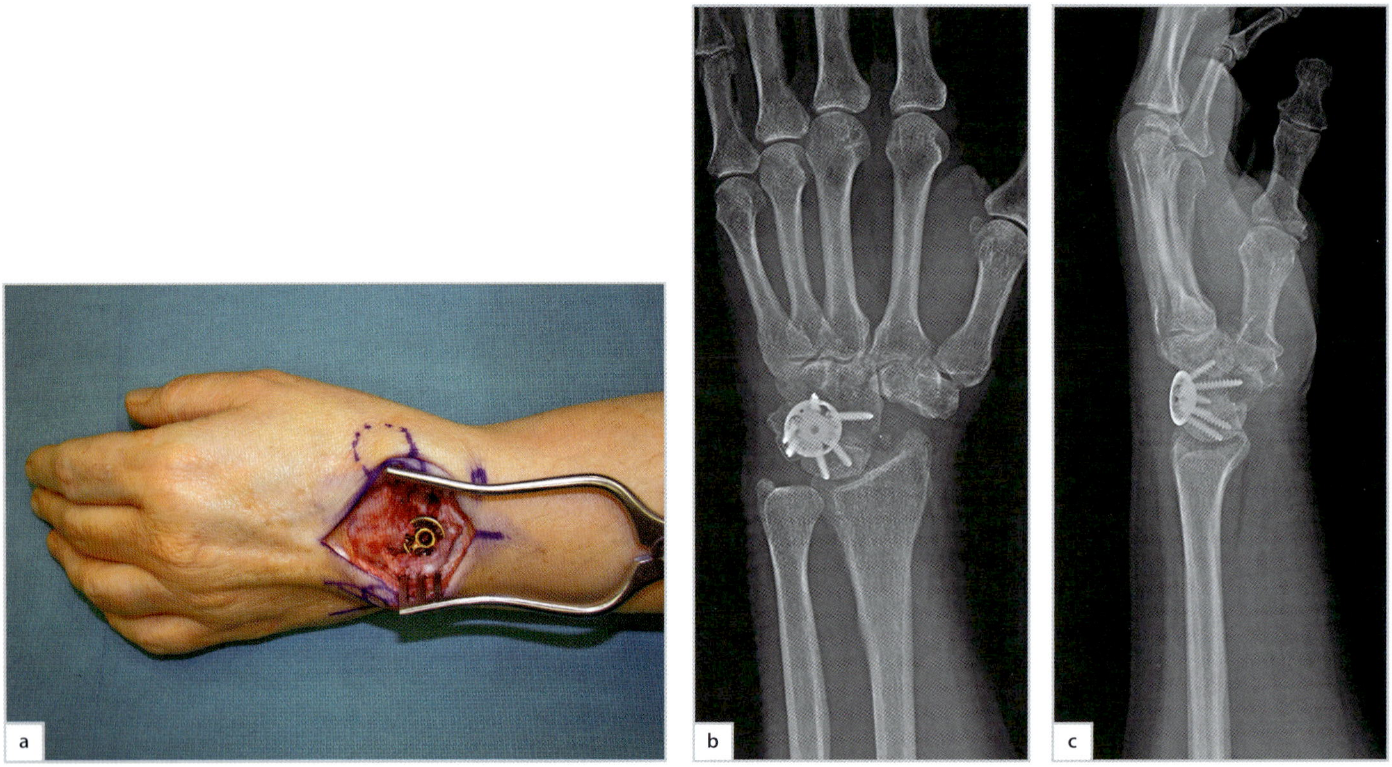

Figure 25.20 (a–c) Four-corner arthrodesis with plate fixation.

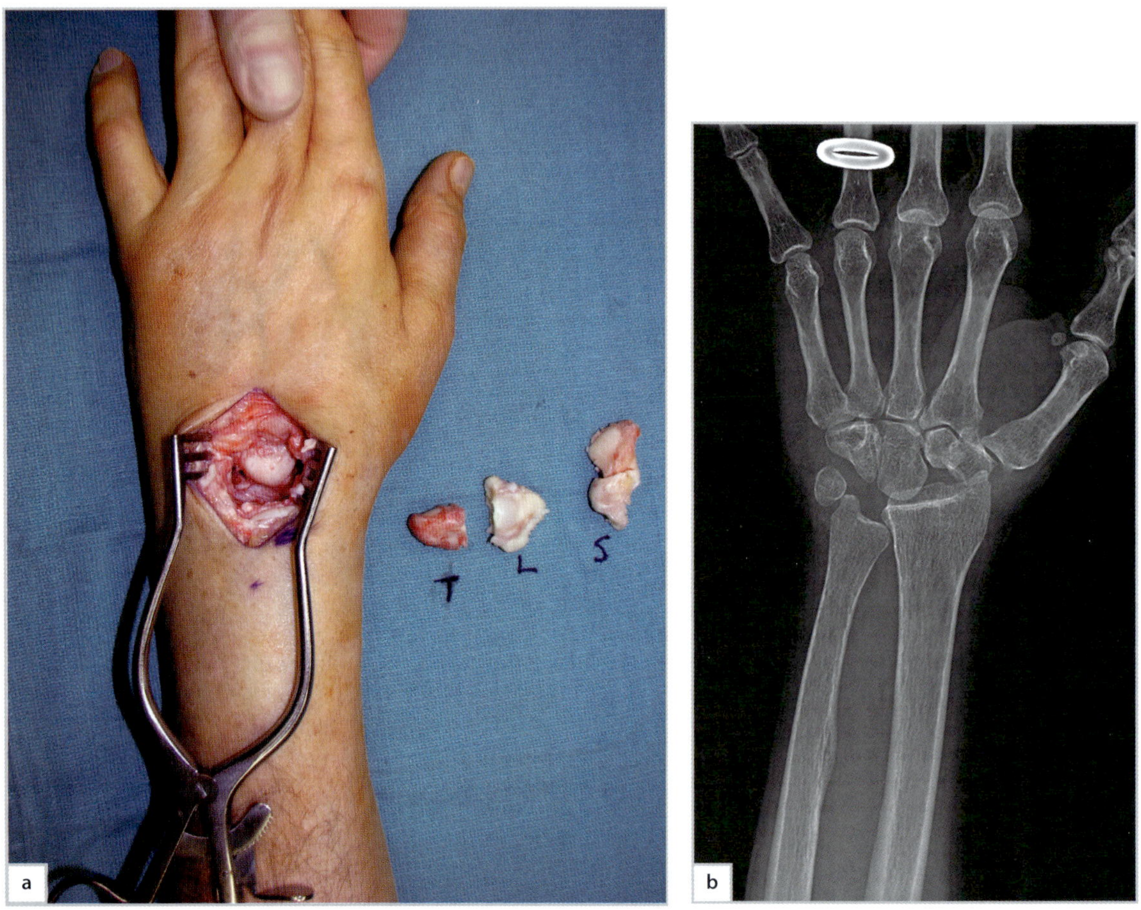

Figure 25.21 (a and b) Proximal row carpectomy for advanced wrist arthritis.

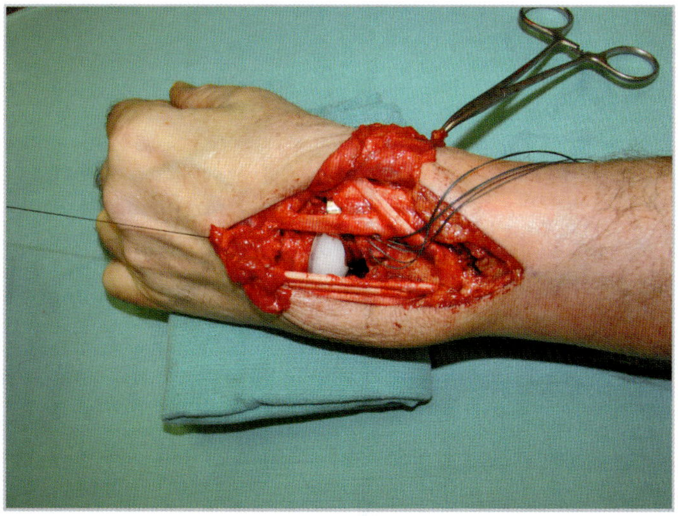

Figure 25.22 Total wrist arthroplasty for advanced wrist arthritis.

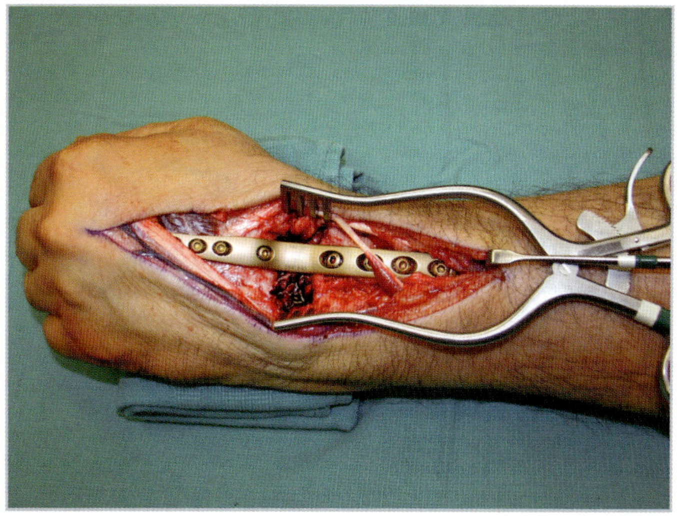

Figure 25.23 Wrist arthrodesis with plate fixation for advanced wrist arthritis.

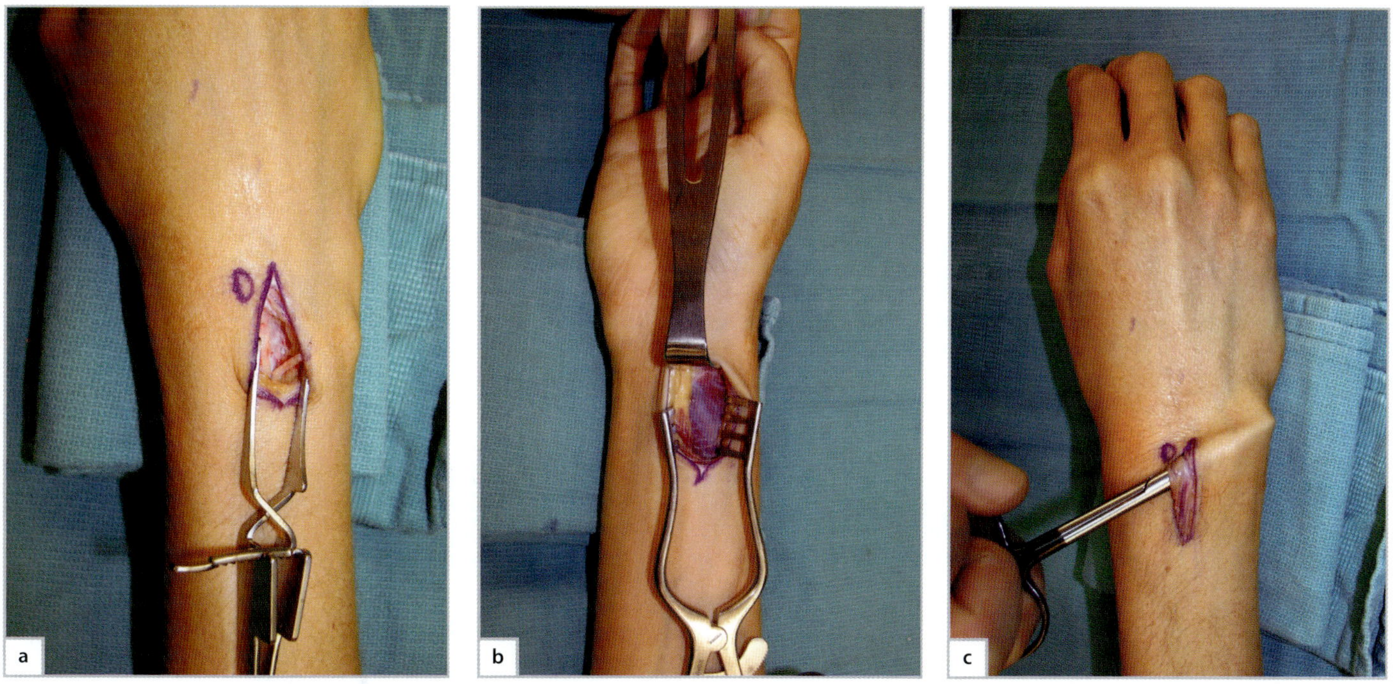

Figure 25.24 (a–c) Wrist denervation for palliation of chronic wrist pain related to wrist arthritis.

Tendon rupture

Tendon rupture occurs among patients with RA due to abrasion over bone prominences (e.g. scaphoid resulting in FPL rupture or extensor tendon rupture over distal ulna) or due to synovial invasion of the tendon resulting in attenuation and rupture. Tendon rupture over the distal ulna most commonly occurs in an ulnar to radial direction, beginning with the extensor tendon to the little finger. Treatment involves bony debridement (e.g. distal ulna excision), synovectomy, and tendon transfer (**Figure 25.30a–d**).

- The little finger extensor typically ruptures first and is the most commonly ruptured tendon. The cause of rupture, such as a bony prominence from the ulna, must be removed to prevent further rupture, and the tendons must be examined more proximally to ensure that they are intact. In general, primary tendon repair is not appropriate, and tendon transfer should be performed. Common transfers include:
  - Ring and little finger extensor tendon rupture: Extensor indicis proprius (EIP) transfer
  - Ring, little, and middle finger rupture: EIP and extensor digitorum communis transfer or flexor digitorum superficialis (FDS) from middle or ring finger
  - EPL rupture: EIP transfer

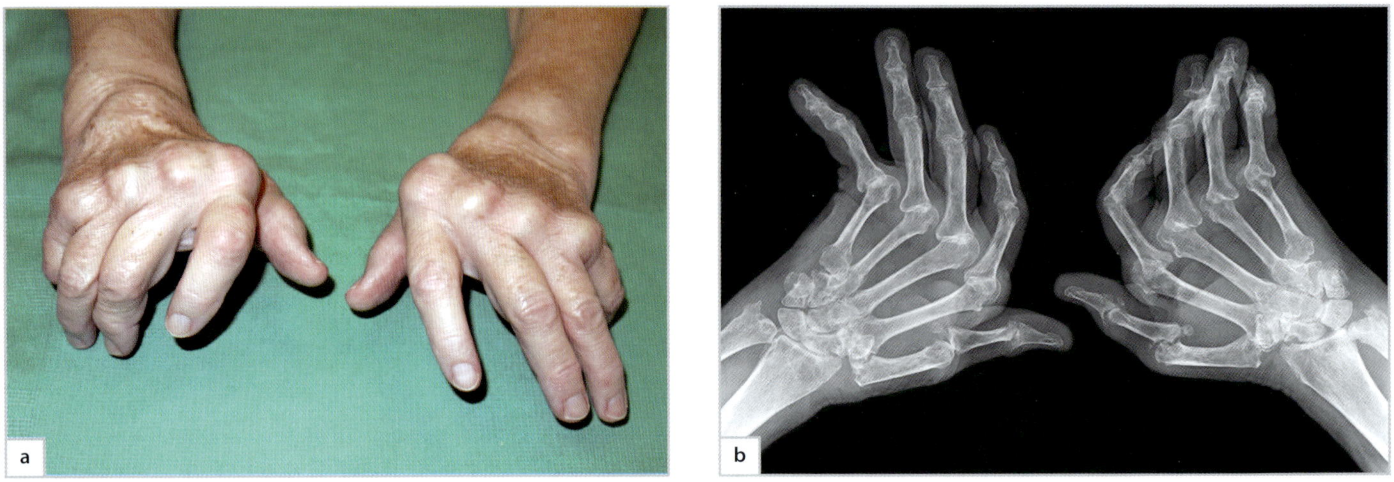

Figure 25.25 (a) Classic hand deformity related to rheumatoid arthritis including ulnar drift and volar subluxation of the metacarpophalangeal joints. (b) Joint destruction at the wrist and metacarpophalangeal joints related to rheumatoid arthritis.

Digital deformities

Swan-neck and boutonnière deformities of the digits are common among patients with RA due to progressive soft tissue laxity. Swan-neck deformities are functionally limiting because of impaired flexion of the PIP joint, whereas boutonnière deformities are largely aesthetic because the finger is already flexed at the PIP joint and can achieve good grip. In general, soft tissue reconstruction can be attempted for flexible deformities, whereas joint arthroplasty or arthrodesis is indicated for fixed deformities.

- Swan-neck deformities (**Figure 25.31**):
  - Limit grip and flexion due to hyperextension of the PIP joint
  - Causes:
    - Volar MCP joint synovitis: Attenuation of the volar plate, flexor tenosynovitis, intrinsic muscle adhesions, and contracture
    - Dorsal MCP joint synovitis: Rupture of the extensor tendon insertion on the base of the middle phalanx
    - Volar PIP joint synovitis: Attenuation of the transverse retinacular ligaments, dorsal translation of the lateral bands, and FDS rupture
    - Dorsal DIP joint synovitis: Rupture and proximal migration of the terminal tendon and oblique retinacular ligament
  - Treatment depends on the anatomic cause of the deformity:
    - DIP joint: Arthrodesis can correct the mallet deformity
    - PIP joint:
      1. Flexible deformity – Ulnar intrinsic release, volar plate advancement, FDS tenodesis, lateral band release, Littler oblique retinacular ligament reconstruction
      2. Fixed deformity – Silicone implant arthroplasty or arthrodesis.
         - MCP joint: Silicone arthroplasty can rebalance the extensor tendon apparatus and improve intrinsic tightness after joint subluxation is corrected
- Boutonnière deformities (**Figure 25.32**):
  - Caused by synovitis of the PIP joint resulting in attenuation of the central slip, subluxation of the lateral bands, and contraction of the retinacular ligaments
  - In general, boutonnière deformities are difficult to correct and do not typically pose a functional limitation. For flexible deformities treatment includes joint synovectomy, reinforcement of the central tendon, and dorsal centralization of the lateral bands. Synovectomy may be performed to prevent boutonnière deformities if synovitis persists for several months. For fixed deformities that are bothersome to the patient, silicone implant arthroplasty or arthrodesis may be considered

Thumb deformities

- Swan-neck deformity:
  - Characterized by MCP joint hyperextension and IP joint flexion due to CMC joint deformity
  - Treatment includes either tendon arthroplasty or arthrodesis
- Boutonnière deformity (**Figure 25.33**):
  - Characterized by MCP joint flexion and IP joint hyperextension due to MCP joint destruction
  - Treatment includes MCP joint fusion using plates or wires with bone grafting to rebalance the extensor tendon mechanism

OTHER ARTHROPATHIES

Systemic lupus erythematoses (SLE)

Systemic lupus erythematoses is a multisystem disease that frequently involves the joints and hands. It is more common in females and African Americans and has an age of onset of 15–25 years. Diagnosis is made by the presence of a constellation of physical signs and symptoms. SLE manifestations in the hand include symmetric joint swelling, pain, stiffness, joint deformities, and Raynaud phenomena. Unlike rheumatoid arthritis, joint manifestations of SLE are marked by tenosynovitis and ligamentous and volar plate laxity without joint destruction, and patients may present with swan-neck deformities, boutonnière deformities, and wrist subluxation. Passively correctable deformities should initially be managed by splinting, until these deformities represent a significant functional impairment and prior to the development of fixed deformities. Soft tissue reconstruction has a high rate of recurrence, and arthroplasty and arthrodesis may be more appropriate depending on the clinical scenario, despite the lack of bony destruction in these patients.

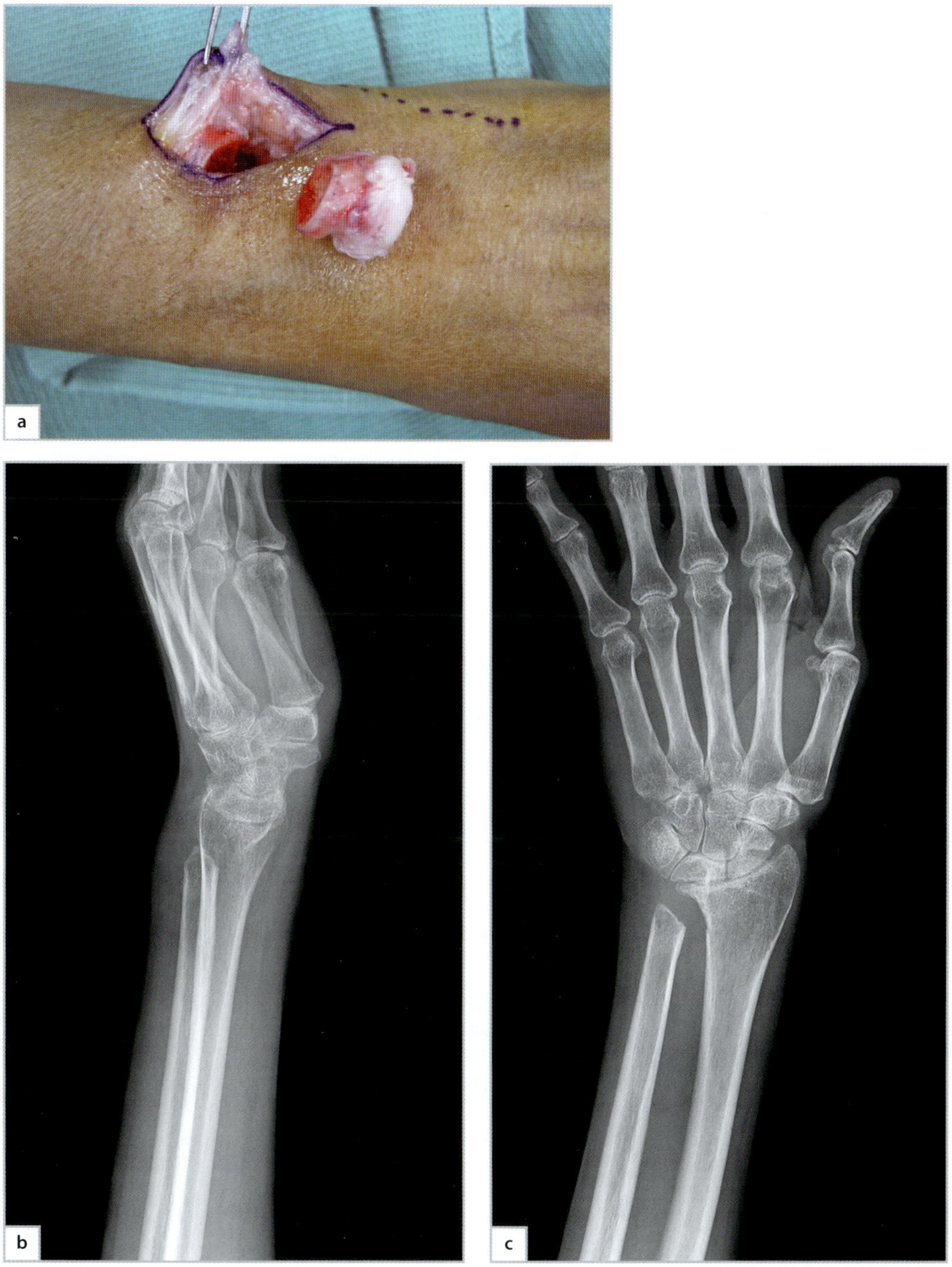

Figure 25.26a and b Distal ulna resection for rheumatoid arthritis (Darrach procedure). Reproduced from Shady R, Chung K. Applying evidence in the care of patients with rheumatoid hand and wrist deformities. Plast Reconstr Surg 2013; 132:885-97, with permission from Wolters Kluwer Health.

Wrist

Wrist deformities due to SLE include ulnar translocation, supination of the carpus, and dislocation of the carpus. Radial-sided and total wrist fusions are appropriate depending on the extent of dislocation, and distal ulna resections may be performed for supination deformities. However, arthroplasty procedures are contraindicated in patients with wrist deformities given the lack of soft tissue stability.

Digital deformities

Digit deformities that are the hallmark of SLE include ulnar deviation and volar subluxation at the MCP joint, resulting in loss of active extension. However, passive extension is maintained early on, and patients are able to maintain active finger flexion. Over time though, the extensor tendons sublux over the metacarpal heads, and thinning of the joint capsule, shortening of the ulnar intrinsic muscles, and the development of hyperextension 'swan neck' deformities at the PIP joint may also occur. Although soft tissue reconstruction can be considered in patients with digital deformities, there is a high rate of recurrence, and MCP silicone arthroplasty is indicated for patients with recurrent deformities. At the thumb, the MCP and EPL often sublux, and a flexion deformity develops at the thumb MCP joint with collateral ligament instability. In response to this change, the distal phalanx and IP joint develop a hyperextension deformity, and treatment involves MCP joint fusion.

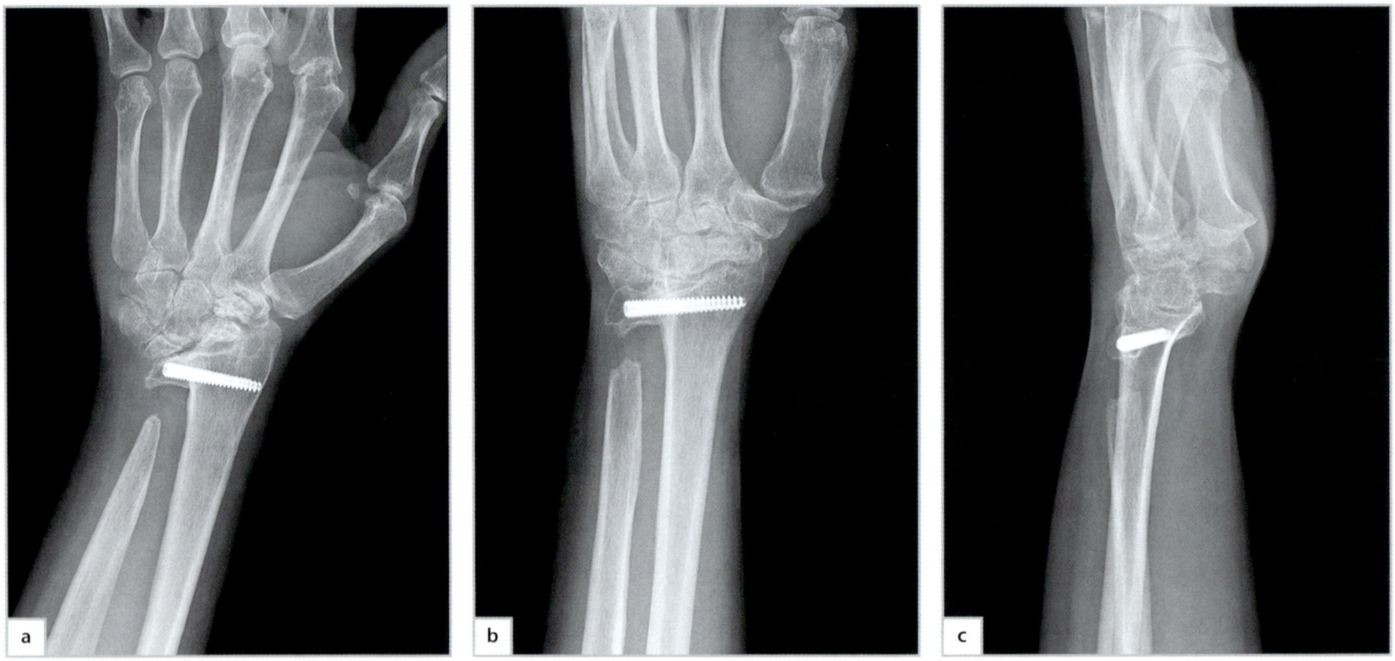

Figure 25.27 (a–c) Shelf arthroplasty for chronic wrist arthritis related to rheumatoid arthritis.

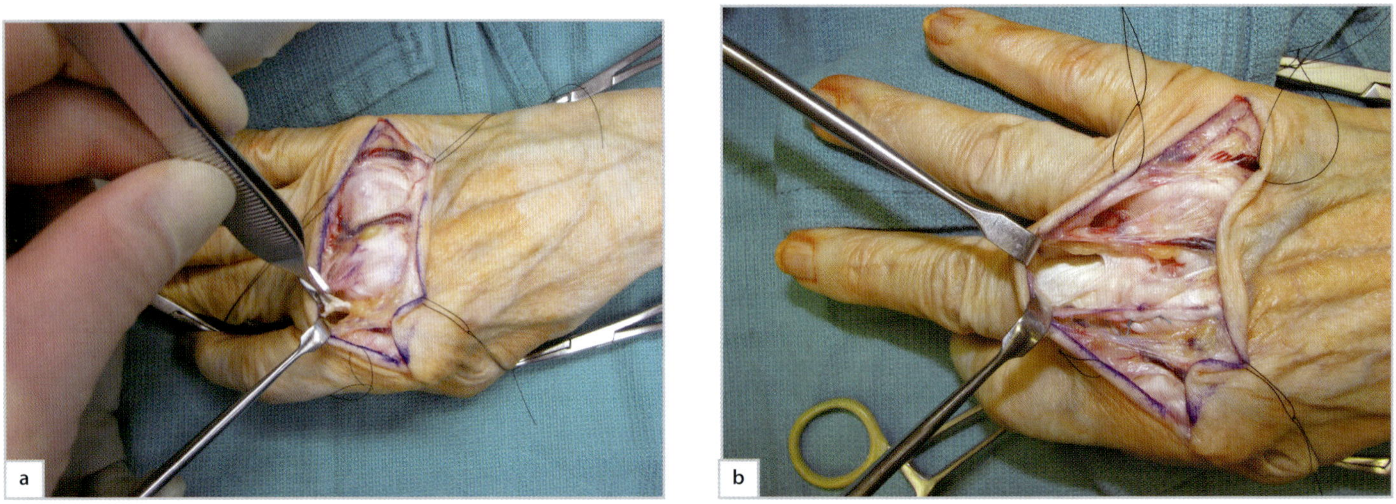

Figure 25.28 (a and b) Cross intrinsic transfer for ulnar drift of digits at the metacarpophalangeal joint related to rheumatoid arthritis.

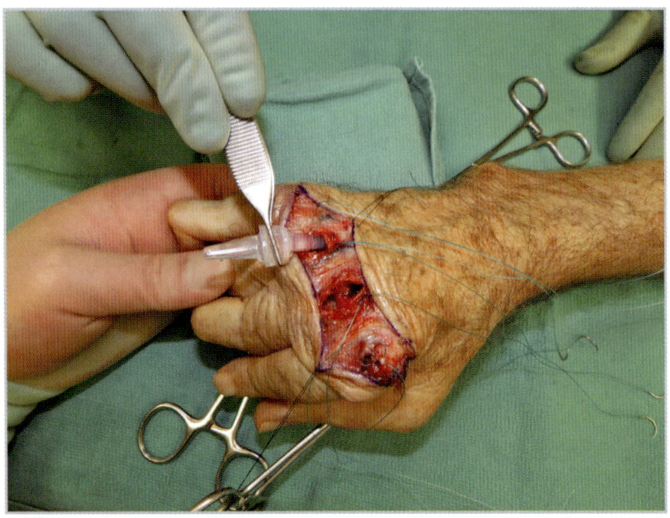

Figure 25.29 Silicone metacarpophalangeal arthroplasty for rheumatoid arthritis.

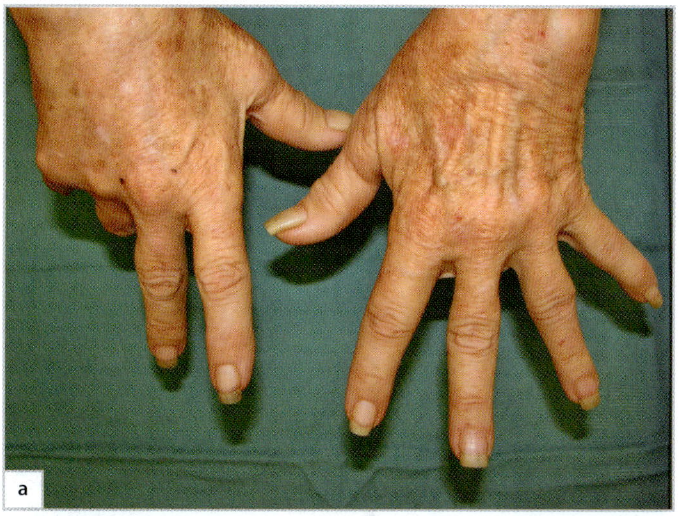

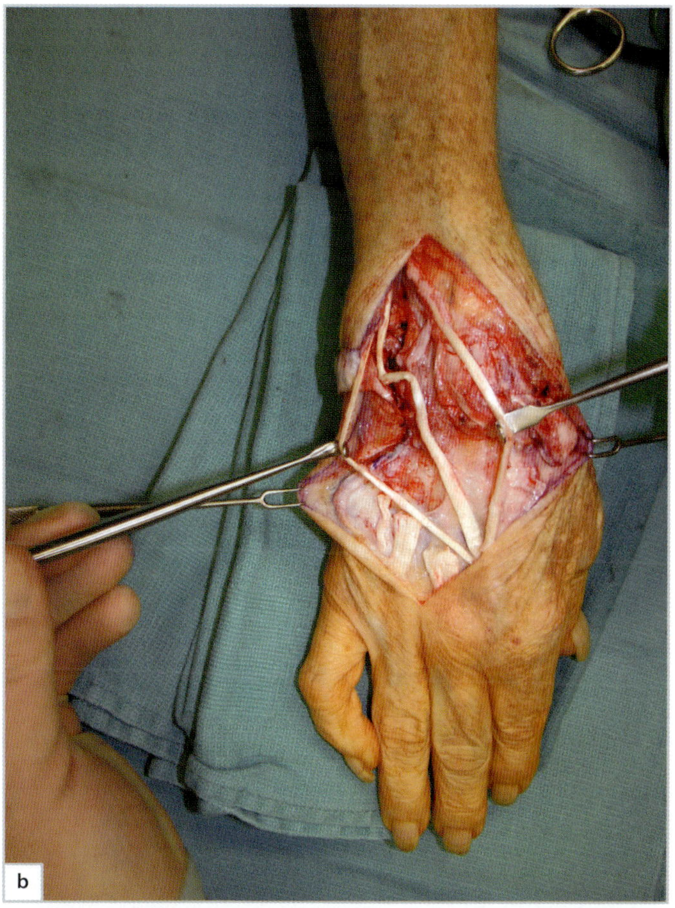

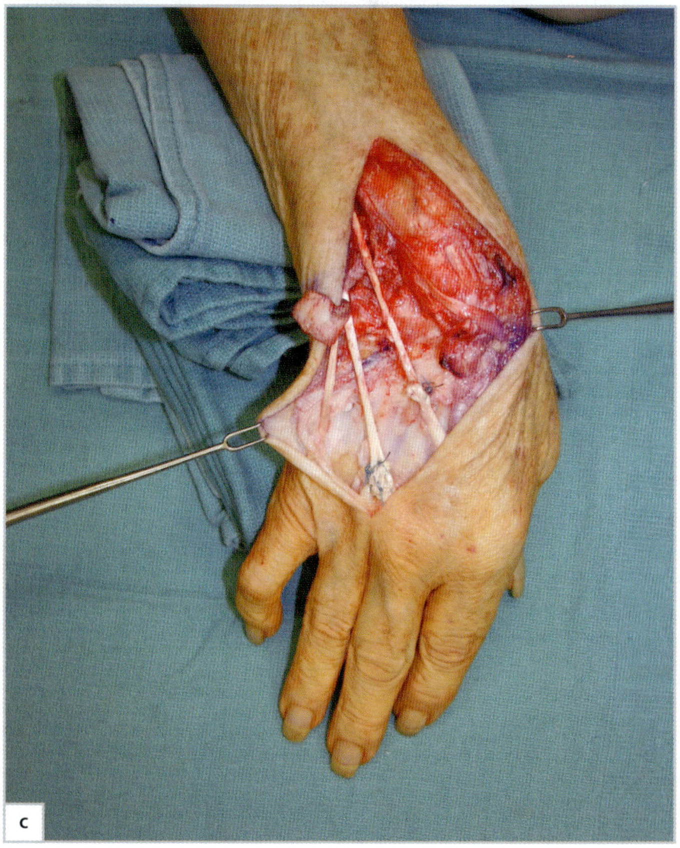

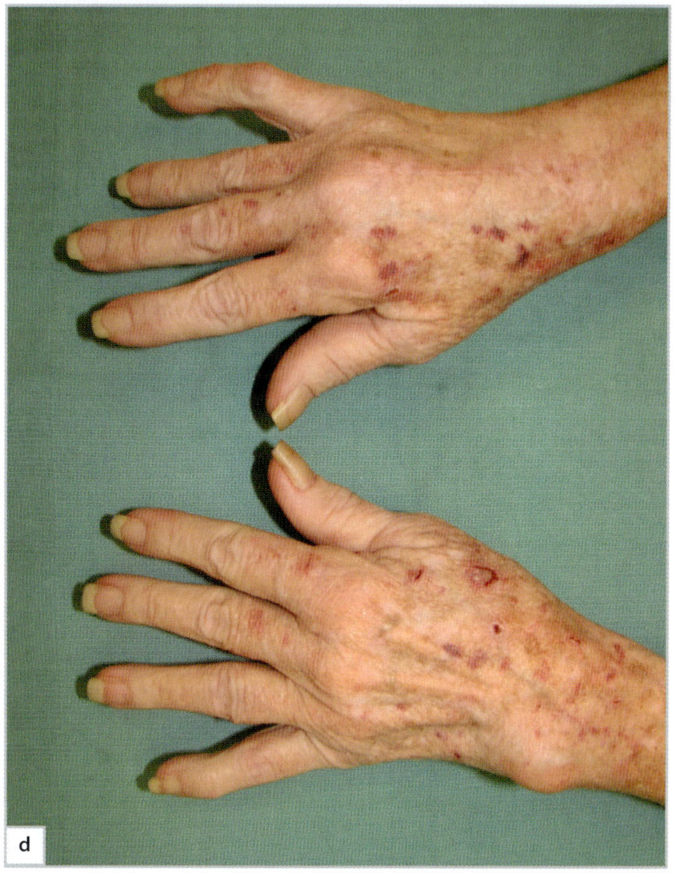

Figure 25.30a and b Extensor tendon rupture due to rheumatoid arthritis. (c and d) Extensor tendon rupture due to rheumatoid arthritis reconstructed with tendon transfer.

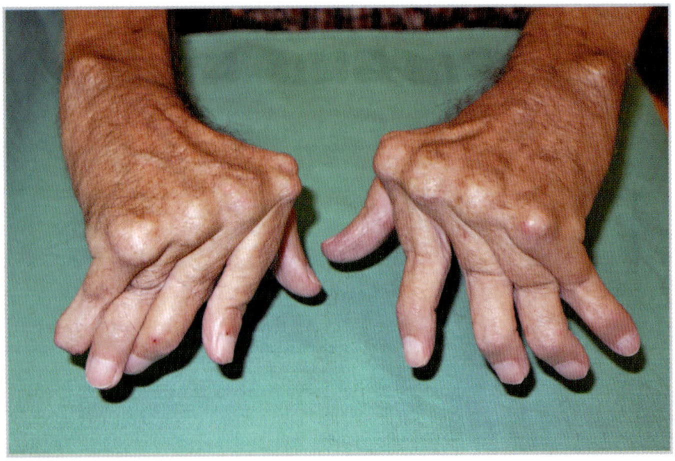

Figure 25.31 Swan-neck deformities of the fingers caused by rheumatoid arthritis.

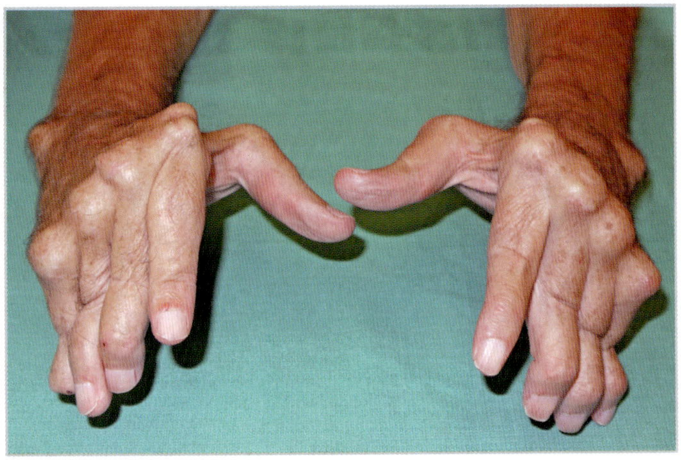

Figure 25.33 Boutonnière deformity of the thumb due to rheumatoid arthritis.

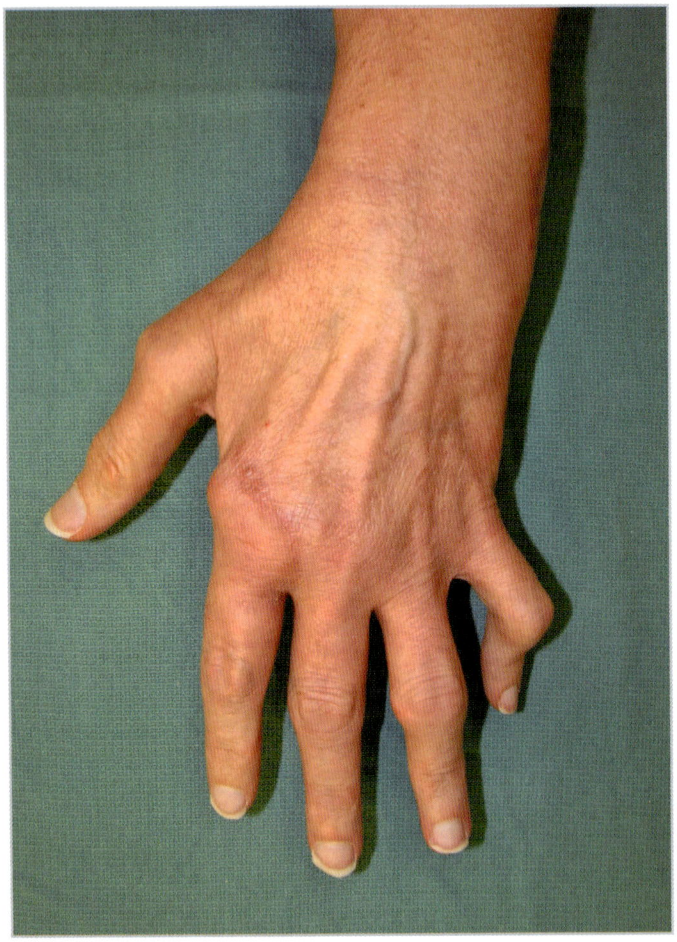

Figure 25.32 Boutonnière deformity of the little finger due to rheumatoid arthritis.

Scleroderma

Systemic sclerosis (**Figure 25.34**) results from progressive vessel and connective tissue fibrosis that involves multiple organ systems, and it is more frequent in females than in males. Patients commonly present with Raynaud phenomena, and prolonged circulation impairment over time leads to tissue loss at the distal fingers. Sclerodactyly refers to the appearance of the digits, which become atrophied with thin, shiny, sclerotic skin. Most commonly, patients present with digital ulceration and vascular insufficiency, but patients also develop joint contractures and calcinosis of the soft tissue. Digital ulceration should be managed with wound care and will often improve or heal with appropriate conservative management. Patients often benefit from occupational therapy to preserve joint range of motion. Calcinosis is best managed by surgical debridement, with the wound left open to heal by secondary intention, or closed loosely.

Digital deformities

Scleroderma can result in PIP joint flexion contractures with extensor tendon rupture and soft tissue loss, resulting in joint infection and osteomyelitis. In response to the PIP joint contracture, the MCP joint hyperextends, and flexion becomes increasingly difficult as patients develop an extension contracture at the MCP joint. Treatment includes:

- PIP joint fusion in patients with fixed flexion contractures
- Extension contractures of the MCP joint can be treated with resection arthroplasty through a volar approach

Psoriatic arthritis

Inflammatory arthritis (**Figure 25.35a** and **b**) affects approximately 5% of patients with psoriasis, and joint changes include bony destruction, nail pitting, onycholysis, and osteolysis. Digital deformities can range from shortening caused by bony collapse

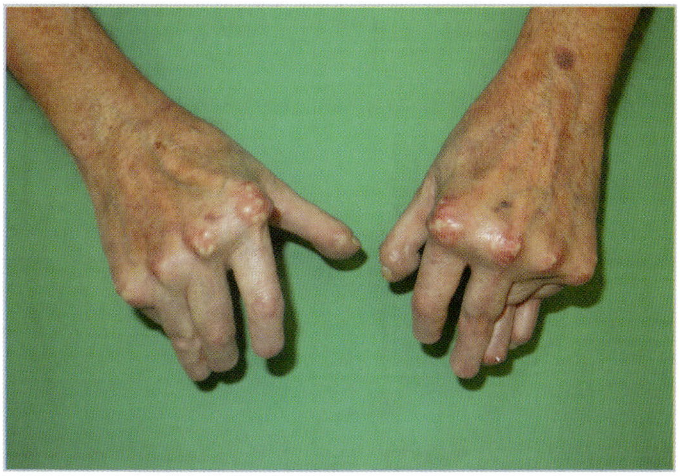

Figure 25.34 Systemic sclerosis of the hand.

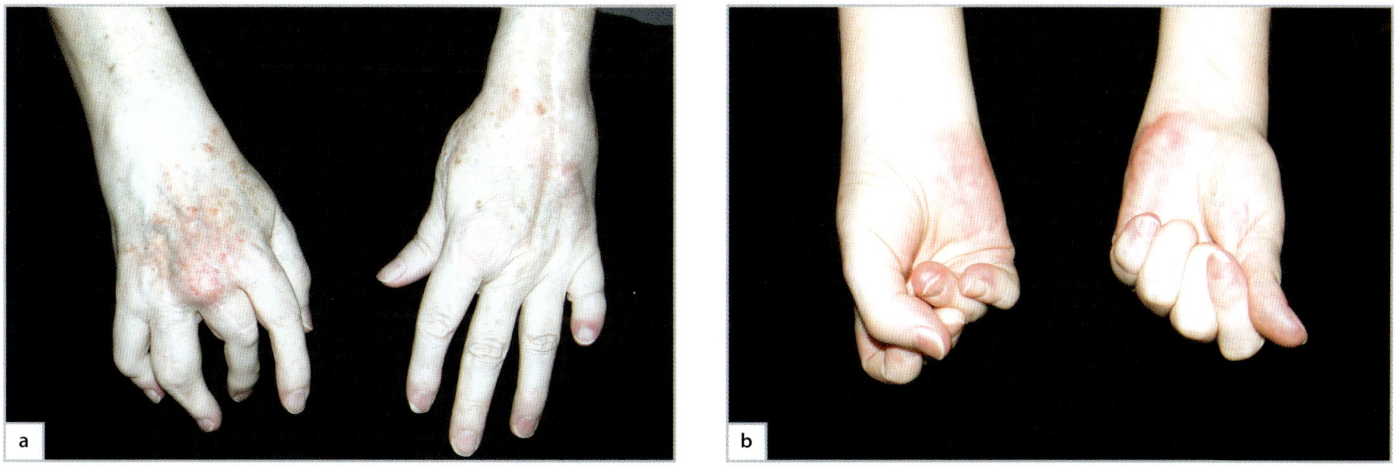

Figure 25.35a and b Psoriatic arthritis of the hand.

to spontaneous joint fusion and are typically asymmetric among hands. Patients with severe cases of the disease can develop arthritis mutilans with complete collapse of the digits, or 'opera glass hands.' In these patients, joint fusion and bone grafting is indicated to prevent further joint collapse. Digital deformities include flexion deformities of the PIP joint with MCP joint hyperextension, and MCP joint arthroplasty can improve range of motion in these patients. Thumb deformities include MCP flexion and IP joint hyperextension, which are treated with arthrodesis.

SUMMARY

- Osteoarthritis is the most common type of arthritis in the hand and wrist, but inflammatory conditions should be considered in the differential diagnosis
- Nonoperative treatment strategies should be attempted prior to surgical intervention for the majority of patients
- The goals of surgical therapy are to relieve pain, correct digital deformity, and maintain as much joint motion as possible. However, few patients will experience an improvement in joint function. Arthroplasty can retain joint motion, and it is preferred for PIP and MCP joint degenerative disease, particularly for ulnar-sided digits. However, there must be adequate bone stock and ligamentous stability to support an implant
- Inflammatory arthritis is less common, but the hand and wrist manifestations are often encountered by hand surgeons. Surgical intervention can improve pain, appearance, and function in patients who suffer symptoms while maintained on a stable medical regimen

SUGGESTED READING

Cohen MS, Kozin SH. Degenerative arthritis of the wrist: proximal row carpectomy versus scaphoid excision and four-corner arthrodesis. J Hand Surg Am 2001; 26:94–104.
The authors follow a cohort of patients who underwent either a scaphoid excision and four-corner arthrodesis or proximal row carpectomy (PRC) for scapholunate advanced collapse arthritis with more than 2-year follow-up. At follow-up, both procedures retain motion at the wrist with few subjective or objective differences.

Eaton RG, Littler JW. Ligament reconstruction for the painful thumb carpometacarpal joint. J Bone Joint Surg Am 1973; 55:1655–1666.
This seminal paper describes the use of the flexor carpi radialis to reconstruct the volar beak ligament for symptomatic thumb carpometacarpophalangeal arthritis in 18 patients with up to 5-year follow-up.

Goldfarb CA, Stern PJ. Metacarpophalangeal joint arthroplasty in rheumatoid arthritis. A long-term assessment. J Bone Joint Surg Am 2003; 85-A:1869–1878.
This study represents one of the longest assessments of silicone metacarpophalangeal arthroplasty for rheumatoid arthritis, with over 14 years of follow-up. The authors describe the durability of arthroplasty at final follow-up, with an implant fracture rate of 63%. Only 38% of patients describe satisfaction with their hand function, and only 22% of patients were pain free at the final follow-up.

Ono S, Shauver MJ, Chang KW, Chung KC. Outcomes of pyrolytic carbon arthroplasty for the proximal interphalangeal joint at 44 months' mean follow-up. Plast Reconstr Surg 2012; 129:1139–1150.
This paper highlights clinical outcomes from 13 patients and 21 arthroplasties with greater than 3 year follow-up, and underscores the prevalence of complications with this technique.

Swanson AB. Flexible implant arthroplasty for arthritic finger joints: rationale, technique, and results of treatment. J Bone Joint Surg Am 1972; 54:435–455.
This study represents one of the earliest single center experiences of silicone arthroplasty for proximal interphalangeal and metacarpophalangeal joint arthritis and reviews indications and surgical techniques.

Weilby A. Tendon interposition arthroplasty of the first carpo-metacarpal joint. J Hand Surg 1988; 13:421–425.
This paper describes the technique of trapeziectomy, abductor pollicis longus imbrications and suspension using a strip of flexor carpi radialis in over 100 thumbs with 6 month follow-up.

Chapter 26 Hand tumors

Mark Puhaindran

INTRODUCTION

Soft tissue tumors of the hand and upper extremity are common problems encountered by hand surgeons in their clinical practice. The vast majority of these tumors are benign such as ganglia, giant cell tumors (GCTs) of the tendon sheath, and lipomas, with malignant tumors rarely encountered. Most of these tumors can be treated with simple excision and minimal sequelae. However, one needs to be suspicious of all masses because inappropriately performed biopsies and excisions of malignant tumors can result in unnecessary amputations.

BENIGN TUMORS

Ganglions

These mucin-filled cysts are the most commonly encountered tumors in the hand. These cysts frequently present between the second and fourth decade, although ganglions can occur at any age. Ganglion cysts can arise from almost any joint within the hand and wrist. The most commonly encountered are dorsal wrist ganglions (approximately 70%), followed by volar wrist ganglions (approximately 20%), and then ganglions arising from the flexor tendon sheaths and mucous cysts (**Figure 26.1**) arising from the distal interphalangeal joints. Up to 50% of ganglions resolve on observation, with higher rates seen in children. Treatment options include aspiration or surgical removal, which can be performed using open or arthroscopic techniques. Recurrence rates of up to 40% have been reported after surgical excision.

Soft tissue tumors

Pigmented villonodular synovitis (PVNS)

These tumors are known by various terms, including GCTs of the tendon sheath, fibrous xanthoma, or localized nodular synovitis. The second most common soft tissue tumor seen in the hand after ganglions, these tumors are normally firm, nodular, and nontender and can be present for long periods of time before medical attention is sought. PVNS occasionally causes pressure erosions of the underlying bone that can be detected on plain radiographs (**Figure 26.2**). Marginal excision is typically the treatment of choice for these tumors. Recurrence rates of 9–27% have been reported after excision, thought to be due to the presence of satellite nodules that are not completely excised during surgery

Factors associated with local recurrence include

- The presence of degenerative joint disease
- Involvement of the distal interphalangeal joint
- Radiographic evidence of pressure erosion of the bone
- Involvement of the flexor or extensor tendons, or joint capsule

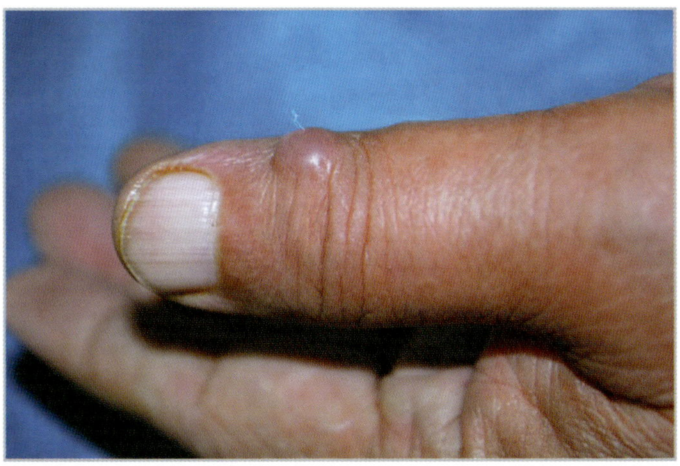

Figure 26.1 Mucous cyst.

Epidermal cysts

Epidermal inclusion cysts are thought to result from the traumatic implantation of epithelial cells into the soft tissue or even bone. Over a period of months to years, these cells grow and produce a painless lump. Occasionally, the mass may be painful and erythematous. Epidermal inclusion cysts are frequently seen over the fingertips and can even be seen in the stumps of amputated fingers. On examination, cysts in the soft tissue will be firm, well circumscribed, and slightly mobile. Cysts that involve the bone can appear as a primary bone tumor – fixed to the bone, and with a lytic appearance on X-ray, and can be mistaken for infectious or malignant processes. Marginal excision is an effective treatment for epidermal cysts, and has a minimal risk of local recurrence.

Lipomas

Lipomas are benign proliferations of mature adipocytes and can occur anywhere in the body. Although these tumors can grow to a large size, they do not invade local tissues. One should be cautious of large tumors as they could actually be liposarcomas. Rapid growth or local tissue invasion are also warning signs of possible malignancy. Marginal excision of lipomas is often curative, with a very low risk of local recurrence after complete excision.

Vascular tumors (described in Chapter 24)

Hemangiomas

These are vascular tumors caused by neoplastic proliferation of the endothelium during a child's development. Their development goes through three phases: (1) Proliferating phase, before the age of 1 year, (2) involuting phase, between 1 and 5 years, when the tumor begins to regress, and (3) involuted phase, after 5 years, when the tumor reaches its stable size. Hemangiomas do not undergo malignant change; however, excision can be considered during the involuted phase (e.g. when there is ulceration and bleeding or if it interferes with function).

Vascular malformations

These are nonneoplastic vascular tumors that can affect the arteries, veins, capillaries, and lymphatics, or any combination of them. Vascular malformations do not regress spontaneously and therefore require

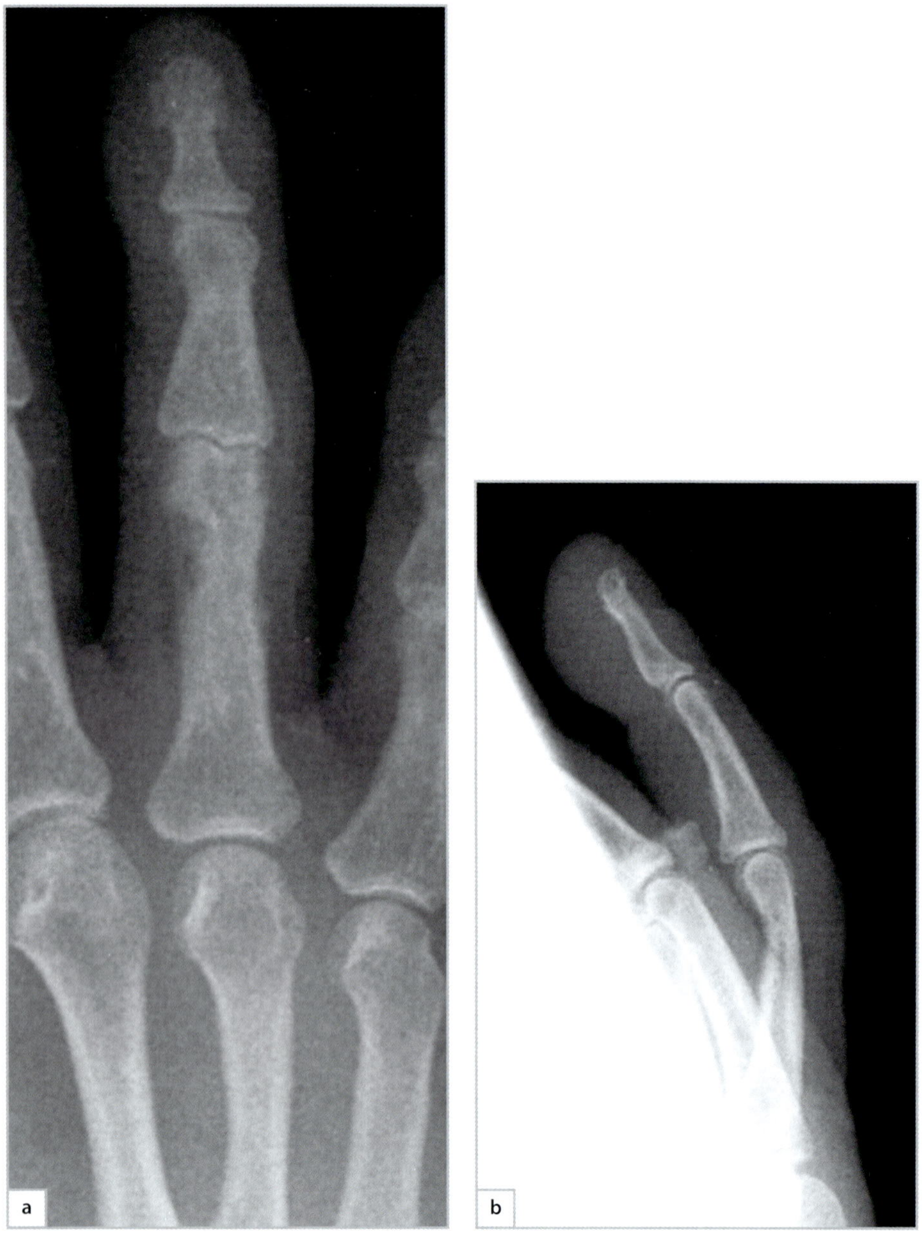

Figure 26.2 (a and b) X-ray showing bony erosion by pigmented villonodular synovitis.

treatment. Conservative treatment modalities include splinting and the use of compressive garments. Embolization or surgical excision can be considered for those that fail conservative management.

Nerve tumors

Schwannomas

Schwannomas, also known as neurilemomas, are common nerve tumors seen in the upper extremity. They arise from Schwann cells and are slow growing and well-circumscribed masses that often grow eccentrically within a peripheral nerve (**Figure 26.3**). Patients often present with a painless mass, although they occasionally present due to radiating pain triggered by contact or even neurological deficits. Nerve preserving excisions can be performed for most schwannomas, but interfascicular dissection under magnification is often required. Postoperative loss of function has been reported in 2.5–30% of patients, and local recurrence after tumor excision is rare. It should be noted that cases of malignant transformation of schwannomas have been reported.

Neurofibromas

Neurofibromas arise within nerve fascicles and are typically more difficult to excise than schwannomas, with greater rates of postoperative neurological deficits after excision. Solitary neurofibromas are occasionally encountered, but patients with multiple neurofibromas are more commonly seen, especially in the setting of neurofibromatosis (Von Recklinghausen disease) (**Figure 26.4**). In these patients, excision should be reserved for enlarging plexiform neurofibromas, causing a progression of sensory and/or motor deficits, or in tumors where malignant transformation is suspected.

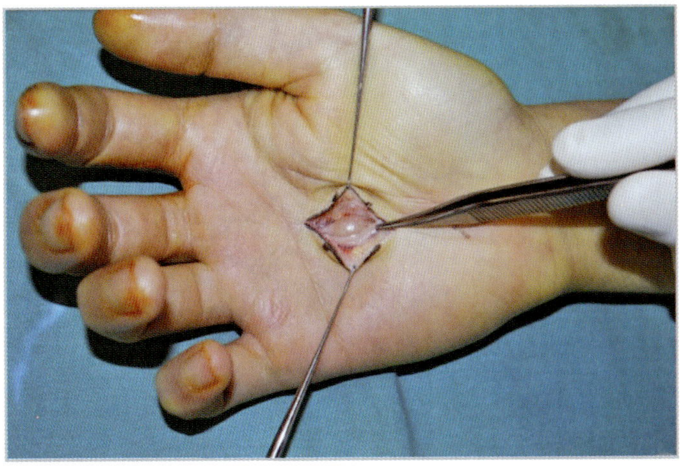

Figure 26.3 Schwannoma.

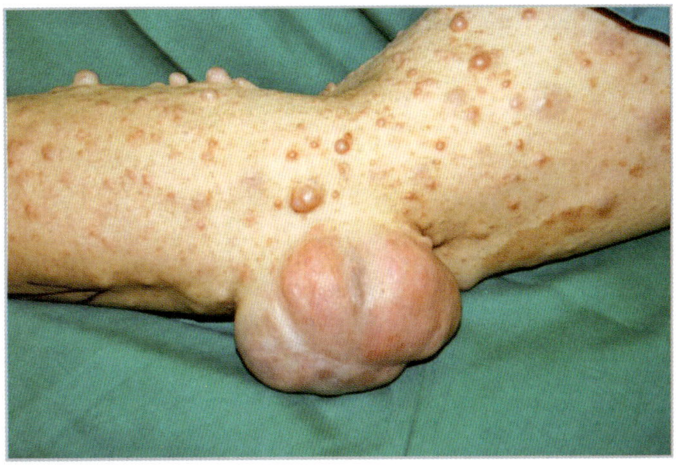

Figure 26.4 Neurofibroma.

Bone and cartilage tumors

Enchondroma

Enchondromas are benign hyaline cartilage tumors found in the bone medullary cavity. They account for up to 25% of all benign bone tumors, with 40% of all enchondromas occurring in the hand, making them the most common primary bone tumor in the hand. Most patients present between the second and fourth decade, but the age distribution varies widely. Enchondromas are most often seen in the proximal phalanges, followed by the middle phalanges, and then the distal metacarpals. Most cases are solitary, although multiple lesions are associated (**Figure 26.5**).

The timing of definitive surgical treatment when patients present with pathologic fractures is controversial. Some surgeons advocate early treatment and mobilization; however, this can be associated with a higher rate of complications compared with delayed surgery. Delayed surgery allows fracture healing, which provides stability for grafting and early mobilization. Studies thus far have not demonstrated whether the material used to fill the defect (autograft bone, allograft bone, cement, or synthetic bone substitutes) influences long-term stability or local recurrence risk. Irrespective of the treatment protocol, the local recurrence rate after curettage and bone grafting is 5%. Although the risk of malignant transformation of solitary lesions is small, malignant transformation can occur in up to one third of patients with Ollier disease, and the risk is even higher with Maffucci syndrome.

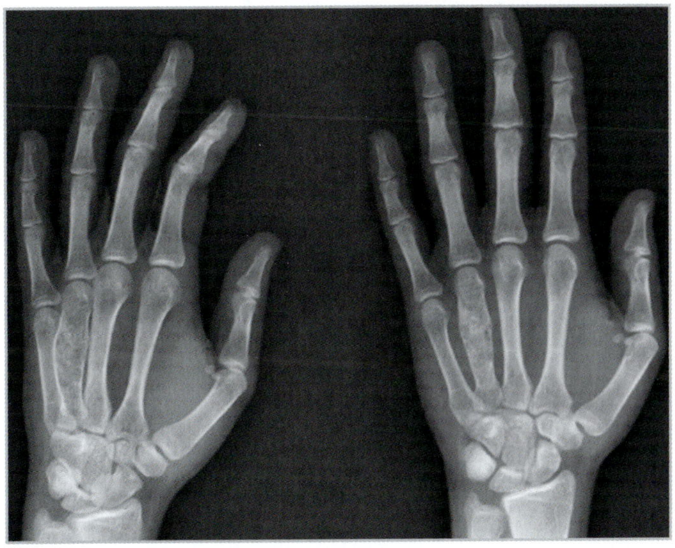

Figure 26.5 X-ray enchondroma of the 4th metacarpal.

Giant cell tumor

Giant cell tumors of the bone are rare in the hand. Although <2% of all GCTs occur in the hand, the distal radius is the third most common site for these tumors. Patients often present between the third and fourth decades of life, and GCTs are slightly more common in females. GCTs are typically seen in the epiphysis and metaphysis, although in the hand they can be seen in the diaphysis as well. The X-ray appearance is lytic with a narrow zone of transition (**Figure 26.6**).

Although GCTs are considered benign tumors, 2% metastasize to the lung at an average of 3–4 years after initial diagnosis. Local tumor recurrence, surgical manipulation, and a distal radius primary tumor are associated with an increased risk of metastasis. The main objective of treatment for a GCT is to prevent local tumor recurrence. The local recurrence rate in the hand after curettage and bone grafting without local adjuvant therapy is up to 80%. Local recurrence rates of <25% have been reported with curettage, high-speed burring, and local treatment with an adjuvant (phenol) at other sites, and this regimen is recommended in the hand as well.

Aneurysmal bone cyst

Aneurysmal bone cysts (ABCs) are benign cystic bone lesions composed of blood-filled spaces separated by connective tissue septa that contain a mixture of fibroblasts, giant cells, and woven bone. They can arise primarily (primary ABC) or in association with other benign or malignant bone tumors (secondary ABC). Although typically benign, rare cases of malignant transformation have been reported. ABCs normally affect people in the first two decades of life, and exhibit no sex predilection. These tumors tend to occur in the metaphysis of the long bones and are rarely seen in the hand, but when they do occur, are often seen in the metacarpals and phalanges. Patients commonly present with pain and swelling, and radiographs reveal an expansile lytic lesion (**Figure 26.7**). Magnetic imaging resonances (MRIs) show multiple fluid levels characteristic of ABCs, but the physician must also investigate for a primary lesion.

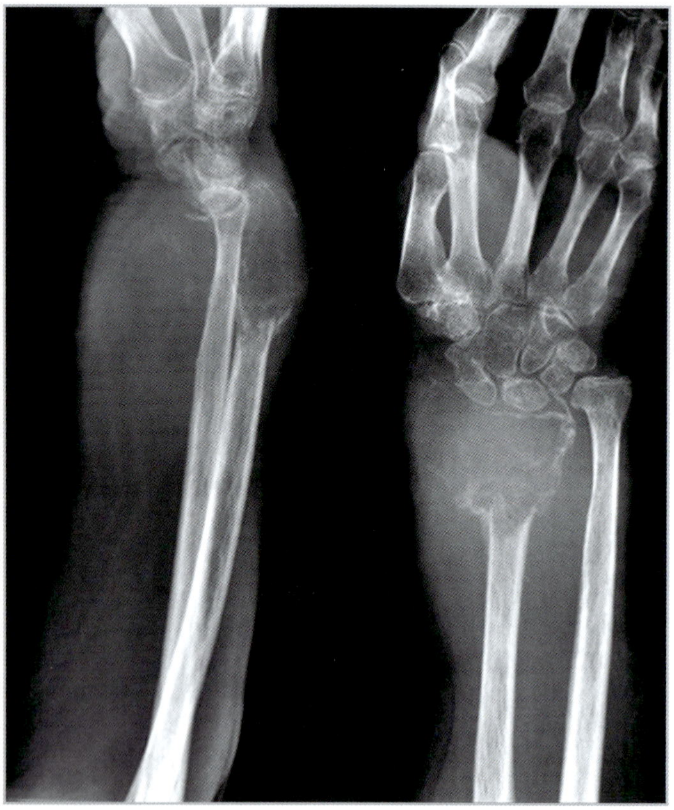

Figure 26.6 X-ray showing a giant cell tumor of the distal radius

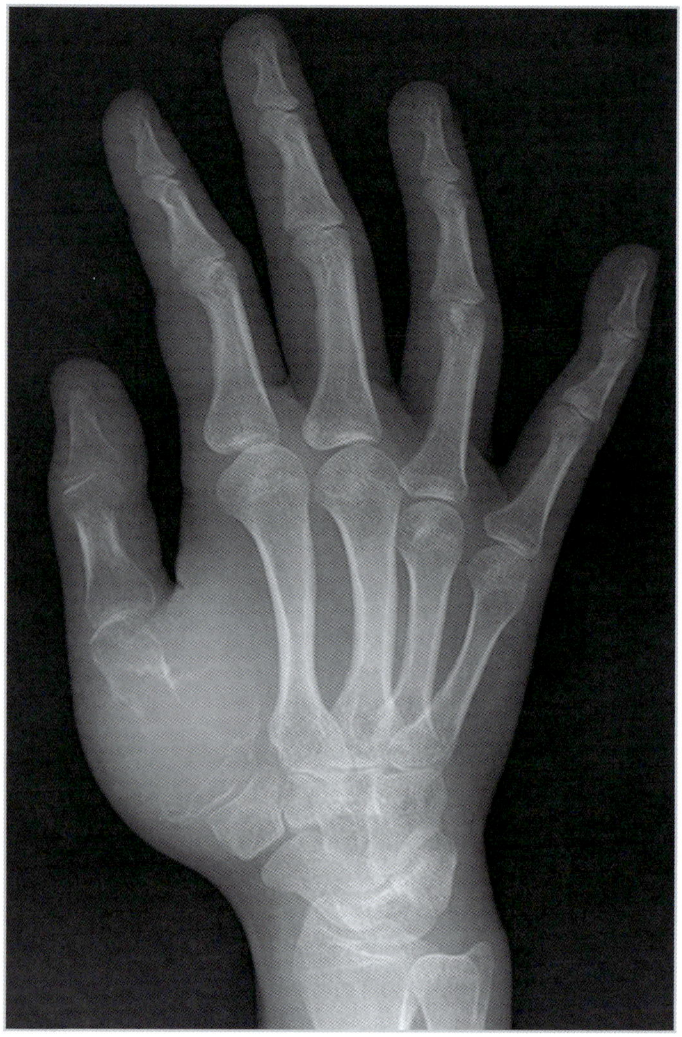

Figure 26.7 X-ray showing aneurysmal bone cyst in the first metacarpal base.

Historically, ABCs treated with curettage and bone grafting alone had a local recurrence rate of up to 70%. This can be reduced by adding high-speed burring and liquid nitrogen, followed by bone grafting or cementing of the defect. Care should be taken when using these adjuvant treatments in skeletally immature patients due to the risk of physeal injury. Wide en bloc resection is generally reserved for lesions where there is insufficient bone stock to allow an intralesional procedure and subsequent reconstruction.

Osteoid osteoma

Osteoid osteomas are uncommon benign osteoblastic tumors that account for approximately 10% of benign bone tumors. They consist of an area of osteoid tissue surrounded by a rim of sclerotic bone and are typically < 2 cm in size. Children and adolescents are the most commonly affected patients, and frequently present with pain that is initially intermittent and worsening symptoms at night, but can progress to continuous pain that affects sleep. This pain can be well controlled with anti-inflammatory medications. Rarely, patients present with painless lesions in the hand that enlarge or deform the bone. The X-ray appearance is characterized by dense cortical sclerosis with a radiolucent nidus, but osteoid osteomas can also have a lytic or mixed appearance.

Conservative treatment with anti-inflammatory medications can be attempted, provided that the diagnosis can be confidently made based on the clinical signs and radiographic appearance. More invasive alternatives include radiofrequency ablation or surgical curettage and bone grafting, which has the added advantage of enabling histologic confirmation of the diagnosis. Osteoid osteomas have limited growth potential, and therefore, local recurrence after surgical treatment is rare.

MALIGNANT TUMORS

Skin tumors

Squamous cell carcinomas

Squamous cell carcinomas are the most common primary malignancy in the hand (**Figure 26.8**). Predisposing factors include excessive sun exposure, immunosuppression (e.g. transplant patients), and exposure to carcinogens. During clinical evaluation, the depth and extent of the lesion should be assessed, and the patient should also be evaluated for regional lymph node involvement and presence of other tumors. If the tumor appears to be extensive on clinical assessment, further imaging should be considered.

Surgical treatment involves complete excision of the tumor with negative margins (circumferential and deep), which can be assessed intraoperatively using frozen section analysis, or postoperatively. Generally, margins of 4–6 mm are recommended. Reconstruction can be decided upon once complete excision based on established clear margin of the pathology specimen is confirmed. Other local treatment options include electrodessication and cryotherapy, or application of topical agents such as 5-flourouracil, although the cure rates are

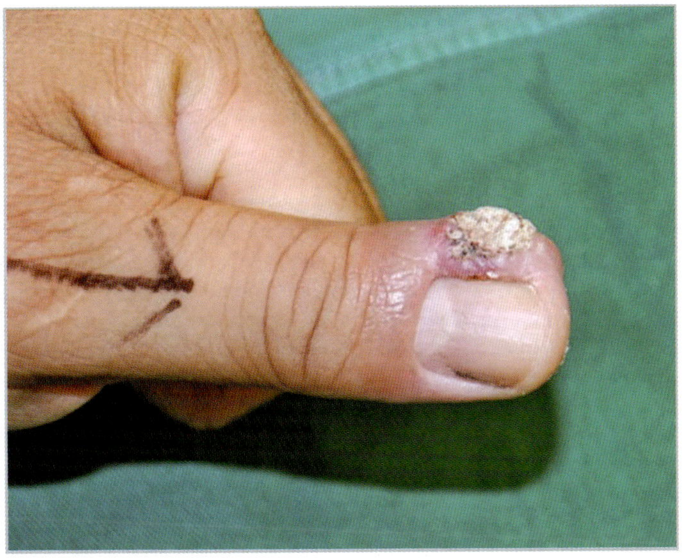

Figure 26.8 Squamous cell carcinoma.

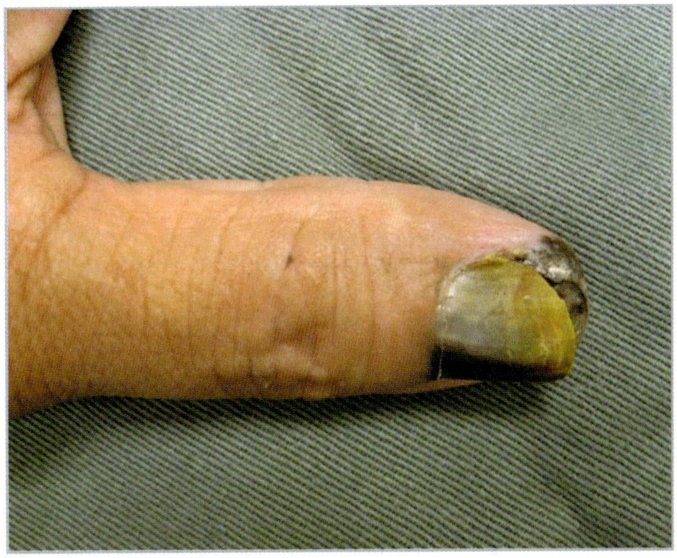

Figure 26.9 Subungual melanoma.

lower for these treatments. If surgery is not an option for a patient, radiotherapy can be used for local control of the tumor. Should lymph node disease be detected, it has to be addressed either surgically, with a block dissection, or with radiotherapy.

Basal cell carcinoma

Basal cell carcinomas (BCCs) are slow growing tumors that originate from the keratinocytes of the basal epithelium. Although they tend to be locally aggressive, BCCs rarely metastasize. There are four different subtypes: (1) nodular, (2) superficial, (3) pigmented, and (4) sclerosing. Nodular BCCs are the most common form of this tumor, whereas sclerosing are the most aggressive. Complete excision with negative margins is required for all types of BCC, and a cure rate of >95% can be expected.

Melanomas

Melanomas are aggressive skin tumors that arise from melanocytes and are responsible for 1–2% of all cancer deaths in the United States. Two percent of melanomas occur in the hand, of which half are subungual melanomas (**Figure 26.9**).

These are the main types of melanoma:

- Superficial spreading
- Nodular
- Acral lentiginous
- Lentigo maligna

During clinical evaluation, the regional lymph nodes should be examined, as well as the entire body, looking for other suspicious lesions and signs of distant metastases

Melanomas follow a series of progression:

- Dysplasia
- Radial growth phase
- Vertical growth phase
- Metastasis

Survival is correlated with the depth of invasion of the tumor (Breslow depth) and the presence of metastasis. The recommended surgical margins required are also dependent on the depth of the tumor (**Table 26.1**). When performing a biopsy, it is recommended that the full depth of the lesion be taken by including all of the fat layer to assess the depth of invasion. It is recommended that sentinel lymph node biopsies are performed to assess for lymph node involvement, which, in turn, will aid in prognostication for the patient.

Table 26.1 Melanoma recommended margins

Thickness	Recommended margin (cm)
In situ	0.5–1.0 cm
<1 mm	1 cm
1-2 mm	1–2 cm
2.01–4 mm	2 cm
>4 mm	2 cm

Soft tissue sarcomas

Sarcomas originate from the embryonic mesodermal layer, and >50 histological subtypes have been described. It was once believed that soft tissue sarcomas of the hand had a poorer prognosis than elsewhere in the extremities, but more recent publications indicate that the reverse may be true, suggesting patients with tumors of the hand have better survival than those with similar tumors at other sites. The work-up for patients with soft tissue sarcomas includes X-ray and MRI to assess the local extent of the disease, and a computed tomographic (CT) scan of the thorax to look for distant metastases.

Care should be taken when performing biopsies, because inappropriately performed biopsies can lead to unnecessary amputations. Some considerations include

- Ideally, biopsies should be performed by the surgeon who will perform the definitive resection
- Longitudinal incisions should be used and placed in line with the intended limb salvage incision. These need to be excised along with the tumor during definitive resection
- The most direct route to the tumor should be used, and exposure of vital structures such as nerves and vessels should be avoided during the biopsy as they will potentially be contaminated
- Specimens should be sent for frozen section analysis to ensure that lesional tissue has been obtained, as well as for cultures

taken prior to antibiotic administration should an infection be suspected
- Meticulous hemostasis must be ensured prior to closure and narrow wound closure used
- Drains, if required, should be placed in line with the incision, because the drain track will also need to be excised during tumor resection

Surgery is the mainstay of treatment for soft tissue sarcoma, and being able to achieve negative resection margins during surgery appears to be especially important in the hand. Adjuvant treatment with radiotherapy can be used to reduce the rate of local recurrence, and chemotherapy may help improve the overall survival in selected patients.

Bone and cartilage tumors

Chondrosarcoma

Chondrosarcomas are the most common primary malignant bone tumor of the hand. However, chondrosarcomas constitute < 2% of all primary cartilaginous bone tumors of the hand. Differentiating an enchondroma from a chondrosarcoma in the hand can be difficult, because more cellular atypia is accepted in enchondromas of the hand than at other sites. Bone cortical destruction and/or a soft tissue mass are features suggestive of a chondrosarcoma. Chondrosarcomas of the hand can arise from preexisting enchondromas and appear to be locally aggressive tumors with a high rate of local recurrence after curettage alone, but they rarely metastasize. The work-up for chondrosarcomas (and other malignant bone tumors) includes X-rays and MRI to assess the extent of local disease and a bone scan and CT scan of the thorax to look for possible distant metastasis.

It is still unclear whether curettage with or without local adjuvant treatment is superior to wide excision and/or amputation, as the risk of local recurrence must be balanced against functional loss and life expectancy, especially because chondrosarcoma tends to occur in older patients. Examination of the entire lesion is important to exclude more rare tumors such as dedifferentiated chondrosarcoma or chondroblastic osteogenic sarcoma, which require more aggressive treatment and carry a worse prognosis. Surgery remains the mainstay of treatment for chondrosarcoma; radiotherapy and chemotherapy are generally ineffective against it.

Osteogenic sarcoma

Primary osteogenic sarcomas of the hand are rare, accounting for as few as 0.2% of all cases of osteosarcoma. The prognosis for osteosarcomas of the hand is typically better than that at other sites, because tumors in the hand are often low-grade tumors. Wide excision of high-grade osteosarcoma is essential because positive margins are strongly correlated with local recurrence, which carries a poor prognosis. The benefit of chemotherapy with doxorubicin, cisplatin, and high-dose methotrexate in improving survival for patients with high-grade osteosarcoma is well established. However, its role in treating osteosarcoma of the hand is not clear, although it is probably beneficial for patients with high-grade tumors. Preoperative chemotherapy has the potential benefit of shrinking the tumor to preserve critical structures during surgical resection, but this must be restarted soon after surgery, preferably within 21 days, because delays reduce overall survival for patients.

Ewing sarcoma

Ewing sarcoma of the hand is rare, and the survival appears to be no different from that in other extremity sites. Both primitive neuroectodermal tumors, Ewing sarcoma, and Askin tumors have been classed together as Ewing sarcoma family tumors, given the similar histologic appearance, molecular translocations, and response to treatment. Treatment includes a combination of systemic chemotherapy and local therapy. The ideal method of achieving local control – whether radiotherapy alone, surgery alone, or combined modalities – has yet to be definitively established, although surgery is preferred in situations when complete tumor resection can be achieved with minimal functional loss.

Hand metastases

Hand metastases constitute an estimated 0.1% of all osseous metastases. The most common primary site is the lung, which accounts for about 40% of cases, followed by renal and breast primary cancers. The true incidence of hand metastases may be higher because many patients with minimal symptoms go unnoticed. Hand metastases can present insidiously and mimic infections, and they are sometimes the initial presentation of an occult malignancy. Treatment options include palliative radiation as well as amputations for fungating lesions. In addition, systemic treatment with bisphosphonates can reduce skeletal events for other sites of bone metastases.

SUGGESTED READING

Angelides AC, Wallace PF. The dorsal ganglion of the wrist: its pathogenesis, gross and microscopic anatomy, and surgical treatment. JHSA 1976; 1:228–235.
This article presents the author's experience in treating 500 dorsal wrist ganglions over a 25-year period. In it, the anatomy and pathogenesis are discussed, as well as the surgical treatment.

Flynn CJ, Danjoux C, Wong J, et al. Two cases of acrometastasis to the hands and review of the literature. Curr Oncol 2008; 15:51–58.
This article presents two cases of hand metastases and also reviews previous publications on hand metastases.

Kim DH, Murovic JA, Tiel RL, et al. A series of 397 peripheral neural sheath tumors: 30-year experience at Louisiana State University Health Sciences Center. J Neurosurg 2005; 102:246–255
This is possibly the largest series of peripheral nerve sheath tumors from a single center. The authors discuss their approach to both benign and malignant tumors, as well as the outcomes achieved from treatment.

Mankin HJ, Mankin CJ, Simon MA. The hazards of the biopsy, revisited. Members of the Musculoskeletal Tumor Society. J Bone Joint Surg Am 1996; 78:656–663.
This article, and update on a previous one published by the same group of authors, highlights the potential complications of biopsies performed for malignant tumors of the musculoskeletal system, emphasizing the need for careful planning and execution of these important procedures.

Moore JR, Weiland AJ, Curtis RM. Localized nodular tenosynovitis: experience with 115 cases. J Hand Surg Am 1984; 9:412–417.
In this article, the authors present their experience in treating 115 lesions in 112 patients over a period of 26 years. They discuss the clinical presentation and surgical treatment and present their outcomes after a long period of follow-up as well as suggestions to reduce the rates of local recurrence.

Ogose A, Unni KK, Swee RG, et al. Chondrosarcoma of small bones of the hands and feet. Cancer 1997; 80:50–59.
In this article, the authors presented the experience in their institution when managing patients with chondrosarcomas involving the hand and feet. The authors advocated an aggressive surgical approach, since many patients treated with currettage developed local tumor recurrence while those treated with en bloc resections had lower rates of recurrence.

Puhaindran ME, Rohde RS, Chou J, et al. Clinical outcomes for patients with soft tissue sarcoma of the hand. Cancer 2011 1; 117:175–179.
This article presents the largest series of soft tissue sarcomas of the hand surgically treated at a single center. In this article, importance of achieving negative resection margins and the morbidity of inappropriately performed biopsies are discussed.

Chapter 27 Contracture

Hari Venkatramani (27.2), Praveen Bhardwaj (27.2), Shady A. Rehim (27.1), Teemu Karjalainen (27.3), Kevin C. Chung (27.1)

27.1 THE STIFF DIGIT

Finger stiffness is a frequently encountered complication of acute and chronic conditions that affects hands and digits, often presenting a challenge to both patients and operating surgeons. A sound knowledge of relevant anatomy and the pathogenesis involved with the development of stiffness is required to reach the correct diagnosis and to formulate an appropriate management plan. In addition, a patient's education and compliance with hand therapy to maintain active and passive range of motion is essential to achieve good final outcomes.

TERMINOLOGY

The following terms are applicable to various conditions that result in stiff fingers and are sometimes used incorrectly or misinterpreted.

- Stiffness: Refers to a reduction in the range of motion of a joint
- Deformity: An alteration in the normal size or shape of a body part
- Lag: A limitation in the range of active joint motion, usually resulting from an injury to the motors (extensors or flexors). The passive range of motion is normal. Patients can have an extension lag (inability to actively extend the joint, but the joint has full passive extension) or flexion lag (inability to actively flex the joint, but the joint has full passive flexion)
- Contracture: A limitation in joint movement (both active and passive) resulting from scarring or shortening of structures (skin and subcutaneous tissue, tendons, muscle/ligaments, and/or capsules) that crosses a joint. Patients can have an extension contracture (the joint may be extended or hyperextended further but does not flex) or a flexion contracture (the joint may be flexed further but does not extend). If patients are unable to extend and flex the joint and the joint is fixed in one position, it is termed as fixed contracture. The joint may be fixed in flexion (fixed flexion contracture) or extension (fixed extension contracture)
- Ankylosis: The restriction of joint motion due to destruction of the joint surface. This may result in fibrous tissue bridging the articular surfaces (fibrous ankylosis) as seen in rheumatoid arthritis (RA) or bony bridging (bony ankylosis) commonly seen in osteoarthritis. There is no motion (active or passive) in a fixed contracture and in an ankylosed joint. The difference between a fixed contracture and ankylosis is that a fixed contracture can result from many causes, including ankylosis, and the joint may be normal in a fixed contracture. However, in ankylosis, the joint is completely destroyed
- Intrinsic-plus hand (**Figure 27.1**): Characterized by flexion of the metacarpophalangeal (MCP) joint and extension of the interphalangeal (IP) joints. This usually results from intrinsic muscle shortening/tightness. Common causes of intrinsic tightness include trauma, ischemia, fibrosis, RA, and spasticity
- Intrinsic-minus hand (**Figure 27.2**): Characterized by hyper-extension of the MCP joint and flexion of the IP joints giving rise to the characteristic claw hand appearance. This is secondary to intrinsic muscle weakness and unopposed extension of the MCP joints and flexion of the IP joints by the long extensors and flexors, respectively. Common causes include trauma, burns, and paralysis

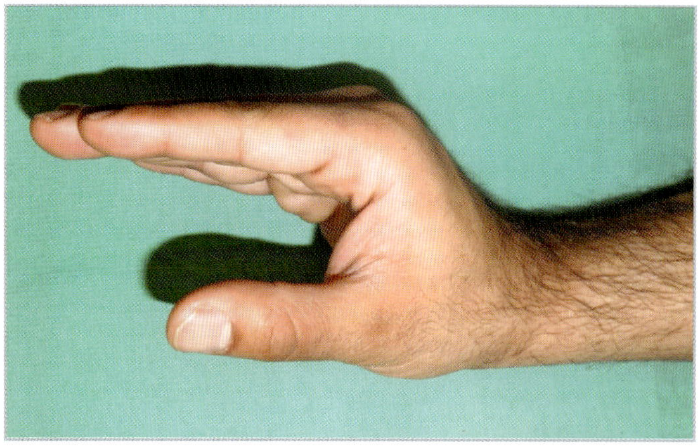

Figure 27.1 Functional position of the hand: slight wrist extension, metacarpophalangeal joint in 70°–90° of flexion and full extension of the interphalangeal joints. This is also the position of an intrinsic-plus hand.

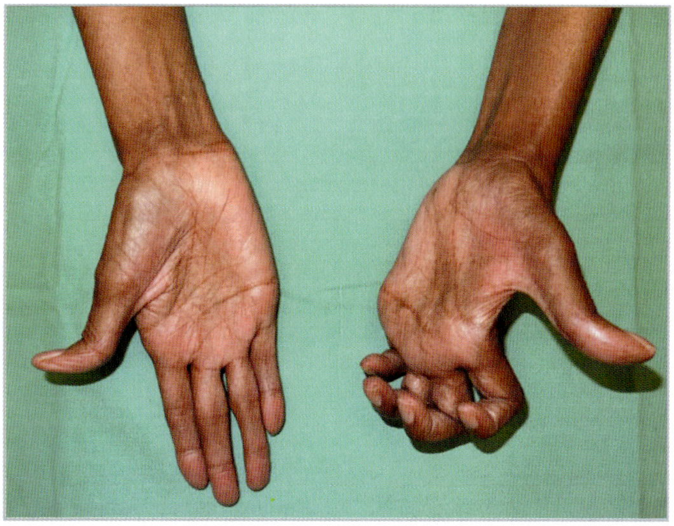

Figure 27.2 Claw hand deformity/intrinsic-minus hand: extension of metacarpophalangeal joints and flexion of interphalangeal joints.

- Lumbrical plus finger: Characterized by paradoxical extension of the IP joints while attempting to flex the fingers. This usually occurs after division of the flexor digitorum profundus (FDP) distal to the origin of the lumbricals. Retraction of the FDP increases tension on the lumbrical muscle belly, and as the patient attempts to flex the finger, traction on the proximal aspect of the divided FDP creates further tension on the lumbricals, resulting in extension of the IP joints instead of flexion.
- Functional position of the hand (**Figure 27.1**): A position in which the hand can be safely immobilized for a period of time without development of significant stiffness or loss of function. This is

achieved by positioning the wrist in slight extension, MCP joints in 70°–90° of flexion, and extension of the proximal interphalangeal (PIP) and distal interphalangeal (DIP) joints. Flexion of the MCP joint keeps collateral ligaments tight, thus preventing shortening/contracture. Extension of the PIP joint prevents formation of adhesions at the volar plate and check rein ligaments, preventing flexion contracture.

ETIOLOGY

The etiology of finger stiffness is diverse and may involve multiple structures:

- Skin and fascia
  - Dupuytren contracture
  - Burn scars and contracture
  - Rheumatoid variants, e.g. scleroderma/calcinosis
- Tendons
  - Tenosynovitis (e.g. RA, infection)
  - Tendon rupture/laceration
  - Volkmann contracture
  - Intrinsic muscle tightness
  - Spasticity
- Joints
  - Arthritis: RA, psoriasis, scleroderma, osteoarthritis, gout, and septic arthritis
  - Fractures (intra-articular fractures >extra-articular fractures)
  - Joints dislocation
  - Bony block exostosis
- Others
  - Chronic regional pain syndrome
  - Neurological and congenital causes of stiffness

PATHOGENESIS

Finger stiffness may develop secondary to edema, skin contractures, tendon adhesions, musculotendinous contractures, capsular contractures, arthrofibrosis, or through combinations of any of these conditions. Ultimately, the finger gets 'stuck' in a position that has a limited range of motion and develops subsequent deformities. Apart from etiology, the following factors and deformities are commonly associated with stiff fingers:

Edema

This is the most common cause of finger stiffness after acute injury. Edema results in a sequence of biological and mechanical factors that contribute to the development of stiffness. Initially, the inflammatory response from an injury leads to accumulation of fluid rich in proteins, cytokines, and inflammatory cells. Organization of fibrin leads to adhesions in tendons and surrounding structures as well as interstitial scarring. In addition, the accumulation of fluid within synovial and joint spaces limits the excursion of a joint's capsule, as well as the surrounding ligaments and tendons. With continued edema, a progressive increase of hydrostatic pressure within joint spaces will lead to hyperextension of the MCP joints and secondary flexion of the PIP joints. If this is not resolved or left untreated, shortening of collateral ligaments and secondary contractures will occur, resulting in an established deformity.

Skin contractures

Skin tightness/contracture commonly develops secondary to Dupuytren disease or burn injuries. However, there are other causes of skin contractures (e.g. connective tissue diseases such as scleroderma). A Dupuytren contracture is defined as a fibromatosis of the palmar and digital fascia that can cause digital flexion contractures. The pathological process involves the differentiation of fibroblasts to contractile myofibroblasts, deposition of type III collagen, and the expression of multiple growth factors and interleukins. Clinically, the condition begins as a palmar nodule(s) and progresses to form pathological cords with flexion deformities that mainly involve MCP and PIP joints. Over time, secondary contractures of the underlying structures develop, which include retraction of the flexor tendons, attenuation of the extensor tendons, and articular and periarticular contractures.

Regarding burn injuries, these can be superficial limited to the skin or deep, which cause shrinkage of the underlying tendons, ligaments, or joint capsules. In acute burns, finger stiffness commonly occurs due to immobilization, pain, and edema. In the chronic phase, hypertrophic scarring or retraction of skin grafted areas often result in the development of adhesions and contractures, which limit finger mobility.

Tenosynovitis

Tenosynovitis is usually a consequence of RA or infections and often results in pain, swelling, and a decreased range of movement. Tenosynovitis develops due to proliferation and inflammation of the synovial sheath around the extensor and flexor tendons, resulting in the development of adhesions that limit gliding movements of the affected tendons.

Boutonnière deformity (Figure 27.3)

This deformity is characterized by flexion of the PIP joint and hyperextension of the DIP joint. Common causes include RA, trauma, and burns. The pathogenesis of boutonnière deformity is primarily due to a central slip disruption. Rupture/elongation of

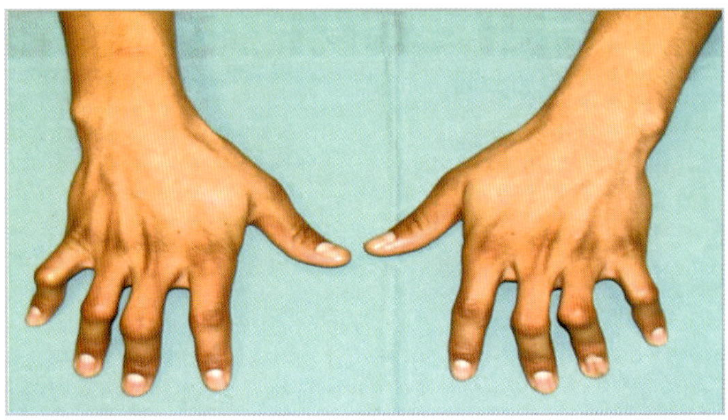

Figure 27.3 Boutonnière deformity in a rheumatoid hand showing flexion of the proximal interphalangeal joints and hyperextension of the distal interphalangeal joints.

the central slip results in a lack of PIP joint extension. Attenuation of the extensor mechanism and triangular ligament causes volar subluxation of the lateral bands. When the lateral bands migrate volar to the axis of rotation of the PIP joint, this leads to PIP joint flexion instead of extension. In addition, this results in increased tension on the distal aspect of the lateral bands, causing hyperextension of the DIP joint. If the condition is not resolved or left untreated, chronic boutonnière deformity develops with secondary changes of the following structures:

- Compensatory hyperextension of the MCP joint
- Fixed flexion contracture of the PIP joint
- Shortening of the oblique retinacular ligament, which maintains hyperextension of the DIP joint

Swan-neck deformity (Figure 27.4)

This deformity is characterized by hyperextension of the PIP joint and flexion of the DIP joint. The pathogenesis primarily involves laxity or avulsion of the PIP joint volar plate (e.g. dorsal dislocation or synovitis), which results in joint hyperextension. Likewise, flexor digitorum superficialis (FDS) rupture causes joint hyperextension due to unopposed action of the extensor tendons. Swan-neck deformity may also develop secondary to deformities of the MCP or DIP joint, which may lead to compensatory changes and imbalance of forces acting on the PIP joint. For example, mallet deformity (extensor tendon disruption at the DIP joint) causes a proximal shift of the extension forces on the PIP joint, resulting in joint hyperextension, while the DIP joint remains in flexion. At the MCP joint, volar subluxation or flexion secondary to intrinsic muscle tightness may result in compensatory hyperextension of the PIP joint. In addition, intrinsic tightness of the lateral bands may cause further extension of the PIP joint.

Mallet deformity

This deformity is characterized by flexion of the DIP joint due to a disruption of the terminal extensor tendon +/- bony avulsion. The DIP joint is flexed due to the unopposed action of the FDP. Chronic mallet deformity may lead to swan-neck deformity in the presence of volar plate laxity of the PIP joint. It may also contribute to boutonnière deformity secondary to disruption of the triangular ligament, resulting in volar subluxation of the lateral bands in the presence of a central slip disruption.

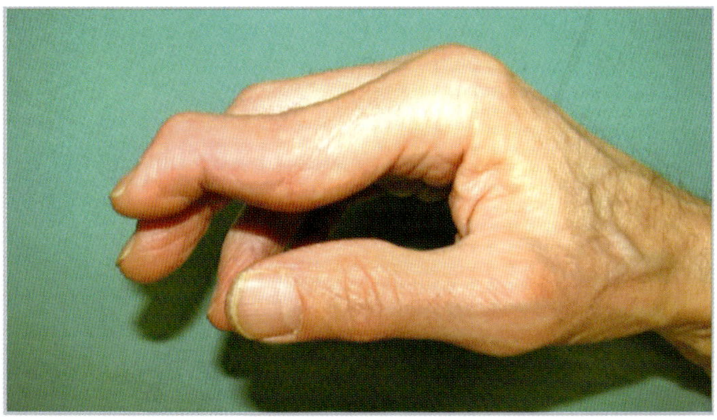

Figure 27.4 Swan-neck deformity in a rheumatoid hand, showing hyperextension of the proximal interphalangeal joint and flexion of the distal interphalangeal joint.

CLINICAL EXAMINATION

On physical examination of the fingers, one must try to answer the following questions to identify the source of stiffness:

Is stiffness due to contracture of the skin and fascia?

- Look for gross deformity (flexion or extension deformity)
- Assess skin quality, blanching, hypertrophic scarring, and availability of healthy surrounding skin
- Palpate palmar skin to assess for the presence of firm cords or nodules
- Cords and nodules of a Dupuytren contracture are usually adherent to the skin (i.e. not mobile with finger flexion or extension)
- Assess active and passive range of movement. A decrease of passive more than active movement may indicate underlying joint contractures
- If the skin and fascia are not involved look for other sources of stiffness

Is stiffness due to musculotendinous or joint contracture?

Decrease of active movement more than passive movement is more likely a musculotendinous problem (e.g. tendon adhesions or muscle tightness). Assuming it is a musculotendinous problem, next try to differentiate whether the stiffness is due to extrinsic or intrinsic muscle tightness.

- Extrinsic tightness:
  - Flexor tightness: To test for flexor tightness place the wrist and MCP joints in extension and passively extend the IP joints; increased resistance on passive extension indicates flexor tightness. Repeat the test after flexing the wrist and MCP joints. If no resistance is met or the fingers can be fully extended then it is flexor tightness
  - Extensor tightness: To test for extensor tightness, place the wrist and MCP joints in flexion and passively flex IP joints; increased resistance on passive flexion indicates extensor tightness. Repeat the test after extending the wrist and MCP joints. If no resistance is met or the fingers can be fully flexed then it is extensor tightness
- Intrinsic tightness:
  - Finochietto–Bunnel test (**Figure 27.5**): To test for intrinsic muscle tightness, extend the MCP joint and passively flex the PIP

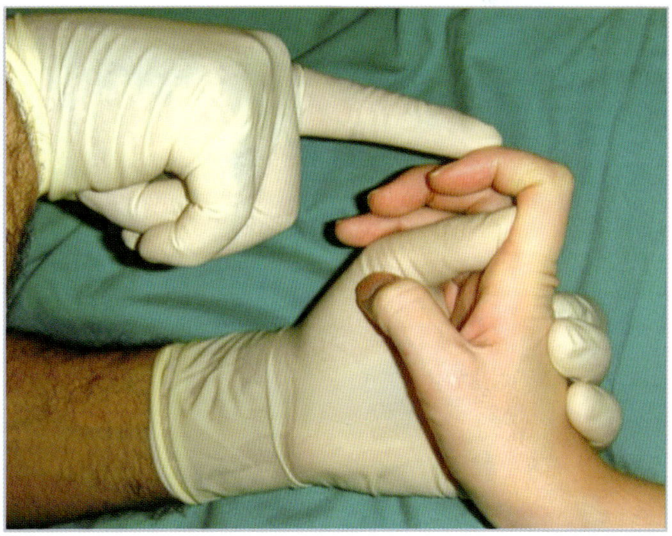

Figure 27.5 Finochietto–Bunnel test: extend the metacarpophalangeal joint and passively flex the interphalangeal joints. Increased resistance indicates intrinsic muscle tightness.

joint; increased resistance indicates intrinsic muscle tightness/contracture. Repeat the test with the MCP joint in flexion (relaxes intrinsic muscles), and if no resistance is met then it is intrinsic tightness. It is worth noting that if you are still unable to flex the PIP joint after MCP joint flexion, this may be due to extrinsic extensor tightness or capsular contracture (see above)

- Elson test (**Figure 27.6**): Used to test central slip integrity. Ask the patient to flex the PIP joint 90° over a table edge and assess PIP joint extension against resistance. A positive test is considered when there is weakness of PIP joint extension and full extension or hyperextension of the DIP joint due to a shift in the extension forces onto the lateral bands
- Landsmeer test: To test for oblique retinacular ligament tightness, extend the PIP joint and passively flex the DIP joint; increased resistance indicates oblique retinacular ligament tightness. Flex the PIP joint and repeat the test and if no resistance is met, it is oblique retinacular ligament tightness
- If muscles and tendons are not involved, look for other sources of stiffness

Is stiffness due to joint contracture?

- Limited passive movement of joint in flexion and extension indicates joint contracture.
  - Measure degree of joint contracture using goniometer
  - Repeated measurements help to monitor progression of contracture or deformity
  - On longstanding disease, assess proximal and distal joints for secondary or compensatory deformities
  - Note specific patterns of joint deformities (e.g. RA)

INVESTIGATIONS

Radiographic investigations may help identify the cause of stiffness, especially if it is due to arthritis, fracture/dislocation, or bony block.

Laboratory

- Routine bloods (complete blood count, urea and electrolytes)
- Inflammatory markers (erythrocyte sedimentation rate and C-reactive protein)
- Uric acid (gout), RA factor, and antinuclear antibodies scleroderma (anti scl-70)

Radiological

- X-ray:
  - Look for fractures, malunions, dislocations, and exostosis
  - Helps diagnose arthritis (RA, psoriasis, or osteoarthritis)
- Ultrasonography:
  - Tendon rupture
  - Ligamentous injury
- Magnetic resonance imaging

TREATMENT

Nonoperative

- Edema control: Elevation and compression bandages, adequate pain control, and gentle mobilization decrease edema and help to prevent the development of stiffness
- Scar management: Scar massage, compression garments, and silicone gel therapy are commonly used techniques to soften and flatten scar tissue as well as mobilize skin and subcutaneous tissue to prevent the formation of adhesions
- Splinting: Applies tension/traction force to remodel joint contractures
  - Static splint (**Figure 27.7**):
    - Holds joint in one position (does not allow any movement). Is applied continuously (e.g. mallet splint) or intermittently in between exercises. Static splints are often used to provide support or to preserve a degree of mobility gained by other methods
  - Serial static splint:
    - These are plaster casts or thermoplastic splints, which are usually reserved for severe contractures. Serial splints are used to maintain the finger or joint in one position; these splints are typically molded to apply maximal tension/stretch on the finger or joint. With gradual stretch of the underlying contracture, the splint is replaced by another to accommodate for the new position and maintain tension
  - Dynamic splint (**Figure 27.8**):
    - This type of splint is designed to apply constant force while preserving joint mobility, achieved by using elastic bands and spring coils (e.g. Capener splint, short dorsal outrigger splint). Dynamic splints are worn by patients during the day and replaced at night by a static splint to avoid splint displacement
  - Static progressive splint (**Figure 27.9**):
    - This splint is similar to dynamic splint in construct; however, the force applied is not dynamic, and the tension can be adjusted using a small adjustment screw (e.g. joint-jack splint). Although static progressive splints hold the joint at a maximal stretch, the difference between static progressive and serial static splints is that serial static splints apply an equal amount of force on the whole finger, whereas static progressive splints concentrate force on certain areas of the finger, typically joint contractures

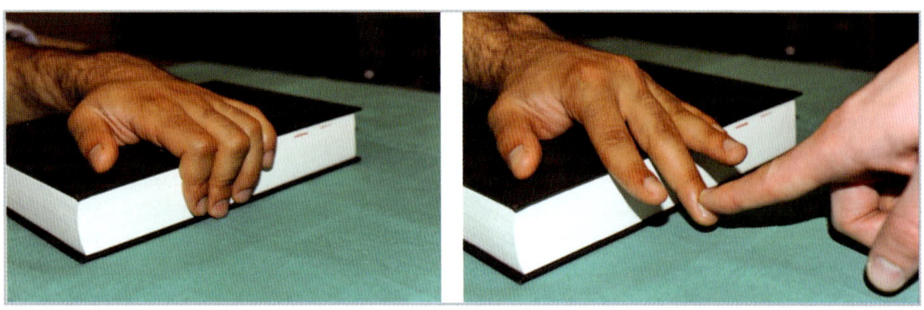

Figure 27.6 Elson test: patient is asked to flex proximal interphalangeal (PIP) joint 90° over the table edge, and the central slip is assessed as the patient extends the PIP joint against resistance.

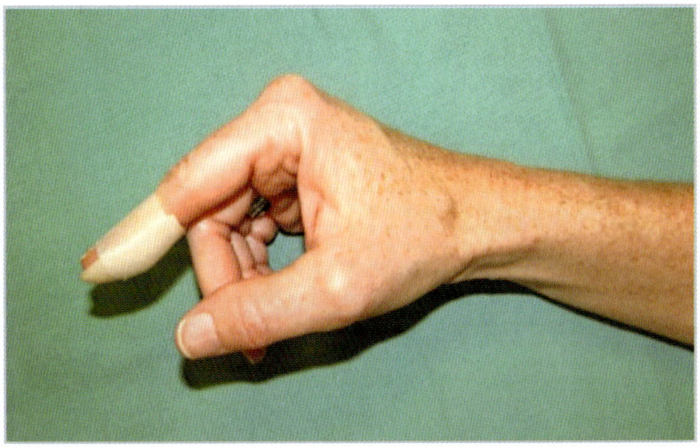

Figure 27.7 Mallet splint: worn for 6 weeks continuously then for another 2 weeks at night time. Patients should be instructed to keep the distal interphalangeal joint straight while replacing or cleaning the splint especially in the first 6 weeks after injury.

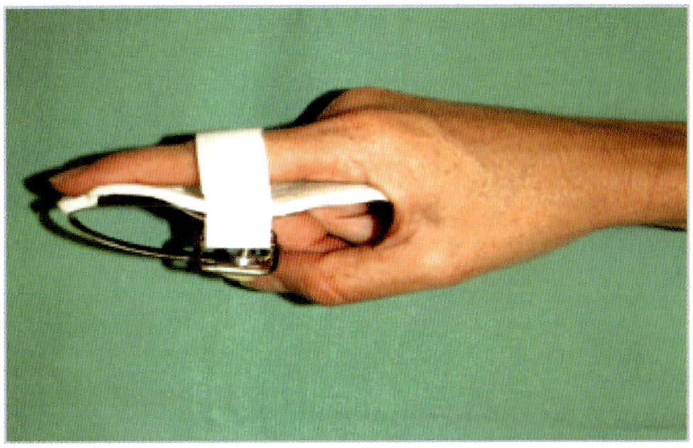

Figure 27.9 Joint-jack (serial progressive finger splint) with a small screw to adjust tension on the joint contracture.

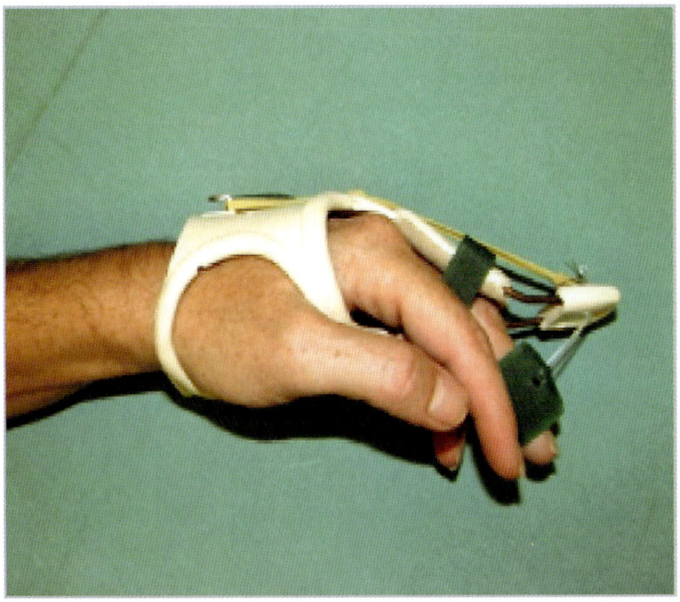

Figure 27.8 Dynamic extension splint allows active flexion and passive extension of the finger joints.

Operative treatment

Surgical treatment is indicated for those who are nonresponsive or fail to progress with nonoperative management. As always, surgery should be tailored to a patient's needs and function. Treatment of finger stiffness should follow a logical sequence of releasing and reconstructing the different finger structures that have resulted in a stiff finger. A single or multistage procedure may be required.

Scar release

Scar release (e.g. z-plasty) or scar resurfacing (skin grafts) helps to release the tension imposed by tight skin. When there are other factors causing superficial tightness of the skin and fascia (e.g. Dupuytren contracture), fasciotomy, fasciectomy or dermatofaciectomy, and skin grafts can be performed.

Tenolysis

- Flexor tenolysis: Expose the flexor tendons using Bruner or midlateral incisions, locate the level of adhesions, and then incise the flexor sheath without damaging pulleys system. Use a circumferential sharp dissection to free extratendinous and intertendinous adhesions and then pass a nonabsorbable suture under the tendons (in areas of limited access) to release any remaining adhesions
- Extensor tenolysis: After a dorsal skin incision, free any adhesions between the skin and extensor tendon. Use sharp dissection to release adhesions along the lateral bands and then dissect between the tendon and bone. Free adhesions along the way up to the terminal tendon if required while preserving the central slip. If necessary, perform dorsal capsulotomy to enable more flexion of the finger

Intrinsic release

- Distal intrinsic release: This technique functions to release intrinsic tightness that is causing PIP joint extension. Depending on the intrinsic muscles involved, a unilateral or bilateral release can be performed. Use a midaxial incision and release the oblique fibers and lateral bands (extending PIP joint) while preserving the central slip and the transverse fibers of the extensor mechanism
- Proximal intrinsic release: This technique releases intrinsic tightness that causes MCP joint flexion. Use a dorsal skin incision over the MCP joint and then release the intrinsic muscles proximal to the MCP joint to release the contracture

Correction of boutonnière and swan-neck deformities

The surgical correction of these deformities depends on the classification of the deformity itself, and this, in turn, depends on the degree of joint flexibility. In general, if the underlying joint is severely damaged and fixed, then arthroplasty or arthrodesis is the most appropriate treatment option. However, if there is a degree of flexibility, soft tissue reconstructive options should be considered.

- Boutonnière deformity: The aim of surgery is to correct the PIP joint flexion and DIP joint extension associated with boutonnière deformity. The DIP joint extension can be corrected by extensor tenotomy, which is achieved by dividing the extensor tendon to allow for DIP joint flexion while preserving the oblique retinacular ligament in order to maintain the capacity for DIP joint extension. Correction of PIP joint flexion is achieved by a central slip reconstruction (shortening) and dorsal mobilization of the lateral bands.
- Swan-neck deformity: The aim of surgery is to correct DIP joint flexion and PIP joint hyperextension associated with swan-neck deformity. This can be achieved by various procedures:
  - FDS tenodesis: The proximal slip of the FDS is divided proximally, leaving the distal end attached. The FDS is then reattached proximally to the A1 pulley or anchored to the bone with the PIP joint in 30° of flexion
  - Retinacular ligament (Littler) reconstruction: This procedure simultaneously corrects PIP joint hyperextension and restores extension of the DIP joint. The ulnar lateral band is divided proximally, leaving the distal end attached. The lateral band is then mobilized under Cleland ligament volar to the axis of rotation of the PIP joint and sutured proximally to the flexor sheath. Tension is adjusted so that it allows for simultaneous PIP joint flexion and DIP joint extension. Note these steps resemble the pathogenesis of boutonnière deformity described earlier
  - Secondary/primary deformities of MCP joint and DIP joint may require arthroplasty or arthrodesis

Joint release

- MCP joint extension contracture:
  - Make a longitudinal skin incision on the dorsum of the MCP joint, followed by a longitudinal split of either the radial or ulnar sagittal band and retraction of the extensor tendon to expose the joint capsule. Release the collateral ligaments partially from the metacarpal head, and then flex the MCP joint, maintaining the position with a transarticular K-wires if required. Finally, repair the sagittal band and splint the MCP joint in flexion
- PIP joint flexion contracture (**Figure 27.10**):
  - Make a Bruner incision, divide the flexor sheath at A3, and retract the tendons of the FDS and FDP to expose the volar plate. Release the volar plate and check-rein ligaments, as well as the collateral and accessory ligaments if required. Try and preserve the articular branch of the digital artery that runs in this vicinity. If the passive movement is still limited, divide the oblique retinacular ligament and any other tight structures to gain further motion
- PIP joint extension contracture (**Figure 27.11**):
  - After an S-type skin incision, incise the interval between the central tendon and each lateral band to allow the lateral band to migrate volarly after the release, expose, and incise the dorsal capsule of the PIP joint transversely while preserving the central slip. Pass a small elevator within the joint to free it from intra-articular adhesions. Release the collateral ligaments if passive flexion is still limited

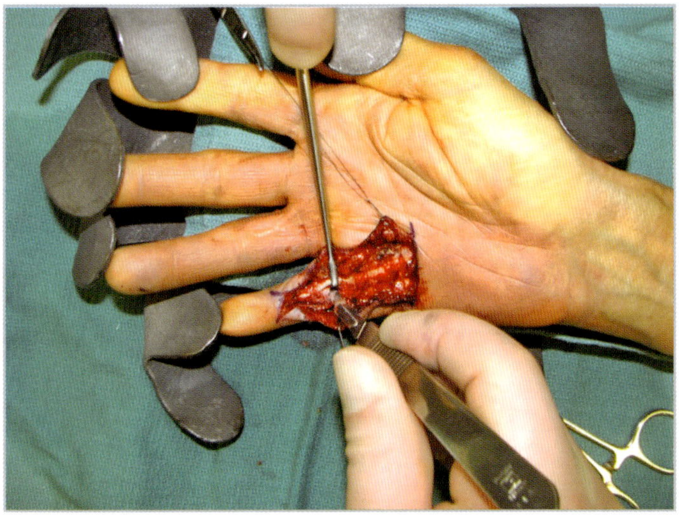

Figure 27.10 Release of proximal interphalangeal joint flexion contracture.

External traction device (Ex-fix)

This treatment method is used to correct PIP joint flexion contractures. The metal frame is fixated to the metacarpal bone below and to the middle phalanx above the PIP joint. A constant distractive force is then applied, which gradually straightens the joint contracture.

Arthroplasty

This procedure is performed when joint mobility is required to decrease pain and improve function. The presence of competent musculotendinous structures and good bony stock to seat the implant are prerequisites for a successful arthroplasty procedure. The indications of joint arthroplasty include joint pain, stiffness (e.g. arthritis), and joint incongruity (e.g. fractures/dislocations), and arthroplasty may be performed with or without the use of a prosthetic material.

- Types:
  - Volar plate arthroplasty: The two techniques for volar plate arthroplasty are Eaton/Tupper arthroplasty, both of which describe volar plate advancement. The volar plate is detached from its distal end and advanced to reconstruct the surface of the damaged joint
    - Eaton–Malerich arthroplasty involves advancement of the distal end of the volar plate to cover part of the articular surface using pull-out wires that are threaded through the substance of the middle phalanx and secured over dorsum of the finger
    - Tupper arthroplasty uses a similar technique; however, it involves interposition of the volar plate between the MCP joint articular surfaces
  - Replacement arthroplasty: Joint replacement or resurfacing using synthetic material.
    - Silicone elastomer arthroplasty: Involves excision of the articular surfaces and replacement with an implanted silicone spacer
    - Pyrolytic carbon arthroplasty: Involves joint replacement using a metallic alloy prosthesis or carbon implants

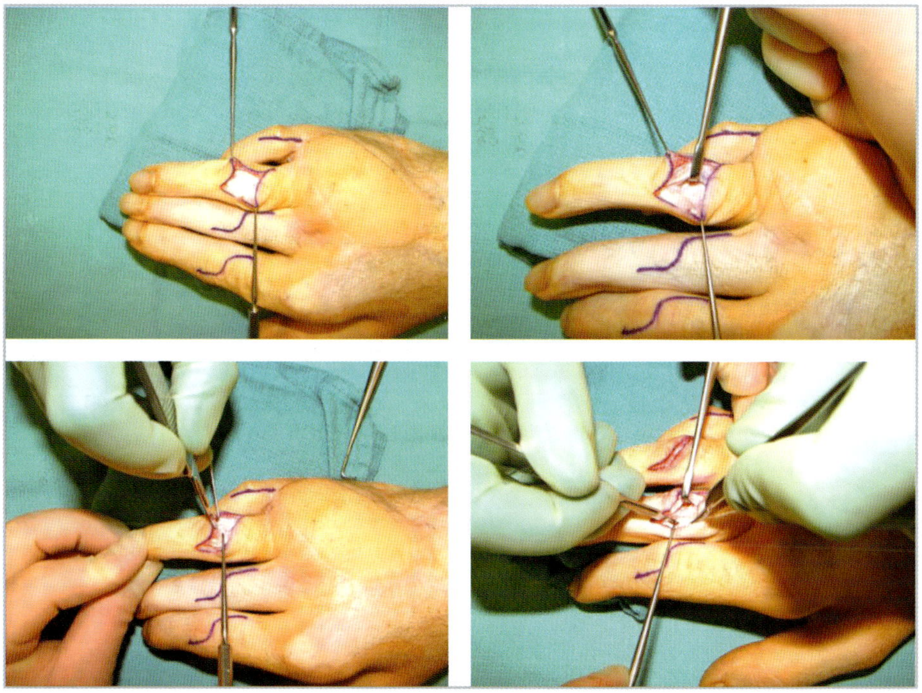

Figure 27.11 Release of proximal interphalangeal joint extension contracture.

SUGGESTED READING

Brüser P, Poss T, Larkin G. Results of proximal interphalangeal joint release for flexion contractures: midlateral versus palmar incision. J Hand Surg Am 1999; 24:288–294.

A comparative retrospective study of 45 digits to compare two surgical techniques of PIP joint release (midlateral vs. palmar incision). At a long-term follow-up, ROM was significantly better in the midlateral incision group than in the palmar incision group.

Giudice ML. Effects of continuous passive motion and elevation on hand edema. Am J Occup Ther 1990; 44:914–921.

A study evaluating the efficacy of the use of continuous passive motion (CPM) of the digits in combination with limb elevation to reduce hand edema. Results showed CPM with limb elevation was a more effective treatment for the reduction of hand edema than limb elevation alone.

Glasgow C, Fleming J, Tooth LR, Hockey RL. The Long-term relationship between duration of treatment and contracture resolution using dynamic orthotic devices for the stiff proximal interphalangeal joint: a prospective cohort study. J Hand Ther 2012; 25:38–46.

A prospective study to examine the long-term relationship between weeks of treatment using dynamic orthoses and contracture resolution, in both flexion and extension deficits of the PIP joint. Results showed a significant improvement of both flexion and extension PIP joint contractures; however, PIP joints respond faster and better to treatment than extension contractures (12 vs. 17 weeks of treatment).

Houshian S, Gynning B, Schrøder HA. Chronic flexion contracture of proximal interphalangeal joint treated with the compass hinge external fixator. A consecutive series of 27 cases. J Hand Surg Br 2002; 27:356–358.

A case series assessing the efficacy of an external hinge fixator to treat chronic PIP joint flexion contractures.

Weeks PM, Wray RC Jr, Kuxhaus M. The results of non-operative management of stiff joints in the hand. Plast Reconstr Surg 1978; 61:58–63.

A retrospective review of hand rehabilitation programs utilized in a large number of patients that presented with stiff joints and opted for nonoperative treatment. Results showed excellent functional improvement of the hand following this treatment protocol

27.2 VOLKMANN ISCHEMIC CONTRACTURE

The Volkmann ischemic contracture (VIC) is a condition occurring at the end stage of an unrecognized or inadequately treated compartment syndrome, first described by a German surgeon Richard von Volkmann in 1881. The irreversible muscle ischemia causes necrosis of the muscles and nerve damage, and subsequent contracture of the forearm, wrist, and hand (**Figure 27.12a** and **b**). There are numerous causes of compartment syndrome, but irrespective of the cause the condition leads to common sequelae: fibrosis of the nonviable tissues (e.g. muscles and nerves) resulting in contractures and nerve deficits. Early diagnosis of compartment syndrome and timely intervention can prevent VIC through a careful examination of the clinical signs (as described in Chapter 9), the 'six Ps': pain, pressure, paresthesia, pallor, pokilothermia, and pulselessness.

PATHOGENESIS

The increase of pressure in the rigid osseofascial compartment results in the rise of compartment pressure, which reduces capillary perfusion below a level necessary for tissue survival.

Effect on muscles

Experimental studies have shown irreversible changes in muscles after 4 hours of ischemia and sustained ischemia causes muscle necrosis. The necrotic muscles eventually become fibrotic through fibroblastic proliferation, and the fibrous tissue shrinks in both longitudinal and horizontal planes, causing deformities of the forearm and hand. The maturation of the fibrotic tissue occurs over 6 months to 1 year, and therefore, the deformities may be progressive until this time.

Effect on nerves

Experimental studies have shown irreversible changes of nerve tissues 8 hours after initial ischemia. Nerves can be affected by two mechanisms:

1. Vascular: Due to the initial primary insult and secondarily because of diminished circulation due to surrounding fibrosis
2. Mechanical: Fibrosis compressing the nerve and impaired nerve function because of inability of the nerves to glide in a fibrotic tissue bed

There are three stages of clinical presentation:

1. Initial stage (vascular crisis)
2. Stage of progressive fibrosis and paralysis
3. Stage of established contractures (VIC)

PATHOLOGY

Deeper muscles of the forearm (FDP, especially the middle and ring) are the most vulnerable muscles, followed by the flexor pollicis longus (FPL) and the FDS and wrist flexors. The extensor muscles may also be involved in severe cases of compartment syndrome. The maximum damage to the muscles occurs in the middle of the muscle belly, as explained by the Seddon ellipsoid infarct concept (**Figure 27.13**). With progressive damage, nerves become markedly constricted and atrophied. It is worth noting that the median nerve is always more severely affected than the ulnar nerve.

EVALUATION

The clinical presentation of VIC has a broad spectrum, depending on the extent of muscle and nerve involvement, although the evaluation is mainly clinical. The group of muscles involved need to be identified, and muscle contractures should then be differentiated from joint contractures by using the tenodesis test (**Figure 27.14a** and **b**). Active and passive range of motion should be measured and documented to assess the extent of the damage. The status of the

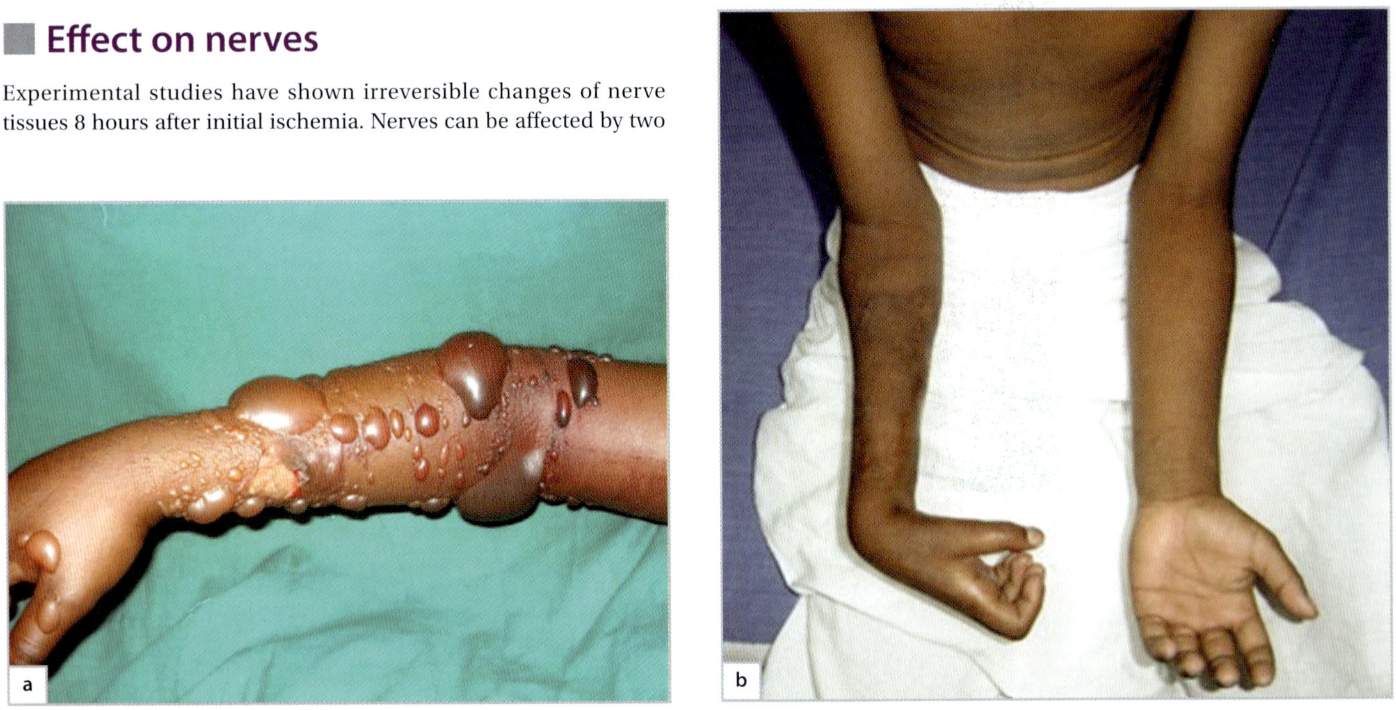

Figure 27.12 (a) Showing the appearance of the hand and forearm in acute compartment syndrome. (b) Showing the appearance of the hand and forearm in established Volkmann ischemic contracture.

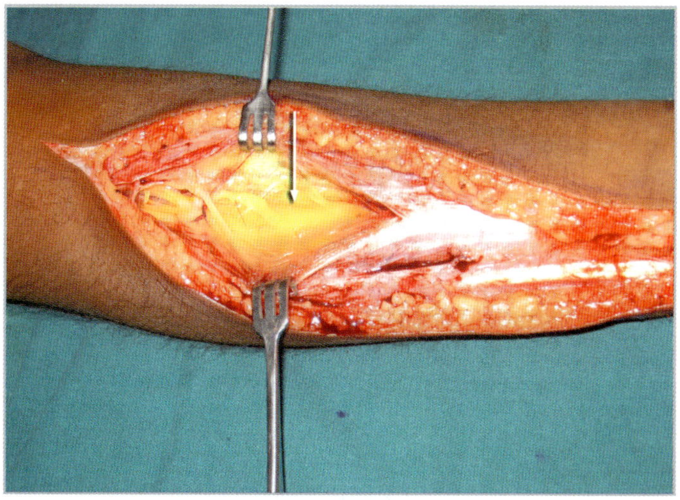

Figure 27.13 The ellipsoid infarct, as described by Seddon, is seen in the center of the flexor muscle mass (arrow).

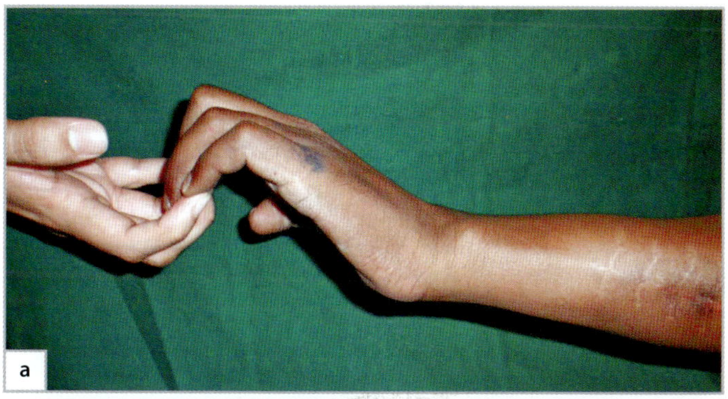

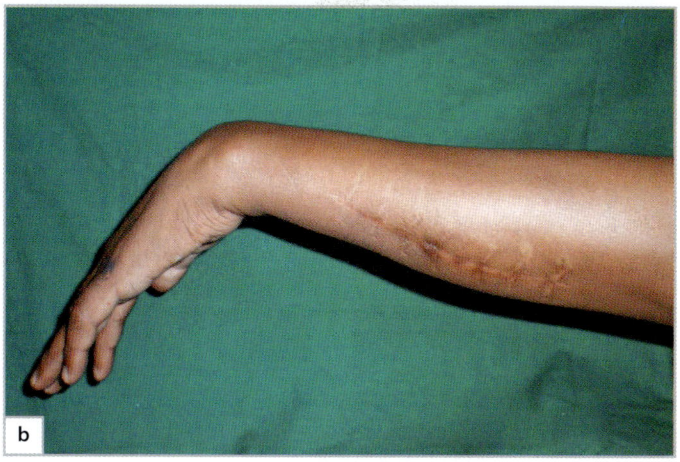

Figure 27.14 (a) The flexion deformity of the fingers following Volkmann ischemic contracture. (b) The flexion deformity in this case is corrected by flexing the wrist (tenodesis test), indicating that it is caused by the tight flexors and that the joints are normal.

intrinsic muscles, ulnar nerve, and median nerve should then be assessed. Contracture of the intrinsic muscles or ulnar nerve damage will result in a claw hand deformity. Similarly, muscle atrophy and wasting to the thenar muscles or median nerve damage will result in weakness of pinch and grip strength as well as thumb opposition. A sensory evaluation by two point discrimination and monofilament testing should be documented for later comparison. In addition, measure the limb length, because the involved limb is usually shorter, especially when the compartment syndrome has occurred in early childhood. X-ray images are important in long standing cases to rule out bone deformation.

CLASSIFICATION

There are three main classification systems widely in use:
1. Holden classification
2. Tsuge classification
3. Zancolli classification

Holden classification (1979)

This system is based on the site of the vascular compression.

Type I

- The cause of compression is proximal to the site of ischemia
- Example – supracondylar fracture resulting in distal ischemic damage

Type II

- There is direct localized compression in the distal segment, resulting in a localized increase in compartmental pressure
- Example – tight bandage applied after forearm fracture

Tsuge classification (1975) [modification of Seddon classification (1964)]

This system is based on the degree of the involvement of muscle groups in the forearm.

Mild type

- Localized
- Involves the deep flexor compartment, more commonly the FDP of the middle and ring fingers and the FPL
- Nerve involvement is absent or insignificant

Moderate type 'classic or typical type'

- Involves all FDP and FPL tendons, with partial involvement of the FDS
- Nerve involvement is always present
- Sensory impairment is more common in the median nerve distribution than the ulnar nerve
- Intrinsic minus deformity is common

Severe type

- Involves all of the digital and wrist flexors and a varying amount of extensor muscles
- Nerve involvement is severe, with total loss of sensation and total intrinsic palsy

Zancolli classification (1979)

This system is based on the degree of involvement of the intrinsic muscles of the hand.
- Type I: Contracture involving forearm muscles with normal intrinsic muscles

- Type II: Contracture involving forearm muscles with paralysis of intrinsic muscles
- Type III: Contracture involving forearm muscles with contracture of intrinsic muscles
- Type IV: Combined type

MANAGEMENT

As with other conditions, each case requires individual analysis of the clinical situation. Treatment depends on the involvement of each of the six components of the forearm, namely, the skin, bones, tendons, joints, nerves, and vessels. There is a broad range of presentation even in each classification type, which precludes treatment based solely on the classification system. The combination of Tsuge classification with Holden classification provides some systematic guide to treatment that can be adapted to each case according to the severity.

Timing of intervention

Seddon advocated a delay of 3 months, whereas Tsuge advocated a delay of 6 months. This delay is mainly promoted to allow the overlying skin to settle well and spontaneous recovery to reach a plateau. This may be a preferred approach in cases with reasonable hand function. On the other hand, some surgeons prefer early intervention in severe cases because with delay, the nerves become thinned due to compression by the fibrosed muscles and further joint stiffness may develop. In patients with severe neuralgic pain, prompt neurolysis and excision of fibrotic tissue has been shown to relieve pain.

Treatment options

The treatment options for VIC range from conservative treatment to surgical intervention such as tenolysis, neurolysis, excision of fibrotic muscle mass, proximal muscle slide, tendon transfer, nerve grafting, and microvascular free-functioning muscle transfer. Prevention of joint stiffness by passive mobilization and splinting is a crucial aspect of management, and static progressive or a combination of dynamic and static splinting will help prevent this occurrence.

Mild type

In mild cases, especially when the patient has presented early, passive stretching exercises and splinting alone may be enough. When there is only involvement of a few deep flexor muscle groups and no sensory or intrinsic loss, fractional release (lengthening the affected muscles by making multiple incisions at the musculotendinous junction) is a very effective form of treatment (**Figure 27.15**). Fractional lengthening may increase the length of the muscle–tendon unit by about 1 cm only. If more lengthening of the tendon is required, z-lengthening should be performed by incising the tendon at proximal lateral and distal medial halves with a lengthening of at least 2.5 cm. However, this technique has the disadvantage of further weakening the already weak muscle.

Moderate type 'classic or typical type'

In cases of Holden type II contractures where the proximal muscle mass is adequate, z-lengthening of the individual tendons may be performed. In patients with a moderate degree of muscle involvement, with good muscle function (good finger flexion) but diffuse contracture of the muscles, a proximal muscle slide procedure (as described by Page and later modified by Scaglietti) can be performed:

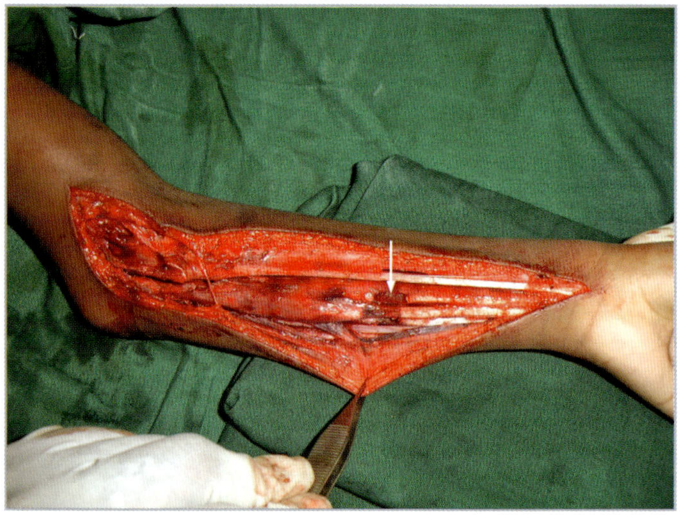

Figure 27.15 Intraoperative picture showing the fractional lengthening of the flexor tendons in mild type of Volkmann ischemic contracture (black arrow).

- The flexor-pronator muscle mass is slid from its proximal insertion and the deformity is corrected (**Figure 27.16**)
- This operation can be combined with neurolysis if nerve involvement is present preoperatively

Most of the other patients with moderate involvement will require a two-stage approach:

- Two-stage approach
  - The first stage involves adequate debridement of the fibrous tissue followed by tenolysis and neurolysis to free up tendons adhesions as well as median and ulnar nerves. Begin by making a wide exposure through a curved volar incision at the forearm. Do not dissect through scarred tissue, because this may precipitate an iatrogenic nerve injury. Thus, it is advisable to locate the nerve at a distant site that is relatively normal, either proximal or distal to the affected area, then follow the nerve to the site of contracture. After debridement of all nonviable tissue, reassess the defect and the degree of soft tissue loss to consider future reconstructive options that may be performed during the second stage
  - In the second stage, if the existing skin coverage is not supple or if secondary tendon and nerve reconstruction is needed, it is preferable to provide soft tissue coverage via a flap

One may encounter three situations related to the management of muscle involvement:

1. Satisfactory muscle mass exists proximally after excising the fibrotic muscle and scar tissue, and there is adequate continuity between the existing muscle mass and the tendons emerging from them. In this situation, tenolysis, fractional/Z-lengthening, and neurolysis will provide good results (**Figure 27.17a–f**).
2. The whole muscle mass is pale and fibrotic with no healthy contractile tissue left on the flexor side but with no involvement of the extensor compartment. In such cases, tendon transfer using the functioning extensor muscles can be performed. Transfer of the extensor carpi radialis longus to the FDP and brachioradialis to FPL can restore function (**Figure 27.18**)
3. The whole of the flexor muscle mass is fibrotic and nonfunctional and the extensor compartment is also partly or completely involved. In such situations, a microvascular free-functioning muscle

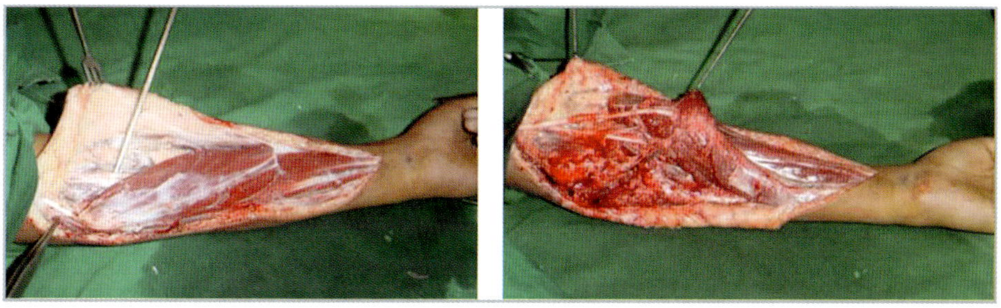

Figure 27.16 Intraoperative photograph showing the proximal muscle slide combined with neurolysis performed for a case of moderate type of involvement in Volkmann ischemic contracture.

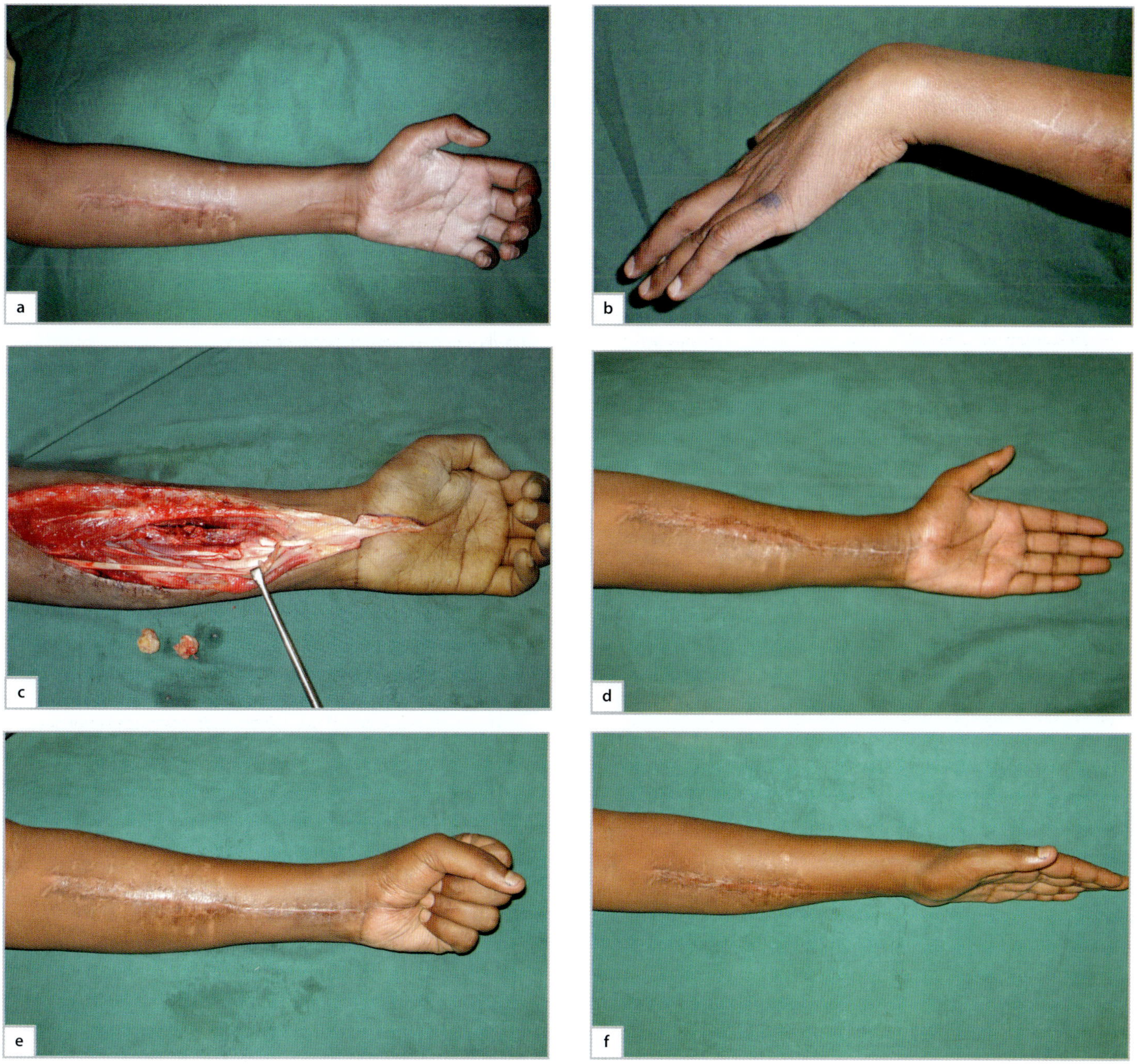

Figure 27.17 (a and b) Preoperative picture showing contracture of the finger flexors. Patient also had median and ulnar nerve involvement with sensory deficit and intrinsic muscle paralysis. (c) Intraoperative picture showing the excised fibrotic and necrotic tissue. This was accompanied by tenolysis, fractional lengthening, and neurolysis of the median and ulnar nerves. (d–f) Postoperative result showing the full range of flexion and extension of the fingers. This patient also had excellent recovery of the median and ulnar nerves after neurolysis.

transfer to enable finger flexion can provide a functional hand (**Figure 27.19a–f**)

Management of nerves is usually challenging, as it requires intraoperative decision making, which requires experience. The intraoperative grading of the nerve lesion and its corresponding management as described by Gulgonen can be a very useful guide.

Severe type

These patients will always require a two-stage approach. The nerves will have segmental scarring, severe thinning, or disruption, and they would require segmental excision and interfascicular nerve grafting (**Figure 27.20a** and **b**). Due to the significant involvement of the extensor muscles, the most suitable option to restore finger flexion is a free-functioning muscle transfer. The muscles that can be used as free-functioning muscle include the gracilis, latissimus dorsi, and rectus femoris.

The steps for free-functioning muscle transfer are as follows:

- The first step involves exploration of the flexor aspect of the forearm and distal arm, and the identification of vessels suitable for anastomosis
- The anterior interosseous nerve is generally spared in the ischemic contracture and is available to power the free-functioning muscle transfer
- The surgeon must strive to restore the appropriate length of the transferred muscle for adequate tensioning and minimize the ischemia time. If the patient is treated appropriately, this procedure can provide a functional hand (**Figure 27.19a–f**)

In long-standing cases with fixed contracture at the wrist, fusion of the wrist joint after proximal row carpectomy allows correction of the wrist deformity and provides shortening to address the contracted flexor muscles.

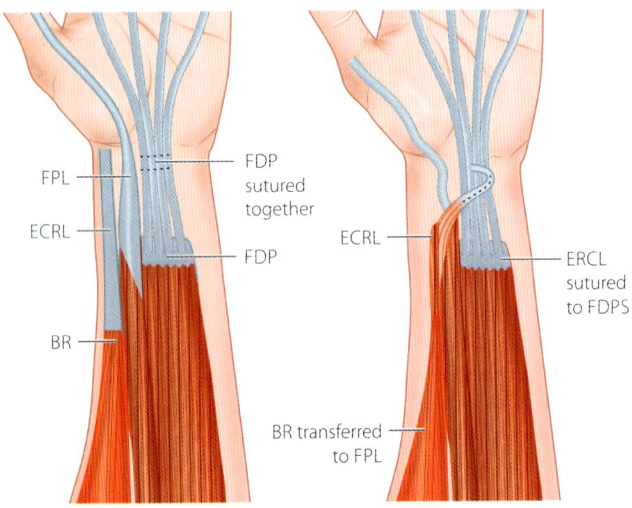

Figure 27.18 Tendon transfer, from the extensor carpi radialis longus (ECRL) to flexor digitorum profundus (FDP). BR, brachioradialis; FPL, flexor pollicis longus.

Intrinsic function

The presence of intrinsic function greatly influences the functional outcome of the hand. If neurolysis is performed early, the intrinsic muscles can recover in mild to moderate cases and in some cases with severe nerve involvement. The presence of intrinsic function greatly improves the outcome of a tendon transfer or free muscle transfer and adds substantially to the level of hand function that can be achieved. Hence, early neurolysis must be considered in all cases. Thumb opposition can be restored by extensor indicis proprius opponensplasty.

EXPECTED OUTCOMES

The final outcome depends on the severity of the initial contractures, timing of intervention, severity of nerve involvement, restoration of muscle power, and dedicated participation in the hand rehabilitation program. The best results are achieved when the decompressed nerve has recovered providing good sensation and intrinsic recovery, there are no contractures, and flexor motor power can be provided by the transfer of good extensor muscles or a free-functioning muscle transfer.

SUMMARY

Prompt recognition and treatment of acute compartment syndrome is the key to prevent VIC, and therefore, high-risk injuries such as supracondylar fractures of the humerus in children or immediate vascular repair should be closely monitored. Treatment of an established contracture is complicated and depends on many variables; however, early neurolysis and appropriately staged reconstruction can provide a useful functional hand.

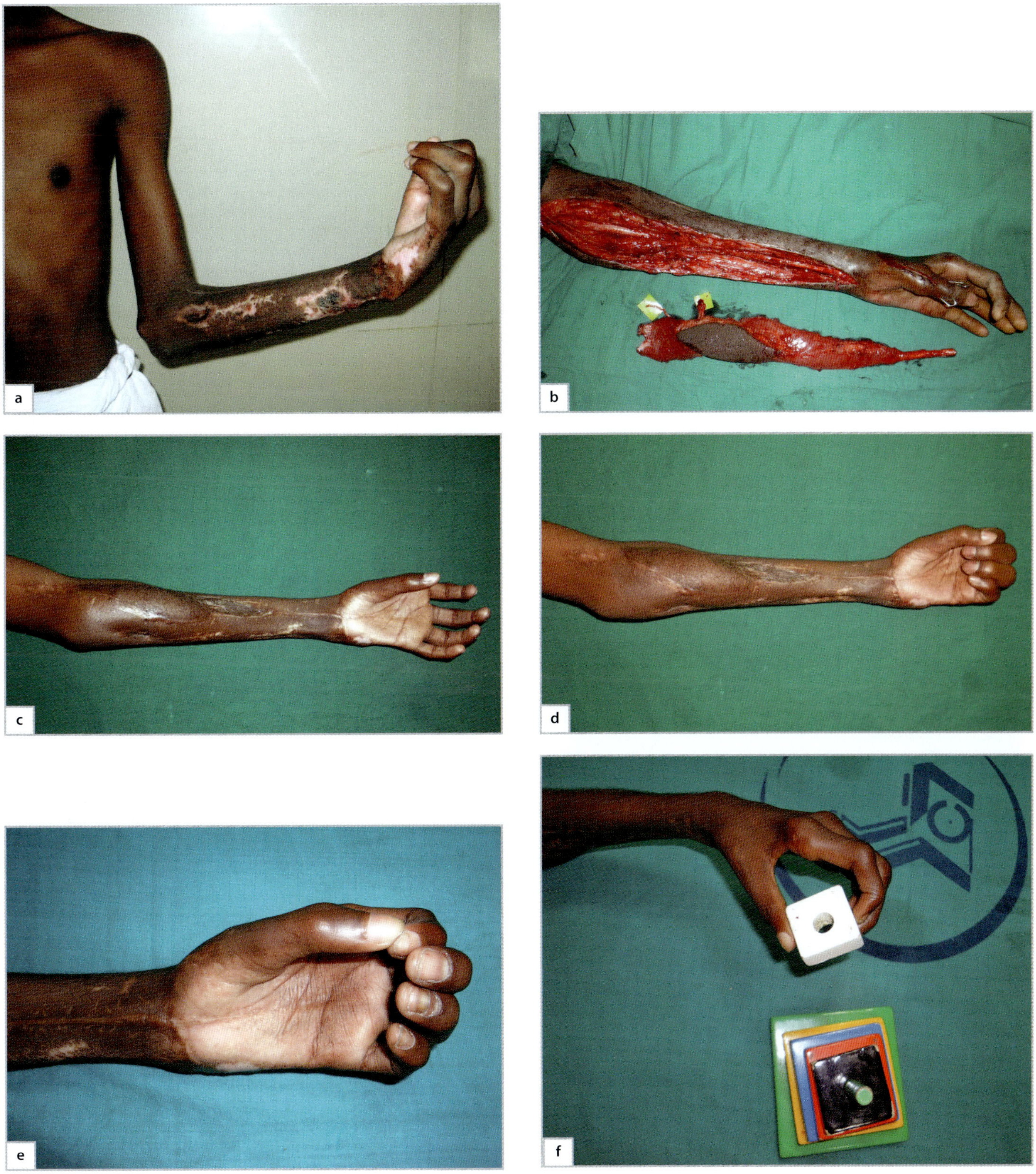

Figure 27.19 (a) Preoperative picture of patient with severe type of Volkmann ischemic contracture with involvement of both the flexor and extensor compartments. (b) Free-functioning gracilis muscle used to restore finger flexion. The muscle was innervated by the anterior interosseous nerve. (c–f) Eighteen-month follow-up pictures showing good flexion of the fingers, as well as good pinch and hand function.

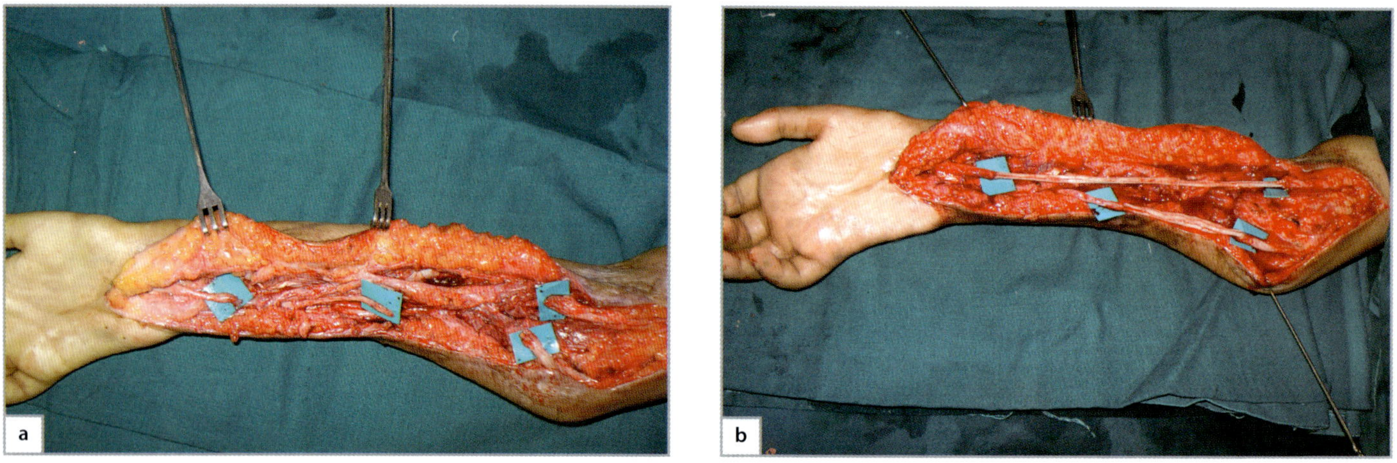

Figure 27.20 (a) Segmental excision of the scarred and thinned median and ulnar nerves and the resultant gap. (b) The segmental loss at the median and ulnar nerves bridged by interfascicular nerve grafts using the sural nerve.

SUGGESTED READING

Hovius S, Ultee J. Volkmann ischemic contracture. Prevention and treatment. Hand Clin 2000; 16:647–657.

This article provides guidelines that are useful in preventing Volkmann ischemic contractures. It also provides treatment protocols for the management of this disabling condition.

Matsen FA, Winquist RA, Krugmire RB. Diagnosis and management of compartment syndrome. J Bone Joint Surg 1980; 62A:286–291.

This is a classic article related to the measurement of compartment pressure for the diagnosis of compartment syndrome. It defines the indications of the compartment pressure measurement and its clinical implications.

Oishi SN, Ezaki M. Free gracilis transfer to restore finger flexion in Volkmann ischemic contracture. Tech Hand Up Extrem Surg 2010; 14:104–107.

This article describes the two-stage approach the authors follow for severe type of involvement in Volkmann ischemic contracture (i.e. initial muscle debridement and later free-functioning gracilis muscle transfer to achieve finger flexion). We have found this approach very useful.

Stevanovic M, Sharpe F. Management of established Volkmann's ischemic contracture of the forearm in children. Hand Clin 2006; 22:99–111.

This article describes the treatment options for Volkmann ischemic contractures. The authors recommend muscle slide operations for mild and moderate cases and wide excision and functional free muscle transfer to limit injury to the nerves in severe cases.

Sundararaj GD, Mani K. Pattern of contracture and recovery following ischemia of the upper limb. J Hand Surg 1985; 10B:155–161.

This is one of the largest series on Volkmann ischemic contractures, describing the different patterns of ischemic contractures seen in this condition. The study documented that sensory recovery could occur even after total ischemic degeneration of the nerves, but motor recovery does not occur.

27.3 DUPUYTREN CONTRACTURE

Dupuytren disease is benign fibromatosis of the palmar and digital fascia of the hand. It sometimes affects plantar fascia of the foot (Ledderhose disease) and penis (Peyron disease).

ETIOPATHOGENESIS

- Epidemiology
  - Dupuytren disease is believed to have autosomal dominant inheritance pattern with variable penetrance. Several genes are either upregulated or downregulated in the diseased tissue. The genetic defect is not of collagen production but of fibroblast density and activity
  - Affects mainly northern European descendants
  - Incidence rises sharply in men in their fifth decade and in women in their sixth decade. Male to female ratio is approximately 1:6 but the ratio approaches 1:1 with increasing age
  - Onset in young age, strong family history, bilateral disease with skin involvement and ectopic presentation (feet, penile) predicts aggressive disease with high probability of recurrence. It is referred to as a diathesis group
  - Associated with smoking, alcohol use, heavy manual labor, diabetes, and epilepsy
- Pathogenesis
  - Local tissue ischemia is believed to trigger proliferation of fibroblasts and differentiation into myofibroblasts. Myofibroblasts are able to contract and produce collagen, which leads to the development of the contracting cords
  - Three phases, which can overlap, can be distinguished both histologically and macroscopically
    - In proliferation phase the amount of myofibroblast arises and the first nodules are formed
    - In involutional phase, the myofibroblasts organize and form thicker nodules and longitudinal cords, which contract and cause the extension deficit. The cords usually follow the normal anatomical structure of the palmar fascia
    - In residual phase the cords are thick scar like tissue with low cellular density and activity

PATHOANATOMY

- The abnormal activity of fibroblasts causes typical cords based on the normal anatomy of the palmar aponeurosis. The cords are named after the normal fascial bands from which they originate (**Figure 27.21**).

CLASSIFICATION

- Tubiana classification
  - Stage 1: Contracture of 0°–45°
  - Stage 2: Contracture of 45°–90°
  - Stage 3: Contracture of 90°–135°
  - Stage 4: Contracture >135°
- Complete Tubiana classification also takes into account degree of the distribution of lesions and condition of the skin but is complex for clinical use

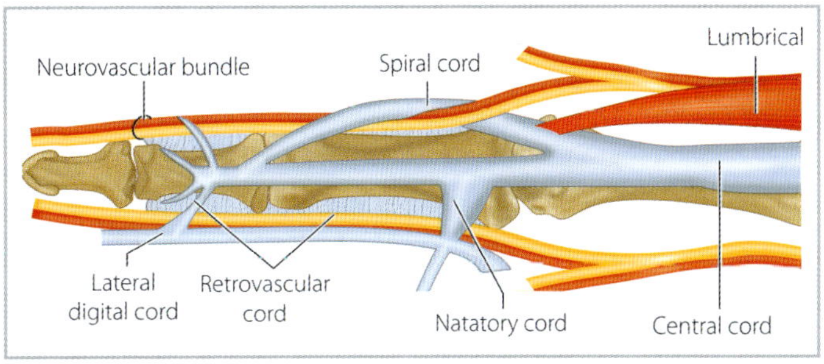

Figure 27.21 Pathoanatomy.

CLINICAL PRESENTATION

- Initially, the disease presents with palmar nodules, which typically occur in the two ulnar rays of the hand. In the proliferation phase, the patient may complain of pain of the nodules. The pain usually resolves when the disease progresses
- Usually, patients seek treatment when total passive extension deficit (TPED) starts to limit hand function. Typically patients complain inability to open the hand properly and difficulties putting the hand inside gloves or to pockets
- Typically, MCP joints are first affected.

EVALUATION

- Inspection and palpation of the cords
  - Affected rays
  - Identify the cords that limit the extension and impede function
    - Typically, there is a central cord that contracts the MCP joint
    - Interdigital soft tissue mass with PIP-joint contracture suggests presence of a spiral cord
    - Recurrence in the fifth-ray PIP joint is typically caused by ulnar abductor digiti minimi cord
- Tight adherence of the cords to overlying skin predicts the need of dermofasciectomy and consecutive skin grafting or flap. Greater TPED also predicts need for a skin graft.
  - Measure the extension deficit of the MCP joint and the PIP joint when the MCP joint is held flexed and extended.
    - A fixed PIP-joint contracture when MCP joint is flexed predicts PIP-joint capsular contracture
    - DIP-joint hyperextension is a sign of retrovascular and lateral cords and secondary extensor imbalance
    - Table top test: Test is positive when hand cannot be held flat upon the table palm down
    - Tissue biopsy or imaging modalities are not required for the diagnosis

TREATMENT OPTIONS

- There is no cure for the disease itself. The aim of the treatment is to improve the extension deficit either by breaking or removing the contracted cords
- The indication for treatment is a contracture, which causes a functional deficit. Indication therefore depends on the patient's needs. Usually, a 30° contracture of the MCP joint and 20° contracture

of the PIP joint are considered indication for intervention. Some patients such as musicians and workers with need for climbing may require earlier intervention.

- The treatment options include
  - Percutaneous needle fasciotomy (PNF).
    - Minimally invasive procedure, which can be performed under local anesthesia in-office. Best suited for MCP-joint contracture of elderly people. Central cord is easy to break and common digital nerve lies deep and lateral in respect of the cord in the palm level. PNF is not suitable for postsurgical scarring
    - Use small volume of 1–2% lidocaine to the skin and a 25-gauge needle. Avoiding digital nerve block may be useful because when the nerve is not blocked, the patient feels if the needle hits the nerve. Push the needle through the cord and retrieve the needle immediately when the resistance decreases. Continue pushing the needle through the cord in different angles until no cord can be felt. Sweeping the needle tip helps to feel for any remaining strings of the cord. After most of the cord is cut by the needle, the cord can be broken by gentle passive extension. Usually, fasciotomy needs to be done in two or three levels to achieve optimal result. Tourniquet is not needed. Active range of motion and night splinting can be commenced immediately. Splinting is usually continued for 3 months
    - Primary result is usually almost complete release in the MCP-joint contracture. PIP joint is more difficult to release and 50–90% of improvement of TPED can be expected primarily
    - The recurrence rate is higher compared with open fasciectomy. The recurrence depends on the definition of the recurrence and on the follow-up time and is 50–66% within the first 3–5 years. Recurrence occurs more commonly in young patients. Up to 65% of the patients have been reported to require further intervention
    - Complications include skin tears (3–16%), infections (2%), nerve injury (1–3%), most of which are temporal neurapraxia
  - Open fasciotomy
    - Open fasciotomy is a historical treatment and is not widely used anymore. It is performed similarly to percutaneuos fasciotomy but with a scalpel
  - Collagenase injection
    - A novel medical office based nonsurgical approach to Dupuytren contracture. Its efficacy is comparable with other treatment modalities but because of the high cost of the drug the cost-effectiveness of collagenase injection requires further evaluation
    - Collagenase clostridium histiolyticum lyses type I collagen, and this leads to disruption of the cord. Because the collagenase only lyses type I collagen, it does not damage nerve or artery walls
    - Injection (0.58 mg) is given into the cord without anesthesia. Do not inject in areas, where skin is tightly adhered to the skin to avoid skin rupture. The finger is straightened the following day in local anesthesia. Night splinting is commenced immediately. Injection can be repeated
    - An efficacy study showed a reduction of TPED to a mean of 7° in the MCP-joint and 22° in the PIP joint. Seventy-seven percent of treated MCP joints and 40% of the PIP joint achieved <5 degrees TPED after 1–3 injections
    - Most patients report at least one minor adverse effect, which does not require treatment. Minor adverse effects include hematoma, swelling, bruising, injection site pain, pruritus lymphadenopathy, and skin laceration. Major collagenase-related adverse effects were reported in 0.9% of the patients including flexor tendon rupture (0.6%) and CRPS (0.3%)
  - Open limited fasciectomy
    - Standard treatment of Dupuytren contracture. The purpose of the limited fasciectomy is to remove the part of the palmar and digital fascia, which is causing the contracture
    - Usually, plexus or general anesthesia is used. The procedure can also be performed under Bier block or local anesthesia. The use of a tourniquet is recommended
    - Skin incisions (**Figure 27.22**) are made and skin flaps raised in the subcutaneous plane. Extreme care should be taken in the proximal digital flexor crease, where the spiral cord may have dislocated the neurovascular bundle (NVB) superficial to the fascia and towards the midline. Multiple transverse incisions, which are left open, have also been used
    - The cord is transected proximally and intermetacarpal NVB is identified. The proximal end of the cord is then lifted up cutting the vertical bands of McGrouther and connections to the flexor tendon sheath. The flexor tendon sheath should be preserved intact in view of potential skin grafting. The cord is dissected free proximal to distal until it is completely removed and the finger can be straightened
    - The NVB is kept visible and protected throughout the procedure. If the NVB is difficult to identify in the base of the finger when progressing proximal to distal direction, it can be identified distally and then followed proximally. Do not continue cutting the cord fibers unless you know exactly in which plane the NVB lies

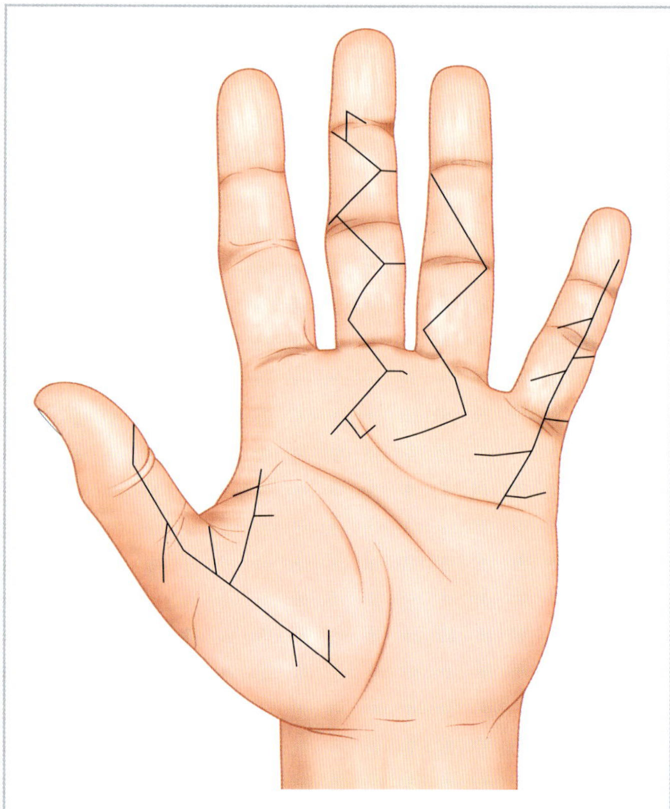

Figure 27.22 Skin incisions for open limited fasciectomy.

- Contracted PIP-joint capsule can limit extension after complete excision of the cords. If severe (stage III–IV) capsular contracture exists, full range of motion of the PIP joint cannot usually be achieved and maintained postoperatively. In these cases, it may be wise to accept 30–40° residual contractures. Prefasciectomy soft tissue distraction with external fixation system may be useful to gain better range of motion
- If the PIP joint cannot be extended after complete excision, gentle passive mobilization should be tried first. The purpose of mobilization is to break thin articular adhesions but not the contracted collaterals
- If the contracture cannot be relieved with mobilization, capsuloligamentous release can be considered. However, there is evidence that in severe contracture, capsuloligamentous release does not have a significant effect on the final range of motion. Accessory collateral and checkrein ligaments are released in capsuloligamentous release. Full release of the volar plate can lead to PIP joint locking in hyperextension and should be avoided if possible
- If the skin cannot be closed when the finger is fully extended, a full thickness skin graft is used. Skin grafts serve as firebreak and may reduce the chance of recurrence. However, in the only prospective randomized study, skin grafting did not seem to have significant effect on the joint angles in 3-year follow-up

– Open radical fasciectomy
  - Radical fasciectomy was proposed for the treatment to decrease recurrence of the diseases. However, the recurrence rate appears to be similar and complication rates significantly higher when compared with limited fasciectomy. Therefore, it should not be performed

SUGGESTED READING

Andrew JG. Contracture of the proximal interphalangeal joint in Dupuytren disease. J Hand Surg Br 1991; 16:446–448.

Breed CM, Smith PJ. A comparison of methods of treatment of pip joint contractures in Dupuytren's disease. J Hand Surg Br 1996; 21:246–251.

Weinzweig N, Culver JE, Fleegler EJ. Severe contractures of the proximal interphalangeal joint in Dupuytren's disease: combined fasciectomy with capsuloligamentous release versus fasciectomy alone. Plast Reconstr Surg 1996; 97:560–566.

These three studies address the problem of PIPJ contracture. Andrews et al. show with amputated severely affected by Dupuytren's contracture fingers that contracture full release can be achieved by excision of the accessory collateral ligaments and only a few fingers needed further volar plate release. Breed and Smith retrospectively compared the efficacy of gentle mobilization to release. They found that best results were achieved when gentle passive mobilization was sufficient. Weinzweig et al. compared fasciectomy and capsuloligamentous release to fasciectomy alone in severe contractures and found that despite the initial result, the long-term extension deficit was similar between the groups. Capsuloligamentous release did not improve the final result.

Chiu HF, McFarlane RM. Pathogenesis of Dupuytren's contracture: a correlative clinical-pathological study. J Hand Surg Am 1978; 3:1–10.

Craft RO, Smith AA, Coakley B, et al. Preliminary soft-tissue distraction versus checkrein ligament release after fasciectomy in the treatment of Dupuytren proximal interphalangeal joint contractures. Plast Reconstr Surg 2011; 128:1107–1113.

This non randomized study compares the results of fasciectomy and checkrein release to soft tissue distraction with external fixator (Digit Widget) followed by fasciectomy. Patients who had prefasciectomy soft tissue distraction gained significantly more extension (54° vs. 36°). Moreover, 3/17 patients in soft tissue distraction achieved full extension and did not require fasciectomy at all. This method can be particularly useful in recidive surgery and cases with severe contracture.

Hueston JT. The table top test. Hand 1982; 14:100–103.

Hueston JT. 'Firebreak' grafts in Dupuytren's contracture. Aust N Z J Surg 1984; 54:277–281.

In these two classical papers, Hueston describes table top test and suggests that a positive test an indication for surgery. In the other paper, he suggests that a skin graft serves as a firebreak zone and reduces the risk for recurrence. This was further supported by Tonkin et al (see later).

Hurst LC, Badalamente MA, Hentz VR, et al. Injectable collagenase clostridium histolyticum for Dupuytren's contracture. N Engl J Med 2009; 361):968–979.

This randomized double-blind controlled study evaluated the efficacy of collagenase injection. Collagenase showed significantly better improvement in extension compared to placebo.

Pess GM, Pess RM, Pess RA. Results of needle aponeurotomy for Dupuytren contracture in over 1,000 fingers. J Hand Surg Am 2012; 37:651–656.

The authors describe their results and share their vast experience and technical tips for successful percutaneous needle fasciectomy.

Tonkin MA, Burke FD, Varian JP. Dupuytren's contracture: a comparative study of fasciectomy and dermofasciectomy in one hundred patients. J Hand Surg Br 1984; 9:156–162.

The authors found 46.5% recurrence rate after excision compared to no recurrence in those patients receiving a firebreak skin graft.

Tubiana R. Evaluation of deformities in Dupuytren's disease. Ann Chir Main 1986; 5:5–11.

Tubiana's classification system of Dupuytren's contracture is described in this paper in detail.

Ullah AS, Dias JJ, Bhowal B. Does a 'firebreak' full-thickness skin graft prevent recurrence after surgery for Dupuytren's contracture? a prospective, randomised trial. J Bone Joint Surg Br 2009; 91:374–378.

The authors did not find difference in recurrence rate of patients receiving skin graft and not receiving skin graft in this prospective randomized trial. This may be due to the wide inclusion criteria.

Chapter 28 Complex regional pain syndrome

Sandeep J. Sebastin

DEFINITION

Complex regional pain syndrome (CRPS) is a condition of the limbs characterized by pain that is out of proportion (in duration or degree) to the usual course for a particular lesion. The pain is regional (not limited to the nerve territory) and associated with motor, sensory, sudomotor, vasomotor, and/or trophic limb changes (**Figure 28.1**).

KEY MILESTONES

- 1864 – Silas Weir Mitchell: First detailed description and coined the term 'Causalgia'
- 1900 – Sudeck: Described post-traumatic atrophy of bone (Sudeck atrophy)
- 1916 – Rene Leriche: Linked sympathetic nervous system to causalgia
- 1946 – Evans: Introduced the term 'reflex sympathetic dystrophy' (RSD)
- 1986 – Roberts: Used the term 'sympathetically mediated pain' (SMP) to describe RSD
- 1994 – IASP (International Association for the Study of Pain) introduced the term CRPS, subdivided it into two types (CRPS I and II), and proposed diagnostic criteria
- 2003 – IASP introduces modified clinical diagnostic criteria

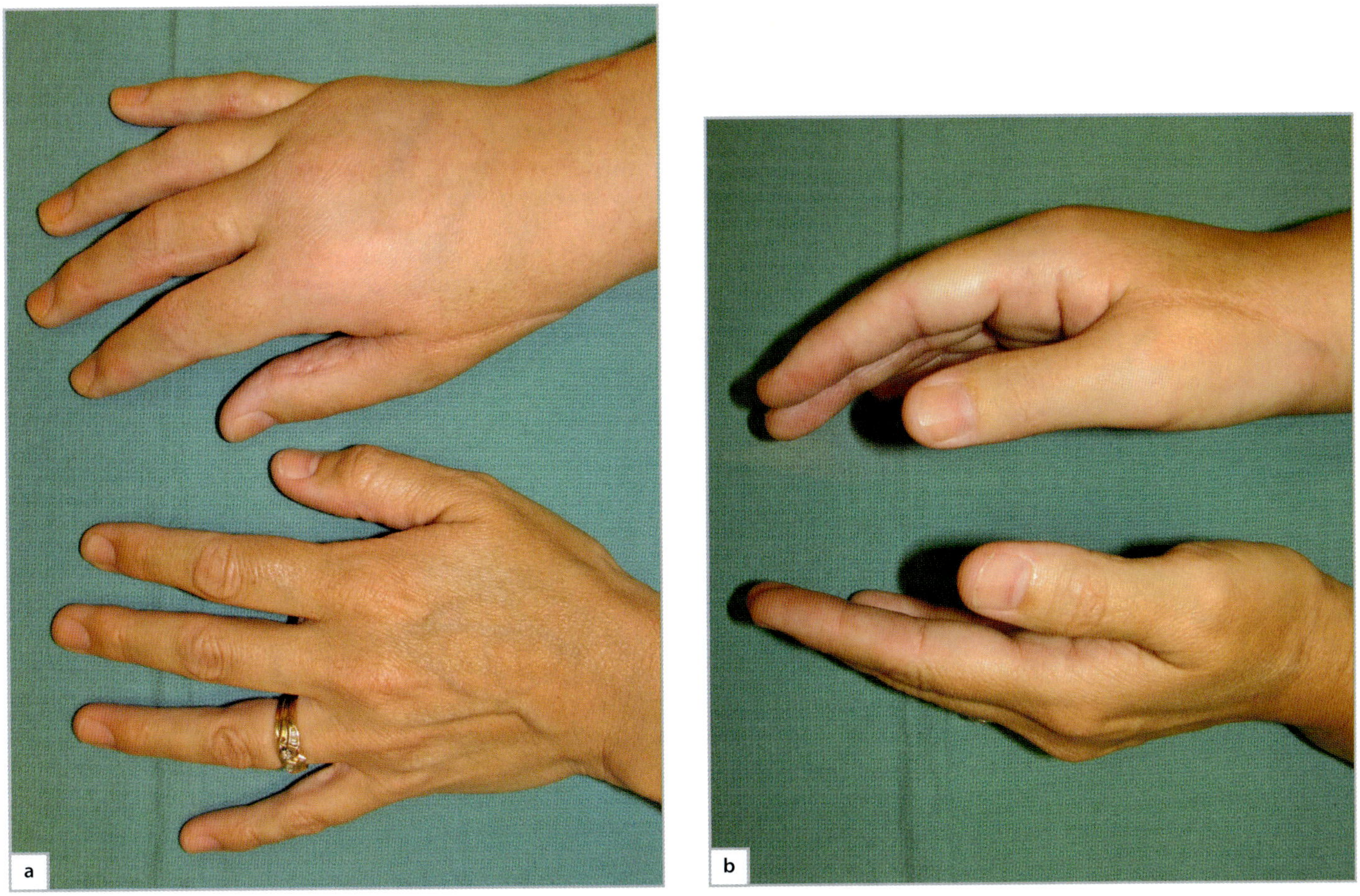

Figure 28.1 Patient with CRPS in the right hand. Notice the swelling and slightly 'shiny' appearance.

INCIDENCE

CRPS is an uncommon disease with a prevalence of <2%. A higher incidence of CRPS is reported in patients between the ages 40–49 years and in women (76%). The upper extremity is affected twice as commonly as the lower limb, and a fracture is the most common trigger (46%). In 10–26% of patients with CRPS, no precipitating factors can be found. No correlation to diabetes, smoking, or alcohol has been found. The incidence of recurrent CRPS I is 1.8% per year, and 50% are spontaneous recurrences. The common hand conditions associated with CRPS include

- Dupuytren contracture (4.5–40%)
- Distal radius fractures (22–39%) (comminuted intra-articular fractures, associated ulnar styloid fractures, closed reduction, and casting)
- Carpal tunnel surgery (2–5%)

PATHOPHYSIOLOGY

Most patients (90%) with CRPS have history of an initiating noxious event (trauma/ischemia/nerve compression). However, it is unclear why only some patients develop CRPS. Multiple mechanisms are believed to be involved in the development of CRPS, including

- Inflammation (edema, redness, hyperthermia, and impaired function)
- Alterations in cutaneous innervation (lower density of small fibers – C and Aα)
- Central and peripheral sensitization (persistent noxious input from tissue damage/nerve injury mediated by neuropeptides like substance P and bradykinin)
- Altered function of the sympathetic nervous system
- Lower levels of circulating catecholamines, increased levels of local and systemic inflammatory cytokines (tumor necrosis factor-α, interleukin-1, -2, and -6), and lower systemic levels of anti-inflammatory cytokines (interleukin-10)
- Genetic factors (HLA-b62 and HLA-DQ8 alleles)
- Psychological factors (anxiety, anger, and depression)

DIAGNOSTIC CRITERIA

The CRPS is a clinical diagnosis based on patient symptoms and signs elicited on physical examination. The symptoms and signs in the various categories have been tabulated in **Table 28.1**. The 1994 IASP diagnostic criteria are as follows:

- Continuing pain, which is disproportionate to any inciting event
- Must report at least one symptom in three of the four categories [sensory, vasomotor, sudomotor (edema), and motor (trophic)]
- Must display at least one sign at time of evaluation in two or more categories [sensory, vasomotor, sudomotor (edema), motor (trophic)]
- There is no other diagnosis that better explains the signs and symptoms

If seen without 'major nerve damage' diagnoses CRPS I; if seen in the presence of 'major nerve damage' diagnoses CRPS II.

STAGING

Three stages of progression based on the duration of symptoms have been described. Although it is not necessary for each patient to develop all stages or for these stages to progress in a sequential fashion, recognizing the stage and the predominant complaint can help with managing this condition.

- Stage I (acute stage: 0–3 months): Pain/sensory abnormalities (e.g. hyperalgesia, allodynia), signs of vasomotor dysfunction, and prominent edema and sudomotor disturbance
- Stage II (dystrophic stage: 3–9 months): More pain/sensory dysfunction, continued evidence of vasomotor dysfunction, with development of significant motor/trophic changes
- Stage III (atrophic stage: 9–18 months): Decreased pain/sensory disturbance, continued vasomotor disturbance, and markedly increased motor/trophic changes

Table 28.1 Symptoms and signs of complex regional pain syndrome. Reproduced with permission from: Sebastin SJ. Complex regional pain syndrome. Indian J Plast Surg 2011; 44:298–307

Diagnostic category	Symptom	Sign
Sensory	Continous burning pain in the distal part of the affected extremity Pain is disproprtionate in intensity to the inciting event and usually increases when the extremity is in a dependal position. Sensory abnormalities are most pronounced distally, and have no consistent spetial relationship to individual nerve terrorioties or to the site of the inciling lesion.	Stimules-evolved pains include mechanical and thermal allodynin and/or hyperplgesia, and deep somatic allodynia (pain due to touching the joints and movement of joints).
Vasomotor	Reports of temperature asymmetry Reports of skin color changes/asymmetry	Evidence of temperature asymmetry Evidence of skin color changes/ asymmetry
Sudomotor Edema	Reports of edema Reports of motor dysfunction Weakness Tremor Dyslomnia Coordination deficits Disturbed body perception of the affected extremity Reports of trophic changes Hair Nail Skin	Evidence of decreased range of motion Evidence of motor dysfunction Weakness Tremor Dyslomnia Coordination deficits Evidence of trophic changes Hair Nail Skin Osteoporosis

APPROACH TO A PATIENT WITH CRPS

History

In patients with a suspected diagnosis of CRPS, history of the period prior to surgery should be obtained to determine any preexisting conditions, past traumatic injuries, or pain issues. Preexisting subclinical problems can be exacerbated in the perioperative period. One should ascertain the time of onset of symptoms relative to surgery. The symptoms of CRPS (pain, numbness, swelling, stiffness, etc) are often nonspecific and frequently seen in most postoperative patients. It is, therefore, important to evaluate the response of patients to standard treatment of these symptoms. Patients with CRPS often do not respond to narcotics, are irritable, do not cooperate with therapy, resist returning to work, and often adopt a protective posture to guard the affected extremity.

Physical examination

The affected extremity should be exposed to allow a full examination from the neck downwards. The examination should be carried out at rest, during activity, and during ambulation. The three goals of physical examination include

1. Comparison of the affected extremity against the unaffected limb and the preoperative examination
2. To determine evidence of sensory, vasomotor, sudomotor/edema, and motor/trophic signs diagnostic of CRPS (**Table 28.1**)
3. To identify any possible nerve injuries. The commonly reported nerve injuries associated with CRPS include the superficial branch of the radial nerve near the radial styloid, the palmar cutaneous branch of the median nerve near the wrist crease, and the dorsal branch of the ulnar nerve close to the ulnar styloid

The extremity examination should also include assessment of skin integrity, range of motion, joint stability, motor power, and neurologic and vascular functions.

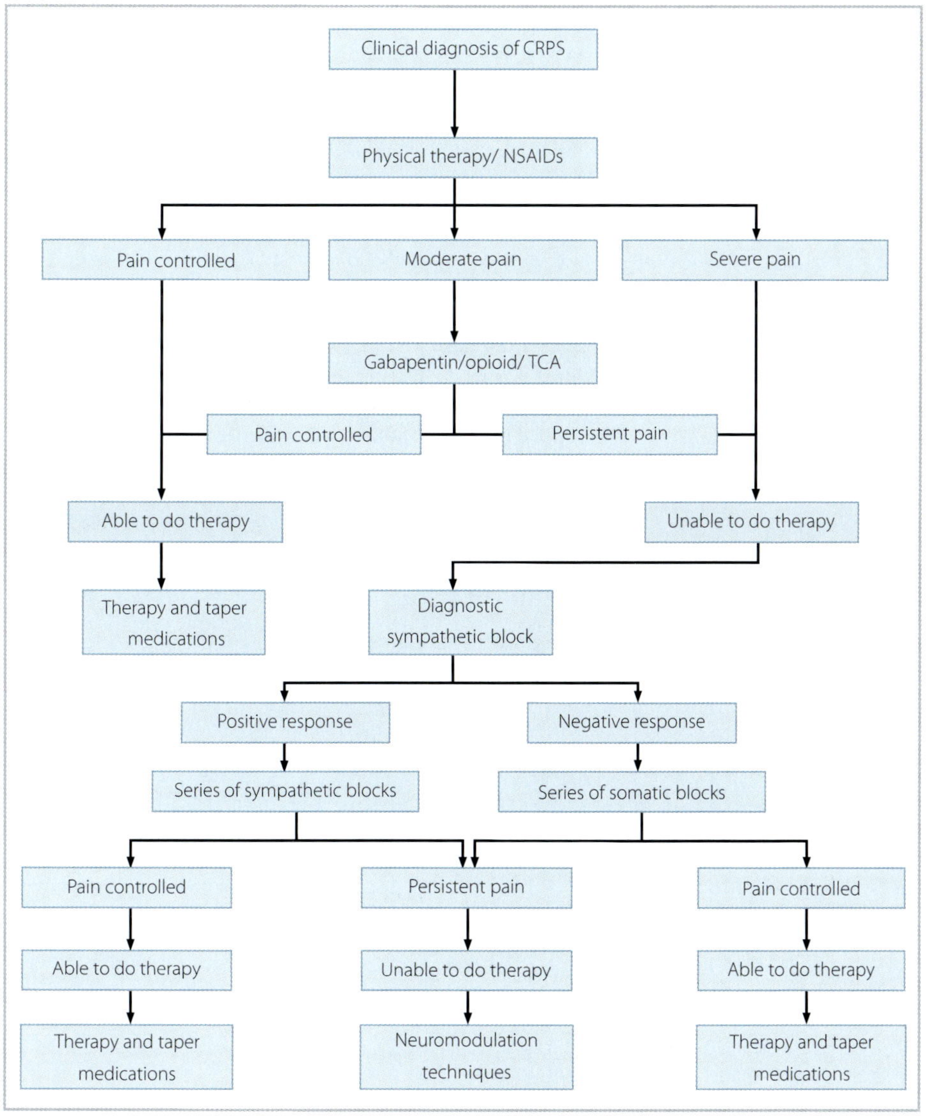

Figure 28.2 Algorithm for the treatment of CRPS.

Investigations

CRPS is a diagnosis of exclusion. Investigations are performed to rule out other causes or to complement the diagnostic criteria. The investigations to rule out other conditions include

- Complete blood count, erythrocyte sedimentation rate, C-reactive protein, and serum autoantibodies to rule out infections and rheumatological conditions
- Electrodiagnostic studies to rule out peripheral neuropathy, entrapment neuropathies, or nerve injury
- Radiographic studies such as magnetic resonance imaging to rule out bone or soft tissue pathology

The investigations performed to complement a diagnosis of CRPS include

- Plain radiography: Serial examination can reveal periarticular osteopenia and patchy osteoporosis
- Bone scans: Evidence of vasomotor instability and abnormal patterns of flow distribution in the first and second phase (blood pool and blood phase) and increased periarticular uptake in the third phase (scan phase). Band-shaped increased radionuclide accumulation in the metacarpophalangeal and interphalangeal joints of the affected extremity during the scan phase is characteristic for CRPS
- Bone densitometry: Lowered bone mineral density and bone mineral content in affected limbs. Can be used to monitor treatment efficacy
- Thermography: A difference of 1.0°C between symmetrical points on the affected and contralateral extremity is considered significant
- Sweat testing: Subjective sweat testing (starch-iodine test) or quantitative sweat production tests can be performed to demonstrate excessive sweating in this condition
- Sympathetic blocks: Sympathetically mediated pain (SMP) (RSD) may be differentiated from sympathetically independent pain (SIP) by an intravenous injection of phentolamine (α1- and α2-adrenergic receptor blocker) that results in pain relief in patients with SMP. Another option is to perform a sympathetic block [upper limb = stellate ganglion/upper thoracic; lower limb = lumbar paravertebral] using a local anesthetic. In patients who respond during the block, pain is relieved, whereas motor function is retained.

Treatment

The aims of treatment are pain control followed by recovery of limb function. An early referral to a pain specialist and a multidisciplinary approach (hand surgeon, hand therapist, anesthetist, and psychologist) is required for optimum outcomes. An algorithm for the treatment of CRPS is depicted in **Figure 28.2**.

- Physical therapy: This is the first line treatment for CRPS. As the patient improves, therapy becomes more aggressive. However, therapy must not exacerbate the pain. If it leads to escalation of pain, it must be given up
  - Immobilization and splinting
  - Elevation, massage, and gentle range of motion
  - Other modalities such as contrast baths (alternating heat and cold), H-wave therapy, and a stress loading program of traction and compression exercises have also been shown to be effective in CRPS
  - Pain control: The severity of pain determines the selection of treatment modality. The different modalities of pain control include
  - Pharmacologic therapy: Useful in patients with mild to moderate pain
    - Traditional nonsteroidal anti-inflammatory drugs [ibuprofen or COX-2 inhibitors (celecoxib)]: Useful in the acute stage
    - Opioids (metamizole, hydrocodone, or oxycodone): Consider these in patients with more severe pain to allow participation in therapy
    - Other drugs: Gabapentin, calcium modulating drugs (nifedipine, amlodipine, calcitonin, and bisphosphonates), and free radical scavengers. Bisphosphonates (alendronate, pamidronate, and clodronate) have demonstrated statistically significant pain reduction in patients with CRPS. Promising results have been seen with the use of free radical scavengers [topical application of 50% dimethylsulfoxide and oral *N*-acetylcysteine (NAC)]. The use of vitamin C (500 mg/day) has been shown to decrease the incidence of CRPS in patients with distal radius fractures. There is also anecdotal evidence for the efficacy of antidepressants (amitriptyline, nortriptyline, and doxepin), anticonvulsants (phenytoin), opioids, topical capsaicin, and transdermal lignocaine patches
    - The dosage and major complications of the use of the common pharmacologic agents have been summarized in **Table 28.2**
- Regional anesthesia techniques: These are useful in patients with moderate to severe pain that do not respond to pharmacologic therapy
  - Sympathetic nerve block: Useful in patients who have marked improvement after a diagnostic sympathetic block

Table 28.2 Pharmacotherapy for complex regional pain syndrome Reproduced with permission from: Sebastin SJ. Complex regional pain syndrome. Indian J Plast Surg 2011; 44:298–307

Drug	Dosage (mg)		Side-Effects
	Initial dose	Maintenance dose	
Oxycodone	10 mg tid	10–80 mg tid	Nausea, dry mouth, nives, nallucination
Gabapentin	100 mg tid	300–600 mg tid	Ataxia, dizziness, somnoience, purpure, fatigue
Nifedipine	10 mg tid	10–30 mg tid	Headache, postural hypotension
Alendronate	40 mg OD	40 mg OD	Nausea, dizziness, heartburn, jaw numbness
Amitriptyline	10 mg ON	25–75 mg ON	Drowsiness
Prednisone	30 mg tid	Tapering dose	Adrenal suppression, avascular necrosis
Phenytoin	50 mg OD	50–100 mg tid	Ataxia, liver damage, convulsion
Pregabain	50 mg tid	50–200 mg tid	Dizziness, somnoience, peripheral oedema
Fluoxetine	20 mg OD	20–80 mg OD	Headache, postural hypotension

- Combined somatic and sympathetic nerve block: Useful in patients who do not respond to the diagnostic sympathetic block

Physical therapy should be initiated immediately after the block. A series of daily or every alternate day blocks using local anesthetic agents is usually required for 1–3 weeks.

- Neuromodulation: This involves modulation of central pain pathways by delivery of an electrical current or chemical application to the central neural axis. Neuromodulation techniques include spinal cord and peripheral nerve stimulation, transcutaneous electrical nerve stimulation, and intrathecal injection of baclofen, clonidine, or opioids. These techniques are invasive and should be reserved for patients in whom other measures have failed
- Surgery: The benefit of surgical (or chemical) sympathectomy in CRPS has not been confirmed by controlled studies. These procedures are associated with significant complications. However, surgery has a role in management of nerve-related nociceptive foci. The most common neural diagnoses contributing to CRPS include:
  - Neuroma
  - Neuroma-in-continuity
  - Secondary compression neuropathies

One needs to address the nerve, the underlying tissue bed, and the overlying skin/scar. The nerve should be explored by an extensible incision, freed of all adhesions, and evaluated using appropriate magnification. A complete release of the involved nerve should be performed in patients with secondary compression neuropathies. Internal neurolysis should be avoided.

In patients with a nerve transection or a neuroma-in-continuity, a tension-free repair should be performed and nerve grafts used, if required. Sural nerve grafts are preferred to medial or lateral antebrachial cutaneous nerves to avoid creating another nociceptive focus in the same extremity. Local fat, muscle, or fascial flaps can be used to resurface a scarred bed. The nerve repair site can be wrapped using a vein graft or an artificial conduit. The adhesions between the skin and nerve can be managed by a Z-plasty, local transposition flaps, or a distant flap. It is important to secure meticulous hemostasis and avoid the use of constrictive postoperative dressings.

SUMMARY

A diagnosis of CRPS should be made cautiously

An early diagnosis and treatment increases the likelihood of a successful outcome

One must look for an underlying nerve-related nociceptive focus and treat it early before it gets to the complex phase

Mild cases respond to physical therapy, whereas moderate cases may require adjuvant analgesics, such as gabapentin and/or an antidepressant medication

Patients with severe pain and/or sympathetic dysfunction require regional anesthetic blockade to participate in physical therapy

A small percentage of patients with refractory, complex pain will require long-term multidisciplinary treatment, including physical therapy, psychological support, and pain-relieving measures

SUGGESTED READING

Harden RN, Bruehl S, Stanton-Hicks M, Wilson PR. Proposed new diagnostic criteria for complex regional pain syndrome. Pain Med 2007; 8:326–331.
This article reports the progress in the international effort to develop a more accurate and valid diagnostic criteria for complex regional pain syndrome (CRPS). It summarizes the latest international consensus group's action in Budapest, Hungary, to approve and codify empirically validated, statistically derived revisions of the International Association for the Study of Pain criteria for CRPS.

Li Z, Smith BP, Tuohy C, et al. Complex regional pain syndrome after hand surgery. Hand Clin 2010; 26:281–289.
This article describes the common causes of CRPS in the upper limb and an approach to the patient with upper limb CRPS.

Marinus J, Moseley GL, Birklein F, et al. Clinical features and pathophysiology of complex regional pain syndrome. Lancet Neurol 2011; 10:637–648.
This article summarizes the pathophysiological mechanisms involved in the development of CRPS.

Rho R, Brewer R, Lamer T, Wilson P. Complex regional pain syndrome. Mayo Clin Proc 2002; 77:174–180.
This article provides an excellent summary of the treatment modalities for CRPS. The treatment algorithm given in this chapter has been adapted from this article.

Index

Note: Page numbers in **bold** or *italic* refer to tables or figures respectively.